D1757508

Visit our website

to find out about other books from W.B. Saunders
and our sister companies in Harcourt Health Sciences

Register free at
www.harcourt-international.com

and you will get

- the latest information on new books, journals and electronic products in your chosen subject areas

- the choice of e-mail or post alerts or both, when there are any new books in your chosen areas

- news of special offers and promotions

- information about products from all Harcourt Health Sciences companies including W. B. Saunders, Churchill Livingstone, and Mosby

You will also find an easily searchable catalogue, online ordering, information on our extensive list of journals...and much more!

Visit the Harcourt Health Sciences website today!

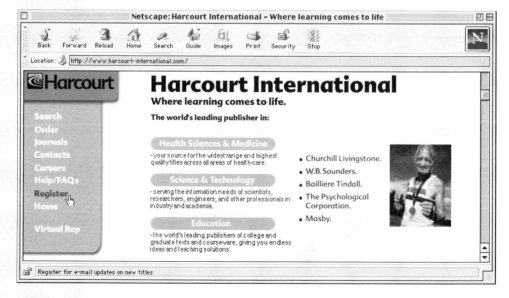

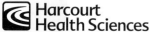

Management of Infections in Immunocompromised Patients

Commissioning Editor: Deborah Russell
Project Development Manager: Francesca Lumkin
Project Manager: Cheryl Brant
Senior Project Manager: Helen Sofio
Designer: Ian Spick

Management of Infections in Immunocompromised Patients

Michel P. Glauser MD

Chief, Division of Infectious Diseases, Department of
Internal Medicine, Centre Hospitalier Universitaire
Vaudois, Lausanne, Switzerland

Philip A. Pizzo MD

Physician-in-Chief and Chair, Department of Medicine,
Children's Hospital;
Thomas Morgan Rotch Professor, Department of
Pediatrics, Harvard Medical School Boston, MA, USA

W.B. Saunders Company Ltd

London   Edinburgh   New York   Philadelphia   St Louis   Sydney   Toronto   2000

WB SAUNDERS
An imprint of Harcourt Publishers Limited

© Harcourt Publishers Limited 2000

 is a registered trademark of Harcourt Publishers Limited

The right of Michel P. Glauser and Philip A. Pizzo to be identified as editors of this
work has been asserted by them in accordance with the Copyright, Designs and
Patents Act 1988

First published 2000
Reprinted 2000

ISBN 0 7020 2506 2

British Library Cataloguing in Publication Data
A catalogue record for this book is available from the British Library

Library of Congress Cataloging in Publication Data
A catalog record for this book is available from the Library of Congress

Note
Medical knowledge is constantly changing. As new information becomes available, changes in
treatment, procedures, equipment and the use of drugs become necessary. The
editors and the publishers have taken care to ensure that the information given in this text is
accurate and up to date. However, readers are strongly advised to confirm that the information,
especially with regard to drug usage, complies with the latest legislation and standards
of practice.

The
Publisher's
policy is to use
paper manufactured
from sustainable forests

Printed in the United Kingdom

Contents

Contributors

Sarah Alexander, MD
Fellow in Pediatric Oncology, Children's Hospital, Boston and Dana Farber Cancer Institute, Boston, MA, USA

Jacques Bille, MD
Head, Clinical Microbiology Laboratory, Institute of Microbiology, CHUV, Lausanne, Switzerland

Eómilio Bouza, MD, Phd
Professor, Clinical Microbiology and Infectious Diseases Department, Hospital General Universitario "Gregorio Maranón", Madrid, Spain

Raleigh A. Bowden, MD
Medical Director, Cancer Program, Providence Seattle Medical Center; Affiliate Associate Member, Fred Hutchinson Cancer Research Center, Seattle; Clinical Associate Professor of Medicine and Pediatrics, University of Washington, Seattle, WA, USA

Thierry Calandra, MD
Attending Physician, Division of Infectious Diseases, Department of Internal Medicine, CHUV, Lausanne, Switzerland

Michel P. Glauser, MD
Chief, Division of Infectious Diseases, Department of Internal Medicine, CHUV, Lausanne, Switzerland

Michael D. Green, MD, MPH
Associate Professor of Pediatrics and Surgery, University of Pittsburgh School of Medicine; Division of Allergy, Immunology, Infectious Diseases, Children's Hospital of Pittsburgh, Pittsburgh, PA, USA

Gilbert Greub, MD
Clinical Fellow, Division of Infectious Diseases, Department of Internal Medicine, CHUV, Lausanne, Switzerland

Andrew Koh, MD
Fellow in Infectious Diseases and Hematology/Oncology, Department of Medicine, Children's Hospital, Boston, MA, USA

Taco W. Kuijpers, MD PhD
Department of Pediatrics, Academic Medical Center, Amsterdam, The Netherlands

Peter K. Linden, MD
Associate Professor of Anesthesiology/Critical Care Medicine and Metidine, Division of Critical Care Medicine, University of Pittsburgh Medical School, Pittsburgh, PA, USA

Marian Michaels, MD, MPH
Associate Professor of Pediatrics and Surgery, University of Pittsburgh School of Medicine; Division of Allergy, Immunology, Infectious Diseases, Children's Hospital of Pittsburgh, Pittsburgh, PA, USA

Patrician Munoz, MD PhD
Associate Professor, Clinical
Microbiology and Infectious
Diseases Department,
Hospital General Universitario
"Gregorio Maranón", Madrid, Spain

Philip A. Pizzo, MD
Thomas Morgan Rotch Professor,
Department of Pediatrics, Harvard
Medical School; Physician-in-Chief and
Chair, Department of Medicine,
Children's Hospital, Boston, MA, USA

Kenneth V. I. Rolston, MD
Professor of Medicine, Chief, Section of
Infectious Diseases, The University of
Texas MD Anderson Cancer Center,
Houston, TX, USA

Eric Rosenberg, MD
Instructor in Medicine, Infectious
Disease Unit, Massachusetts General
Hospital, Harvard Medical School,
Boston, MA, USA

Robert H. Rubin, MD
Gordon and Marjorie Osborne Professor
of Health Sciences and Technology and
Professor of Medicine, Harvard Medical
School and the Harvard-MIT Division
of Health Sciences and Technology;
Chief of Surgical and Transplant
Infectious Disease, Massachusetts
General Hospital, Boston, MA, USA

Velma P. Scantlebury, MD
Associate Professor of Surgery, Thomas
E. Starzl Transplantation Institute,
University of Pittsburgh School of
Medicine, Pittsburgh, PA, USA

Michael C. Sneller, M.D.
Chief, Immunologic Diseases Section,
Laboratory of Immunoregulation,
National Institute of Allergy and
Infectious Diseases, National Institutes
of Health, Bethesda, MD, USA

Jos W. M. van der Meer, MD PhD
Professor of Medicine, University
Medical Center St. Radboud
Nijmegen, Nijmegen, The Netherlands

Miriam Weinberger, MD
Senior Consultant and Head, Infections
in the Immunocompromised Host
Service Rabin Medical Center, Petach-
Tikva, Sackler School of Medicine,
Tel-Aviv University, Tel-Aviv, Israel

Preface

During the past three decades we have both had the opportunity to participate in the changes which now guide the management of infections in immunocompromised patients. When we began our careers in infectious diseases and oncology, we encountered cancer patients who developed fever and neutropenia with defined sites of infection, predominantly with Gram-negative bacteria. Moreover, infectious complications represented the leading cause of morbidity and mortality in both adults and children receiving antineoplastic chemotherapy. The traditional principles of infectious disease management in immunocompetent patients often proved inadequate in these patients and, as a consequence, a group of physician-scientists with backgrounds in oncology and infectious diseases emerged to create new treatment and preventive strategies for these patients. Moreover, parallel with the challenge of infections in oncological patients, infectious diseases specialists were faced with a growing number of patients undergoing immunosuppressive therapy for autoimmune diseases or following various organ transplants. These patients also presented a number of infections that were new in their mode of presentation and/or in their etiologies.

In the intervening years, management approaches once deemed novel or even heretical have become standard modern practice for the immunocompromised patient. At the same time, changes have continued to unfold: shifts in the organisms associated with infection; new insights into the risk factors leading to various infectious complications; better understanding of microbial pathogenesis; new diagnostic tools; the development of potent new antimicrobial agents; the discovery of biological modifiers that either bolster or improve muted host defenses, or selectively depress various arms of immunity; and the emergence of new categories of immunocompromised hosts due to both the underlying disease and its treatment(s).

We have approached the practical management of infections in immunocompromised hosts through our respective research efforts in Europe and the United States of America. We have shared our laboratory and clinical research findings and the management approaches they delineated in the literature and at scientific meetings. Because of the mass of data that has emerged and the sometimes bewildering and confusing recommendations that unfolded, we decided to develop a practical guide that addressed the most common problems and questions that arise in the management of the immunocompromised patient. That led us to develop the *Management of Infections in Immunocompromised Patients*.

Our specific goal was to develop a book that would be useful at the bedside and in the acute management of immunocompromised patients. Accordingly, we chose to divide the book into two parts. The first part is a series of tables that codify relevant information regarding the host defense systems and alterations in compromised hosts along with the major microorganisms responsible for infection, the microbiologic and nonmicrobiologic evaluation of the immunocompromised patient irrespective of the specific type of immunodeficiency, and a practical guide to the antimicrobial management of these patients. To accomplish these goals, we asked colleagues to prepare detailed tables that could be used alone or in conjunction with chapters focusing on specific immunocompromised hosts or disease states.

In order to address specific disease states or problems in more detail, we invited a group of international experts to prepare focused chapters but with a common format. Each author was asked to address the specific questions related to the clinical presentation and evaluation of the patient, the risk factors leading to infection, and the specific management of the patient, including the major potential sites of infection. The format we chose was a question and answer dialogue aimed at providing practical answers to specific problems. We asked our expert authors to base their answers and recommendations on their personal experience as well as their synthesis of the literature and the clinical studies that are currently available. We chose authors whose knowledge would capture both published and unpublished data and whose communication skills and experience would reflect what is known and what remains to be determined. We sought a guide that was not just an authoritative review but that was an informed and practical management tool. Since our authors are extremely experienced and respected experts in their fields, we have deliberately accepted that preventive, diagnostic or therapeutic recommendations might slightly differ from one chapter to the other, thus reflecting uncertainties that still prevail in the management of immunocompromised patients.

In the *Management of Infections in Immunocompromised Patients*, we decided to focus on primary immunodeficiency states, aplastic anemia, hematological and solid tumor malignancies and the management of patients receiving nonneoplastic immunosuppressive therapies. We also included the practical management of patients undergoing bone marrow transplantation as well as those receiving various solid organ transplants. Because of its special challenges, we elected to not include the report of AIDS patients in this volume. In each chapter authors followed the same format and responded, wherever possible and relevant, to the same list of questions. This allows readers to rapidly seek advice that is clinically relevant and that, at the bedside, can help in the management of the specific patient being cared for. Because we wanted each chapter to be comprehensive for a given type of immunocompromised state, we chose a format that largely avoids references to other chapters. This carries with it the fact that there are often repetitions or redundancies between chapters. This format was unanimously agreed upon by all the authors. Of course to make this information relevant, we needed to assure that the information is current. Our colleagues understood that and worked diligently to provide their submissions in a remarkably rapid manner. We owe them our sincere thanks for their many efforts and for their willingness to respond to our seemingly endless queries and demands for additional information.

Because our project engaged editors an ocean away and authors from many different countries, we benefited from coordination and modern communications. Indeed it is hard to imagine carrying out such as project without the Internet and Email. We also benefited from enormously helpful assistants. Ms Renée Senti provided a central coordinating role. From her office in Lausanne, Switzerland, she served as a vital conduit between the editors and authors. We are deeply grateful to her. We are also enormously appreciative of Ms Sharon Olsen who worked in our Boston office and who also played a critically important role in communications and production. Naturally, none of this would be possible without the vision and support from WB Saunders.

We recognize that the *Management of Infections in Immunocompromised Patients* is not a traditional rendition or a secure recast. Our intention is to provide a new and useful guide to clinicians so that they can benefit from the advice of international experts and, with that, improve the care and practical management of their patients. We hope that our goal has been achieved.

Michel P. Glauser, M.D.   Philip A. Pizzo, M.D.
Lausanne, Switzerland   Boston, MA, USA

March 2000

Abbreviations

ADA	adenosine deaminase deficiency
ADD	adenosine deaminase deficiency
AIDS	acquired immune deficiency syndrome
ALG	antilymphocyte globulin
ALT	alanine transaminase
ANA	antinuclear antibody
ATG	antithymocyte globulin
BAL	bronchoalveolar lavage
bid	twice daily
BLS	bare leukocyte syndrome
BMT	bone marrow transplant
BPI	bactericidal-permiability-increasing protein
BSI	bloodstream isolates
CD	cluster of differentiation
CDI	clinically documented infection
CF	cystic fibrosis
CGD	chronic granulomatous disease
CMI	cell-mediated immunity
CMV	cytomegalovirus
CMV-IVIG (CytoGam®)	cytomegalovirus intravenous immunoglobulin (CytoGam®)
CNS	central nervous system
CoagNS	coagulase-negative staphylococci
CR	complement receptor
CRP	C-reactive protein
CSF	cerebrospinal fluid
CT	computed tomography
CVC	central venous catheter
CVID	common variable immune deficiency
DFA	direct fluorescent assay
DNA	deoxyribonucleic acid
EBV	Epstein–Barr virus
EIA	enzyme immunoassay
ELISA	enzyme-linked immunosorbent assay
EMB	ethambutol
EORTC	European Organisation for Research and Treatment of Cancer
ESBL	extended-spectrum β-lactamase
FACS	fluorescent-activated cell sorting
5–FU	5-fluorouracil
FUO	fever of unknown origin
G-CSF	granulocyte colony-stimulating factor

GGT	γ-glutamyltranspeptidase
GISA	glycopeptide intermediate *Staphylococcus aureus*
GM-CSF	granulocyte–macrophage colony-stimulating factor
GSD-1b	glycogen storage disease 1b
GVHD	graft-versus-host disease
HBcAb	hepatitis B core antibody
HBeAg	hepatitis B e antigen
HBsAg	hepatitis B surface antigen
HDM	host defense mechanism
HEPA	high-efficacy particulate air
HHV	human herpesvirus
Hib	*Haemophilus influenzae* type b
HIM	hyper IgM syndrome
HIV	human immunodeficiency virus
HLA	human leukocyte antigen
HSV	herpes simplex virus
IATCG	International Antimicrobial Therapy Cooperative Group
IDSA	Infectious Diseases Society of America
IFN	interferon
Ig	immunoglobulin
IL	interleukin
INH	isoniazid
IPA	invasive pulmonary aspergillosis
KGF	keratinocyte growth factor
LAD	leukocyte adhesion deficiency
LAK	lymphokine-activated killer
LAM	leukocyte adhesion molecule
LBP	LPS-binding protein
LPS	lipopolysaccharide
LRTI	lower respiratory tract infection
MALT	mucosa-associated lymphoid tissue
MBL	mannan-binding lectin
MBP	mannan-binding protein
M-CSF	macrophage colony-stimulating factor
MDI	microbiologically documented infection
MHC	major histocompatibility complex
MRI	magnetic resonance imaging
MRSA	methicillin-resistant *Staphylococcus aureus*
MRSE	methicillin-resistant *Staphylococcus epidermidis*
NADPH	nicotinamide adenine dinucleotide phosphate
NK	natural killer
oid	once daily
OLB	open lung biopsy
PBSCT	peripheral blood stem cell transplantation
PCP	*Pneumocystis carinii* pneumonia
PCR	polymerase chain reaction
PML	progressive multifocal leukoencephalopathy

PMN	polymorphonuclear neutrophil
PPD	purified protein derivative
PTLD	posttransplant lymphoproliferative disease
RSV	respiratory syncytial virus
RTI	respiratory tract infection
RUQ	right upper quadrant
SAP	serum amyloid protein
SBD	selective bowel decontamination
SCF	stem cell factor
SCN	severe congenital neutropenia
SCID	severe combined immune deficiency
SGOT	serum glutamic–oxaloacetic transaminase
SGPT	serum glutamic–pyruvic transaminase
SLE	systemic lupus erythematosus
SMX	sulfamethoxazole
Th	T-helper cell
tid	three times daily
TLR	toll-like receptors
TMP	trimethoprim
TNF	tumor necrosis factor
UNOS	United Network of Organ Sharing
URI	upper respiratory infection
UTI	urinary tract infection
VATS	video-assisted thorascopic surgery
VRE	vancomycin-resistant enterococci
VREF	vancomycin-resistant *Enterococcus Faecalis*
WAS	Wiskott-Aldrich syndrome
XHM	X-linked hyper IgM syndrome
XLA	X-linked agammaglobulinemia
VZIG	varicella zoster immune globulin
VZV	varicella zoster virus

Part I

General Principles

1

Practical Guide to Host Defense Mechanisms and the Predominant Infections Encountered in Immunocompromised Patients

Thierry Calandra

1.1 COMPONENTS OF THE NATURAL HOST DEFENSE SYSTEM AGAINST INFECTION

Component	Factor	Effect or function
1. ANATOMIC BARRIERS		
1.1. Skin	Physical environment: • Dryness • Low pH • Temperature <37 °C	Unfavorable growth conditions for bacteria
	Squamous cells: desquamation	Clearance of bacteria
	Sudoriparous and sebaceous glands: • Sweat • Free fatty acids	Unfavorable growth conditions for bacteria
	Microflora	Colonization resistance
1.2. Mucous membranes	Mucus layer: • Glycoproteins • Secretory IgA	Physical barrier Binding of microbes
	Ciliated cells: • Mucociliary motion (respiratory tract) • Peristalsis (gastrointestinal tract)	Clearance of trapped bacteria
	Secretory cells: production of peptides with antimicrobial activity (defensins)	Inhibition of growth, killing of bacteria
	Body fluids (tears, saliva, nasal secretions, mucus, lysosomal granules): lysozyme	Disruption of peptidoglycan of bacterial cell walls

Component	Factor	Effect or function
	Saliva, milk: • Lactoperoxidase • Lactoferrin, transferrin	Production of superoxide radicals Inhibition of bacterial growth Deprive bacteria of iron Inhibition of bacterial growth
1.3. Gastrointestinal tract	Stomach: • Low pH • Proteolytic enzymes	Bacterial killing
	Small intestine: • Bile salts • Peristaltic flow	Disruption of bacterial membrane Elimination of bacteria
	Colon: endogenous flora (anaerobes)	Colonization resistance
1.4. Genitourinary tract	Bladder: • Low pH • Urine flow	Unfavorable growth conditions for bacteria Flushing effect
	Vagina: • Low pH • Endogenous flora	Unfavorable growth conditions for bacteria Colonization resistance
2. IMMUNE SYSTEM **2.1. INNATE IMMUNITY** *2.1.1. Soluble proteins* Complement	C3a, C4a, C5a, C3b C5–C9	Attraction and activation of phagocytes Opsonization of bacteria Membrane attack complex (lysis of certain pathogens and cells)
Acute-phase proteins	C-reactive protein (CRP)	Opsonization of bacteria and enhancement of phagocytosis; activation of complement (binds to C1q)
	Serum amyloid protein (SAP) Mannan-binding lectin (MBL)	Activates complement Opsonization of bacteria; activation of complement
	LPS-binding protein (LBP)	Amplifies host responses to endotoxin (LPS), transfers LPS to lipoproteins
2.1.2. Cells Polymorphonuclear leukocytes (PMN, neutrophil)	Oxidative products: • Superoxide • Hydrogen peroxide Nonoxidative products: • Lysozyme • Lactoferrin • Elastase • Cathepsin G • Bactericidal–permeability-increasing protein (BPI)	Phagocytosis and killing of bacteria Recruitment of inflammatory cells (monocytes, lymphocytes)
Monocytes/ macrophages	Products of macrophages: • Complement components (C2, C3, C4, C5)	Phagocytosis and killing of bacteria Induction of inflammatory response

	• Lysozyme • Cytokines and chemokines • Growth factors • Nitric oxide • Platelet-activating factor • Oxygen metabolites • Fibronectin • Proteases	Antigen processing and presentation
Natural killer cells	Perforin Granzymes	Killing of antibody-coated target cells (antibody-dependent cell-mediated cytotoxicity)
2.1.3. Receptors CD14 (soluble and membrane-associated; expressed on myeloid cells – monocytes, macrophages and PMN)	***Ligand*** Microbial products (LPS)	***Function*** Binds microbially derived products and mediates cellular activation (myeloid cells, epithelial and endothelial cells)
Toll-like receptors (TLR2, TLR4) (expressed on lymphocytes, monocytes and macrophages)	Endotoxin (LPS-LBP complexes) Peptidoglycan, lipoteichoic acids, lipoproteins, lipoarabinomannan	Signaling receptor activated by LPS-LBP complexes; response enhanced by CD14
Mannose receptors	Carbohydrates	Involved in targeting antigens to MHC class II
Complement receptors: CR1 CR2	C3b, C4b C3bi, C3dg	Clearance of immune complexes B-cell activation; targeting of immune complexes
CR3	C3bi, LPS, fibrinogen	Adhesion (PMN, monocytes) Phagocytosis
2.2. ADAPTIVE IMMUNITY ***2.2.1. Cellular immunity*** T lymphocytes: CD4+ Th1 cells	***Effector molecules*** Cytokines: IFNγ, GM-CSF, TNFα, Fas ligand, CD40 ligand	 Activation of macrophages (microbicidal activity)
CD4+ Th2 cells	Cytokines: IL-4, IL-5, IL-10 CD40 ligand	Activation of B lymphocytes (antibody production)
CD8+ T cells	Perforins Granzymes Fas ligand Cytokines: IFNγ, TNFα, TNFβ	Cytotoxicity
2.2.2. Humoral immunity B lymphocytes	***Effector molecules*** Immunoglobulins	 Neutralization of pathogens and toxins Opsonization of bacteria Complement activation

1.2 DEFECTS OF THE NATURAL HOST DEFENSE SYSTEM AND THEIR PREDOMINANT ASSOCIATED INFECTIONS

Component	Host defense defects or conditions predisposing to infection	Increased susceptibility to infections caused by
1. ANATOMIC BARRIERS		
1.1 Skin	*Underlying diseases:* Tumors Skin diseases *Iatrogenic factors:* Puncture (fingerstick, venipuncture, marrow aspiration) Intravascular catheters Surgical wounds Wound dressings Radiation therapy Trauma (hematomas) Burns	Staphylococci Streptococci Corynebacteria Gram-negative bacilli (*Pseudomonas aeruginosa*) *Candida* spp.

1.2 Mucous membranes	*Underlying diseases:*
	Tumors
	Ulcerations (aphthae, mucositis, infections:
	  herpes sunplex virus, adenovirus)
	
	Iatrogenic factors:
	Mucositis, ulcers (chemotherapy, radiation
	  therapy)
	Bleeding
	Surgery
	Catheters (urinary tract)
	Endoprosthesis (esophagus)
		Viridans streptococci
		Coagulase-negative staphylococci
		Enterococcus spp.
		Anaerobes
		Enterobacteriaceae
		Pseudomonas spp.
		Herpes simplex virus
		Candida spp.

2. IMMUNE SYSTEM **2.1 INNATE IMMUNITY**		
2.1.1 Complement	*Complement deficiencies:* – Classic pathway (C1qrs, C2, C4) – Alternate pathway (properdin, factor D) – C3 – Terminal pathway (C5-C9) *Deficiencies in plasma or membrane* *proteins regulating complement activation:* – Factor H – Factor I – Complement receptor type 3	*Streptococcus pneumoniae* *Haemophilus influenzae* *Neisseria meningitidis* (especially serogroup: W135, X, Y) *Staphylococcus aureus* (CR3) *Pseudomonas* spp. (CR3)

2.1.2 Cells
Polymorphonuclear
leukocytes (PMN, neutrophil)
	Quantitative defects:
	Granulocytopenia (<1000/ml)
	
	– Infantile or familial benign
	  granulocytopenia (low risk)
		Viridans streptococci
		Staphylococcus aureus
		Coagulase-negative staphylococci
		Gram-negative bacilli (*Escherichia coli*,
		  Klebsiella spp., *Pseudomonas* spp.)

– Cyclic neutropenia	*Candida* spp.
– Infiltration of marrow by tumor cells	*Aspergillus* spp.
– Aplastic anemia	
– Myelodysplastic syndromes	
– Immunologically mediated	
(drugs, leukemia, lymphoma)	
– Hypersplenism	
– Chemotherapy	
– Radiation therapy	

Qualitative defects:
- Leukocyte adhesion deficiency (LAD)
- Chédiak–Higashi syndrome
- Hyperimmunoglobulinemia E with impaired chemotaxis (Job syndrome)
- Chronic granulomatous disease (CGD)
- Glucose 6-phosphate dehydrogenase deficiency
- Myeloperoxidase deficiency
- Specific granule deficiency
- Impairment of phagocytosis and chemotaxis (leukemia)
- Chemotherapy
- Radiation therapy

2.2 ADAPTIVE IMMUNITY

2.2.1 Cellular immunity

Primary deficiencies:

- Severe combined immune deficiency (SCID)
- Adenosine deaminase deficiency (ADA)
- Pure nucleoside phosphorylase deficiency
- Major histocompatibility complex (MHC) deficiency
- CD3, CD4, CD8 deficiencies
- T-cell signaling defect
- X-linked hyperIgM syndrome (XHM)
- Wiskott–Aldrich syndrome
- Ataxia telangectasia
- Natural killer cell deficiency

Secondary deficiencies:
- Malnutrition

- Malignancies (thymoma, Hodgkin disease, hairy cell leukemia)
- Chemotherapy
- Radiation therapy
- Immunosuppressive therapy: (corticosteroids, azathioprine, methotrexate, cyclosporin, tacrolimus, rapamycin, antilymphocyte serum, monoclonal antibodies: anti-T cells, anti-IL-2)
- Infections: viral (HIV, measles, CMV, EBV, HHV-6, influenza, RSV, lymphocytic choriomeningitis virus), parasitic (leishmaniasis, leprosy, malaria, trypanosomiasis)

Viruses:
Herpes simplex virus
Varicella zoster virus
Cytomegalovirus
Epstein–Barr virus
  (B-cell lymphoproliferative disorders)

Bacteria:
Mycobacterium tuberculosis
Atypical mycobacteria
Legionella spp.
Listeria monocytogenes
Salmonella typhi

Fungi:
Candida spp.
Histoplasma capsulatum
Cryptococcus neoformans

Parasites:
Pneumocystis carinii
Toxoplasma gondii
Cryptosporidium spp.
Leishmania

Component	Host defense defects or conditions predisposing to infection	Increased susceptibility to infections caused by
2.2.2 Humoral immunity	*Primary deficiencies:* – X-linked agammaglobulinemia – Transient hypogammaglobulinemia – Common variable immunodeficiency – X-linked hyperIgM syndrome – Selective IgA and IgG deficiencies – Severe combined immunodeficiency – Wiskott–Aldrich syndrome – Ataxia telangectasia *Secondary deficiencies:* – Malignancies (multiple myeloma, Waldenström disease, chronic lymphatic leukemia, lymphoma, lymphosarcoma, thymoma) – Nephrotic syndrome – Severe burns – Protein-losing enteropathies – Splenectomy – Bone marrow transplantation	*Streptococcus pneumoniae* Other streptococci *Haemophilus influenzae* *Neisseria meningitidis* *Capnocytophaga canimorsus* *Pneumocystis carinii* (XHM)

1.3 PREDOMINANT MICROORGANISMS CAUSING INFECTIONS IN THE IMMUNOCOMPROMISED HOST IN RELATION TO THE NATURAL HOST DEFENSES, MODE OF ACQUISITION AND RISK FACTORS

Microorganism	Natural host defenses	Mode of acquisition and predisposing factors	Patients at risk
Gram-positive cocci *Staphylococcus aureus* Coagulase-negative staphylococci	Skin Skin-associated lymphoid tissue (lymphocytes, monocytes, cytokines, immunoglobulins) Mucous membranes Mucosa-associated lymphoid tissue (MALT) Phagocytosis (PMN, macrophages) Complement-mediated lysis	Colonization of: • Skin • Mucosal surface (nares, oropharynx, vagina) • Gastrointestinal tract (feces) Factors predisposing to infection: • Loss of skin and mucous membrane integrity – Wounds (surgery, biopsy, punctures) – Ulcerations (chemotherapy) – Burns (radiotherapy) – Indwelling catheters – Skin diseases • Presence of foreign bodies (intravascular catheters, wound dressing) • Granulocytopenia (disease and treatment associated)	Patients with indwelling catheters Patients with cancer (solid tumors, hematologic malignancies, lymphomas) Transplant patients (BMT, solid organ transplants) Immunosuppressed patients (corticosteroids, cyclosporin A, tacrolimus, azathioprine, methotrexate, etc.)

		• Humoral and cellular immune dysfunctions (immunosuppression, chemotherapy, radiotherapy)	

Viridans streptococci
Group A streptococci
Streptococcus pneumoniae
 	
Enterococcus faecalis
Enterococcus faecium
	Skin
	Mucous membranes
	Humoral immunity (Ig)
	Phagocytosis
	  (PMN, macrophages)
	Complement
		Ecological niches:
		• Viridans streptococci
		  (oral cavity – part of the
		  normal flora)
		• Group A streptococci
		  (skin and oropharynx –
		  few carriers)
		• *S. pneumoniae* (nasopharynx
		  – part of the normal flora;
		  many carriers)
		• *E. faecalis, E. faecium*
		  (colon – part of the normal flora)
		
		Factors predisposing to infection:
		• Granulocytopenia
		• *S. pneumoniae*: young age,
		  alcoholism, splenectomy or
		  functional asplenia, humoral
		  immune dysfunction,
		  complement deficiency (C2)
		• Viridans streptococci: mucositis,
		  oral herpetic ulcers, treatment
		  with fluoroquinolones, high-
		  dose cytosine arabinoside C,
		  antacids
			Viridans streptococci:
			• Patients with
			  granulocytopenic
			  cancer (hematologic
			  malignancies,
			  solid tumors),
			  especially
			  those with mucositis
			
			S. pneumoniae:
			• Patients with humoral
			  immune dysfunction
			• Splenectomized
			  patients,
			  functional asplenia
			• Patients with multiple
			  myeloma, Hodgkin
			  disease
			• HIV-infected patients
			
			Enterococcus spp.
			• Solid organ transplant
			  patients (liver,
			  pancreas, small
			  bowel, kidney)
			• Patients with cancer
			  + BMT (not a
			  frequent
			  cause of infection)

Gram-positive bacilli
Nondiphtheria
corynebacteria
(*Corynebacterium
jeikeium, C. urealyticum,
C. minutissimum,
C. haemolyticum,
C. pseudotuberculosis,
C. pyogenes*)
	• Skin
	• Mucous membranes
		Skin and oropharynx
		  (part of the normal flora)
		
		Factors predisposing to infection:
		• Granulocytopenia
		• Prolonged hospitalization
		• Prior antibiotic therapy
		• Loss of skin integrity
		• Foreign material (intravascular
		  devices, shunts, prosthetic valves)
		• Immunosuppression (steroids)
		• Urologic procedure or
		  genitourinary disorder
		  (*C. urealyticum*)
			Patients with cancer
			Transplant patients
			  (BMT, solid organ)

Bacillus cereus		Acquisition via contaminated food:
		• Transient colonization of
		  gastrointestinal tract
		  (usually <4 days)
		• Dissemination to bloodstream
		  and CNS
			Patients with cancer
			  and transplant
			  (BMT, solid organ)

Microorganism	Natural host defenses	Mode of acquisition and predisposing factors	Patients at risk
		Factors predisposing to infection: • Granulocytopenia • Prior antibiotic therapy	
Nocardia asteroides	Cell-mediated immunity • PMN and macrophages • Activated lymphocytes Humoral immunity: minor role (resistance against filamentous form)	Acquired from environment (soil) Transmission: • Airborne (lung) • Ingestion (gastrointestinal tract) • Trauma, surgery (skin)	Patients with solid organ transplant Patients with lymphoma Immunosuppressive therapy (corticosteroids) HIV-infected patients Patients with chronic granulomatous disease Patients with dys-gammaglobulinemia
Gram-negative cocci *Neisseria meningitidis* *Neisseria gonorrhoeae*	Humoral immunity Complement (C5–C9)	• Colonization of mucosal cells (nasopharynx, urogenital epithelia: role of pili) • Resistance to phagocytosis (capsule) • Dissemination to bloodstream	Patients with deficiency of terminal complement pathway
Intracellular bacteria *Listeria monocytogenes*	Cell-mediated immunity • T-cells • NK cells • Activated macrophages	• Ingestion of contaminated water or food (fecal carriage 1–5%) • Invasion of macrophages • Predisposing factors: all therapies associated with impairment of cellular immunity	All immuno-compromised patients (corticosteroids, cyclosporin A, tacrolimus, azathioprine, methotrexate, etc.)
Salmonella spp.	Humoral (antibodies to O, Vi antigens) Cell-mediated immunity (*S. typhi*)	• Ingestion of contaminated food (poultry, eggs, dairy products) • Direct fecal-oral contact (children) • Chronic carrier (rate 1–5%)	HIV-infected patients Transplant patients Patients with leukemia, lymphoma Patients with chronic granulomatous disease Patients with sickle cell disease
Mycobacterium tuberculosis Atypical mycobacteria	Cell-mediated immunity	*M. tuberculosis:* Reactivation of dormant foci Rarely reinfection Atypical mycobacteria: Exogenous acquisition (environment) Nosocomial infections (infected instruments, solutions or equipment)	HIV-infected patients (atypical mycobacteria – disseminated infections) Transplant patients (BMT and solid organ) Immunosuppressive therapy (corticosteroids)

Legionella pneumophila	Cell-mediated immunity Cytokine-activated monocytes and alveolar macrophages Activated PMN	Acquired from environment (water) • Aerosols (air-conditioning system, humidifiers, tap water, showers, etc.) • Transient colonization (<60 min) of oropharynx after gargling with contaminated water (risk of aspiration) Predisposing factors: • Alcoholism • Diabetes • Old age • Smoking • Granulocytopenia • Renal failure (end-stage)	Patients with hematologic malignancy Renal transplant patients Patients with lung cancer HIV-infected patients Immunosuppressive therapy (corticosteroids)
Gram-negative bacilli *Escherichia coli* *Klebsiella pneumoniae* *Pseudomonas aeruginosa*	Humoral immunity (antibodies to O, K or H antigens) Complement-mediated bacterial killing Phagocytosis (PMN, macrophages)	Endogenous flora of the gastrointestinal tract (Enterobacteriaceae) Acquisition from environment and food (*P. aeruginosa*) Colonization of oropharynx, perineum, urinary tract Predisposing factors: • Granulocytopenia • Alcoholism • Diabetes • Chronic obstructive pulmonary disease • Broad-spectrum antibiotics	Patients with cancer (hematologic malignancy, solid tumors) Transplant patients (BMT, solid organ)
Haemophilus influenzae	Mucosal immunity (prevention of attachment) Humoral immunity Complement-mediated opsonization and killing Phagocytosis (PMN, macrophages)	Part of the normal bacterial flora (prevalence of pharyngeal carriage 1–5%) Asymptomatic colonization (person-to-person transmission)	Splenectomized patients Patients with functional asplenia (sickle cell anemia) Antibody deficiency syndromes Complement deficiency Hodgkin disease
Anaerobes *Bacteroides* spp.	Humoral immunity (IgM antibodies to strain- specific determinants) Complement-mediated opsonization (classic and alternate pathway) Phagocytosis (PMN, macrophages) Cell-mediated immunity (*B. fragilis*) (animal models)	Predominant constituents of normal bacterial flora (oral cavity, tonsils, colon, vagina)	Infrequent cause of infection even in patients with granulocytopenic cancer and solid organ transplant (liver, small intestine, pancreas)

Microorganism	Natural host defenses	Mode of acquisition and predisposing factors	Patients at risk
Clostridium difficile	Normal anaerobic flora of colon Mucosal immunity Humoral immunity (total IgG levels, antibodies to toxins A and B)	Part of the normal intestinal flora Development of infection after exposure to antibiotics Acquisition of toxigenic *C. difficile* strains (nosocomial transmission: infected patients, healthcare workers or contaminated environment)	Patients with granulocytopenic cancer (especially those with gastrointestinal and pelvic tumors)
Clostridium septicum and other clostridia		Risk factors for enterocolitis: granulocytopenia, mucositis, cytotoxic chemotherapy	Same as *C. difficile*
Yeasts and yeast-like organisms *Candida* spp.	Intact skin and mucosal membranes PMN Cell-mediated immunity • Monocytes/macrophages • Lymphocytes	Normal commensal of oropharynx, gastrointestinal tract and female genital tract Most frequent source of infection: • Endogenous flora • Hospital environment • Colonization of intravascular and urinary tract catheters	Patients with granulocytopenia and cancer Transplant patients (BMT, solid organ) Immunosuppression (corticosteroids, cyclosporin A, tacrolimus, azathioprine, methotrexate, etc.)
Cryptococcus neoformans	PMN Cell-mediated immunity • Alveolar macrophage • T-cells (CD4+), NK cells Humoral immunity (anticapsular antibodies)	Acquired from environment (airborne) No predisposing factors in 50% of cases	HIV-infected patients Patients with acute lymphocytic leukemia, lymphoma, Hodgkin disease Transplant patients
Histoplasma capsulatum	PMN Cell-mediated immunity • Macrophages • CD4+ T-cells >CD8+ T-cells	Inhaled from environment in endemic areas (USA – Mississippi, Missouri and Ohio valleys; Caribbean; Central and South America; Africa; southern Asia) Reactivation in immunocompromised host (rarely)	Immunocompetent or immunocompromised host (HIV-infected patients, patients with Hodgkin disease or lymphocytic leukemia, immunosuppressed patients) infected in endemic areas
Blastomyces dermatitidis	PMN (phagocytosis and killing of conidia) Cell-mediated immunity • Alveolar macrophages (phagocytosis and killing of conidia) • T-cells	Inhaled from environment (riverbank soil) Pulmonary infection, lympho-hematogenous dissemination Endemic areas (USA – Great Lakes, Mississippi valley and southeast; Canada – Ontario, Quebec, Manitoba; sporadic cases in South America, Europe, Africa and Asia)	Mainly an infection of immunocompetent host Disseminated infections in immunocompromised host infected in endemic areas: • HIV-infected patients • Transplant patients

			Immunosuppressed patients (steroids, cytotoxic drugs)
Coccidioides immitis	PMN Cell-mediated immunity • Macrophages • NK cells • CD4+ T-cells (Th1 subset)	Inhalation of arthroconidia (soil, fomites) Endemic area (positive skin test in 70–90% of long-term residents) (southwestern USA, northern Mexico, limited areas of Central and South America) Cutaneous inoculation (laboratory) Rare cases of person-to-person transmission Asymptomatic infections (60% of cases) to disseminated infections after hematogenous spread from pulmonary focus Reactivation in immunocompromised host	Mainly an infection of immunocompetent host Disseminated infections in immuncompromised host infected in endemic areas: • HIV-infected patients • Patients with solid organ transplant • Immunosuppressed patients (corticosteroids, cytotoxic drugs) • Congenital immune defects • Patients with cancer
Molds *Aspergillus* spp. *Rhizopus* spp. *Absidia* spp. *Mucor* spp.	PMN Cell-mediated immunity • Alveolar macrophages • T-cells (possibly)	Acquired from environment (community, hospital, ?water) Routes of transmission: airborne, contact (skin, wound) Predisposing factors: • Granulocytopenia • Immunosuppressive therapy (corticosteroids, cyclosporin A, tacrolimus, azathioprine, methotrexate, etc.) • Diabetes (mucorales)	Patients with granulocytopenic cancer (leukemia, lymphoma) Transplant patients (BMT, solid organ) Immunosuppressed patients HIV-infected patients Patients with chronic granulomatous disease
Atypical fungi *Pneumocystis carinii*	Cell-mediated immunity • Alveolar macrophages Humoral immunity	Environmental source and patient-to-patient transmission Transmission is airborne Reactivation of latent infection or reinfection	Premature, debilitated infants Patients with primary immunodeficiency Patients with cancer Patients with solid organ transplant (especially lung) HIV-infected patients Immunsuppressed patients
Protozoa *Toxoplasma gondii*	Cell-mediated immunity • Alveolar macrophages • CD8+ T-cells (immuno-competent host) • CD4+ T-cells (immunocompromised host)	Transmission of infection: • Ingestion of food containing cysts and oocysts • Contact with cat feces • Transplacental (in utero and at delivery)	HIV-infected patients Patients with solid organ transplant Immunosuppressed patients (lymphoproliferative

Microorganism	Natural host defenses	Mode of acquisition and predisposing factors	Patients at risk
	• Macrophages, NK cells, LAK cells	• Transfusion of blood, leukocytes, organ transplantation (heart)	diseases: Hodgkin disease, lymphoma; hematologic malignancy)
	Humoral immunity (immunoglobulin and complement)	Asymptomatic infection in most cases Disease by reactivation of latent infection or acquisition from	Neonates
	Cytokines (IFNγ, IL-12, TNFα)	exogenous source	
Cryptosporidium parvum	Humoral immunity (secretory antibodies; ?antibody-dependent cytotoxicity) Cell-mediated immunity (CD4+ T-cells, IFNγ)	Transmission of infection: • Contaminated water • Human to human (daycare, household contact, healthcare workers, hospitalized patients) Asymptomatic carrier state Infection in immunocompromised patients: ?reactivation or reinfection	HIV-infected patients Immunosuppressed patients Patients with: • Severe combined immunodeficiency • Immunoglobulin deficiency
Helminths *Strongyloides stercoralis*	Cell-mediated immunity (adult and larval worms) Humoral immunity (secretions of infective larvae): minor role	Soil contaminated with free-living form Route of infection: • Skin contact (filariform larvae) • Gastrointestinal tract, perianal area (larvae) = autoinfection Immunocompetent host: asymptomatic infection Immunocompromised host: hyperinfection syndrome (fatal) Endemic areas: Central and South America, central and southern Africa, southern Asia; sporadic cases in other countries	Patients with leukemia or lymphoma Immunosuppressed patients (corticosteroids) HIV-infected patients who sojourned in endemic areas
Viruses Herpes simplex virus (HSV)	Nonspecific host defenses: • Cornified epithelium • Intact mucous membranes • Monocytes/macrophages • Cytokines (IFNα) Humoral immunity (complement-dependent neutralizing antibodies, antibody-dependent cellular cytotoxicity): prevention of establishment, localization of primary infection and prevention of dissemination	Reservoir of virus: latently infected adults (50–90% of population) Spread by close personal contact Vertical transmission Recurrence by reactivation of latent infection	Primary infection: • Newborns • Malnourished children • Patients with alterations of skin or mucous membrane (ulcers, burns, skin diseases) • Patients with measles • HIV-infected patients • Patients with cancer • Immunosuppressed patients • Patients with selected immunodeficiencies (WAS)

	Cell-mediated immunity (T-cells, NK cells): • Prevention of cell-to-cell transmission • Eradication of infected cells		Reactivated infection: • Transplant patients (solid organ, BMT) • Patients with cancer (leukemia, lymphoma, solid tumors) • HIV-infected patients
Varicella zoster virus (VZV)	Cell-mediated immunity (T-cells, NK cells): • Limit progression of infection Humoral immunity: • Prevention of primary infection • No impact on reinfection or reactivation	Transmission by direct contact or airborne (droplets of nasopharyngeal secretions) Primary infection: varicella Latent infection (dorsal spinal ganglia) Reactivation: zoster, usually localized, may be disseminated (viremia) in the immunocompromised host	Primary infection (varicella): • Patients with leukemia, BMT • Immunosuppressive therapy Reactivated infection: • Patients with BMT, Hodgkin disease (30–50% within a year) • Patients with cancer (leukemia, lymphoma, solid tumors)
Cytomegalovirus (CMV)	Cell-mediated immunity (cytotoxic T-cells, NK cells): • Impact on outcome of infection • Role in pathogenesis of CMV disease	Transmission (person to person): • Pregnancy, perinatal period • Blood transfusion • Transplantation Portal of entry: upper respiratory tract, gastrointestinal tract, genital tract Site of replication: unknown CMV induces immunosuppression Latency in tissues (PMN, monocytes, macrophages) Reactivation and/or reinfection in immunocompromised host	Neonates Transplant patients (solid organ: liver, heart, lung > kidney; BMT) HIV-infected patients Immunosuppressed patients (cytotoxic drugs, cyclosporin A, tacrolimus, corticosteroids: cofactor; antilymphocyte antibodies) Patients with graft-versus-host disease
Epstein-Barr virus (EBV)	Cell-mediated immunity: T-cells required for controlling infection, limit proliferation of B-cells	Transmitted by intimate contact (oropharyngeal secretions of infected individuals, blood transfusion) Infection of B cells and pharyngeal epithelial cells Dissemination via blood Depression of nonspecific cell-mediated immunity during acute infection	Reactivation of EBV and EBV-related lymphoproliferative disease: • Transplant patients (solid organs and BMT) • Patients with AIDS • X-linked lympho-proliferative diseases

Microorganism	Natural host defenses	Mode of acquisition and predisposing factors	Patients at risk
Adenovirus	Humoral immunity (neutralizing antibodies prevent from symptomatic infection) Cell-mediated immunity (role unclear)	Spread from person to person Transmission by: • Inhalation (respiratory tract) • Direct contact (eye) • Fecal–oral route Route of infection not clearly identified for urogenital infections Target: epithelial cells (lytic infection) Latency: lymphoid cells (tonsils), other cells or tissues	Severe primary infection: • Patients with severe combined immunodeficiency • X-linked lymphoproliferative disease Reactivation and disseminated disease: • Patients with AIDS • Transplant patients

AIDS, acquired immune deficiency syndrome; BMT, bone marrow transplant; CD, cluster of differentiation; CNS, central nervous system; HIV, human immunodeficiency virus; IFN, interferon; Ig, immunoglobulin; IL, interleukin; LAK, lymphokine-activated killer; NK, natural killer; PMN, polymorphonuclear neutrophil; Th, T helper cell; TNF, tumor necrosis factor.

Practical Guide to Diagnostic Procedures in Immunocompromised Patients

Jacques Bille and Sarah Alexander

2.1 MICROBIOLOGIC DIAGNOSTIC PROCEDURES

The laboratory diagnosis of infections in immunocompromised patients encompasses several challenging problems. The sample techniques often require invasive procedures, and in order to detect the broadest range of pathogenic microorganisms the selection method to be applied to a specimen is very complex. Finally, the interpretation of the results according to the type and severity of immunosuppression is difficult, in particular the assessment of the clinical significance of the microorganisms detected.

In order to make a rapid diagnosis, the diagnostic procedures require constant collaboration between the clinicians and the clinical microbiologists. The correlation between microbiology and histopathology is also particularly important. To address these questions, the tables in section 2.1 have been divided into three parts: Table A lists the sites of recovery of microorganisms; Table B lists the preferred diagnostic procedures; and Table C lists the diagnostic procedures according to the sites of recovery.

Table A. Sites of recovery of microorganisms

	Sites and modes of recovery	
Organism	**Most common**	**Other**
BACTERIA		
Legionella	Lower respiratory tract system (LRTS)	Blood, urine (antigen)
Bartonella	Blood	LN
Nocardia	LRTS, skin	CSF, wounds, blood, brain
Mycobacteria		
Mycobacterium tuberculosis	LRTS	CSF, urine, tissues, gastric lavage, blood
Other spp.	LRTS	CSF, urine, tissues, wounds, feces, blood
Ureaplasma	Urogenital	Joints
Mycoplasma	LRTS	Throat swabs, blood, joint fluid, wounds, bone,
Campylobacter	Feces	Brain
Clostridium difficile	Feces	Blood
FUNGI		
Candida	Multiple (mucosae, skin, blood)	iv catheter-tip, urine, deep organs
Cryptococcus	CSF	Blood, LRTS, skin

Organism	Sites and modes of recovery	
	Most common	**Other**
Aspergillus	LRTS	Sinuses, skin biopsy, deep tissues (brain, kidney, heart)
Phaeohyphomycoses, dematiaceous fungi[a]	Soft tissues (mycetomas)	Sinuses, LRTS, joints, brain
Dimorphic fungi[b]	LRTS	Wound, blood (*Histoplasma*)
Penicillium marneffei	LRTS	Blood, skin, liver, BM
Pneumocystis carinii	LRTS	
Dermatophytes	Hair, nails, skin lesions	
Fusarium	Blood	Skin, LRTS, brain
Malassezia	Blood	LRTS, skin
VIRUSES		
Cytomegalovirus	PBLC	Urine, throat wash, saliva, BAL
Herpes simplex virus	Vesicles	Mouth wash, mouth scraping, blood, tissues, CSF, brain biopsy
Varicella zoster virus	Vesicles	Tissues, skin scrapings
Epstein–Barr virus	Blood, PBL	Throat wash
Human herpesvirus 6	PBLC	Saliva, CSF
Human herpesvirus 8	PBLC	Biopsy, skin lesions, lymphoid tissue, BM
Parvovirus B19	Blood	Nasal or throat wash, amniotic fluid
Papillomavirus	Tissue	
Polyomavirus	Urine	Blood, CSF
Influenza	Nasopharyngeal aspirate	Throat swab
Respiratory syncytial virus	Nasal aspirate or wash	
Adenovirus	Nasopharyngeal aspirate	Eye, stool or rectal swab, urine, tissues
Hepatitis B virus	Blood	Liver tissue
Hepatitis C virus	Blood	
Enterovirus	Rectal or throat swab	Nasal wash, CSF, blood, urine
Rotavirus	Stool	
PARASITES		
Entamoeba	Stool	Liver, lung cyst or biopsy, skin
Cryptosporidium	Stool	Liver bopsy, LRTS, duodenal aspirate
Isospora/Cyclospora	Stool	
Giardia	Stool	Duodenal aspirate or biopsy
Microsporidia	Stool	Brain, kidney, muscle, liver, spleen, eye (cornea, conjunctiva), sinuses, LRTS
Plasmodium spp.	Blood	BM aspirate, CNS
Babesia	Blood	BM
Leishmania	Extraintestinal (multiple)	BM, liver biopsy, LN, spleen, skin, blood
Toxoplasma gondii	Extraintestinal (multiple)	Brain, liver, spleen, heart, CSF, blood, BM, LRTS, LN, eyes
Strongyloides stercoralis	Stool (fresh)	Duodenal aspirate, LRTS

[a] *Bipolaris, Exophiala, Scedosporium, Sporothrix;* [b] *Histoplasma, Blastomyces, Coccidioides.*

BAL, bronchoalveolar lavage; BM, bone marrow; CNS, central nervous system; CSF, cerebrospinal fluid; LRTS, lower respiratory tract specimen; LN, lymph nodes; PBL, peripheral blood lymphocytes; PBLC, peripheral blood leukocytes.

Table B. Methods of detection and identification of microorganisms

Organism	Detection	Methods of choice for			Serology*
		Identification	Quantification	Other methods	
BACTERIA					
Conventional (Gram-positive cocci, Gram-negative bacilli)	Gram stain	Culture			
Legionella	IF (DFA)	Culture		DNA amplification (R), Ag (urine)	Yes
Bartonella	DNA amplification (R)	Culture			Yes
Nocardia	Gram, modified ZN	Culture			
Mycobacteria	ZN, AR	Culture		DNA amplification, adenosine deaminase (in CSF)	
Ureaplasma		Culture		DNA amplification (R)	Yes
Mycoplasma	DNA amplification (R)	Culture		DFA, Ag	Yes
Campylobacter		Culture		DNA amplification (R)	
Clostridium difficile	Ag (toxin)	Culture		Cytopathic effects in cell culture	
FUNGI					
Candida	mi: direct examination (KOH, Calcofluor white, Gram) hist: MSS, PAS	Culture		Mannan antigen (R), metabolites (arabinitol serum/creatinine ratio) (R), β glucan (R), PCR (R)	Yes (Ab–Ag) (R)
Cryptococcus neoformans	mi: cf. Candida + India ink hist: mucicarmin stain	Culture		Antigen	
Aspergillus	mi: cf. Candida hist: MSS, PAS	Culture		Galactomannan antigen (R), PCR (R)	Yes (Ab–Ag) (R)
Phaeohyphomycoses, dematiaceous fungi	mi: cf. Candida histopatology	Culture			
Dimorphic fungi	mi: cf. Candida histopathology	Culture		Ag, Wright stain, Giemsa stain	Yes (s),

Organism	Detection	Methods of choice for			Serology*
		Identification	Quantification	Other methods	
Penicillium marneffei	mi: cf. *Candida*	Culture		(*Histoplasma*), nucleic acid probes (on cultured isolates)	Yes (R)
Pnuemocystis carinii	mi: MSS, Giemsa toluidine blue, IF				
Dermatophytes	mi: KOH or NaOH solution, Calcofluor white, Congo red	PCR (R) Culture			
Fusarium	mi: cf. *Candida*	Culture			
Malassezia	mi:cf. *Candida*	Culture			
VIRUSES					
Cytomegalovirus	IF, histopathology	Cell culture (sv)	Quantitative RT-PCR (R) antigenemia assay (pp65), pp 67 mRNA (R)		Yes (s)
Herpes simplex virus	IF, histopathology	Cell culture (sv)		PCR (R)	Yes (s)
Varicella zoster virus	IF	Cell culture (sv)		PCR (R)	Yes (s)
Epstein–Barr virus	IF, in situ hybridization		Cell-free DNA in serum (R)	PCR (R)	Yes (s)
Human herpesvirus 6	In situ hybridization	Cell culture		PCR (R)	Yes (s)
Human herpesvirus 8	In situ hybridization			PCR (R)	
Parvovirus B19	PCR (R), histopathology			EM, hybridization	Yes
Papillomavirus	In situ hybridization			PCR (R)	Yes
Polyomavirus (JC, BK)	In situ hybridization, histopathology			PCR (R), EM	
Influenza	IF, EIA	Cell culture		RT-PCR (R)	Yes
Respiratory syncytial virus	IF, EIA	Culture		RT-PCR (R)	Yes
Adenovirus	IF, EIA	Culture		EM, PCR (R)	Yes

Organism	Microscopy / Molecular	Culture	Antigen detection / Other	Serology*
Hepatitis B virus	PCR		IF, in situ hybridization, Ag (Ag)	<u>Yes (s)</u>
Hepatitis C virus	<u>RT-PCR</u>			<u>Yes (s)</u>
Enterovirus	<u>RT-PCR (R)</u>	Cell culture	EIA	Yes
Rotavirus	EIA		EM, PCR (R)	Yes
PARASITES				
Entamoeba	mi: wet mount, trichrome		Adhesin Ag (EIA), PCR (R), culture	Yes
Cryptosporidium	mi: wet mount, modified acid-fast smear, IF		Oocyst Ag (EIA)	
Isospora/Cyclospora	mi: wet mount, modified acid-fast smear			
Giardia	mi: wet mount, trichrome, IF		GSA G5 glycoprotein Ag (EIA)	
Microsporidia	mi: modified trichrome, acid-fast stain, Calcofluor, Giemsa; hist: MSS, PAS		EM	
Plasmodium spp.	mi: Giemsa, thick and thin smear		Histidine-rich protein 2 Ag, PCR (R)	
Babesia	mi: Giemsa, thick and thin smear			
Leishmania	mi: Giemsa, thick and thin smear		Buffy coat smear, culture, PCR (R)	Yes
Toxoplasma gondii	mi: Giemsa		Tissue culture, animal inoculation, PCR (R)	Yes (s)
Strongyloides stercoralis	mi: wet mount histopathology		Harada–Mori filter, paper-strip culture	

Methods underlined are the most accurate or preferred methods, particularly in the context of an immunocompromised host.

*Classic serology is of notoriously low sensitivity in immunocompromised patients; however, it could be used in conjunction with antigen detection (Ab–Ag) or to identify latent infection (s = serostatus).

Ab, antibody; Ag, antigen; AR, auramine–rhodamine stain; CSF, cerebrospinal fluid; DFA, direct fluorescent antibody; DNA, deoxyribonucleic acid; EIA, enzyme immunoassay; EM, electron microscopy; hist, histopathology; IF, immunofluorescence; KOH, potassium hydroxide; mi, direct microscopy; mRNA, messenger ribonucleic acid; MSS, methenamine silver stain; NaOH, sodium hydroxide; PAS, periodic acid–Schiff; R, research method; RT-PCR, reverse transcription polymerase chain reaction; sv, shell vial; ZN, Ziehl–Neelsen stain.

Table C. Diagnostic procedures according to site of infection

Procedure	Details	Comments
BLOODSTREAM INFECTIONS		
Common procedure		
BC	Two or three separate samples (20–30 ml each) divided in equal volume in two bottles (aerobic and anaerobic) from peripheral vein and catheter entry site (all channels) Manual or automated blood culture monitoring for an incubation period of 5–7 days	
Special procedures		
Catheter-related bacteremia	Quantitative BC from catheter exit site(s) compared with peripheral BC	A ratio of 4–10 between the number of CFU in blood taken by catheter and that in blood taken from the periphery is suggestive of catheter-related bacteremia
Particular organisms		
Filamentous fungi	Special BC system (lysis–centrifugation) and/or special fungal BC media Prolonged incubation (up to 6 weeks for *Histoplasma*)	Standard BC are sufficient for the detection of yeasts (*Candida* and *Cryptococcus*) and some filamentous fungi (*Fusarium*)
Bartonella	Special BC system (lysis–centrifugation) Prolonged incubation (up to 6 weeks)	*Bartonella* is difficult to recover from BC
Mycobacteria	Special BC system Prolonged incubation (up to 6 weeks)	Use of radiometric or nonradiometric automated monitoring BC system has considerably reduced the time to positivity
CENTRAL NERVOUS SYSTEM INFECTIONS		
Common procedures		
CSF, brain biopsy	Gram stain of (cyto)centrifuged CSF or of tissue, bacterial culture (aerobic and anaerobic) for an incubation time of 5 days	
Special procedures		
Particular organisms		
Nocardia	Direct examination (modified ZN stain), culture	
M. tuberculosis	AFB smear, culture (6–12 weeks) PCR (R)	Needs a large volume of CSF due to low numbers of organisms
Cryptococcus neoformans	India ink direct examination of (cyto)centrifuged CSF, fungal culture, Ag detection (CSF and serum)	Ag level useful for monitoring therapy
Candida, Aspergillus	Stain of (cyto)centrifuged CSF or tissue, fungal culture CSF Ag (R), PCR (R)	Usually low sensitivity due to paucity of organisms

Herpes simplex virus	PCR (R)	PCR for HSV in CSF is considered the 'gold standard'
Cytomegalovirus	PCR (R)	
Epstein–Barr virus	PCR (R)	
Enteroviruses	PCR (R)	

LOWER RESPIRATORY TRACT INFECTIONS

Sputum, bronchial aspirate or brushing, BAL, lung biopsy	Direct examination (Gram stain) Assess quality (for sputum specimen only) Culture for aerobic bacteria (quantitative for BAL) Culture for anaerobic bacteria (only on biopsies)	Quality determined by absence or low number of epithelial cells and high number number of WBC (not always present in neutropenic patients) Usual threshold for quantitative cultures for BAL $\geq 10^5$ CFU (only for nonobligatory pathogens)

Special procedures

Legionella	IF (DFA), culture on selective and nonselective media, PCR (R) Ag (urine)	Always combine several methods to increase the sensitivity
Nocardia	Direct examination (modified ZN), culture	
Chlamydia	IF (DFA) (R), culture, PCR (R)	
Mycobacteria .	Direct examination (ZN, AR), culture for mycobacteria, PCR	
Mycoplasma	Culture on special media, PCR (R)	
Fungi	Direct examination (KOH, GMS, Calcofluor) Culture for yeasts and fungi Ag for *Aspergillus* (R), PCR (R)	
Pneumocystis carinii	Direct examination (MSS, IF) PCR (R)	Induced sputum not very sensitive in nonHIV-infected patients
Viruses	Cytology, culture (sv) (HSV, CMV, adenovirus, RSV, influenza virus, VZV), PCR (R)	

UPPER RESPIRATORY TRACT INFECTIONS

Sinusitis	Direct examination (Gram, MSS or Calcofluor stain) of sinus aspirate and/or mucosal biopsy Culture for aerobes, anaerobes and fungi	Nasal wash or scraping could be indicative of an etiology (particularly filamentous fungi)
Otitis media	Direct examination (Gram) of middle ear fluid (tympanocentesis) Culture for aerobes, anaerobes, fungi	
Conjunctivitis	Direct examination (Gram) of secretions Culture for bacteria and viruses	
Pharyngitis Infection of the mouth	Direct examination of secretions (Gram stain, KOH preparation, Calcofluor)	

Procedure	Details	Comments
	Tzanck preparation Culture for bacteria (group A streptococci, other), yeasts (*Candida*) and viruses (EBV, adenovirus, influenza, HSV)	
GASTROINTESTINAL TRACT INFECTIONS		
Esophagitis	Direct examination of mucosal scrapings or biopsy for bacteria (Gram), fungi (Calcofluor), for HSV and CMV (IF) Culture for bacteria, yeasts and viruses (sv)	
Intestinal infection Colitis	*Intestinal biopsies:* Direct examination (histopathology) for viruses (CMV, EBV, adenovirus) Culture for viruses *Stool:* Direct examination for ova and parasites Culture for common enteropathogens (*Clostridium difficile*) Ag detection of C. *difficile* toxin Rotavirus direct detection (EM, EIA), PCR (R)	

Ag, antigen; AR, auramine–rhodamine stain; BAL, bronchoalveolar lavage; BC, blood culture; CFU, colony-forming units; CMV, cytomegalovirus; CSF, cerebrospinal fluid; DFA, direct fluorescent antibody; EBV, Epstein–Barr virus; EIA, enzyme immunoassay; EM, electron microscopy; HIV, human immunodeficiency virus; HSV, herpes simplex virus; IF, immunofluorescence; KOH, potassium hydroxide; MSS, methenamine silver stain; PCR, polymerase chain reaction; RSV, respiratory syncytial virus; sv, shell vial; VZV, varicella zoster virus; WBC, white blood cells; ZN, Ziehl–Neelsen stain.

2.2 NONMICROBIOLOGIC DIAGNOSTIC PROCEDURES

Clinical diagnosis	Evaluation technique	Comments
Respiratory tract		
Otitis media	Radiographic 1) CT	Primarily a clinical diagnosis, but radiology may provide supporting evidence
	– opacification of middle ear cleft	May reveal evidence of disease extension (e.g. mastoiditis, malignant otitis externa)
	Invasive 1) myringotomy/tympanocentesis	Provides for identification of pathogens when there is a failure of empirical therapy

Sinusitis	Radiographic	
	1) Plain film	
	– mucosal thickening, sinus opacification with or without air fluid levels	High incidence of transient or nonspecific abnormalities in patients with acute upper respiratory tract symptoms A negative exam may obviate need for further radiologic evaluation
	2) CT	More specific and sensitive than plain films Useful for preoperative mapping before endoscopic surgery
	– mucosal thickening, sinus opacification with or without air fluid levels	Usually secondary to acute bacterial infection often following upper respiratory viral infection
	– evidence of bony destruction with loss of outline of bony wall, osteolysis	Secondary bacterial osteomyelitis, rhinocerebral invasion by *Aspergillus* or mucormycosis
	Invasive techniques	
	1) biopsy/endoscopic surgery	Required for definitive diagnosis of pathogen, important for *Aspergillus* and mucormycosis, where surgical debridement may be required
Upper respiratory tract infection	Radiographic	
	1) Chest radiography	Screen for clinically asymptomatic lower tract disease Provides baseline evaluation in the event of clinical progression
Lower respiratory tract infection	Radiographic	
	1) Chest radiography	Low yield in the absence of respiratory symptoms, but may provide baseline image Radiography patterns that are not specific for infectious pathogens but can be suggestive:
	– focal infiltrate	Bacterial (Gram-positive and negatives), fungal (*Aspergillus*, *Cryptococcus*), viral (RSV, parainfluenza, adenovirus), parasitic (*P. carinii* (rarely))
	– nodular abnormalities	Bacterial (*S. aureus*, *Nocardia*, *Legionella*), fungal (*Cryptococcus*, *Aspergillus*, *Mucor*, *Candida*), mycobacteria (miliary tuberculosis), atypical mycobacteria
	– diffuse interstitial	Viral (CMV, HSV, VZV, RSV, parainfluenza, influenza, adenovirus), protozoa (*P. carinii*, *T. gondii*), bacterial (*Mycoplasma*, *Chlamydia*), fungal (*Aspergillus*, *Candida*, *Cryptococcus*, *Histoplasma*)
	– air crescent sign	*Aspergillus*
	– upper lobe involvement with cavity formation	Tuberculosis, although findings may be limited in the immunocompromised host
		Common noninfectious causes of pulmonary infiltrates include congestive heart failure, drug- or radiation-induced pneumonitis, bronchiolitis obliterans, alveolar hemorrhage, pulmonary infarction, progressive neoplastic disease

Clinical diagnosis	Evaluation technique	Comments
	2) Chest computed tomography (CT) (similar pattern of disease as chest radiography)	Provides additional information regarding pattern, extent of disease and response to therapy May detect small nodules not visible on plain film Provides guidance for biopsy target areas
	Invasive techniques 1) Fiberoptic bronchoscopy with bronchoalveolar lavage (BAL)	Sensitivity for the diagnosis of *Aspergillus* depends of the clinical situation (e.g. the presence of hyphae in association with symptoms is highly suggestive, however, the absence of hyphae does not rule out the diagnosis) Potential for oropharyngeal contamination of culture material (e.g. by bacteria, *Candida*, HSV)
	2) Transbronchial biopsy	Provides small pathologic specimens for histopathology, increasing the diagnostic yield for specific infections over BAL alone (e.g. CMV infection) Procedure limited by refractory thrombocytopenia, size of scope in pediatric patients
	3) Video-assisted thorascopic surgery (VATS)	Direct visualization of macroscopic surface lesions Decreased postoperative recovery time compared with open procedures Procedure limited by refractory thrombocytopenia, thoracic size in young pediatric patients
	4) Open lung biopsy	Considered the gold standard, able to obtain the largest sample of diseased tissues Direct visualization of the diseased tissues, limited by refractory thrombocytopenia Indicated in patients with nondiagnostic bronchoscopy with worsening clinical condition despite empirical therapy
	5) Transthoracic needle biopsy	Indicated in patients with accessible peripheral lung nodules, usually done under CT guidance, limited by refractory thrombocytopenia
	6) Thoracocentesis	Diagnostic and/or therapeutic for pleural effusions/empyema
Gastrointestinal tract Esophagitis/gastritis	Radiographic 1) Barium swallow	Less sensitive than direct visualization May provide evidence of mucosal irregularity, ulcerations suggestive of *Candida*, HSV, CMV or bacterial infection

	Invasive techniques	
	1) Endoscopy	Direct visualization, gross appearance may provide information re pathogen: HSV – friable mucosa, diffuse ulcerations, vesicular lesions; CMV – often large discrete ulcerations in the distal esophagus; *Candida* – white plaques with mucosal irregularity
		Washings and biopsy material for culture and histopathology
Small bowel disease/colitis	Radiographic	
	1) Plain film	
	– fuzzy mucosal edges, loss of haustral markings	Nonspecific evidence of bowel inflammation
	– air–fluid levels, dilation	Evidence of ileus or obstruction
	– visible 'free air'	Evidence of perforation
	2) Barium follow through exam/ contrast enema	Enema is contraindicated in a neutropenic host
	– small bowel fold edema, haustral loss	Can provide suggestive evidence of mucosal ulcerations, bowel edema
	3) CT	
	– bowel wall thickening, fluid-filled loops	Suggestive of colitis, may be infectious or noninfectious (e.g. GVHD, chemotherapy or radiation effects)
	– cecal bowel wall thickening, pericolic edema and focal pneumotosis	Suggestive of typhlitis
	– significant mesenteric and retroperitoneal adenopathy	Associated with *Mycobacterium avium-intracellulare* colitis
	– adenopathy, extranodal enhancing mass lesions, may involve multiorgans	Consistent with posttransplant lymphoproliferative disease
	Invasive techniques	
	1) Rectal biopsy	Minimally invasive
		Pathology may represent entire colonic process (i.e. evaluation for CMV or GVHD)
	2) Colonoscopy	Direct visualization of areas of involvement
		Biopsy for pathologic identification of grossly abnormal areas
Hepatitis/ hepatic infection	Radiographic	
	1) Ultrasonography (US)	US is commonly used as an initial screen for parenchymal pathology
	– homogenous disease	Most commonly viral (hepatitis viruses A, B, C, delta agent, HSV, CMV, EBV, VZV, coxsackie and adenovirus)
	– focal/multifocal disease	Bacterial, parasitic (*P. carinii*, *T. gondii*), fungal (*Candida*)
		Hepatosplenic candidiasis is a unique syndrome in neutropenic patients, visualized with resolution of neutropenia (rarely diagnosed during neutropenia)

Clinical diagnosis	Evaluation technique	Comments
	2) CT (similar pattern of disease as US)	CT must be done with and without contrast for maximizing sensitivity Useful for following response of disease to therapy
	3) MRI (similar pattern of disease as US)	MRI may provide earlier detection and characterization of small focal lesions than US or CT (e.g. in the detection of hepatosplenic candidiasis)
	Invasive techniques 1) Transcutaneous liver biopsy	Important for the confirmation of pathogen Significant risk of procedure associated bleeding in coagulopathic patients Specimens for culture stains and pathology Usually US guided
	2) Transjugular liver biopsy	Alternative to transcutaneous biopsy in coagulopathic patients, provides smaller tissue sample
	3) Laparoscopic liver biopsy	Visualize and target surface macroscopic lesions
	4) Open liver biopsy	May be required if other procedures are nondiagnostic and clinical suspicion for infection remains high
Cholangitis	Radiographic 1) US	May reveal thickened gallbladder wall, stones or sludge, gallbladder wall, pericholecystic fluid, dilatation of the intra- and extra-hepatic bile ducts
	2) CT	Similar to US
	3) Hepatobiliary scintigraphy	Sensitive for biliary leak (post liver transplant)
	Invasive techniques 1) Endoscopic retrograde cholangiopancreatography (ERCP)	May provide evidence of stricture formation or focal dilatation associated with infection Bile sampled for culture and stain, ampullary biopsy for histopathology Contraindications include refractory coagulopathy, severe neutropenia.
Perirectal cellulitis	Radiographic 1) CT	Can aid in defining lesion, ability to assess potential abscess formation Assess response to therapy
Cardiovascular system Endocarditis	Radiographic 1) Transthoracic US 2) Transesophageal US	May reveal valvular lesions, vegetations More sensitive than the transthoracic approach

Septic thrombophlebitis	Radiographic	Most often associated with indwelling vascular catheter Radiographic evaluation often useful in determining extent of disease, informing potential need for thrombolysis and/or systemic anticoagulation and management of indwelling catheters
	1) Venography	Best resolution of venous anatomy, filling defects and obstruction
	2) CT with contrast	Less sensitive for partial obstruction of vascular lumen
	3) MR venography	May be limited by availability
	4) US with Doppler	Less sensitive for partial obstruction of vascular lumen
Skin and soft tissue infection		
Skin Infection	Radiographic 1) CT	Assess depth of penetration and whether there is an underlying inflammatory process
	Invasive techniques	Cutaneous manifestations of infection may represent primary skin infection or dissemination Typical skin findings for specific organisms may be absent in the immunocompromised host
Soft tissue infection	Radiographic 1) Plain film	Limited sensitivity, can be used to evaluate for soft tissue gas
	2) CT – edematous enlarged muscle, with or without localized fluid or air collections	Consistent with pyomyositis, fasciitis
	– well-defined fluid density collection with enhancing rim	Abscess
	3) MRI	Most sensitive technique for the definition of soft tissue pathology
	4) US	Useful for the evaluation of potential vascular compromise (compartment syndrome)
	Invasive techniques – biopsy, drainage, debridement	Specimens for culture, stain, histopathology May be required emergently (i.e. fasciitis)
Bone and joint infection		
Osteomyelitis	Radiographic 1) Plain film	Findings not apparent for several weeks into disease course Disease pattern depends somewhat on the patient's age (e.g. in long bones, metaphyseal involvement is more common than epiphyseal involvement in children compared to adults)

Clinical diagnosis	Evaluation technique	Comments
	2) CT	Can detect soft tissue changes associated with acute osteomyelitis Useful for the evaluation of bony changes of chronic osteomyelitis
	3) MRI	Most sensitive for soft tissue and medullary changes in bone infection
	4) Tc-99m bone scan	Valuable in early diagnosis, can be positive as early as 48 h from onset of disease Sensitive but not specific (tumors, trauma, infection may have similar appearances) Useful for the evaluation of multifocal disease
	5) In-111 white blood cell scan	Variable sensitivity, better in long bones, limited availability
	Invasive techniques 1) Bone biopsy	Needle or open procedure, often fluoroscopically, US or CT guided
Septic arthritis	Radiographic 1) Plain film	May reveal evidence of asymmetric joint space, displacement of fat lines
	2) US	Rapid and sensitive means for evaluation of joint effusion Often used for guidance of drainage procedures
	3) MRI	Useful for the evaluation of involvement of contiguous cartilage and bone
	Invasive techniques 1) Aspiration	Must be done emergently to preserve joint function, particularly for infection of the hip joint Diagnostic evaluation with Gram stain and culture, cell count with differential and glucose
Central nervous system Meningitis	Radiographic 1) CT	Done before lumbar puncture if there is concern regarding possible increased intracranial pressure May define complications of an inflammatory meningeal process: obstructive or communicating hydrocephalus, venous sinus thrombosis or subdural collections
	Invasive techniques 1) Lumbar puncture	Specific culture Nonspecific: cell count, Gram stain, latex agglutunation or rapid diagnostic studies, PCR, cytology, glucose, protein, lactate

Encephalitis/brain abscess	Radiographic	
	1) CT	In general, MRI is more sensitive and specific for parenchymal processes
	2) MRI	
	– focal or multifocal lesions with contrast ring enhancement	Pyogenic abscess, fungal, mycobacterial or parasitic disease (especially toxoplasmosis), also lymphoma
	– linear contrast enhancement outlining ventricular wall, may reveal intraventricular septations	Ventriculitis/ependymitis associated with spontaneous or iatrogenic rupture of abscess cavity
	– temporal lobe disease with signal on T2-weighted images, may have evidence of hemorrhage with increased signal on T1-weighted images	Suggestive of herpes simplex virus encephalitis
	– diffuse white matter increased signal intensity on T2-weighted images, ependymal enhancement	Nonspecific, but may be consistent with CMV
	– evidence of demyelination with increased signal of T2-weighted images in widespread multifocal pattern	Consistent with progressive multifocal leukoencephalopathy
	Invasive techniques	
	1) Lumbar puncture	Similar screening evaluation as meningitis
	2) Brain biopsy	Specimens for culture, stains and pathology Therapeutic in some situations (abscess drainage, removal of a single lesion)
Genitourinary system		
Pyelonephritis	Radiographic	
	1) US	Often performed as the initial screen for parenchymal involvement
	– increase in renal size, generalized increased echogenicity	
	2) CT	
	– enlarged kidneys, caliceal distortion loss of corticomedullary differentiation, delayed contrast enhancement, focal defects	CT with contrast may be more sensitive than US
Renal abscess	1) US	May provide guidance for needle aspiration percutaneous drainage
	– hypoechoic mass(es) often with irregular border	Often multiple abnormal foci, especially in fungal disease
	2) CT	May define areas of abscess formation more clearly
	– low attenuation foci with surrounding rim enhancement	

Practical Guide to Antimicrobial Agents Commonly Used in the Immunocompromised Patient

Gilbert Greub, Andrew Koh and Thierry Calandra

ANTIMICROBIAL AGENTS COMMONLY USED IN THE IMMUNOCOMPROMISED PATIENT

Antimicrobial agent	Dosage and route of administration		Comments
	Adults	Children	
ANTIBACTERIAL AGENTS			
Penicillins			
penicillin G	1–4 million units q 4–6 h iv (max. daily dose 24 million units)	100,000–400,000 units/kg/24 h q 4–6 h (max. 24 million units/24 h)	
amoxycillin	0.5–2.0 g q 6–8 h iv (max. daily dose 12 g)	20–50 mg/kg/24 h q 8 h po, (max. 2–3 g/24h)	
ampicillin	0.5–2.0 g q 6–8 h iv (max. daily dose 12 g)	Mild-moderate infection 100–200 mg/kg/24 h q 6 h im/iv Severe infections 200–400 mg/kg/24 h q 4–6h (max. 12g/24h)	
Extended-spectrum penicillins			
ampicillin–sulbactam	1.5–3.0 g q 6 h iv	100–200 mg/kg/24 h q 6 h iv/im (dosed as ampicillin), (max. 8 g of ampicillin/24 h)	
amoxycillin–clavulanate	1.2–2.2 g q 6–8 h iv	<3 months:30 mg/kg/24 h q12 h po; >3 months: 20–40 mg/kg/24 h q 8 h po or 25–45 mg/kg/24 h q 12 h po, (max. 2 g/24 h)	
oxacillin	1.0–2.0 g q 4h iv	100–200 mg/kg q 4–6 h iv	
cloxacillin, dicloxacillin	6.25–25 mg/kg q 6 h po	50–100 mg/kg/24 h q 6 h (max. 4 g/24 h)	
flucloxacillin	0.5–2.0 g q 4–6 h iv (max. 12 g/24 h)	6.25–12.5 mg/kg q 6–8 h po	
nafcillin	20–50 mg/kg q 4 h iv	Mild-moderate infection: 50–100 mg/kg/24 h q 6 h iv/im Severe infection: 100–200 mg/kg/24 h q 4–6 h iv/im 50–100 mg/kg/24 h q 6 h po	
mezlocillin	3–4 g q 4–6 h iv	200–300 mg/kg/24 h q 4–6 h iv/im	Association with an aminoglycoside advisable for severe Gram-negative infections, especially those caused by *Pseudomonas aeruginosa*
azlocillin	50–75 mg/kg q 6 h iv	50–75 mg/kg q 4–6 h iv	
piperacillin	3–4 g q 4–6 h iv	200–300 mg/kg/24 h q 4–6 h iv (max. 24 g/24h) CF: 350–600 mg/kg/24 h q 4–6 h im/iv (max. 24 g/24 h)	
piperacillin–tazobactam	3.375–4.5 g q 6 h iv	All doses based on piperacillin component <6 months 150–300 mg/kg/24 h q 6–8 h iv >6 months 300–400 mg/kg/24 h q 6–8 h iv	
ticarcillin–clavulanate	3.1 g q 4–6 h iv	200–300 mg/kg/24 h q 4–6 h im/iv (max. 24 g/24 h) CF: 300-600 mg/kg/24 h q 4–6 h im/iv (max. 24 g/24 h)	

Antimicrobial agent	Dosage and route of administration		Comments
	Adults	Children	
Carbapenems			
imipenem–cilastatin	0.5–1 g q 6 h iv	4 weeks–3 months: 100 mg/kg/24 h q 6 h iv >3 months: 60–100 mg/kg/24 h q 6 h iv (max. 4 g/24 h)	Imipenem may cause seizures (especially in elderly patients and in case of renal failure, prior seizures, or cerebrovascular disease)
meropenem	1 g q 8 h iv	>3 months and children: Mild to moderate infections: 60 mg/kg/24 h q 8 h iv (max. 3 g/24 h) Meningitis & severe infections: 120 mg/kg/24h q 8 h iv (max. 6 g/24 h)	Less likely to cause seizures than imipenem
First-generation cephalosporin			
cefazolin	1 g q 8 h iv	>1 month: 50–100 mg/kg/24 h q 8 iv/im (max. 6g/24 h)	
Second-generation cephalosporins			
cefuroxime	0.75–1.5 g q 8 h iv	75–150 mg/kg/24 h q 8 iv/im (max. 6 g/24 h)	
cefoxitin	2 g q 6–8 h iv	80–160 mg/kg/24 h q 4–8 h iv/im	
Third-generation cephalosporins			
ceftriaxone	1–2 g/24 h iv	50–75 mg/kg/24 h q 12–24 h iv/im Meningitis (including penicillin resistant pneumococci): 100 mg/kg/24 h q 12 h iv/im (max. 4 g/24 h)	Enterobacteriaceae with inducible extended-spectrum β-lactamases should be considered resistant to third-generation cephalosporins
cefotaxime	1–2 g q 4–6 h iv (max. daily dose 12 g)	<50 kg: 100–200 mg/kg/24 h q 6–8 h iv/im Meningitis: 200 mg/kg/24 h q 6 h iv/im >50 kg: 1–2 g/dose q 6–8 h (max. 12 g/24 h)	
ceftazidime	2 g q 8 h iv (max. daily dose 8 g)	90–150 mg/kg/24 h q 8 h iv/im Meningitis 150 mg/kg/24 h q 8 h iv/im CF 150 mg/kg/24 h q 8 h iv/im	
Fourth-generation cephalosporin			
cefepime	1–2 g q 8–12 h iv (max. daily dose 6 g)	>2 months: 100–150mg/kg/24 h q 8–12 h iv/im (max. 6 g/24 h)	
Monobactam			
aztreonam	0.5–2 g q 6–8 h iv (max. daily dose 6 g)	90–120 mg/kg/24 h q 6–8 h iv/im CF: 150–200 mg/kg q 6–8 h (max. 8 g/24 h)	Spectrum of activity limited to Gram-negative bacteria. Safe for patients with allergy to penicillins or cephalosporins
Macrolides			
erythromycin	0.25–0.5 g q 6–8 h po 0.25–0.5 g q 12 h iv	Oral: 30–50 mg/kg/24 h q 6–8 h (max 2g/24 h) iv: 20–50 mg/kg/24 h q 6 h (max. 4 g/24 h)	Possibility of drug interactions. Active against atypical mycobacteria
clarithromycin	0.25–0.5 g q 12 h po 0.5–1 g q 12 h iv	15 mg/kg q 12 h po	Clarithromycin is more active than erythromycin against Gram-positive bacteria
azithromycin	0.5 g on day 1, then 0.25 g/24 h po 0.5 g/24 h iv	OM or community acquired pneumonia (≥ 6 months): 10 mg/kg/dose q 24 h po (max. 500 mg), then 5 mg/kg/24 h q 24 h po (max. 250 mg) for days 2–5 MAC prophylaxis: 20 mg/kg/dose q 7 days po (max. 1200 mg/dose)	Azithromycin is more active than erythromycin against Gram-negative bacteria
Aminoglycosides Conventional dosage:			
gentamicin	Loading dose 2 mg/kg, then 1.7 mg/kg q 8 h	6–7.5 mg/kg q 8 h iv/im	Most often used in combination with other antibiotics (penicillins, cephalosporins, carbapenems, monobactams, glycopeptides)
tobramycin	Loading dose 2 mg/kg, then 1.7 mg/kg q 8 h	3–6 mg/kg/24 h q 8 h	
amikacin	7.5 mg/kg q 12 h iv	15–22.5 mg/kg/24 h q 8 h iv/im	
netilmicin	Loading dose 2 mg/kg, then 2 mg/kg q 8 h	3–7.5 mg/kg/24 h q 8–12 h iv/im	

Once-daily dosage: gentamicin	5 mg/kg q 24 h iv	1 month–10 years: 7.5 mg/kg/24 h q 24 h; ≥ 10 years 6 mg/kg/24 h q 24 h	
tobramycin	5 mg/kg q 24 h iv	4 mg/kg/24 h q 24 h	
amikacin	6.5 mg/kg q 24 h iv	No data for children	
netilmicin	15 mg/kg q 24 h iv	No data for children	
Glycopeptides vancomycin	0.5–1 g q 12 h iv 125 mg q 6 h po (*Clostridium difficile* colitis)	40 mg/kg/24 h q 6–8 h iv CNS infection: 60 mg/kg/24 h q 6 h iv	Risk of hypotension, red-neck syndrome in case of rapid infusion (< 60 min)
teicoplanin	Loading dose 6–12 mg/kg q 12 h (day 1), then 6–24 mg/kg q 24 h	10 mg/kg/dose q 12 h iv/im for 3 doses, then 6–10 mg/kg/24 h q 24 h iv/im	Alternative to vancomycin for patients with impaired renal function. Less likely to cause red-neck syndrome than vancomycin
Fluoroquinolones ciprofloxacin	0.25–0.75 g q 12 h po 0.2–0.4 g q 8–12 h iv	20–30 mg/kg/24 h q 12 h po (max 1.5. g/24 h) 10–20 mg/kg/24 h q 12 h iv (max. 800 mg/24h)	Not recommended for therapy in children (potential risk of cartilage toxicity). New quinolones (sparfloxacin, levofloxacin) have activity against streptococci and anaerobes
levofloxacin	0.25–0.5 g/24 h po/iv	Undetermined for children	
ofloxacin	0.2–0.4 g q 12 h po/iv	Undetermined for children	
sparfloxacin	First dose: 0.4 g, then 0.2 g/24 h iv	Undetermined for children	
Sulfonamides + trimethoprim trimethoprim (TMP) sulfamethoxazole (SMX) (TMP–SMX = cotrimoxazole)	2–20 mg/kg/24 h (TMP) po/iv divided q 6, 8 or 12 h Single-strength tab.: 80 mg TMP/400 mg SMX Double-strength tab.: 160 mg TMP/800 mg SMX UTI, otitis media: 160 mg TMP/800 mg SMX q 12 h *Pneumocystis carinii*: 2 × 160 mg TMP/800 mg SMX q 8 h	Dosing based on TMP Minor infections: 8–10 mg/kg/24 h q 12h iv/po Severe and PCP: 20 mg/kg/24 h q 6–8h iv/po PCP prophylaxis: 5-10 mg/kg/24 h q 12h po/iv; 150 mg/m²/24 h q 12 h for 3 consecutive days/week (max. 320 mg/24 h) PCP treatment:20 mg/kg/ 24 h divided q 6-8 h po/iv	
sulfadoxine/pyrimethamine	PCP prophylaxis : sulfadoxine 0.5–1 g po weekly + pyrimethamine 25–50 mg po weekly	No data for children	
sulfadiazine	0.5–1 g q 6 h po	Congenital toxoplasmosis: 100 mg/kg/24 h q 12 h po × 12 months Toxoplasmosis: 100–200 mg/kg/24 h q 6 h po × 3–4 weeks	High blood and CSF levels. First choice as single-agent therapy for nocardiosis infection and in combination for toxoplasmosis of CNS. Prescribe folinic acid to prevent pyrimethamine toxicity
sulfisoxazole	1–2 g q 6 h po	OM prophylaxis: 50 mg/kg/dose q 24 h po Rheumatic fever prophylaxis: <27 kg: 500 mg po q 24 h ≥ 27 kg: 1000 mg po q 24 h Meningococcus prophylaxis (for susceptible strains) <1 yr: 500 mg po q 24 h × 2 days 1–12 yrs: 500 mg po q 12 h × 2 days >12 years 1 g po q 12 h × 2 days	
sulfadiazine + pyrimethamine	Pyrimethamine: 50–100 mg q 12 h (day 1), then 25–100 mg/24 h Sulfadiazine: 1–1.5 g q 6 h	15 mg/m² or 1 mg/kg q 12 h during 2 days, then q 24 h	
Miscellaneous clindamycin	0.15–0.45 g q 6 h po 0.15–0.9 g q 8 h iv	10–30 mg/kg/24 h q 6–8 h po 25–40 mg/kg/24 h q 6–8 h iv/im	Given in combination with primaquine for treatment of *P. carinii* pneumonia
metronidazole	0.25–0.5 g q 6–8 h po 0.5–1 g q 12 h iv (max. daily dose 4 g) 7.5 mg/kg q 6 h iv	Anaerobic infection: 30 mg/kg q 6 iv/po, (max. 4 g/24 h) *C. difficile*: 30 mg/kg/24 h q 6 h po/iv (iv may be less efficacious) × 10 days	Excellent activity against anaerobes. Intravenous therapy for patients with toxic megacolon

Antimicrobial agent	Dosage and route of administration		Comments
	Adults	**Children**	
rifampicin	10 mg/kg q 24 h	Daily dose: 10–20 mg/kg/24 h q 12–24 h iv/po Twice weekly therapy: 10–20 mg/kg/24 h po twice weekly (max. 600 mg/24 h)	Numerous drug–drug interactions
doxycycline	First day: 0.1 g q 12 h, then 0.1–0.2 g q 12–24 h po/iv	Initial ≤ 45 kg: 5 mg/kg q 12 h po/iv × 1 day, (max. 200 mg/24 h) >45 kg: 100 mg q 12 h po/iv × 1 day Maintenance: ≤ 45 kg 2.5–5 mg/kg/24 h q 12–24 h po/iv >45 kg 100–200 mg q 24 h q 12 h po/iv	
mupirocin	q 8 h topically	Apply q 8 h topically × 5–14 days	Alternative for tt of impetigo; eradication of nasal carriage of MRSA
colistin	Aerosol: 75–150 mg q 12 ho	5–15 mg/kg/24 h q 6–8 h po	Per os for selective bowel decontamination or in aerosol for *Burkholderia cepacia*
chloramphenicol	0.25–0.5 g q 6 h po 0.5–1 g q 6 h iv	50–75 mg/kg/24 h q 6 h po Meningitis: 75–100 mg/kg/24 h q 6 h iv (max.4 g/24 h)	Side effects: anemia, aplastic anemia, anaphylactic reactions
quinupristin + dalfopristin	7.5 mg/kg q 8 h iv		
ANTIFUNGAL AGENTS ***Amphotericin B*** conventional formulation	0.5–1 mg/kg/24 h iv (4–6 h infusion)	Amphotericin B: Test dose: 0.1 mg/kg/dose iv (max. 1 mg) Initial dose: 0.5 mg/kg/24 h over 2 h Increment: increase as tolerated by 0.25–0.5 mg/kg/24 h q 24–48 h Maintenance: 0.25–1 mg/kg/24 h q 24 h or 1.5 mg/kg/dose q 48 h (max 1.5 mg/kg/24 h)	Test dose of 1 mg (hypersensitivity reactions)
lipid formulations: • amphotericin B lipid complex (Abelcet, Amphotec)	3–5 mg/kg/24 h iv	2.5–5 mg/kg q 24 h	Hydration with saline (before and after infusion) may help reduce nephrotoxicity
• liposomal amphotericin B (AmBisome)	3–5 mg/kg/24 h iv (2 h infusion)	Infusion rate: administer dose over 2 h; infusion may be reduced to 1 h if well tolerated	
Azoles itraconazole	100–200 mg q 12–24 h po	3–5 mg/kg q12–24h Dosages as high as 5–10 mg/kg/24 h have been used for aspergillus prophylaxis in chronic granulomatous disease	Poor bioavailability. Very high protein binding. Very weak penetration into CSF. Several drug interactions (life-threatening arrhythmias). Active against *Aspergillus* spp.
ketoconazole	200–400 mg/24 h po	>2 years 3.3–6.6 mg/kg q 24 h po (max. 800 mg/24 h q 12 h)	Absorption reduced by antacids (omeprazole and cimetidine). Not recommended in immunocompromised patients
fluconazole	400–800 mg/24 h po/iv (up to 1600 mg)	3–13 years: Loading dose: 10 mg/kg iv/po Maintenance: begin 24 h after loading dose, 3–6 mg/kg/24 h q 12 h iv/po	Good penetration in CSF. Liver toxicity (increase level of ASAT)
voriconazole	6 mg/kg q 12 h for day 1, then 4 mg/kg q 12 h iv 200 mg q 12 h po	No pediatric data	Active against yeasts, *Aspergillus* spp., *Fusarium*; iv and po formulations available. Available through clinical trials and for compassionate use

nystatin	0.1–1.0 million units q 6-8 h po	Preterm: 0.5 ml (50, 000 units) to each side of mouth q 6 h Term 1.0 ml (100,000 units) to each side of mouth q 6 h Children: 4–6 ml (400,000–600,000 units) swish and swallow q 6 h	
Miscellaneous 5-fluorocytosine (flucytosine)	50–100 mg/kg q 6 h po/iv	Neonates: 80–160 mg/kg/24 h q 6 h po Children: 50–150 mg/kg/24 h q 6 h po	Given in association with amphotericin B (cryptococcosis). Rapid development of resistance when given alone. Adverse effects: myelosuppression (monitor blood levels)
ANTIVIRAL AGENTS acyclovir	200–800 mg 2–5 times daily po 5–10 mg/kg q 8 h iv	HSV: iv: 750–1500 mg/m^2 q 8 h × 7–14 days po: 1000 mg 3–5 times/24 h × 7–14 days HSV prophylaxis: iv: 750 mg/m^2/24 h q 8 h during risk period po: 600–1000 mg/24 h divided 3–5 times/ 24 h during risk period Varicella zoster: iv: 30 mg/kg/24 h or 1.5 g/m^2 q 8 h × 7–10 d po: 250–600 mg/m^2 dose 4–5 times/24 h CMV prophylaxis: iv: 1500 mg/m^2/24 h q 8 h during risk period po: 800–3200 mg/24 h q 6–24 h during risk period Max. dose of oral acylcovir in children: 80 mg/kg/24 h.	Higher doses required for treatment of VZV than for HSV. Nephrotoxicity
valacyclovir	Genital herpes: 1 gm/dose q 12 h po × 10 days Recurrent genital herpes: 500 mg q 12 h po × 5 days Suppressive therapy: 500–1000 mg/dose q 12 h po Zoster 1 g po q 8 h × 7 days within 48–72 h of onset of rash	No data for children	Bioavailability better than that of acyclovir
famciclovir	Herpes zoster: 500 mg q 8 h po × 7 days Genital herpes simplex: 125 mg q 12 h po × 5 days Recurrent mucocutaneous herpes in HIV pts: 500 mg q 12h	No data for children	
ganciclovir	1 g q 8 h po (with food) 5 mg/kg q 12 h for 14 days (5 mg/kg/24 h for maintenance therapy)	>3 months Induction: 10 mg/kg/24 h q 12h iv (14–21 days) Maintenance: 5 mg/kg/dose q 24 h iv or 6 mg/kg/dose q 24 h iv for 5 days/week	Adverse effects: granulocytopenia, thrombocytopenia, fever, nausea, vomiting
foscarnet	CMV retinitis: Induction: 60 mg/kg/24 h q 8 h × 14–21 days Maint.: 90–120 mg/kg/24 h Acyclovir-resistant HSV infection: 40 mg/kg q 8 h 40–60 mg/kg/dose q 12 h for up to 3 weeks or until lesions heal.		Nephrotoxicity and electrolytes disturbances are common. Use lower dose (40 mg/kg q 8 h) to treat HSV or VZV infection
ribavirin	RSV: aerosol (6g/24 h at 20 mg/ml 18 h/day x 3–7 days or 6 g/24 h at 60 mg/ml for 2 h every 8 h) 3 days, given as aerosol Hepatitis C: in combination with interferon alfa 2b at 3 million units 3 times/ week sc	Continuous: aerosol 12–18 h daily for 3–7 days. The 6 g ribavarin vial is diluted in 300 ml preservative-free steril water to a final concentration of 20 mg/ml	

Antimicrobial agent	Dosage and route of administration		Comments
	Adults	**Children**	
	<75 kg: 1000 mg/24 h po (400 mg a.m 600 mg p.m.) >75 kg: 600 mg q 12 h po	Intermittent: aerosol 2 g over 2 h q 8 h for 3–7 d The 6 g ribavarin vial is diluted in 100 ml preservative-free steril water to a final concentration of 60 mg/ml. Use not recommended in patients with endotracheal rubes	
amantadine	100 mg q 12 h	Influenza A prophylaxis and treatment: 1–9 yr: 5–9 mg/kg/24 h q 12–24 h po (max. 150 mg/24 h) >9 yr (<40 kg): 5 mg/kg/24 h q12–24 h po, (max. 200 mg/24 h) >9 yr (>40 kg): 200 mg/24 h q 12–24 h Symptomatic treatment: continue for 24–48 h after disappearance of symptoms	CNS toxicity (anxiety, difficulty concentrating, light-headedness). Reduced dosage in the elderly or in patients with prior seizures or psychiatric disorders
rimantadine	100 mg q 12 h	Prophylaxis: <10 yr: 5mg/kg/24h q24h po (max.150mg/24h) >10 yr: 100 mg q 12 h po Treatment: <10 yr: 5 mg/kg/24 h q 12–24 h po (max. 150 mg/24 h) >10 yr (<40 kg): 5 mg/kg/24 h q 12–24 h po >10 yr (>40 kg):100 mg q 12–24 h po	
lamivudine	150 mg q 12 h po	3 months-12 yrs: 4 mg/kg/dose q 12 h (max. 150 mg/dose) Adolescents and adults: <50 kg: 2 mg/kg/dose q 12 h po ≥ 50 kg: 150 mg/dose q 12 h po	Early failure due to viral mutation; should be used in combination with interferon alpha (HBV)
interferon α2a or 2b	3 million units 3 times/week im or sc (hepatitis C) 30–35 million units/week im or sc (hepatitis B) 30–36 million units 3–7 ×/week im or sc (Kaposi sarcoma)	Chronic Hepatitis B and Hepatitis C: 3 million IU 3 times/week for 6 months	Adverse effects: fever, myalgia, headache (i.e. flu-like syndrome)
TUBERCULOSTATIC AGENTS			
ethambutol	15–25 mg/kg as single po dose; 50 mg/kg/dose twice weekly up to a max. of 2.5 g/24 h	15 mg/kg/24 h q 24 h po	
isoniazid	5 mg/kg q 24 h po	Prophylaxis: Infant and children: 10–15 mg/kg/dose (up to 300 mg) q 24 h po or 20–40 mg/kg/dose (up to 900 mg) twice weekly po after one month of daily therapy Treatment: Infant and children: 10–15 mg/kg/dose (up to 300 mg) q 24 h po or 20–30 mg/kg/dose (up to 900 mg) po twice weekly with rifampin With INH-resistant TB: discuss with health department or consult infectious disease specialist.	
rifampicin	10 mg/kg q 24 h po	Daily: 10–20 mg/kg/24 h q 12–24 h iv/po Twice weekly: 10–20 mg/kg/24 h q 24 h po (max. 600 mg/24 h) Twice weekly dosing may be used after 1–2 months of daily treatment.	
streptomycin	15 mg/kg q 24 h im	Daily therapy: 20–40 mg/kg/24 h q 24 h im (max. 1 g/24 h) Twice weekly: 20–40 mg/kg/24 h im (max. daily1.5 g/ dose)	
pyrazinamide	15–30 mg/kg q 24 h po	Daily therapy: 20–40 mg/kg/24 h q 12–24 h po (max. 2 g/24 h) Twice weekly: 50–70 mg/kg/dose q 24 h (max. 4 g/dose)	

OTHER ANTI-MYCOBACTERIAL AGENTS			
rifabutin	Adolescents and adults: 300 mg po qd or 150 mg po q 12 h with or without azithromycin with food	MAC prophylaxis for first episode of opportunistic disease in HIV: < 6 yr: 5mg/kg/24h q 24h po (max 300mg/24h) > 6 yr: 300 mg q 24 h po with food MAC prophylaxis for recurrence of opportunistic disease in HIV (in combination with a multidrug regimen which includes a macrolide antibiotic): Infants and children: 5 mg/kg po q 24 h (max. 300 mg/24 h) MAC treatment: 5–10 mg/kg/24 h q 24 h po (max. 300 mg/24 h)	
clofazimine	50–100 mg q 24 h po	1 mg/kg/24 h po × 1 dose	
dapsone	100 mg q 24 h	PCP prophylaxis: >1 month: 2 mg/kg/24 h q 24 h po (max. 100 mg/24 h) Leprosy: 1–2 mg/kg/24 h q 24 h po for a minimum of 3 years (max. 100 mg/24 h)	
ANTIPARASITIC AGENTS			
trimethoprim (TMP) + sulfamethoxazole (SMX) (cotrimoxazole)	*P. carinii:* 2 × 160 mgTMP/ 800 mg SMX q 8 h	3 mg/kg (TMP) + 15 mg/kg (SMX) q 8 h iv	
sulfadiazine + pyrimethamine	Pyrimethamine: 50–100 mg q 12 h, then 25–100 mg/24 h Sulfadiazine: 1–1.5 g q 6 h	Pyrimethamine: Congenital toxoplasmosis Load: 2 mg/kg/24 h q 24 h po × 2 days Maintenance: 1 mg/kg/24 h q 24 h po × 2–6 months, then 1 mg/kg /24 h q 24 h po 3 times weekly to complete 12 months Toxoplasmosis Load: 2 mg/kg/24 h q 12–24 h po × 3 days (max.100 mg/24 h) Maintenance: 1 mg/kg/24 h q 12–24 h po × 4 weeks (max. 25 mg/24 h) Sulfadiazine: Congenital toxoplasmosis: 100 mg/kg/24 h q 12 h po × 12 months Toxoplasmosis: 100–200 mg/kg/24 h q 6 h po × 4 weeks	Combination for CNS *Toxoplasma gondii* infections Use of folinic acid is mandatory to prevent pyrimethamine toxicity
primaquine	*P. carinii:* 15 mg q 24 h	0.3 mg/kg/24 h q 24 h po × 14 days	In association with clindamycin
pentamidine	Treatment: 4 mg/kg/24 h iv for 21 days Prophylaxis: 300 mg aerosol q 4 weeks	PCP: Prophylaxis: 4 mg/kg/dose q 2–4 w im/iv or ≥ 5 yr 300 mg in 6 ml aerosol q 4 weeks Therapy: 4 mg/kg q 24 h im/iv × 14–21 days Trypanosomiasis: Prophylaxis: 4 mg/kg/24 h im q 3–6 month Therapy: 4mg/kg q 24 h iv/im × 10 days Leishmaniasis: 2–4 mg/kg/dose q 24–48 h im × 15 doses (max. single dose 300 mg)	*P. carinii:* alternative therapy for patients intolerant to TMP–SMX
atovaquone	750 mg q 12 h po × 21 days	30–45 mg/kg q 24 h po	
thiabendazole	25 mg/kg q 12 h po for 2–10 days	50 mg/kg/24 h q 12 h (max. 3 g/24 h) Duration in consecutive days: Strongyloides × 2 days (5 days for disseminated disease) Intestinal nematodes × 2 days Cutaneous larva migrans × 2–5 days Visceral larva migrans × 5–7 days Trichinosis × 2–4 days	

Antimicrobial agent	Dosage and route of administration		Comments
	Adults	**Children**	
mebendazole	100–200 mg q 12 h po for 3–20 days	Pinworms: 100 mg po once, repeat in 2 weeks if not cured Hookworms, roundworms (*Ascaris*), and whipworm (*Trichuris*): 100 mg q 12 h po × 3 days, repeat in 3–4 weeks if not cured. Capillariasis: 200 mg q 12 h po × 20 days	
albendazole	400 mg q 12–24 h po	10 mg/kg/24 h q 12 h po × 2 doses	
tinidazole	2 g × 1 day po	50–60 mg/kg/24 h q 24 h po	
metronidazole	250–750 mg/kg 3–5 times/24 h po 7.5 mg/kg q 6 h iv	Amebiasis: 35–50 mg/kg/24h q 8h po × 10 days Giardiasis: 15 mg/kg/24 h q 8 h po × 6 days Trichomoniasis: 15mg/kg/24 h q 8h po × 7 days	
ivermectin	150 µg/kg po	Cutaneous larva migrans, scabies or strongyloidiasis: 0.2 mg/kg po one, (200 µg/kg/dose q 24 h po × 2 days can be used for strongyloidiasis) Onchocerciasis: 0.15 mg/kg once po	For eye involvement due to *Onchocerca volvulus*, pre-treatment with prednisone 1 mg/kg advisable
paromomycin	500-750 mg q 6-8h po Cryptosporidial diarrhea : 1.5–3 g q 4–8 h po, duration from 10–14 days to 4–8 weeks	Intestinal amebiasis: 25–35 mg/kg/24 h q 8 h po × 5–10 days Tapeworms (*T. saginata, T. solium, D. latum, D. caninum*): 11 mg/kg/dose q 15 minutes × 4 doses Tapeworm (*Hymenolepis nana*): 45 mg/kg/dose q 24 h po 5–7 days	
quinidine gluconate	15 mg/kg over 4 h (first dose), then 7.5 mg/kg over 4 h q 8 h iv	10 mg/kg iv for one hour, then 0.02 mg/kg/min in continuous IV infusion until oral therapy can be started	
quinine sulfate praziquantel	600 mg/24 h q 8 h po Schistosomiasis: 20 mg/kg q 8–12 h po × 1 day	25 mg/kg/24 h in 3 doses po/iv for 7–12 days Schistosomiasis: 20 mg/kg/dose q 8–12 h po × 1days Flukes: 25 mg/kg/dose q 8 h po × 1 day (X 2 days for *P. westermani*) Cysticercosis: 50 mg/kg/24 h q 8 h po × 15 d (dexamethasone may be added to regiment of 2–3 days to minimize inflammatory response) Tapeworms: 5–10 mg/dose once (25 mg/dose once for *H. nana*)	
quinacrine	100 mg q 8 h po	2 mg/kg q 8 h po (max. 100 mg q 8 h)	

ASAT, aspartate aminotransferase; CF, cystic fibrosis; im, intramuscular; iv, intravenous; MAC, *Mycobacterium avium* complex; max., maximum; OM, otitis media; PCP, *Pneumocystis carinii* pneumonia; po, by mouth; q, every; sc, subcutaneous; tab., tablets.
Adapted from Freifeld AG, Walsh TJ and Pizzo PA (1997) Infections in cancer patients. In: de Vita VT Jr, Hellman S and Rosenberg SA (eds) *Cancer: Principles and Practice of Oncology*, 5th edn, pp. 2868–2869, Table 52.3.

Part II

Specific Conditions

Model Template for the Questions to be Answered by Authors

In order to enhance readability and to ensure a consistent approach throughout the book, the editor's recommended that the authors based their chapters on the following template. For a more comprehensive presentation of their topic some of the authors may have deviated from this template by omitting some of the questions, by combining them, or even (e.g. Chapters 1 and 6 of Part 2) by introducing further subheadings within the chapters.

1. Regarding the **clinical presentation and evaluation** of the patient:
   1.1. What are the clinically **predominant modes of presentation** of infection in that specific condition?
   1.2. What are the predominant sites of infection?
   1.3. What are the predominant organisms that contribute (by site)?
   1.4. How do the organisms vary according to various risk factors?
   1.5. How does this differ from other conditions?
            from center to center?/and country to country?
   1.6. What is the appropriate approach to the **initial evaluation** and diagnosis of infection in that condition?
   1.7. How should the evaluation be modified according to the severity of the risk?
   1.8. What are the specific evaluation measures?
   1.9. What **new developments** are going to impact on
      - emerging organisms
      - recognition
      - evaluation
      - diagnosis
      of infection in that condition?

2. Regarding the **risk factors** accompanying each condition:
   2.1. What are the main alterations in host defense mechanisms and what are the appropriate **investigations** to document them?
      How does this differ from other conditions?
   2.2. What are the alterations due to **iatrogenic factors?**
      How does this differ from other conditions?
   2.3. What is the influence of **environmental factors?**
      How does this differ from other conditions?

2.4.   What are the most significant factors that contribute to the risk of infection in patients that condition?

2.5.   What are the specific or nonspecific **measures** aimed at minimizing each of these factors?

2.6.   Are there different **levels of risk** of infection recognized for that condition?

2.7.   How does the level of risk impact on management?

2.8.   What new **developments** are going to impact on minimizing or suppressing the specific risk factors?

3.   Regarding the **surveillance** of patients with each condition:

3.1.   What is the important **premorbid** information to be gathered?

3.2.   What are the **surveillance measures** to be taken when a patient presents with the condition?

3.3.   What are the other **specific measures** to be taken when a patient presents with the condition?

3.4.   What **development(s)** are to be expected for surveillance in patients with the condition?

4.   Regarding the **prevention** of infection in patients with each condition:

4.1.   What approaches, if any, to the prevention of infection should be considered in this group of patients?

4.2.   What are the future challenges and opportunities for reducing the risk of infection?

5.   Regarding the **treatment** of patients with each condition:

5.1.   What is the role of **empirical therapy?**
  – What considerations should direct the decision to start empirical therapy?
  – What considerations should direct the choice of antimicrobials?
  – What duration of treatment should be considered?
  – What events should direct change of empirical therapy?
  – What algorithm could be proposed?

5.2.   What is the appropriate approach to the patient with the condition and evidence of:
  a) upper respiratory tract infection?
    – sinuses
    – ear external otitis
    – middle ear infections
    – eye
    – throat
    – teeth and gingiva
  b) lower respiratory tract infection?
  c) gastrointestinal infection?
  d) genitourinary tract infection?
  e) cardiovascular system infection?
  f) musculoskeletal infection?
  g) skin infection?
  h) central nervous system infection?

       i) foreign body in place?

       j) abdominal infections?

5.3. What is the appropriate approach to the patient with the condition and evidence of **bacteremia,** with or without site of infection?

       a) Gram-positive bacteremia

       b) Gram-negative bacteremia

       c) anaerobic infection

       d) mixed or polymicrobial bacteremia

       e) bacteremia with a defined primary site of infection

5.4. What is the appropriate approach to the patient with the condition and evidence of a **viral infection?**

       a) herpes viruses

       b) respiratory viruses

       c) enteroviruses

       d) hepatitis

       e) others

5.5. What is the appropriate approach to the patient with the condition and evidence of a **fungal infection?**

       a) *Candida*

       b) *Aspergillus*

       c) *Cryptococcus*

       d) *Mucor*

       e) others

5.6. What is the appropriate approach to the patient with the condition and evidence of a **parasitic infection?**

       a) *Pneumocystis carinii*

       b) *Toxoplasma gondii*

       c) *Strongyloides stercoralis*

       d) *Cryptosporidia, Isospora, Cyclospora*

       e) others

5.7. What is the role of **nonantiinfective interventions** (including reducing or altering immunosuppression) in the management of established infection?

Infections in Patients with Primary (Congenital) Immunodeficiencies

Jos W M van der Meer and Taco W Kuijpers

INTRODUCTION

Primary immunodeficiencies are a group of rare congenital disorders in which the host defense is defective. Primary immunodeficiencies impact one or more components of the effector mechanisms of the host defense. The congenital forms of primary immunodeficiency usually become manifest in early childhood, although symptoms may sometimes be vague so that the diagnosis of a congenital immunodeficiency is made only after a series of recurrent infections. The prognosis for a number of primary immunodeficiency disorders has improved considerably over the past decades, and many patients now survive to adulthood.

In recent years the pathogenesis and molecular defects of several primary immunodeficiency disorders have been unraveled.

When should a primary immunodeficiency be considered?

A primary immunodeficiency should be considered if a patient suffers or has suffered from:

- Recurrent infection: Specifically, the number of infections is increased according to the age of the patient and the severity and pattern of infection. Recurrent viral infections in a child who is in a daycare center should not lead to suspicion of an immunodeficiency, but recurrent bacterial infections of the upper and lower airways and a high antibiotic usage (more than four courses a year) should lead to further evaluation.
- Unusual infections, including causative organism or site of infection: Examples that should arouse suspicion include disseminated atypical mycobacterial infection, disseminated staphylococcal infection (e.g. liver abscess), progressive number of warts, or extraintestinal salmonella infection.
- Infections with a severe course, such as disseminated pneumococcal infection or other bacterial infection not responding to appropriate antimicrobial treatment.

Investigation

In the workup of a patient with possible primary immunodeficiency, special attention should be given to:

- Previous history: Evaluation of growth and psychomotor development during childhood. Were milestones attained at the correct age? Are data on linear growth available? Are the infections well documented? What were the causative organisms? Is there a pattern that could suggest a certain host defense defect? Is there histologic confirmation of invasive infection? Were the infections serious (as judged by admissions, need for surgery, drainage and antimicrobial treatment)? What was the response to antimicrobial treatment? Were live vaccines tolerated? Were serologic responses documented?

- Family history: Do other family members have similar problems?
- Physical examination: Has there been normal linear growth? Are there overt or subtle dysmorphic features? What is the nutritional status? Is there weight loss? Are there skin lesions (eczema, scars, wound healing, pigment changes)? Are there mucosal abnormalities (periodontal and dental disease, ulcerations, candidiasis, aphthous lesions)? Are there tonsils? Are there visceral abnormalities (especially liver, spleen and lymph nodes) or perianal abnormalities? Are there any muscular or joint complaints? Are there suspicious neurologic signs (vision, hearing loss, tactile sensibility, cerebellar or motor function)?

Differential diagnosis

The clinician should also consider possibilities other than immunodeficiency. For example, can the symptoms or could the clinical picture be explained by:

- Anatomic abnormalities (e.g. bronchiectasis, bronchogenic cysts, hidradenitis, foreign body)
- Functional abnormalities (e.g. ciliary dyskinesia and cystic fibrosis)
- Unusual exposure (e.g. *Pseudomonas* skin infection due to whirlpool exposure, histoplasmosis due to exposure to bats, travel to (sub)tropical areas)
- Iatrogenic problem (e.g. mycobacterial infection due to contaminated injection fluids)
- Unusual behavior or factitious disorder (e.g. skin lesions within the reach of the dominant arm).

Type of primary immunodeficiency

If nonimmunologic possibilities are excluded, the clinician should focus on the type of primary immunodeficiency that is most likely? Importantly, the clinician should be aware of the fact that certain host defects predispose to certain infections (as will be detailed below). In this respect, the following questions become very relevant:

- Which line of defense (humoral or cellular) is affected?
- Is this a defect of the nonspecific or specific host defense?

From these considerations, the following categories can be distinguished:

I Humoral aspecific primary immunodeficiency	Complement deficiencies
II Humoral specific primary immunodeficiency	Immunoglobulin deficiencies
III Cellular aspecific immunodeficiency	Phagocytic and natural killer cell deficiencies
IV Cellular specific immunodeficiency	T-cell and macrophage defects

Combined immunodeficiencies are being dealt with under category IV.

In addition, there are a number of developmental defects and autoimmune syndromes without major dysmorphic features, accompanied by immunodeficiencies. These are beyond the scope of this book. Chronic mucocutaneous candidiasis, a group of heterogeneous disorders with different underlying defects (T-cell defects, phagocyte defects), will not be discussed separately. As mentioned above, the molecular and genetic background of a large number of congenital primary immunodeficiencies is now known and is rapidly expanding.

I HUMORAL ASPECIFIC PRIMARY IMMUNODEFICIENCY

A. COMPLEMENT DEFICIENCIES: THE ALTERNATE ROUTE AND EARLY FACTORS OF THE CLASSIC PATHWAY

It should be remembered that the alternate route and the classic route of complement represent different ways to initiate the complement cascade. Both activation routes yield activated C3, after which both pathways are the same. The alternate route can be activated in the absence of specific antibodies. For example, lipopolysaccharide and other repetitive exogenous molecules (e.g. teichoic acid of several Gram-positive bacteria) as well as endogenous molecules [C-reactive protein (CRP) and fibrillar β-amyloid] can start the cascade. In contrast, the classic route of activation is initiated by binding of C1q to immunoglobulin bound to antigen. The classic route can also be initiated in an immunoglobulin-independent fashion by the acute-phase reactant mannan-binding protein (MBP), which binds to various microorganisms, yeast and fungi, or by activated factor XII.

The redundancy in both pathways probably explains why not all deficiencies are accompanied by infection. The major deficiencies that lead to infection are factor B and D in the alternate route, and C1q, C2, C3 and C3b inactivator in the classic route. Recent data demonstrate that deficiency of MBP is also associated with increased susceptibility to (bacterial) infections, such as pneumococcal or meningococcal disease. Because the lack of activated C3 (especially the lack of generation of C3b, a major opsonin for encapsulated bacteria) predominates the susceptibility of infection, the consequences of defects in either route are discussed together.

I REGARDING THE CLINICAL PRESENTATION AND EVALUATION OF THE PATIENT

I.I What are the clinically predominant modes of presentation of infection in patients with deficiency of early complement components?

Patients generally present with recurrent or severe respiratory tract infections, otitis and sinusitis, usually starting in early childhood. Lupus syndromes [sometimes antinuclear antibody (ANA) negative] and glomerulonephritis may also be associated with complement deficiencies, some of which are not associated with a significant host defense defect (Table 1.1). The pathogenesis of these lupus syndromes has not been fully elucidated, but solubility of circulating immune complexes could play a role. In addition, deposition of classic components of complement, such as C1q and C4, appears to play a role in receptor-mediated clearance of apoptotic cells; when these complement factors are absent, apoptotic cells are not cleared appropriately. The surface blebs of apoptotic cells contain subcellular and nuclear material that could serve as autoantigens, and thereby lead to autoimmunity.

I.2 What are the predominant sites of infection?

Ears, sinuses, upper and lower airways and lungs are the major sites of infection. Patients may also present with meningitis or bacteremia.

Table 1.1 Clinical consequences of deficiency of early complement components

Complement factor deficiency	Infection	Lupus erythematosus	Glomerulonephritis	Other
MBP	++	?		
C1q	+	++	+	SCID (?)
C1		++	+	
C1s		+		
C1 inhibitor				Angioedema
C4	+	++	±	
C2	++	+	±	Polymyositis
C3	++	+	+	Cirrhosis
Factor I (C3b inactivator)	++			
Factor H	+		++	IgA nephropathy
Factor D	++			
Properdin	++			
C5	++	+		
C6	+			
C7	+			Raynaud disease
C8	+			
C9	±			

++, common; +, occurs but not in all individuals with the defect; ±, less common. MBP, mannan-binding protein; SCID, severe combined immune deficiency.

1.3 What are the predominant organisms that contribute (by site)?

The predominant causative organisms are encapsulated bacteria, especially *Streptococcus pneumoniae*, *Haemophilus influenzae* and *Neisseria meningitidis*.

1.4 How do the organisms vary according to various risk factors?

As the complement system has its greatest impact before specific immunity develops, the status of specific immunity towards the encapsulated microorganisms is particularly important (see also section 4.1). Because of the rarity of most complement defects, it is difficult to compare the risk for infection between the various defects. Nevertheless, patients with deficiency of C3, factor I, factor H or factor B probably have the greatest risk for infections, particularly pneumococcal disease, usually before the age of 3 years. Factor D and properdin defects seem to be associated with a somewhat lower risk, occurring later during childhood.

1.5 How does this differ from other conditions, from center to center, and from country to country?

Deficiencies in the early component of the complement cascades seem to be more prevalent in Caucasians than other racial backgrounds. MBP deficiency represents the most prevailing defect in complement activation among various populations tested. About 3–6% of the Caucasian population has a dysfunctional MBP. In Asian populations, the gene frequency for a functional but lowered expression of MBP is 10%, whereas interregional variance of these gene polymorphisms has been observed among African populations (Kenya and Namibia, about 3%; The Gambia, South African Xhosa, less than 0.1%).

C2 deficiency is the second most common and complete deficiency in Caucasians (1 in 10 000 population), but is absent in Japanese and African American populations. C2, as well as both C4 isotypes and factor B, is located within the so-called class III region of the major histocompatibility complex (MHC) (chromosome 6p21). Approximately 40% of C2-deficient patients develop systemic lupus erythematosus (SLE)-like disease, and 50% develop recurrent infections.

Another frequently encountered complement deficiency in Caucasians consists of a defect in C4. This factor has two isotypes encoded by two distinct loci, *C4A* and *C4B*, with subtle differences. First, electrophoretic mobility differs slightly, and second, transacylation of amino groups of proteins is carried out more efficiently by C4A, and vice versa for hydroxyl groups of (bacterial) polysaccharides by C4B. While a complete C4 deficiency is very rare, individuals homozygous for the *C4A*Q0* or *C4B*Q0* allele are both encountered in about 0.01% of the Caucasian population. Whereas both the extremely rare complete C4 deficiency and the far more common C4A deficiency are associated with SLE-like disease (in 50% and 2–5% of the cases, respectively), homozygous C4B deficiency has been associated predominantly with an increased risk of bacterial infection.

Although rare, a deficiency in properdin is the most prevalent defect of the alternate route, with more than 70 male patients described, mostly Caucasian (chromosome Xp11.3).

With respect to the infectious microorganisms involved, the encapsulated microorganisms are ubiquitous, so that complement-deficient patients throughout the world will have similar presentations. However, the prognosis of such patients is dismal in developing nations.

1.6 What is the appropriate approach to the initial evaluation and diagnosis of infection in patients with deficiency of early complement components?

History, previous disease episodes and contacts with patients with meningococcal disease should be explored. As in all primary immunodeficiencies, the family history is very important. Gram staining and culture of relevant specimens [pus, sputum, cerebrospinal fluid (CSF)] should be performed. Blood cultures should be done when bacteremia is suspected. Antigen tests (urine, CSF) for *S. pneumoniae*, *H. influenzae* and *N. meningitidis* should also be performed. Typing of meningococci is important, because strains with low virulence (serogroups W-135, X, Y, Z, 29E) generally indicate complement deficiency. In addition, radiographs of chest and sinuses are indicated.

1.7 How should the evaluation be modified according to the severity of the risk?

If the patient is acutely ill, immediate diagnostic and therapeutic interventions are indicated (see sections 3.2 and 5.1). If the patient is not acutely ill, the evaluation may be done in an ambulatory setting.

1.8 What are the specific evaluation measures? (see also Chapter 2 in Part 1)

The diagnostic tests given in section 1.6 are important when considering the array of possible infections. To assess the cumulative damage due to recurrent or chronic infections of the respiratory tract, pulmonary function should be measured at regular intervals (approximately once a year). High-resolution computed tomography (CT) should also be performed to assess the presence of bronchiectasis. In childhood, auditory function should be assessed 6 months after meningitis, particularly when *H. influenzae* type b (Hib) or *Pneumococcus* is the causative agent.

If the underlying complement defect has not yet been diagnosed, testing of total hemolytic complement (CH50) to assess the functional quality of the classic route of the complement system, and of the functional integrity of the alternate pathway (AP50), is indicated. As there may be consumption and decreased synthesis of complement during acute infection, these tests should be performed at least 2 weeks after the infection has subsided. When complement function in one of these pathways is defective, measurement of the relevant individual complement factors should be performed in a dedicated laboratory. Following this, investigation at the deoxyribonucleic acid (DNA) level may be appropriate. As these complement deficiencies cannot easily be distinguished from immunoglobulin deficiencies on clinical grounds, and because combined defects occur, an assessment as for immunoglobulin deficiencies is indicated (see below). As indicated in Table 1.1, C1q deficiency may occur together with severe combined immune deficiency (SCID). If the latter is suspected, investigation for cellular immunodeficiency is indicated as well.

1.9 What new developments are going to impact on emerging organisms, recognition, evaluation and diagnosis of infection in patients with deficiency of early complement components?

Rapid diagnostic tools [polymerase chain reaction (PCR), antigen tests] for pneumococci, *H. influenzae* and meningococci should be improved or developed, evaluated, and become generally available.

2 REGARDING THE RISK FACTORS ACCOMPANYING DEFICIENCY OF EARLY COMPLEMENT COMPONENTS

2.1 What are the main alterations in host defense mechanisms and what are the appropriate investigations to document them?

The chance of finding a complement deficiency is generally extremely low, even when there is an apparently unique presentation such as pneumococcal peritonitis. Complement deficiencies are more often diagnosed by screening of idiopathic autoimmune diseases. In patients with infection, microbiologic typing may warrant investigation of complement (see section 1.6). Bacterial infections are usually systemic (septicemia and meningitis), with encapsulated bacteria such as pneumococcal strains and Hib as the major cause of disease, and are more common in childhood than in adolescence or adulthood. Thus, age of onset must be taken into account.

Recurrence of bacterial infection is a reason for screening the complement system, initially with measurement of CH50 and AP50 (see section 1.8). Since acute infection is often accompanied by complement activation, and consumption and decreased synthesis, levels of complement should be determined approximately 2 weeks after recovery. If the levels are abnormal, the concentration of individual complement factors should be measured.

Other aspects of humoral immunity should also be assessed (levels of immunoglobulins and subclasses). Circulating immune complexes and secondary impaired splenic macrophage function may be responsible for both clinical manifestations.

As noted above, MBP polymorphism has been shown to be of importance in the acquisition of (bacterial) infections. Testing for such polymorphism is important, especially when the complement system is normal and a host defense defect is likely, for example because of a positive family history.

2.2 What are the alterations due to iatrogenic factors?
No iatrogenic factors leading to impaired complement function are known.

2.3 What is the influence of environmental factors?
Crowding (military camps, kindergarten) will lead to the acquisition of certain organisms (e.g. meningococci or pneumococci).

2.4 What are the most significant factors that contribute to the risk of infection in patients with deficiency of early complement components?
There is some evidence, especially in adult patients, that the episodes of infection with the encapsulated microorganisms are preceded by viral infections.

2.5 What are the specific or nonspecific measures aimed at minimizing each of these factors?
In view of the above, measures to avoid crowding may be helpful. Other preventive and more specific measures, such as vaccination with conjugate vaccines, may be indicated (see section 4.1).

3 REGARDING THE SURVEILLANCE OF PATIENTS WITH DEFICIENCY OF EARLY COMPLEMENT COMPONENTS

3.2 What are the surveillance measures to be taken when a patient presents with deficiency of early complement components?
When a patient with complement factor deficiency presents, it is reasonable to assess colonization with *S. pneumoniae*, *H. influenzae* (sputum) and *N. meningitidis* (nasopharynx). Radiography of the chest and sinuses is indicated and, when bronchiectasis is suspected, CT of the thorax. Pulmonary function tests should be considered when there is a positive history of respiratory tract infection. A positive history of recurrent or chronic otitis media requires auditory testing in childhood.

3.3 What are other specific measures to be taken when a patient presents with deficiency of early complement components?
If applicable (see Table 1.1), investigation for SLE, vasculitis and glomerulonephritis should be undertaken.

4 REGARDING THE PREVENTION OF INFECTIONS IN PATIENTS WITH DEFICIENCY OF EARLY COMPLEMENT COMPONENTS

4.1 What approaches, if any, to the prevention of infection should be considered in patients with deficiency of early complement components?
Appropriate preventive measures may depend on the complement component that is missing. Morbidity and mortality rates associated with deficiencies of properdin factor I or C3 at an early age are greater than those for C2 and C4, where the risk of infection is less prominent. In view of the limited number of pathogens that are a threat to these patients, vaccination with Pneumovax, Hib conjugate vaccine and meningococcal vaccine should be done and repeated at 2–3-year intervals because of the annual decline in pro-

tective antibody levels. A protective vaccine against group B meningococci is not available and the current pneumococcal vaccine is suboptimal in terms of coverage of serotypes (50–80%) and immunogenicity (polysaccharide versus conjugate vaccine).

The availability of conjugate vaccines can be used to induce efficient antibody responses during the first year of life, whereas the polysaccharide vaccines are effective from the age of 18–24 months onward. In some C2 (and C4)-deficient patients, the production of functional antibodies is impaired, which also may contribute to their increased risk of infection. This may also explain the scattered reports on recurrent infections with Neisserieae strains of an identical serotype spaced by only 1–2 months. The development of antibodies against the missing complement component limits the benefits of plasma transfusions, and in some patients an aggravation of Neisserieae infections has been observed during acute infection.

If vaccination measures have failed, prophylactic antibiotics [e.g. with cotrimoxazole (i.e. trimethoprim–sulfamethoxazole)] may help to prevent recurrent sinopulmonary infections with pneumococci and *H. influenzae*, and may also provide protection against meningococci. The danger of colonization and subsequent infection with resistant strains is real, and should be weighed against the prevalence of such strains in the local environment (e.g. hospital).

4.2 What are the future challenges and opportunities for reducing the risk of infection?

Vaccination with improved pneumococcal vaccine and a meningococcal vaccine providing protection to group B strains could be of help.

In the future, gene therapy will be the ultimate way to reduce the risk of infection.

5 REGARDING THE TREATMENT OF PATIENTS WITH DEFICIENCY OF EARLY COMPLEMENT COMPONENTS

5.1 What is the role of empirical therapy?

Given the severity of the infections, empirical therapy should be directed towards pneumococci, *H. influenzae* and meningococci. When selecting empirical antibiotic therapy, the potential for antibiotic-resistant pneumococci must be considered. In most cases, initial therapy with amoxycillin–clavulanate should prove adequate. Alternatively a cephalosporin (e.g. cefuroxime or ceftriaxone parenterally, or an oral cephalosporin) may be chosen. The choice for the parenteral or the oral route of initial therapy depends on the severity of illness. When the microbiologic results are defined, antibiotic treatment can be streamlined to the simplest regimen possible.

5.2 What is the appropriate approach to the patient with deficiency of early complement components and evidence of:

Upper respiratory tract infection?

The antibiotic policy in upper respiratory tract infection (including sinusitis and middle ear infection) is given in section 5.1. Drainage of sinuses may be necessary.

Lower respiratory tract infection?

The approach in lower respiratory tract infection is the same as in section 5.1. With recurrent lower airway infection, investigation of pulmonary function (including arterial blood gas analysis) and of the presence of bronchiectasis (high-resolution CT of the thorax) is indicated.

Skin infection?
Skin infections are encountered in patients with deficiency of C2 and C4, and in those with discoid lupus lesions. Topical treatment often suffices.

Central nervous system infection?
In case of purulent meningitis, while awaiting the results of the Gram stain and antigen testing, antibiotic coverage should be given for pneumococci, *H. influenzae* and meningococci. Taking into account the considerations outlined in section 5.1, ceftriaxone is the drug of choice.

5.3 What is the appropriate approach to the patient with deficiency of early complement components and evidence of bacteremia, with or without site of infection?
See section 5.1.

5.4 What is the appropriate approach to the patient with deficiency of early complement components and evidence of a viral infection?
If serious viral infection occurs in a patient with a complement deficiency, a concomitant cellular immunodeficiency should be seriously considered.

5.5 What is the appropriate approach to the patient with deficiency of early complement components and evidence of a fungal infection?
If fungemia occurs, additional immune defects should be considered (neutrophil or cellular immune defect).

B. COMPLEMENT DEFICIENCIES: ABNORMALITIES OF THE LATE COMPONENTS OF THE CLASSIC PATHWAY

Once C3 and C5 are activated and split, the terminal components of complement C6 through C9 are activated. They form a channel-like structure (the membrane attack complex) in the membrane of bacteria and somatic cells, which are then killed osmotically. When C6, C7 or C8 is deficient, a membrane attack complex is not formed. Similarly, in C9 deficiency, the complex is not sufficient. In the serum of such patients, meningococci and gonococci are therefore not lyzed by complement.

I REGARDING THE CLINICAL PRESENTATION AND EVALUATION OF THE PATIENT

1.1 What are the clinically predominant modes of presentation of infection in patients with deficiency of late complement components?
Patients may present with fever of unknown origin (recurrent, benign), skin lesions, tenosynovitis, arthritis, arthralgia and meningitis.

1.2 What are the predominant sites of infection?

Infections of the bloodstream and/or the meninges predominate. Skin lesions and arthritis may occur.

1.3 What are the predominant organisms that contribute (by site)?

In carriers, only half of the meningococcal strains are encapsulated and potentially virulent. Of these encapsulated strains, serogroups B and C constitute 30%. Currently, 12 serogroups have been identified, the most commonly isolated being serogroups B and C. In complement-deficient patients, the predominant causative organisms are, however, serogroups W-135, X, Y, Z and 29E; these strains usually contribute to only 2% of all meningococcal disease.

Complement-deficient patients are also susceptible to disseminated *Neisseria gonorrhoeae* infections. Pneumococcal disease should not be underestimated, since it represents some 30% of the infections in these patients.

1.4 How do the organisms vary according to various risk factors?

The severity of the immunodeficiency additionally depends on factors such as Fcγ receptor status, certain MBP gene polymorphisms, or genetic cytokine-response profile (see section 2.1), as has been shown in several infectious diseases among immune-competent individuals, as well as a small group of complement-deficient patients. It is unclear whether these factors have an additional impact on the kind (serotype) of microorganisms that cause the disease. Since the complement system has its greatest impact before specific immunity arises, the status of specific immunity, especially towards *N. meningitidis*, makes all the difference.

1.5 How does this differ from other conditions, from center to center, and from country to country?

In various countries the prevalence of Neisseriaceae infections (both *N. gonorrhoeae* and *N. meningitidis*) varies. The prevalence of capsular types of *N. meningitidis* also varies worldwide, group B being the most prevalent in western Europe, and group A (and C) in other parts of the world (e.g. Africa, South America, Asia). The occurrence of serogroups W-135, X, Y, Z and 29E in complement-deficient patients is unexplained.

1.6 What is the appropriate approach to the initial evaluation and diagnosis of infection in patients with deficiency of late complement components?

Many of the Neisserieae infections in these patients are not particularly serious, pointing to the role played by the membrane attack complex in damaging the host. Thus, in many cases, there is time for the diagnostic process.

In the patient's history, risk factors for sexually transmitted disease should be identified. Previous disease episodes should be asked for, as well as information on contacts with meningococcal disease. As with all primary immunodeficiencies, the family history is very important.

In the patient who presents with fever, subtle skin lesions may be present. These lesions may be macules or papules, petechial or pustular (like a small hemorrhagic blister), the latter occurring in disseminated gonococcal infection, and most often located on the fingers or distal part of the feet. When skin lesions are found, they should be biopsied for Gram staining, culture and histologic examination. Since *Neisseria* (especially *N. gonorrhoeae*) is a somewhat fastidious organism, care should be taken to handle the material properly. Negative results do not rule out neisserial infection. To detect the causative organism, cultures of blood and CSF (in case of meningitis) should be done. Swabs from the nasopharynx, throat and genital sites should be investigated for *Neisseria*. Meningococcal antigen can be detected in CSF, blood and urine. Other valuable serological and molecular techniques are not generally available.

1.7 How should the evaluation be modified according to the severity of the risk?

Dependent on the severity of the clinical presentation, the diagnostic workup should be performed more rapidly. If antibiotics have been started, biopsies of skin lesions may still be valuable.

1.8 What are specific evaluation measures?

See section 1.6. and Chapter 2 in Part 1.

1.9 What new developments are going to impact on emerging organisms, recognition, evaluation and diagnosis of infection in patients with deficiency of late complement components?

Given the difficulty of diagnosing gonococcemia (and sometimes also meningococcemia), better diagnostic tools (PCR, antigen tests) need to be developed and evaluated, and to become generally available.

2 REGARDING THE RISK FACTORS ACCOMPANYING DEFICIENCY OF LATE COMPLEMENT COMPONENTS

2.1 What are the main alterations in host defense mechanisms and what are the appropriate investigations to document them?

In cases where the diagnosis of complement deficiency has not yet been made, measurement of CH50 concentration is indicated. Since acute infection is often accompanied by complement activation and consumption, such measurements should be done after recovery. If an abnormally low CH50 level is found, the concentrations of the individual complement factors should be measured. If relevant (see Table 1.1), assessment for associated conditions should be performed.

2.2 What are the alterations due to iatrogenic factors?

As mentioned, these defects often present with relatively mild *Neisseria* infection. When these patients are given fresh plasma, thereby providing them with the components to build up functional membrane attack complexes, fulminant infection may ensue.

2.3 What is the influence of environmental factors?
2.4 What are the most significant factors that contribute to the risk of infection in patients with deficiency of late complement components?

Dependent on their sexual behavior, patients with these defects have an increased risk of disseminated gonococcal infection. Environmental risk factors for meningococcal disease are crowding (military camps, kindergarten) and travel (to 'meningitis areas'; see section 1.5).

2.5 What are the specific or nonspecific measures aimed at minimizing each of these factors?

Patients with a deficiency of a late complement component should be educated about their condition, paying special attention to the risk of crowding, travel and unprotected sexual practices.

2.6 Are there different levels of risk of infection recognized for patients with deficiency of late complement components?

The FcγR polymorphism mentioned in section 1.4 may be an additional risk factor. The same holds for the MBP polymorphism. Both contribute to the process of opsonophagocytosis.

2.7 How does the level of risk impact on management?

The recurrence rate in defects of the late complement components is about 40%. Vaccination and boosts against meningococci may be of limited value (due to coverage of relevant serogroups or unpredictable immune response). In case of clinical vaccine failure, chemoprophylaxis (penicillin) is the alternative with proven efficacy in these patients.

3 REGARDING THE SURVEILLANCE OF PATIENTS WITH DEFICIENCY OF LATE COMPLEMENT COMPONENTS

3.1 What is the important premorbid information to be gathered?

If available, information on the exact nature of the host defense defect should be gathered. Concomitant risk factors may be the FcγR IIa and MBP gene polymorphisms.

3.2 What are the surveillance measures to be taken when a patient presents with deficiency of late complement components?

Surveillance cultures are of no value because colonization does not necessarily reflect the risk of infection.

3.4 What development(s) are to be expected for surveillance in patients with deficiency of late complement components?

See sections 2.5, 2.7 and 3.1. In addition, vaccination with meningococcal vaccine A/C or ACYW-135 should be given, since vaccination significantly enhances opsonization for phagocytosis and killing by neutrophils. Postvaccine measurement to check for antibody generation and/or opsonic activity is advised. Booster vaccination is recommended on a regular basis (with a 2–3-year interval) because of a normal decline in protective antibody levels. It should, however, be noted that other serotypes also occur in these patients. One prospective study in C6–deficient South African patients showed a protective effect of prolonged penicillin prophylaxis; the availability of conjugate vaccine was limited at that time and further studies are needed. The conjugate vaccines are effectively inducing specific antibody responses with repeated immunizations starting at 2–3 months of age (see also section 4.1 above for patients with deficiency of early complement components). Such antibodies enhance opsonization and phagocytosis, but not serum bactericidal effects.

4 REGARDING THE PREVENTION OF INFECTION IN PATIENTS WITH DEFICIENCY OF LATE COMPLEMENT COMPONENTS

4.2 What are future challenges and opportunities for reducing the risk of infection?

Improved meningococcal vaccines (e.g. conjugate vaccine and vaccines covering the group B meningococcus) as well as a gonococcal vaccine would be a major step forward. Given the low frequency of these deficiencies and the relatively mild infections in many of these patients, it is questionable whether substitution therapy with the missing component (or even gene therapy) will ever be feasible or wise to implement.

5 REGARDING THE TREATMENT OF PATIENTS WITH DEFICIENCY OF LATE COMPLEMENT COMPONENTS

5.1 What is the role of empirical therapy?

Dependent on the severity of disease, empirical antimicrobial treatment should be started. In patients with a known defect and a mild infection there is no reason to withhold treatment after taking material for microbiologic investigation (see section 1.6).

When infection with a gonococcus is suspected or cannot be excluded, treatment with a second- or third-generation cephalosporin (cefuroxime 750 mg iv three times daily or ceftriaxone 2 g iv per day in adults) is first choice. In mild disease, an oral fluoroquinolone derivative (e.g. ciprofloxacin) may suffice.

When meningococcal disease is evident (e.g. meningitis with a positive meningococcal antigen test) benzylpenicillin iv is the drug of choice. The duration of treatment for these disseminated infections is generally 7–10 days. Prevalent resistance patterns may necessitate the use of other antibiotics.

As mentioned in section 2.2, plasma therapy should not be given.

5.2 What is the appropriate approach to the patient with deficiency of late complement components and evidence of:

Genitourinary tract infection?

Gonorrhea should be suspected and treated accordingly (see section 5.1).

Musculoskeletal infection?

Tenosynovitis and arthritis, either purulent or serous, occur in infection with gonococci and meningococci. In case of purulence, drainage is indicated in addition to antibiotics (see section 5.1).

Skin infection?

Skin infection should be considered as disseminated infection, and treated as outlined in section 5.1.

Central nervous system infection?

Meningitis is a major manifestation. See section 5.1.

5.3 What is the appropriate approach to the patient with deficiency of late complement components and evidence of bacteremia, with or without site of infection?

See section 5.1.

5.4 What is the appropriate approach to the patient with deficiency of late complement components and evidence of a viral infection?
If serious viral infection occurs in complement deficiency, a concomitant cellular immuno-deficiency should be seriously considered.

5.5 What is the appropriate approach to the patient with deficiency of late complement components and evidence of a fungal infection?
If fungemia occurs, additional immune defects should be considered (neutrophil defect or cellular immune defect).

5.6 What is the appropriate approach to the patient with deficiency of late complement components and evidence of a parasitic infection?
Not applicable.

5.7 What is the role of nonantiinfective interventions (including reducing or altering immunosuppression) in the management of established infection?
Not applicable.

II HUMORAL SPECIFIC PRIMARY IMMUNODEFICIENCY

Immunoglobulins provide multiple functions including antigen neutralization, comple-ment binding and activation, prevention of adherence of microorganism to (mucosal) cells, opsonization, and arming of killer cells. The major problems that occur in immunoglobulin (Ig) G deficiency is defective opsonization (i.e. the coating of particles, especially encapsulated bacteria, by IgG and/or complement to facilitate phagocytosis) and the inability to prevent adherence of microorganisms to epithelial surfaces (mainly due to lack of IgA). The spectrum of immunoglobulins and the absolute number of lym-phocyte subpopulations permits the categorization of patients into two major groups:
1 Hypogammaglobulinemia
   - early onset
     –X-linked agammaglobulinemia (XLA)
     –other
   - late onset (common variable immune deficiency; CVID)
2 Dysgammaglobulinemia
   - hypogammaglobulinemia with increased levels of IgM (hyperIgM syndrome; HIM)
   - IgG subclass deficiency
   - IgA deficiency

I REGARDING THE CLINICAL PRESENTATION AND EVALUATION OF THE PATIENT

1.1 What are the clinically predominant modes of presentation of infection in patients with immunoglobulin deficiencies?
With the exception of selective IgA deficiency (in which infectious complications may not occur), patients with primary immunoglobulin deficiencies present with recurrent or severe infections. In the congenital (early-onset) forms, infection usually begins at between 3 and 6 months of age (when the maternal IgG has disappeared). In late-onset forms the infectious problems generally start gradually.

Apart from clearcut infections, patients may also present with autoimmune phenomena or manifestations of proliferative disease. This is especially the case in late-onset hypogammaglobulinemia, in which gastric pathology (chronic antrum gastritis, gastric carcinoma, pernicious anemia), benign lymphonodular hyperplasia and malignant B-cell lymphoma (especially in the gastrointestinal tract), thymoma, hypothyroidism, sicca syndrome, vitiligo and sarcoid-like granulomatous disease. In XLA, aggressive colorectal cancer has been observed as an additional complication.

Arthralgia and arthritis may be seen in both late- and early-onset forms of immunoglobulin deficiency. Arthritis may be due to infection (see below). It is not uncommon that the arthritic symptoms and signs respond rapidly to IgG substitution alone; whether such arthritis is noninfectious or represents low-grade infection is generally difficult to discern.

1.2 What are the predominant sites of infection?
The predominant sites of infection are:
- Ear, nose and throat region: otitis, mastoiditis and sinusitis
- Upper respiratory tract: bronchitis
- Lower respiratory tract: pneumonia
- Gastrointestinal tract: gastroenteritis with diarrhea; malabsorption
- Bloodstream
- Meninges: purulent meningitis
- Joints: arthritis

1.3 What are the predominant organisms that contribute (by site)?
- *Streptococcus pneumoniae*
- Encapsulated *Haemophilus influenzae* (especially type b)
- *Campylobacter jejuni*
- *Giardia lamblia*
- *Salmonella* spp.
- *Ureaplasma* and *Mycoplasma* spp.
- *Pneumocystis carinii* (especially in HIM)
- Cytomegalovirus (in cases with thymoma)
- Enteroviruses (especially ECHOvirus)

1.4 How do the organisms vary according to various risk factors?
It is currently unclear why certain patients, even within one family, vary in susceptibility to infection, or differ in their response to immunoglobulin therapy. From a theoretical point of view, the quality of the FcγR's, the residual mucosal immunity and the reactivity of the cellular immune system [including cytokine response profiles as demonstrated for tumor necrosis factor (TNF) α and/or interleukin (IL) 10] may explain such differences. Some cases of common variable immunodeficiency (especially those with thymoma), and hyperIgM syndrome (in which the interaction between CD40 and CD40 ligand is defective, resulting in disturbed T-cell function) have disturbed cellular immunity, with increased risk for certain types of infection (see section 1.3).

1.5 How does this differ from other conditions, from center to center, and from country to country?
The defective mucosal immunity makes the patients vulnerable to gastrointestinal infections. Patients are at greater risk of such infections under circumstances of high microbial pressure and poor hygiene.

1.6 What is the appropriate approach to the initial evaluation and diagnosis of infection in patients with immunoglobulin deficiencies?

When taking the patient's history, information should be sought regarding previous infectious episodes, their sites, course and treatment, as well as the family history for infection, autoimmunity and cancer.

Exposure history should be ascertained. For example, in cases of otitis, sinusitis and respiratory tract infection, the clinician should ask about exposure to respiratory viruses, which can result in secondary bacterial infection. Patients with an enteric problem should be asked about exposure to food that was potentially contaminated.

In patients who present with weight loss and malaise, giardiasis should be suspected, whereas patients with bouts of spiking fever may suffer from transient and recurrent *Campylobacter* bacteremia (sometimes accompanied by erysipelas-like skin lesions).

Patients with complaints about micturition, arthritis and/or unexplained fever should have a workup for *Ureaplasma* and *Mycoplasma* spp. (special culture specimens from urethra, urine and blood). Patients with muscular complaints or symptomatology pointing to central nervous sytem (CNS) pathology should be investigated for enterovirus (ECHOvirus) infection. The physical examination should, dependent on the major complaints, further focus on the pulmonary status, the abdomen or other body sites.

Gram stain and culture of relevant specimens (secretions, sputum, and sometimes CSF) should be performed. Blood cultures should be done when bacteremia is suspected; as mentioned, special techniques may be required to demonstrate *Ureaplasma* and *Mycoplasma* spp. Antigen tests (urine, CSF) for *S. pneumoniae*, *H. influenzae* and *Neisseria meningitidis*, if available, may be of some help. As indicated above, viral cultures should be performed in selected cases. Note that serological examination has little or no value (especially in patients who are being substituted with iv IgG).

Radiography of the chest and sinuses is indicated in most cases.

1.7 How should the evaluation be modified according to the severity of the risk?

If the patient presents with infections caused by intracellular microorganisms, viruses or parasites such as *P. carinii*, abnormalities in cellular immunity should also be tested.

1.8 What are the specific evaluation measures? (see also chapter 2 in Part II)

Recurrent infections in the hypogammaglobulinemic patient, even relatively mild ones, may lead to anatomical damage (especially bronchiectasis) and loss of pulmonary function. High-resolution CT of the thorax is an important tool to evaluate the patient for the presence of bronchiectasis. The efficacy of IgG replacement can be judged by a reduction in the frequency of infection or, for patients with pulmonary infection, evidence of improved respiratory tract function. Gastrointestinal biopsies should be taken for culture and histologic examination in patients with CVID.

See also section 1.6 and Chapter 2, Part I.

1.9 What new developments are going to impact on emerging organisms, recognition, evaluation and diagnosis of infection in patients with immunoglobulin deficiencies?

Rapid diagnostic tools (PCR, antigen tests) for various relevant organisms (encapsulated bacteria, enteric pathogens, *Ureaplasma*, *Mycoplasma*, enteroviruses) should be improved or developed. Note that it may be difficult to establish the microbial cause of enteric illness in some hypogammaglobulinemic patients; even the diagnosis of giardiasis may not be easy. Thus, there is a critical need for new diagnostic techniques.

2 REGARDING THE RISK FACTORS ACCOMPANYING IMMUNOGLOBULIN DEFICIENCIES

2.1 What are the main alterations in host defense mechanisms and what are the appropriate investigations to document them?

As explained in the introduction to this section, the major host defense defects consist of the lack of opsonizing antibodies (in the defense against encapsulated bacteria), the lack of IgA antagonizing adherence of microorganisms (*Giardia lamblia*, *C. jejuni*, *Salmonella* spp.), of bactericidal, complement-binding antibodies (against *C. jejuni* and *Ureaplasma/Mycoplasma* strains) and of enterovirus-neutralizing antibodies. In patients presenting with agammaglobulinemia, secondary hypogammaglobulinemia should be considered. B-lymphocyte malignancies as well as acquired hypogammaglobulinemia due to loss of IgG in stools (exudative enteropathy) or in urine (nephrotic syndrome) should be considered. Anticonvulsive drugs (phenytoin, carbamazepine) may induce a reversible severe hypogammaglobulinemia by a mechanism that is not yet understood.

To document the immunoglobulin deficiency, agar gel electrophoresis and immunoelectrophoresis represent the initial approach. After that, quantitative IgG determinations are performed. In cases with the typical infections seen in hypogammaglobulinemia or dysgammaglobulinemia and relatively normal concentrations of the plasma immunoglobulins, IgG (and IgA) subclass determinations should be carried out. These determinations have to be performed according to the manufacturer's standardization and are not of universal value or applicability. In addition to the serum measurements, IgA levels may be determined in secretions such as saliva or tears; the latter measurements are of little value if serum IgA concentration is low.

Further support for an immunoglobulin disorder and/or a specific antibody response defect may be obtained by determining the humoral reactivity to polysaccharide antigens, such as pneumococcal vaccine (note that reliable quantitative measurements of antibody titers to these antigens are not generally available). To investigate the capacity to form antibodies against protein antigens, the secondary response to tetanus, diphtheria and parenteral poliomyelitis vaccine may be measured; for a primary response, hepatitis B vaccine or rabies vaccine may be used. In addition, levels of the isohemagglutinins may be determined, but the value of this investigation is overestimated.

To establish further the type of immunoglobulin disorder, an assessment of the presence of B lymphocytes and plasma cells in blood and bone marrow should be made. In XLA neither cell types are detectable, whereas in late-onset agammaglobulinemia B lymphocytes are often present and plasma cells are not. When XLA is suspected, a molecular diagnosis (determination of the genetic defect of the Bruton tyrosine kinase) should be performed for genetic counseling. The genetic defects of selective IgA deficiency and CVID are as yet unknown.

In HIM syndrome, the defect of the CD40 ligand should be evident. Determination of the cellular immune status in late-onset agammaglobulinemia is of more scientific interest than clinical relevance.

Before starting on IgG replacement therapy, it is prudent (especially in late-onset agammaglobulinemia and in patients who present with severe combined IgA–IgG subclass deficiency) to check for antibodies against IgA. Such antibodies may elicit severe anaphylactoid reactions during the first iv IgG substitution. Most patients with such antibodies may tolerate subcutaneous IgG (16%) given by slow infusion.

2.2 What are the alterations due to iatrogenic factors?

Antiepileptic drugs, sulfasalazine and nonsteroidal antiinflammatory drugs (NSAID) may induce hypogammaglobulinemia.

2.3 What is the influence of environmental factors?

It is not certain whether episodes of infection with the encapsulated microorganisms are preceded by viral infections. It is wise to avoid crowding since it may lead to the acquisition of respiratory viruses. Because of the undue susceptibility to enteric pathogens (especially *C. jejuni*, *Salmonella* spp. and *G. lamblia*), care with food safety is important. Proper preparation of meat, chicken, eggs, salad and raw vegetables is essential. Water used while camping should be boiled.

2.4 What are the most significant factors that contribute to the risk of infection in patients with immunoglobulin deficiencies?

See section 2.3.

2.5 What are the specific or nonspecific measures aimed at minimizing each of these factors?

In view of section 2.3, avoidance of crowding may be effective. Special care should be taken with regard to the preparation of food (meat, chicken and salad). Patients should be thoroughly counseled about hygiene when they travel to countries with a high risk for enteric infection.

3 REGARDING THE SURVEILLANCE OF PATIENTS WITH IMMUNOGLOBULIN DEFICIENCIES

3.2 What are the surveillance measures to be taken when a patient presents with immunoglobulin deficiency?

When a patient presents with immunoglobulin deficiency, some clinicians believe it is reasonable to culture sputum in order to assess the susceptibility of *S. pneumoniae* and *H. influenzae*. Radiography of the chest and sinuses is helpful and, when bronchiectasis is suspected, CT of the thorax should be performed. Pulmonary function tests should be considered.

Stools should be investigated for *C. jejuni*, *Salmonella* and *G. lamblia*.

3.3 What are the other specific measures to be taken when a patient presents with immunoglobulin deficiency?

Since pulmonary function over time is a good indicator for the success of immunoglobulin replacement therapy, assessment of vital capacity and forced expiratory volume in 1 s (FEV_1) should be done on a regular basis (e.g. once every 2 years) in patients who have had pulmonary infections.

Because of the high incidence of gastric ailments in late-onset hypogammaglobulinemia (antral gastritis, atrophic gastritis, gastric cancer and lymphoma), gastroscopy should be performed. Although the role of *Helicobacter pylori* in these abnormalities is not well established, investigation for this organism should be done (biopsies or urease breath test). Based on the findings at endoscopy, the frequency for subsequent procedures can be determined. Since patients with XLA have an increased risk of recto-colonic cancer, sigmoidoscopy every 3 years is a prudent policy in adults.

4 REGARDING THE PREVENTION OF INFECTION IN PATIENTS WITH IMMUNOGLOBULIN DEFICIENCIES

4.1 What approaches, if any, to the prevention of infection should be considered in patients with immunoglobulin deficiencies?

The main preventive measure in these patients is administration of immunoglobulins, commonly via the intravenous route. The majority of intravenous IgG (IVIG) preparations are safe and of good quality. Although most patients seem to fare well on a dose of 300–400 mg/kg/month, a recent Dutch controlled trial showed that a dose of 600–800 mg/kg/month was superior in terms of prevention of infection. In view of the relatively long half-life of IgG, the dosage interval is generally every 3–4 weeks, with a goal of maintaining the nadir IgG concentration at above 4 g/l.

The side effects are generally mild; the acute effects (malaise, chills and hypotension) are dependent largely on the speed of infusion, and generally disappear when the infusion is temporarily stopped. In many cases, home infusions are feasible. It is important to note that there are differences between batches (of one brand) and between brands in terms of tolerability by individual patients. Some of these differences are due to constituents of the preparations (e.g. the amount of prekallikrein). The pathogenesis of the subacute serous meningitis that may occur with some preparations is unclear. Patients with antibodies against IgA and those whose IgA antibody status is unknown should not receive IVIG. There is experience in such patients demonstrating that slow subcutaneous infusion of 16% IgG (2–3 ml/h) is safe; after a couple of such infusions the antibodies against IgA generally disappear. Most of these patients can then be safely switched to IVIG.

Subcutaneous IgG replacement is not only a preferable method for patients with side effects, but also for young children and adults with poor iv access. The preferred dose is approximately 0.33 ml/kg of the 16% IgG solution, once per week.

Although immunoglobulin replacement is the cornerstone of management in XLA and early- and late-onset agammaglobulinemia, its benefit in patients with IgG subclass deficiency and symptomatic IgA deficiency is much less clear. In these patients, IVIG should be used when antibiotic prophylaxis has failed after a period of 3–6 months.

The use of live polio vaccine should be avoided in these patients because of 'enterovirus-associated' pathology.

Although the majority of patients receiving IVIG do not need prophylactic antibiotics, some patients (especially those with anatomic damage to the respiratory tract) may benefit from antimicrobial prophylaxis. However, the risk of emergence of resistant organisms must be considered, making the use of fluoroquinolone prophylaxis inadvisable.

4.2 What are the future challenges and opportunities for reducing the risk of infection?

There are currently no established vehicles for delivering immunoglobulin replacement to the mucosal surfaces. Therefore, even high-dose IVIG is not as successful in preventing infection as hoped. The development of stable IgA preparations, preferably with specific activities against the major pathogens, that could be applied to mucosal surfaces (e.g. gastrointestinal tract or conjunctivae) could prove beneficial.

5 REGARDING THE TREATMENT OF PATIENTS WITH IMMUNOGLOBULIN DEFICIENCIES

5.1 What is the role of empirical therapy?

Given the severity of the infections, empirical therapy should be directed towards pneumococci and *H. influenzae*, while awaiting the initial microbiologic results. Dependent on results of recent surveillance cultures, and what is known of recent antimicrobial exposure, empirical treatment should be administered. The potential likelihood of β-lactamase-producing *H. influenzae* and penicillin-resistant pneumococci should be considered.

In the majority of cases, initial therapy with amoxycillin–clavulanate is adequate. Alternatively a second- or third-generation cephalosporin may be employed. The choice of parenteral or oral route depends upon the severity of illness. When the microbiologic results are known, the antibiotic regimen should be narrowed to cover the isolated organism. In patients who have not been receiving immunoglobulin infusion, IVIG support should be started (see section 4.1).

5.2 What is the appropriate approach to the patient with immunoglobulin deficiency and evidence of:

Upper respiratory tract infection?

The antibiotic policy in upper respiratory tract infection (including sinusitis and middle ear infection) is given in section 5.1. Drainage of sinuses or the middle ear may be necessary. For appropriate assessment of local invasion, CT or magnetic resonance imaging (MRI) may be necessary.

Some patients suffer from chronic conjunctivitis, which may be difficult to cure. Success may be obtained with a course of antibiotic-containing ophthalmic ointment (e.g. oxytetracyclin), although the effect is often transient.

Lower respiratory tract infection?

The approach to lower respiratory tract infection is the same as that given in section 5.1. With recurrent lower airway infection, the investigation of pulmonary function (including arterial blood gas analysis) and of the presence of bronchiectasis (high-resolution CT of the thorax) is indicated.

In patients with end-stage pulmonary function, lung transplantation should be considered. Until recently, however, few centers were accepting these patients as lung transplant recipients.

Gastrointestinal infection?

The role of *H. pylori* in the gastric pathology of late-onset agammaglobulinemia is not well established. If *Helicobacter* is found, appropriate treatment schedules should be administered, preferably after determination of susceptibility of the organism in vitro. *C. jejuni* may cause acute enteritis and require treatment with a macrolide or (empirically) a fluoroquinolone. In contrast to the immunocompetent individual, who does not carry *C. jejuni* for longer than 16 weeks, patients with agammaglobulinemia are frequent chronic *C. jejuni* carriers. It may be desirable to try to eradicate the asymptomatic carrier state because it may lead to chronic intermittent bacteremia and, on occasion, fatal meningitis. *Salmonella* infection should be treated, preferably with a quinolone (e.g. 500 mg ciprofloxacin bid for an adult) or cotrimoxazole (trimethoprim–sulfamethoxazole). Because of the lack of mucosal and systemic humoral immunity, dissemination may occur. The carrier state may be hard to eradicate, even with prolonged treatment with a quinolone.

Giardiasis may also be difficult to treat. Metronidazole (250 mg tid in adults or 15–30 mg/kg/day in three divided doses for children) or tinidazole (single dose of 2 g in adults) are the drugs of choice in Europe. Prolonged (>3 weeks) or repeated courses harbor the risk of irreversible polyneuropathy. Quinacrine (100 mg tid in adults or 6 mg/kg/day in children in three divided doses for 7 days) is the drug of choice in the US; it is rather poorly tolerated in children.

Genitourinary tract infection?

The major pathogens here are *Ureaplasma urealyticum* and *Mycoplasma* spp. These are hard to treat. Drugs of choice are tetracyclines (e.g. doxycycline in adults) and the newer macrolides (e.g. azithromycin), which are preferred in children.

Musculoskeletal infection?

Pneumococci, *H. influenzae* and *Ureaplasma/Mycoplasma* spp. may cause suppurative arthritis in agammaglobulinemic patients.

Persistent enterovirus infection of the CNS may be accompanied by a dermatomyositis-like illness in agammaglobulinemia (see CNS infection below).

Rarely a skeletal metastatic infection may be seen caused by *C. jejuni* (see section 5.3) or by *Salmonella* spp.

Skin infection?

Persistent enterovirus infection may present as a dermatomyositis-like illness in patients with agammaglobulinemia (see CNS infection below). *C. jejuni* bacteremia may lead to erysipelas-like skin lesions (see section 5.3) A noninfectious pyoderma gangrenosum can occur in patients with agammaglobulinemia and may respond to high-dose IVIG.

Central nervous system infection?

In case of purulent meningitis, while awaiting the results of the Gram stain and antigen testing, antibiotic coverage should be given for pneumococci, *H. influenzae* and meningococci. Ceftriaxone may be the drug of choice.

Another major cause of CNS infection is persistent enterovirus infection, for which high-dose immunoglobulin therapy may provide some benefit. It is probably worthwhile to select batches of immunoglobulin preparations that contain neutralizing antibodies against the causative strain of virus.

5.3 What is the appropriate approach to the patient with immunoglobulin deficiency and evidence of bacteremia, with or without site of infection?

Bacteremia in patients with immunoglobulin disorders may be caused by pneumococci or *H. influenzae*. This should be treated as indicated in section 5.1.

C. jejuni bacteremia may be a cause of recurrent, albeit self-limited, fever. Treatment with a macrolide or quinolone may not be successful. The latter type of drug may lead rapidly to development of quinolone-resistant *Campylobacter*. Recalcitrant cases have been treated successfully with a carbapenem (imipenem 1 g iv bid) and either plasma or an IgM-containing immunoglobulin preparation. The rationale behind the latter approach is that IgM and complement are needed for the bactericidal effect of plasma. Standard preparations of IVIG provide only IgG, which does not give bactericidal activity against *C. jejuni*. Bacteremia with *Ureaplasma/Mycoplasma* spp. may respond poorly to antibiotics and

IVIG. To optimize treatment, antimicrobial susceptibility testing of the causative microorganisms should be performed. In addition, the bactericidal effect of the patient's plasma and that of various IVIG preparations (including preparations containing IgM) should be tested.

5.4 What is the appropriate approach to the patient with immunoglobulin deficiency and evidence of a viral infection?

For enteroviruses, see section 5.2 on CNS infection.

With regard to hepatitis, there are reports of a severe and rapidly progressive course of hepatitis B and C infection in patients with agammaglobulinemia. On the other hand, an indolent course with chronic hepatitis, not really different from that in a normal host, has also been observed. The therapeutic approach should probably be similar to that in the normal host.

5.6 What is the appropriate approach to the patient with immunoglobulin deficiency and evidence of a parasitic infection?

P. carinii pneumonia occurs occasionally in immunoglobulin-deficient patients who have concomitant T-cell immune defects. The approach is identical. Giardiasis may be difficult to diagnose and treat in these patients (see section 5.2 on Gastrointestinal infection). The role of microsporidia and cryptosporidia in patients with hypogammaglobulinemia is not well established (see T-cell and macrophage defects, section 5.2 on gastrointestinal and hepatobiliary infection).

III CELLULAR ASPECIFIC IMMUNODEFICIENCY

In some syndromal forms of primary immunodeficiency (e.g. Chédiak–Higashi syndrome), NK cell function and numbers should be tested to support the diagnosis. Since isolated defects of NK cells are very rare (and the patients seem to suffer almost exclusively from recurrent herpes simplex infections) this section will be limited to a discussion of phagocyte disorders.

PHAGOCYTIC DISORDERS

The professional phagocytic cells, the polymorphonuclear leukocytes (neutrophilic granulocytes, neutrophils) and the mononuclear phagocytes (monocytes and macrophages) make up the most important defense systems against bacteria and fungi.

Strictly, the eosinophilic granulocyte is also a professional phagocyte that serves mainly in defense against metazoa. Eosinophilia is sometimes encountered in patients with phagocyte disorders, probably reflecting a compensatory mechanism.

For optimal defense, the phagocytic precursors of neutrophils and monocyte lineages should proliferate properly, and the cells should mature and gain access to the bloodstream. In the bloodstream, about half of the population of granulocytes adheres to the endothelium (the marginating pool) and subsequently crosses the endothelial layer to gain access to the tissues. In the tissues, the monocytes differentiate into macrophages. During inflammation, proliferation in the bone marrow is augmented and, because of a gradient of chemotactic substances, the phagocytes infiltrate the inflammatory field. The granulocytes arrive earlier than the monocytes. The phagocytes function by ingesting particles (e.g. bacteria, fungi), killing them by means of oxygen-dependent and oxygen-independent mechanisms. In addition the phagocytes are important as secretory cells as they release a large series of inflammatory mediators. Phagocytosis, especially of encapsulated microorganisms is great-ly facilitated by opsonins such as IgG. Since the phagocyte binds the Fc portion of the opsonin with its Fc receptor, the quality of the receptor contributes to the efficiency of phagocytosis. Thus far, defects is Fc receptors and polymorphism in these molecules have not been associated with a clinical syndrome; they appear to act merely as cofactors.

It is clear that each step of the process, from proliferation up to killing, is important for proper defense. A series of molecules (growth factors, adhesion molecules, cytokines, chemokines, complement factors and lipid mediators) is crucial for the orchestration of this program. Defects may occur in each of the steps and almost invariably lead to infection.

For practical purposes, the following classification of primary defects of phagocytes is useful:

1 Quantitative defects
   - Severe congenital neutropenia (SCN) syndromes
     –Kostmann syndrome (autosomal recessive)
     –Granulocyte colony-stimulating factor (G-CSF) receptor mutation (auto-somal dominant, sporadic)
     –chronic idiopathic neutropenia
     –cyclic neutropenia
     –Shwachman–Diamond syndrome
     –Glycogen storage disease 1b (GSD-1b)
2 Qualitative defects
   - Disorders of adherence
     –Leukocyte adhesion deficiency type 1/variant
     –Leukocyte adhesion deficiency type 2
   - Disorders of chemotaxis
     –Chédiak–Higashi syndrome
     –Neutrophil actin dysfunction (variants)
     –Neutrophil-specific granule deficiency
     –Glycogen storage disease 1b (GSD-1b)
     –Papillon–Lefèvre syndrome
     –Wiskott–Aldrich syndrome (WAS)
     –HyperIgE (HIE) recurrent infection syndrome
   - Disorders of phagocytosis
     –Leukocyte adhesion deficiency type 1
     –Neutrophil actin dysfunction (variants)
   - Disorders of microbicidal activity
     –Chronic granulomatous disease (CGD)
     –Chédiak–Higashi syndrome
     –Neutrophil actin dysfunction (variants)
     –Neutrophil-specific granule deficiency
     –(Myeloperoxidase deficiency)

I REGARDING THE CLINICAL PRESENTATION AND EVALUATION OF THE PATIENT

1.1 What are the clinically predominant modes of presentation of infection in patients with phagocytic disorders?

In patients with neutropenia, those with a neutrophil count below 500/mm^3 have a more severe course than patients with a higher count.

Recurrent ear, nose and throat (ENT) infections such as otitis media and lower respiratory tract infections, skin infections, and perianal infiltrates are suspicious of a clinically important neutropenia.

Of interest, some patients are relatively free from infection, despite severe neutropenia as long as skin and mucous membranes are intact. Moreover the circulating pool of neutrophils represents only a fraction of the total pool. The latter can be assessed by measuring the concentration of a neutrophil-specific, surface-derived antigen in plasma or serum (e.g. soluble FcRγIII).

Patients with primary defects of phagocyte function usually present with recurrent or severe infection from a very early age. Often the inflammatory response is blunted (no infiltrate, 'cold abscesses') and this may lead to a delay in diagnosis despite overwhelming infection. Eczema is a common manifestation in patients with phagocyte disorders. Failure to separate the umbilical cord occurs in leukocyte adhesion deficiency and to a lesser extent in the congenital neutropenia syndromes.

The severity and frequency of infection vary with the different syndromes and within the same genetic defect (genotype–phenotype relationship).

In patients with partial leukocyte adhesion defects, the severity of disease is inversely related to the degree of expression of the CD11/CD18 molecules. In Wiskott–Aldrich syndrome there is a progressive course unless it is limited to the X-linked thrombocytopenia (XLT) form. Patients with CGD with residual NADPH (nicotinamide adenine dinucleotide phosphate) oxidase function may have less severe disease than those without any enzyme activity. The latter forms are usually diagnosed before 3 years of age, whereas the former patients, especially those with autosomal forms, are sometimes diagnosed in adulthood. In CGD, granuloma formation, especially in the gastrointestinal, respiratory or urinary tract, may give rise to obstruction.

Gastrointestinal Crohn disease-like granulomatous lesions may also be seen in GSD-1b, a disease characterized by early hepatomegaly, a tendency to hypoglycemia and recurrent infections. A glucose 6–phosphate transport defect goes along with a variable neutropenia and concomitant chemotaxis defect.

Patients with HIE are prone to recurrent (subcutaneous and pulmonary) infections with *Staphylococcus aureus* in the presence of a normal humoral response and intact opsonophagocytosis. Although a defect in neutrophil chemotaxis has been described, this has not been a consistent finding. The primary defect in HIE has not yet been elucidated. These patients can be easily recognized by a distinct physiognomy (coarse facies with hypertelorism, hyperostosis frontalis and a flattened bulky nose), hyperlaxity of joints, an often-delayed dental shedding, osteoporosis and eczema. Many of these abnormalities will not be apparent until adolescence.

The same applies to Papillon–Lefèvre syndrome, in which precocious periodontal disease results in the loss of primary or permanent teeth. Apart from palmoplantar hyperkeratosis, one in five patients suffer from recurrent extraoral infections such as pyoderma and furunculosis, as a consequence of a neutrophil chemotaxis defect. The genetic defect is as yet unknown.

The neutrophil defects such as neutrophil actin dysfunction (NAD) and neutrophil-specific granule deficiency (SGD) are extremely rare and beyond the scope of this chapter.

1.2 What are the predominant sites of infection?
- Skin: pyoderma, impetigo, folliculitis, furunculosis, eczema
- Lymph nodes: suppurative lymphadenitis
- CNS: cerebral abscesses

- Mouth: aphthous ulcers, gingivitis and periodontal disease
- ENT infections (otitis media)
- Upper respiratory tract: bronchitis
- Lower respiratory tract: pneumonia, lung abscess
- Bone: osteomyelitis
- Gastrointestinal tract: gastroenteritis, liver abscess, perianal abscesses
- Joints: suppurative arthritis

1.3 What are the predominant organisms that contribute (by site)?

1 Bacteria
  - *Staphylococcus aureus*, *Streptococcus pyogenes*
  - *Haemophilus influenzae* and *Streptococcus pneumoniae*
  - Enteric Gram-negative bacteria (*Escherichia coli* and *Pseudomonas* spp.)
  - *Salmonella* spp.
2 Fungi
  - *Candida* spp.
  - *Aspergillus* spp.

Note: The granulomatous lesions in CGD do not necessarily represent active infection; they tend to respond to glucocorticosteroids. When infections are present in CGD, they are almost exclusively caused by catalase-positive microorganisms (*S. aureus*, enteric Gram-negative bacteria, *Salmonella* spp., fungi).

The cause of aphthous ulcers is not understood.

Myeloperoxidase deficiency, which is not a particularly rare disorder (incidence 1 in 2000 persons), is not accompanied by infection unless there is a concomitant risk factor such as poorly controlled diabetes; in this case, severe candidal infection may be seen.

1.4 How do the organisms vary according to various risk factors?

As mentioned in section 1.1, different defects may predispose patients to particular microorganisms. Following the success of antimicrobial prophylaxis with cotrimoxazole (trimethoprim–sulfamethoxazole) in CGD, many patients with phagocyte defects have been put on such a regimen. However, fungal infections are seen in these patients.

1.5 How does this differ from other conditions, from center to center, and from country to country?

The nature of the infectious disease depends, to a large extent, on the primary defect. So-called genotype–phenotype relations have an impact on clinical disease expression, as shown for CGD and WAS. Defects (even within one family) have been found to vary due to such polymorphic immune genes as those mentioned above (see Complement deficiencies: abnormalities of the late components of the classic pathway, section 1.4).

1.6 What is the appropriate approach to the initial evaluation and diagnosis of infection in patients with phagocytic disorders?

The patient's history of previous infectious episodes, their sites, course and treatment should be sought. Also the family history is important with regard to susceptibility to infection, as well as contact and exposure history.

In the case of otitis, sinusitis and respiratory tract infection, information should be sought regarding exposure to respiratory viral infections, as these may result in secondary bacterial infection. Patients with an enteric problem should be queried about exposure to food contamination.

The physical examination should focus on the skin, pulmonary status, the abdomen or other body sites, as well as other sites identified by the history.

Gram staining and culture of relevant specimens (secretions, pus, sputum) should be performed; radiography of the chest and sinuses is indicated in most cases. Ultrasonographic investigation of the liver, spleen and kidneys should be performed when a focus of infection is not readily found. Imaging procedures (e.g. bone scan or ^{111}In-labeled IgG scintigraphy) may be of help to find hidden foci of infection.

1.9 What new developments are going to impact on emerging organisms, recognition, evaluation and diagnosis of infection in patients with phagocytic disorders?

Rapid diagnostic tools (e.g. PCR, antigen tests) for various relevant organisms need to be improved or developed.

2 REGARDING THE RISK FACTORS ACCOMPANYING PHAGOCYTIC DISORDERS

2.1 What are the main alterations in host defense mechanisms and what are the appropriate investigations to document them?

As discussed in the introduction to this section, phagocytic cells represent the major host defense system against bacteria and fungi. In patients with lifelong infections that are compatible with a phagocyte disorder (see sections 1.1, 1.2 and 1.3), a specific workup should be done. Since acquired quantitative defects are most prevalent, the total number of leukocytes and the numbers of neutrophils and monocytes should be determined first. Severe congenital neutropenia (SCN) is very rare and is generally detected early in infancy, in contrast to cyclic forms or syndromal forms, in which neutropenia may not be evident from birth.

When suspected, cyclic neutropenia should be evaluated by twice-weekly determination of the number of neutrophils during a 4–6-week period. If there is neutropenia, the bone marrow should be examined for granulocytopoiesis and granulocyte–macrophage colony-forming unit formation in culture. Next, the dynamics of the neutrophils should be tested by injecting G-CSF (10 μg/kg sc), or hydrocortisone (10 mg/kg sc or iv) to mobilize bone marrow reserves of granulocytes. The adrenaline test (0.05 ml/kg of a 1 : 10 000 dilution up to a maximum of 1 ml sc) may be performed to study the marginating capacity.

Measurement of sFcγRIII levels (if available) may be a good indicator of the total neutrophil mass and a predictor of the risk of infection. Patients with plasma concentrations greater than 100 units/ml do not appear to have serious infections.

In some forms of SCN, investigations should be directed towards a mutation of the G-CSF receptor gene (chromosome 1). In these patients, the defect predisposes to a form of myeloid leukemia with an annual cumulative risk of 2%. Bone marrow examination, immunophenotyping and cytogenetics should be performed on a regular basis (once per 1 or 2 years).

Leukocyte morphology should be studied by light microscopy and, if necessary, by electron microscopy.

With regard to qualitative defects, myeloperoxidase staining is easy to perform. In patients with suspected HIE syndrome, serum IgE levels should be measured (although normal levels do not exclude the syndrome). If there is persistent leukocytosis, the diagnosis of leukocyte adhesion deficiency (LAD) should be sought. Patients with LAD type 1 have a mutation in the common component of the integrins, CD18, whereas those with LAD type 2 have defective sialyl–Lewis X (CD15s) surface antigen expression; both molecules are important for margination, adherence to endothelial cells and chemotaxis. Determination of expression of these adhesion molecules can be performed by flow cytometry and fluorescence-activated cell sorting (FACS) analysis. Functional assays are required to confirm the concomitant functional defect, or to identify the variant forms in which expression of the adhesion molecules are normal but dysfunctional.

The function of phagocytes can be studied in vitro: assays for granulocyte aggregation, chemotaxis, phagocytosis and intracellular killing of a relevant microorganism (e.g. *S. aureus*) should be performed. To assess the biochemical aspects of the microbicidal process, analysis of oxygen consumption, superoxide production and hydrogen peroxide production should be performed. If defects are found, further molecular analysis for NADPH oxidase and accessory molecules is indicated.

To obtain insight into the ability of the white blood cells to enter an inflammatory field in vivo, a skin window test (according to Rebuck) or a skin blister test can be done. Since they are difficult to standardize, experience with the assays is needed.

Note that some primary immunodeficiencies (WAS and SCID; see T-cell defects below) may be accompanied by a phagocyte defect.

2.2 What are the alterations due to iatrogenic factors?
Care should be taken not to damage skin and mucous membranes, to avoid indwelling catheters. Drugs that further compromise neutrophil number or function (glucocorticosteroids, colchicine, cyclophosphamide, NSAIDs, IL-2) should be avoided.

2.3 What is the influence of environmental factors?
Patients should be aware of exposure to pathogens such as *Salmonella* spp. (food, pets). It may be also hard to recognize and avoid situations with large numbers of *Aspergillus* spores (e.g. construction, airborne soil and dust).

2.4 What are the most significant factors that contribute to the risk of infection in patients with phagocytic disorders?
See section 2.3. Damage to skin and mucous membranes probably poses the most significant risk.

2.5 What are the specific or nonspecific measures aimed at minimizing each of these factors?
Patients should avoid damage to the skin and mucous membranes. Special care should be taken with regard to preparation of food (meat). Patients should be thoroughly counseled about hygiene when they travel to countries considered to be at high risk for enteric and skin infection. Patients with CGD and other phagocyte defects should try to avoid aerosols that potentially contain fungal spores (e.g. in construction or farming). Patients should also be warned against smoking tobacco (so

as not to compromise pulmonary defense further) or marihuana (to avoid *Aspergillus* spores).

2.6 Are there different levels of risk of infection recognized for patients with phagocytic disorders?
As mentioned in sections 1.1 and 1.3, there is variation in the susceptibility to infection as well as in the age of onset of infections.

2.7 How does the level of risk impact on management?
It is important that patients be educated carefully about risk factors that could result in more serious infections.

3 REGARDING THE SURVEILLANCE OF PATIENTS WITH PHAGOCYTIC DISORDERS

3.2 What are the surveillance measures to be taken when a patient presents with phagocytic disorders?
When a patient who is known to have a phagocyte disorder presents, it may be reasonable to assess colonization with *S. aureus* (swabs of skin lesions, nose, perineum). A chest radiograph is indicated in most patients.

3.3 What are the other specific measures to be taken when a patient presents with phagocytic disorders?
Growth of the patient should be checked. Radiography to detect metaphyseal dysplasia is indicated in patients with a short stature or disproportional growth. When failure to thrive occurs in the presence of loose stools or diarrhea, analysis for malabsorption should be performed. Evaluation of vision, hearing and psychomotor development are part of the investigation.

4 REGARDING THE PREVENTION OF INFECTIONS IN PATIENTS WITH PHAGOCYTIC DISORDERS

4.1 What approaches, if any, to the prevention of infection should be considered in patients with phagocytic disorders?
Hygienic measures, such as oral hygiene, are important in patients with phagocyte disorders. Eczematous lesions should be treated carefully. Attempts should be undertaken to combat staphylococcal carrier state (mupirocin nose ointment and chlorhexidine scrub).

The main preventive measure in patients with symptomatic neutropenia is administration of G-CSF. A starting dose of 5–10 µg/kg sc daily is adequate, and the dose interval can be tapered depending on the number of neutrophils.

In GSD-1b, the functional abnormality seems to improve with G-CSF treatment, as well as the quantitative defect. This is, however, in contrast to Shwachman–Diamond syndrome, where the beneficial effect of G-CSF is marginal.

In patients with CGD, prophylactic cotrimoxazole (trimethoprim–sulfamethoxazole) appears to offer benefit. In these patients, the efficacy of additional interferon-γ prophylaxis has also demonstrated in a controlled trial; the frequency of infection was diminished by 70% and infections were less severe in the interferon-treated group. The recommended dose is 50 µg per m² of body surface given subcutaneously three times per week. Whether patients with phagocyte defects should also receive prophylaxis with itraconazole (100 mg oral solution daily in an adult) against fungal infection (especially aspergillosis) is not firmly established. However, once invasive infection has occurred and been cured, such prophylaxis is recommended to prevent recurrence.

Although allogeneic bone marrow transplantation has been performed in a few patients with CGD, it is generally accepted that the complications of the bone marrow transplantation are still such that this procedure has to be reserved for the worst cases and is not recommended as a general approach.

In patients with less common phagocyte disorders (e.g. Chédiak–Higashi syndrome, HIE and LAD), preventive measures have not been investigated in a systematic fashion. Elements of the management of CGD are generally applied to these patients. Patients with HIE syndrome usually benefit also from antibacterial and antifungal prophylaxis.

4.2 What are the future challenges and opportunities for reducing the risk of infection?

In those disorders in which the gene defect is known, gene transfer is an approach that may become feasible as a therapy in the coming years.

Disadvantages of interferon-γ and G-CSF are that these substances have to be injected. Although the advantages greatly outweigh the disadvantages, long-acting formulations of these products will be a step forward for these patients with chronic disorders.

5 REGARDING THE TREATMENT OF PATIENTS WITH PHAGOCYTIC DISORDERS

5.1 What is the role of empirical therapy?

Under all circumstances adequate culture specimens should be taken, since adequate (usually prolonged) treatment is virtually impossible without knowing the causative microorganism. Given the severity of the infections, empirical therapy in a patient with a phagocyte defect should consist of broad-spectrum drugs to include coverage of *S. aureus* while awaiting the baseline microbiologic results. Dependent on the clinical picture, results of recent surveillance cultures, and what is known of recent exposure to microbes and antimicrobial drugs, an empirical treatment should be selected. If methicillin-resistant *Staphylococcus aureus* (MRSA) is prevalent, a glycopeptide (vancomycin or teicoplanin) should be included in the initial therapy. Since these patients may harbor other organisms as well, coverage for Gram-negative bacilli (*Haemophilus influenzae*, Enterobacteriaceae, *Pseudomonas*) is indicated, for example with a third-generation cephalosporin or a quinolone.

In CGD, the intracellular killing defect should be overcome by giving antibiotics that reach effective concentrations inside the phagocytic cell; to that end antimicrobials such as rifampicin, clindamycin and the quinolones are considered important drugs. If there is reason to suspect fungal infection, an empirical antifungal treatment should be installed (see section 5.5).

There is no reason to withhold surgery for infection (abscesses, osteomyelitis, etc.) in patients with phagocyte defects. Indeed, an even more aggressive defects approach is required to eliminate foci of infection than in patients without such host defense. Selected patients with recurrent infections (e.g. skin or lungs) may be instructed to take adequate specimens for culture (they should be provided with material for that), and thereafter the patient should be started on oral antibiotics at home.

5.2 What is the appropriate approach to the patient with phagocytic disorders and evidence of:

Upper respiratory tract infection?
The antibiotic policy in upper respiratory tract infection (including sinusitis and middle ear infection) is given in section 5.1. While awaiting the microbiologic results, coverage for *S. aureus*, *H. influenzae* and other Gram-negative bacteria should be given. Resistant organisms (MRSA, resistant pneumococci and *H. influenzae*) should be taken into account.

Drainage of sinuses or the middle ear may be necessary. For appropriate assessment of the ENT area, CT or MRI may be necessary. In general there should be a high index of suspicion for fungal infections of the sinuses.

Lower respiratory tract infection?
The approach in lower respiratory tract infection is the same as that given in section 5.1. With recurrent lower airway infection, investigation of pulmonary function (including arterial blood gas analysis) and the presence of bronchiectasis (high-resolution CT of the thorax) is indicated. Here too, there should be a high index of suspicion for fungal infection (especially *Aspergillus* spp.).

Lesions (e.g. abscesses, empyemas, aspergillomas) that are refractory for treatment may need drainage and/or surgery.

In patients with defects of phagocyte function and an infection that does not respond to the above measures, white cell transfusion of G-CSF-treated donors (e.g. a family member) should be considered. The G-CSF-pretreated donor granulocytes are easy to harvest in relatively large numbers and have the advantage of being preactivated. Apart from cost and burden to the donor(s), disadvantages are the side effects (fever and chills, allosensitization).

Gastrointestinal and hepatobiliary infection?
Salmonella infection should be treated, preferably with a quinolone, which should be used long enough to eliminate the carrier state. It must be noted that gastrointestinal granulomas occur in patients with CGD; these are not infectious and may respond to a short course of corticosteroids (prednisone 2 mg/kg for 2 weeks).

Liver abscesses are common in disorders such as CGD, and *S. aureus* is among the most frequent causative organisms. Treatment consists of drainage (echography guided or surgical), adequate antibiotics (see section 5.1) and, if necessary, white cell transfusions (see Lower respiratory tract infection above). Perianal abscesses occur in patients with quantitative and qualitative defects.

Genitourinary tract infection?
The major pathogens are Gram-negative organisms, staphylococci and *Candida* spp.; treatment should be directed towards these organisms. In CGD, bladder granulomas occur, which are not clearly infectious but present as frequency dysuria. They usually respond to a short course of corticosteroids.

Musculoskeletal infection?
Occasionally a pyomyositis may be encountered. When suspected, CT, preferably, or MRI should be performed. After obtaining material for culture, therapy should

be instituted as outlined in section 5.1. The approach in arthritis and osteomyelitis is similar.

As stated in section 5.1, there is no reason to withhold surgery in patients with phagocytic disorders.

Skin infection?
The major cause of skin infection is *S. aureus*, but fungi (*Aspergillus* spp., *Candida* spp.) may also be the cause.

Central nervous system infection?
Metastatic infections (brain abscess, meningitis) may occur in the CNS in patients with phagocytic disorders, but are rare. The causative organisms are the same as those given in section 5.1. Surgical drainage of brain abscesses is necessary. Antibiotic therapy is as discussed in section 5.1. Care should be taken to reach adequate concentrations in the CSF and brain tissue.

Foreign body in place?
Staphylococcus epidermidis is an important pathogen in the presence of a foreign body. Hospital-acquired strains may be methicillin resistant. Also, the intracellular concentrations of the antibiotic may be an issue (see section 5.1). Duration of treatment is dependent on whether the foreign body can be removed.

5.3 What is the appropriate approach to the patient with phagocytic disorders and evidence of bacteremia, with or without site of infection?
Bacteremia in patients with phagocyte disorders is relatively rare.

In several parts of the world, septicemia with *Burkholderia cepacia* has been observed in patients with CGD, with a similar outcome to that in patients with the *B. cepacia* syndrome as a result of underlying cystic fibrosis. The approach is as outlined in section 5.1.

5.5 What is the appropriate approach to the patient with phagocytic disorders and evidence of a fungal infection?
In phagocyte disorders, fungemia is rare. However, deep-seated fungal infections are relatively common. First, the kind of fungus should be established to determine adequate therapy. For infection with *Candida albicans* and most other *Candida* spp., with the exception of *C. krusei* and *C. glabrata*, fluconazole is the drug of choice. For the latter, amphotericin B is still the preferred drug. For *Aspergillus fumigatus*, itraconazole is probably more effective than amphotericin B, but the mode of administration (oral, no licensed parenteral form) as well as the relatively low plasma concentrations are of concern. However, itraconazole does not reach adequate concentrations in the CNS. A newer drug, voriconazole, has activity against *Aspergillus* spp. and can be given orally as well as parenterally with relatively minimal side effects.

There is little experience in patients with phagocyte disorders and liposomal antifungal agents. Optimal supportive treatment is necessary in fungal infections; dependent on the phagocyte defect, G-CSF, interferon-γ and/or granulocyte transfusions may be needed (see section 4.1).

For refractory fungal infections, surgery may be the only solution.

IV CELLULAR SPECIFIC IMMUNODEFICIENCY: T-CELL MACROPHAGE DEFECTS

Within the specific part of the cellular immune system the various T lymphocytes and the antigen-presenting cells (dendritic cells and macrophages) cooperate. The major effector cells are the cytotoxic T lymphocytes and the macrophages. These cells are crucial in the defense against a series of viruses and against the so-called facultative intracellular microorganisms (bacteria such as mycobacteria, *Listeria monocytogenes*, *Salmonella* spp., *Legionella* spp., *Yersinia* spp.; fungi such as *Candida* spp., *Cryptococcus neoformans*, *Aspergillus* spp., *Pneumocystis carinii*; protozoa such as *Toxoplasma gondii*, Microsporidiae and *Leishmania* spp.). In addition patients with defective cellular immunity are vulnerable to infection with *Strongyloides stercoralis*.

Since the help of T lymphocytes is required for optimal specific humoral immunity, patients with T-cell defects almost always have suboptimal antibody responses. However, in quite a number of patients this does not result in overt hypogammaglobulinemia.

When both specific cellular and humoral immunity are found to be defective during infancy (<6–12 months of age), severe combined immune deficiency (SCID) may be diagnosed. If such a combined immune defect is diagnosed later during childhood, it generally constitutes a much less severe syndrome.

The molecular nature of a large number of these immunodeficiencies is now known, and many of the defects appear to reside in the intracellular signal transduction pathway. Primary defects of cellular immunity are very rare (1 in 100 000), compared with incidence for the acquired defects. For practical purposes the following classification of the major primary defects of specific cellular immunity is useful:

1 Severe combined immune deficiency (SCID); early pathology
   - Reticular dysgenesis
   - Recombination activation gene (RAG) 1/2 deficiency
   - Interleukin (IL) 2Rγ deficiency
   - Janus kinase (JAK) 3 deficiency
   - Adenosine deaminase (ADA) deficiency
   - Purine nucleotide phosphorylase (PNP) deficiency
   - T-cell receptor deficiency
   - MHC class II deficiency [bare leukocyte syndrome (BLS) 2]
   - Zeta-associated protein of 70 kDa (ZAP-70) tyrosine kinase deficiency
2 Combined immunodeficiencies or T-cell deficiency; variable severity and pathology
   - Hyper-IgM syndrome (HIM)
   - Ataxia telangiectasia (AT)
   - Nijmegen breakage syndrome (NBS)
   - PNP deficiency
   - IL-2Rα deficiency
   - MHC class I deficiency (BLS-1)
   - Wiskott–Aldrich syndrome (WAS)
3 Macrophage/cytokine defects
   - Interferon (IFN) γ receptor deficiency
   - IFNγ deficiency
   - IL-12 receptor deficiency
   - IL-12 deficiency

I REGARDING THE CLINICAL PRESENTATION AND EVALUATION OF THE PATIENT

1.1 What are the clinically predominant modes of presentation of infection in patients with T-cell defects?

Patients with primary defects of cellular immunity usually present with recurrent or severe infection from a very early age.

Congenital infection with or without malformations or dysmorphic features must be distinguished from the primary congenital SCID syndromes by early screening for TORCHES (toxoplasmosis, rubella, cytomegalovirus, herpes simples virus, Epstein–Barr virus, syphilis). Metabolic disease may be accompanied by a temporary defect in immunity and should be considered (e.g. leukopenia/lymphopenia in organic acid metabolism or orotic aciduria). The immunodeficiency-associated alopecia and eczematous dermatitis of Omenn syndrome (SCID variant) may look very similar to the features of severe biotinidase deficiency or an extensive zinc deficiency (e.g. acrodermatitis enteropathica).

In case of a congenital immune defect, the severity and frequency of infection may vary among the different syndromes. Apart from the infections, there is usually failure to thrive and chronic diarrhea. Vaccination with live attenuated viruses (mumps–measles–rubella; MMR) or bacillus Calmette–Guérin (BCG) may result in unexpected, prolonged or disseminated disease.

Many of the syndromes have their own characteristics. In DiGeorge anomaly (DGA), for example, the anomalous development of the third and fourth pharyngeal pouches may result in distinct facial abnormalities, thymus development that is defective or absent, parathyroids that have not developed normally (tetany) and cardiovascular defects.

Lymphoproliferative malignancy may develop in patients with cellular immune defects. In some syndromes, chromosomal instability may result in a generally increased risk of malignancy (lymphoproliferative as well as solid tumors).

Newly described defects are those in which macrophage microbicidal activity is suboptimal because of defects in the signaling by IFNγ or IL-12.

1.2 What are the predominant sites of infection?

The predominant sites of infection are represented schematically in Table 1.2; they are:
- Skin: a variety of skin lesions is encountered in these patients (see Table 1.2 and section 5.2 on skin infection).
- Mouth, pharynx and esophagus: stomatitis, esophagitis
- Lower respiratory tract: pneumonia, pneumonitis, bronchiectasis
- Bone: osteomyelitis
- Gastrointestinal tract: gastroenteritis; hepatitis, liver abscess, cholangitis, colitis
- CNS: meningoencephalitis, focal lesions
- Eyes: endophthalmitis, panophthalmitis

1.3 What are the predominant organisms that contribute (by site)?

The major organisms that cause infection in patients with diminished cellular immunity are presented in Table 1.2. Not all the organisms listed have been encountered in the primary immunodeficiencies, but are included here because they could play a role, based on the similarities with the acquired disorders:
- Viruses: herpes simplex virus, varicella zoster virus (VZV), cytomegalovirus (CMV), Epstein–Barr virus (EBV), human papillomaviruses, papovaviruses (JC virus, BK virus), poliovirus (Sabin vaccine associated), measles virus

Table 1.2 Predominant infections by site in patients with T-cell defects

CNS	Skin	*Aspergillus* spp.
Varicella zoster virus	Herpes simplex virus	*Toxoplasma gondii*
Epstein–Barr virus (lymphoma)	Varicella zoster virus	*Strongyloides stercoralis*
Papovavirus	Human herpesvirus 8	
Measles	Papillomavirus	**Liver**
Poliomyelitis	*Bartonella henselae*	Cytomegalovirus
Nocardia asteroides	Mycobacteria	*Bartonella henselae*
Mycobacteria	*Cryptococcus neoformans*	*Toxoplasma gondii*
Listeria monocytogenes	*Candida* spp.	
Salmonella spp.	*Aspergillus* spp.	**Gastrointestinal tract**
Bartonella henselae	*Histoplasma capsulatum*	Cytomegalovirus
Cryptococcus neoformans	*Strongyloides stercoralis*	Rotavirus
Aspergillus fumigatus		Adenovirus
Zygomycetes	**Lungs**	Enterovirus
Coccidioides immitis	Herpes simplex virus	*Salmonella* spp.
Toxoplasma gondii	Varicella zoster virus	Mycobacteria
Strongyloides stercoralis	Cytomegalovirus	*Cryptosporidium*
	Measles	Microsporidia
Oropharynx/esophagus	*Nocardia asteroides*	
Herpes simplex virus	Mycobacteria	**Bloodstream**
Cytomegalovirus	*Legionella* spp.	*Salmonella* spp.
Candida spp.	*Pneumocystis carinii*	*Campylobacter fetus*
Histoplasma capsulatum	*Histoplasma capsulatum*	*Listeria monocytogenes*
	Cryptococcus neoformans	Mycobacteria
	Coccidioides immitis	

- Bacteria: mycobacteria (tuberculous, BCG and atypical), *Listeria monocytogenes*, *Salmonella* spp., *Legionella* spp., *Yersinia* spp., *Nocardia asteroides*, *Bartonella henselae*, *Campylobacter fetus*
- Fungi (*Candida* spp., *Aspergillus* spp., *Cryptococcus neoformans*, *Coccidioides immitis*, *Histoplasma capsulatum*, *Pneumocystis carinii*)
- Protozoa (*Toxoplasma gondii*, *Cryptosporidium* spp., *Isospora belli*, *Microsporidia* and *Leishmania* spp.)
- Helminths (*Strongyloides stercoralis*)

1.4 How do the organisms vary according to various risk factors?

Defects in cellular immunity, whether congenital or acquired, show a remarkably similar pattern of opportunistic infection. In congenital primary immunodeficiency, the combined cellular and humoral defects may lead to a wide range of infections (see also section on Immunoglobulin deficiencies).

Most herpesviruses are transferred via contact with saliva and oral mucosa. Since small healthy children may excrete large amounts of CMV, they may present a threat for the patient with a cellular immune defect. Close contacts with children in daycare centers and kindergarten may harbor the risk for transmission of rotavirus, respiratory syncytial virus (RSV) and CMV, and the other herpes infections. Patients with defects of cellular immunity are very vulnerable to chickenpox. *Salmonella* spp. may be acquired from food or pets (e.g. reptiles, turtles, pigeons). *Listeria* infection may be acquired from contaminated food products, especially those containing unpasteurized milk (e.g. soft cheese). *Salmonella* spp., *Yersinia* spp. and *C. fetus* may also occur due to contaminated food. *B. henselae* may be acquired from cats. Patients may become infected with *Legionella* through exposure to aerosols containing these microorganisms; this may occur in hotels as well as in hospitals with contaminated water supplies and/or air conditioning systems. Exposure to *Aspergillus* spores may occur in construction work, from aerosols of soil and dust. Cryptococcal infection may be acquired after exposure to bird droppings. *Pseudallescheria boydii* is associated with submersion in contaminated water.

Infection with *T. gondii* may be due to handling or eating uncooked meat or contact with cat feces (as a cat owner or from gardening). *Cryptosporidium* may contaminate potable water and swimming pools. The latter may also be contaminated by *Pseudomonas* or *Legionella* spp.

1.5 How does this differ from other conditions, from center to center, and from country to country?
Patients run more risk for such infections under circumstances of high microbial pressure and poor hygiene. Some microorganisms (*Yersinia enterocolitica* and *Listeria*) are probably more often acquired in a moderate climate, whereas the acquisition of some others is confined to (sub)tropical areas (*Brucella* spp., *Leishmania* spp., *Histoplasma capsulatum*, *Strongyloides stercoralis*).

1.6 What is the appropriate approach to the initial evaluation and diagnosis of infection in patients with T-cell defects?

1.7 How should the evaluation be modified according to the severity of the risk?

1.8 What are the specific evaluation measures? (see also Chapter 2 in Part I)
When taking the patient's history, previous infectious episodes, their sites, course and treatment should be sought. A history of exposure to potentially pathogenic microorganisms should be sought (see sections 1.4 and 1.5). For the current episode it is essential to try to locate the site of the infection by taking a careful history and performing a complete physical examination. Dependent on the location and the risk factors, a differential diagnosis can be made according to the potential causative organism.

The kind of microorganisms that may cause an infection at a certain site dictates the way relevant material from that site should be taken, transported and investigated. In patients with fever without localizing symptoms and signs, an adequate workup for CMV infection should always be done (ideally, antigen testing, PCR, serology and rapid culture from blood and other relevant specimens). In such patients mycobacterial infection (with bacteremia) should also be considered; blood cultures and bone marrow culture in media suitable for the isolation of mycobacteria should be taken.

1.9 What new developments are going to impact on emerging organisms, recognition, evaluation and diagnosis in patients with T-cell defects?
Rapid diagnostic tools (PCR, antigen tests) for various relevant organisms should be improved or developed, evaluated and become generally available.

2 REGARDING THE RISK FACTORS ACCOMPANYING T-CELL DEFECTS

2.1 What are the main alterations in host defense mechanisms and what are the appropriate investigations to document them?

As explained in the introduction to this section, defects of specific cellular immunity are due to defects in T-cell function, i.e. the function of cytotoxic T-cells and/or of T-helper cells. In addition, the function of antigen-presenting cells or the effector function of macrophages may be defective. In patients with lifelong infections that are compatible with a defect of cellular immunity (see sections 1.1, 1.2, 1.3), a specific workup should be done. First, a thorough family history should be taken. The total number of leuko-cytes, the differential and the absolute numbers of T and B lymphocytes and NK cells should be determined; also the T-cell subsets (CD4+ and CD8+) cells should be enumerated.

When presenting at an early age, the possibility of secondary immune dysfunction due to congenital infection, metabolic defects or nutritional factors should be taken into account. Infection with human immunodeficiency virus should also be considered.

Following these studies, a lymphocyte proliferation test, using a mitogen such as phy-tohemagglutinin (PHA), a combination of monoclonal antibodies (such as CD3 and CD28), and one or more relevant antigens (e.g. tetanus or diphtheria before and after a DT booster; *Candida albicans*), should be performed. The possibility of HIM syndrome (X-linked CD40L defect or autosomal recessive defect in CD40 signaling) should be excluded.

Skin tests for cell-mediated immunity with relevant antigens (e.g. PPD, *Candida* anti-gen, *Trichophyton*, tetanus) are optional.

If there are abnormalities in lymphocyte number and function, ADA and PNP levels should be determined, as well as genetic screening for the most common defects (e.g. in IL-2Rγ, JAK-3 or RAG-1/2). Chromosome investigations and investigations of DNA repair should be considered and the maternal cells in the circulation (chimerism) assessed.

In patients with recurrent or refractory infections caused by *Salmonella* spp. or mycobacteria, the IL-12 and IFNγ pathway should be investigated. This is done most easily by exposing peripheral blood mononuclear cells to a stimulus (e.g. endotoxin or CD3/28) and exogenous IL-12 or INFγ, and measuring the subsequent production of IL-12, INFγ, TNFα and IL-6 after 1–3 days of culture.

2.2 What are the alterations due to iatrogenic factors?

Care should be taken not to damage skin and mucous membranes. Drugs that further compromise cellular immunity (e.g. glucocorticosteroids) should be avoided.

2.3 What is the influence of environmental factors?

Patients should be aware of the danger of exposure to pathogens, as discussed in section 1.4.

2.4 What are the most significant factors that contribute to the risk of infection in patients with T-cell defects?

See section 1.4.

2.5 What are the specific or nonspecific measures aimed at minimizing each of these factors?

Although difficult, it is best to keep children out of settings (e.g. daycare, school) where exposure to pathogens (e.g. CMV, RSV, EBV and VZV) may occur. Pets such as cats, reptiles and birds should not be in the homes of patients with cellular immune deficiencies. Potentially contaminated food products, such as those containing unpasteurized milk (e.g. soft cheese) or undercooked meat or poultry, should be avoided. Exposure to construction work, or to aerosols of soil and dust, should be avoided by patients with severe immunodeficiency. Travel to areas of the world with poor hygienic conditions should also be avoided.

2.6 Are there different levels of risk of infection recognized for patients with T-cell defects?

The various primary defects of cellular immunity vary in severity, partly because of differences in the remaining T-cell function and partly because of differences in the quality of B-cell function. This risk can be assessed to some extent with the measurements mentioned in section 2.1.

2.7 How does the level of risk impact on management?

The mainstay of management in these patients is informing them about risks, as detailed in sections 1.4 and 2.5.

2.8 What new developments are going to impact on minimizing or suppressing the specific risk factors?

Restoration of the immunodeficiency (e.g. gene therapy, supplementation with the missing factors) will have a great impact on the specific risk for infection. A detailed discussion is beyond the subject of this chapter.

3 REGARDING THE SURVEILLANCE OF PATIENTS WITH T-CELL DEFECTS

3.2 What are the surveillance measures to be taken when a patient presents with T-cell defects?

When a patient with a primary cellular immune defect presents, a careful examination should guide the kind of evaluation for infection risk that is necessary. Table 1.2 provides some guidance regarding notable infection hazards. Given the extensive array of microorganisms that may cause infection in these patients, surveillance cultures are not worthwhile. Antibody status for CMV, EBV and *T. gondii* should be ascertained, assuming that there is no concomitant antibody deficiency.

4 REGARDING THE PREVENTION OF INFECTIONS IN PATIENTS WITH T-CELL DEFECTS

4.1 What approaches, if any, to the prevention of infection should be considered in patients with T-cell defects?

In addition to the measures presented in section 2 above, antimicrobial prophylaxis [e.g. cotrimoxazole directed against *P. carinii*, oral antifungals against *C. albicans* or

Aspergillus spp., and occasionally chronic suppression of herpesviruses with (val)acy-clovir] may be indicated, based on the nature and severity of the immune defect.

If a patient with an SCID has to wait for allogenic bone marrow transplantation, IVIG substitution against bacterial infections should be combined with the administration of a monoclonal antibody against RSV (15 mg/kg sc, monthly) as a protective measure against deleterious effects during the winter season.

4.2 What are the future challenges and opportunities for reducing the risk of infection?

In disorders in which the gene defect is known, gene therapy is an approach that may become feasible as therapy in the coming years. Attempts to restore ADA deficiency through gene therapy is under evaluation.

5 REGARDING THE TREATMENT OF PATIENTS WITH T-CELL DEFECTS

5.1 What is the role of empirical therapy?

Every attempt should be made to determine the etiology and focus of a fever or infection in the patient with altered cellular immunity. Given the severity of the infections, empirical therapy may be necessary, and may be guided by the site of the infection and the most probable microorganism (Table 1.2).

5.2 What is the appropriate approach to the patient with T-cell defects and evidence of:

Upper respiratory tract infection?

Initially, *P. carinii* pneumonia (PCP) may mimic upper respiratory tract infection. For patients who are not receiving prophylaxis for PCP, chest radiography and blood gas analysis should be performed and, based on the results, bronchoalveolar lavage (BAL) should be carried out. It is important to remember that breakthrough infections with PCP can occur in patients receiving prophylaxis.

For appropriate assessment of the ENT area, CT or MRI may be necessary. In general, there should be a high index of suspicion for fungal infections of the sinuses, and empirical therapy (amphotericin B, as Zygomycetes are not susceptible to azoles) may be needed.

Lower respiratory tract infection?

The approach in lower respiratory tract infection is the same as that outlined in section 5.1. Arterial blood gas analysis and chest radiography are indicated. If PCP is high on the list, a BAL should be done. Empirical therapy directed towards *P. carinii* (high-dose co-trimoxazole) may be started before the BAL.

High-resolution CT may help in the lung differential diagnosis. If BAL and additional investigations do not yield a diagnosis, video-assisted thoracoscopy (VATS) with biopsy or open lung biopsy is required.

Gastrointestinal and hepatobiliary infection?

In patients with diarrhea, stools should be investigated for bacterial pathogens as well as for *Cryptosporidium* and microsporidia. It is often necessary to investigate more than one sample. Microsporidia may also disseminate to almost any organ (in particular lung and brain).

There is no known effective treatment for *Cryptosporidium* and microsporidia, although paromomycin has been used with some success in the former and albendazole in the latter.

In addition, cultures should be sent for bacteriologic and virologic investigation. It is important to realize that CMV infection may occur not only as a generalized enteritis, but also as ulcers (which may bleed or even perforate), localized in the esophagus, stomach, small and large bowel. Endoscopy with biopsy (for histologic culture and/or PCR) is often necessary to make this diagnosis.

In the patient with an enlarged liver and/or liver enzyme abnormalities, the liver should be visualized (ultrasonography, CT) to distinguish between diffuse and localized abnormalities. In the liver, diffuse hepatitis may be due to *T. gondii* and CMV. Mycobacteria may cause granulomatous hepatitis, whereas *B. henselae* causes peliosis hepatis (spaces in the liver filled with blood, mainly described in patients with acquired immune deficiency syndrome). It may be necessary to perform a liver biopsy to diagnose the infection; in peliosis this may be dangerous because of the risk of bleeding. A liver biopsy should be sent for histologic examination and microbiology. Molecular diagnostics may help to distinguish rapidly between the various causative organisms.

Infection with *Mycobacterium tuberculosis* should be treated with rifampicin, isoniazide, pyrazinamide and ethambutol. A fifth drug (amikacin or a quinolone) may be added if multidrug resistance is likely. Infection with atypical mycobacteria requires other drugs: clarithromycin or azithromycin with clofazimine and/or rifabutin.

Skin infection?

The major causes of skin infection are viral infections (herpes simplex, VZV, CMV, mollusca contagiosum, verruca vulgaris); bacterial infections [mycobacterial infection caused by *M. tuberculosis* (lupus vulgaris, tuberculosis miliaris cutis) and by a variety of atypical mycobacteria], bacillary angiomatosis (caused by *B. henselae*); fungal infections (dermatophytosis, candidiasis, cryptococcosis, mucor, aspergillosis, histoplasmosis); protozoal infection (leishmaniasis); and metazoal infection (strongyloidiasis).

Some of these skin infections can be recognized by their typical appearance, but often a biopsy is necessary for confirmation. The biopsy should be sent for microbiologic studies.

Central nervous system infection?

It is important to differentiate between meningitis/meningoencephalitis, encephalitis and focal lesions. Following a careful neurological examination, CT or MRI and a lumbar puncture should be performed. Some of the organisms listed in Table 1.3 typically produce a mening(oencephal)itis, whereas others cause encephalitis or focal lesions.

Focal abnormalities may pose the greatest difficulty in establishing a diagnosis. Often a neurosurgical biopsy is required. Therapy should be directed towards the suspected causative organism.

5.3 What is the appropriate approach to the patient with T-cell defects and evidence of a documented bacteremia, with or without site of infection?

Bacteremia is rare in patients with cellular immunodeficiency disorders. The causative organisms are given in Table 1.2. In most cases the source of the bacteremia or the metastatic infectious foci are a clue to the diagnosis and guide the initial treatment. For initial treatment of *Salmonella* or *Campylobacter* sepsis, a quinolone is the drug of choice, whereas in *Listeria* sepsis, amoxycillin and/or cotrimoxazole is indicated. Since mycobacteria are susceptible to quinolones, culture specimens from blood and other relevant sites should be taken to enable the diagnosis of mycobacterial infection to be made.

Table 1.3 Presentation of CNS infection according to causative organism

Causative organism	Presentation
Viruses	
Varicella zoster virus	M, E
Epstein–Barr virus (lymphoma)	F
Papovavirus	F
Measles	M
Poliomyelitis	F
Bacteria	
Nocardia asteroides	F, (M)
Mycobacteria	M, F
Listeria monocytogenes	M, E, F
Bartonella henselae	M, E, F
Fungi	
Cryptococcus neoformans	M, (F)
Aspergillus fumigatus	M, F
Zygomycetes	F
Coccidioides immitis	M, F
Pseudallescheria boydii	F, (M)
Toxoplasma gondii	F, E
Helminth	
Strongyloides stercoralis	M, F

M, meningitis; E, encephalitis; F, focal infection.

5.4 What is the appropriate approach to the patient with T-cell defects and evidence of a documented viral infection?

Depending on the virus, specific treatment may be given. Herpes simplex and VZV are amenable to treatment with acyclovir and related drugs (valaciclovir and famciclovir). Depending on the clinical condition of the patient and the severity of infection, the drugs should be given parenterally or orally. For oral treatment valaciclovir or famciclovir is the preferred drug since resorption after oral administration is much greater than that of acyclovir; the efficacy of these oral drugs is close to that of iv acyclovir.

In patients with severely impaired cellular immunity, the response of herpes simplex or VZV to acyclovir and analogs may be less rapid than in the normal host. Prolonged exposure to these drugs may lead to resistant virus (mostly based on a loss of viral thymidine kinase). Although such viruses have a decreased virulence they may produce ongoing infection. Treatment with foscarnet iv (which is not dependent on the viral thymidine kinase) is indicated in such cases.

For cytomegalovirus infection ganciclovir iv is first choice. It is important to recognize that the oral formulation of ganciclovir attains a blood concentration that is considerably lower than that of intravenous ganciclovir, and is mainly indicated only for maintenance treatment. Foscarnet is an effective alternative for CMV infection. The wart viruses are not amenable to specific antiviral therapy. Treatment with interferon α or β (systemically or locally) is generally disappointing. Local treatment with laser or liquid nitrogen may be of some help.

5.5 What is the appropriate approach to the patient with T-cell defects and evidence of a fungal infection?

Although candidiasis in patients with defects of specific cellular immunity is generally manifest as a superficial infection, deep-seated candidiasis may occur when patients are given indwelling vascular catheters, parenteral nutrition, corticosteroids and/or broad-spectrum antibiotics. Other deep-seated fungal infections occur in these patients: cryptococcosis, aspergillosis, zygomycosis, histoplasmosis and coccidioidomycosis. For treatment of infection caused by *Candida* species, with the exception of *C. krusei* and *C. glabrata*, fluconazole is the drug of choice. For *C. krusei* and *C. glabrata*, amphotericin B is still the drug of choice. Cryptococcal meningitis should be treated with amphotericin B and 5-fluorocytosine initially. After 2 weeks' treatment, patients may be switched to fluconazole. Maintenance treatment with fluconazole is indicated when the immune defect is not restored.

For *Aspergillus fumigatus*, itraconazole may be more effective than amphotericin B, but the mode of administration (oral, no parenteral form) as well as the relatively low plasma concentrations are of concern. A newer drug, voriconazole, has excellent activity against *Aspergillus* spp.; it can be given orally as well as parenterally and the side effects seem to be mild compared with those of amphotericin B.

Zygomycosis does not respond to azoles; treatment consists of amphotericin B and surgery. For histoplasmosis, amphotericin B is the drug of choice for initial treatment. For maintenance therapy, itraconazole is effective. For coccidioidomycosis, amphotericin B is the drug of choice. Intrathecal amphotericin B therapy is indicated in meningitis caused by this organism. Maintenance therapy is necessary as long as there is an immune defect. Azoles are used for this purpose.

There is little experience with liposomal antifungals in patients with cellular immunodeficiency, but so far the data suggest at least equal efficacy and less toxicity than with plain amphotericin B.

G-CSF or IFNγ may be considered as supportive treatment in poorly responsive fungal disease. For refractory fungal infections, surgery may be the only solution.

5.6 What is the appropriate approach to the patient with T-cell defects and evidence of a parasitic infection?

The treatment of choice in toxoplasmosis is pyrimethamine and sulfadiazine. Patients who do not tolerate the sulfonamides may be given clindamycin instead. There is no known effective treatment for *Cryptosporidium* and microsporidia. For *S. stercoralis*, thiabendazole or ivermectin is the treatment of choice.

REFERENCES

Buckley RH, Schiff SE, Schiff, RI et al. Human severe combined immunodeficiency (SCID): genetic, phenotypic and functional diversity. *J Pediatr* 1997; **130**: 378–387.

Comans-Bitter WM, de Groot R, van den Beemd R et al. Immunophenotyping of blood lymphocytes in childhood. Reference values for lymphocyte subpopulations. *J Pediatr* 1997; **130**: 388–393.

Drogari-Apiranthitou M, Fijen CA, van de Beek D, et al. Development of antibodies against tetravalent meningococcal polysaccharides in revaccinated complement-deficient patients. *Clip Exp Immunol* 2000; **119**: 311–316.

Fijen CA, Kuijper EJ, te Bulte MT et al. Assessment of complement deficiency in patients with meningococcal disease in The Netherlands. *Clin Infec Dis* 1999; **28**: 98–105.

Hermaszewski RA, Webster ADB. Primary hypogammaglobulinemia: a survey of clinical manifestations and complications. *Quart J Med* 1993; **86**: 31–42.

Kuijpers TW, Weening RS, Out TA. IgG subclass deficiencies and recurrent pyogenic infections: unresponsiveness against bacterial polysaccharide antigens. *Allergol Immunopathol* 1992; **20**: 28–34.

Kuijpers TW, Weening RS, Roos D. Clinical and laboratory work-up of patients with neutrophil shortage or dysfunction. *J Immunol Methods* 1999; **232**: 211–229.

Ottenhoff TH, Kumararatne D, Casanova JL. Novel human immunodeficiencies reveal the essential role of Type-I cytokines in immunity to intracellular bacteria. *Immunol Today* 1998: **19**: 491–494.

Roos D, de Boer M, Kuribayashi F et al. Mutations in the X-linked and autosomal recessive forms of chronic granulomatous disease. *Blood* 1996; **87**: 1663–1618.

Schneider PM, Wurzner R. Complement genetics: biological implications of polymorphisms and deficiencies. *Immunol Today* 1999; **20**: 2–5.

Spickett GP, Farrant J, North ME et al. Common varaible immunodeficiency: how many diseases. *Immunol Today* 1997; **18**: 325–328.

Turner, MW. Mannose-binding lectin (MBL) in health and disease. *Immunobiology* 1998; **199**: 327–339.

Chapter 2 — Infections in Patients with Aplastic Anemia

Miriam Weinberger

INTRODUCTION

Aplastic anemia is a rare hematopoietic disorder with an annual incidence of 2–6 per 10^6 population. It is characterized by a hypocellular bone marrow and pancytopenia which is progressive and life-threatening. With supportive therapy alone, up to 80% of patients with severe aplastic anemia may die from the disease within 18–24 months as a result of overwhelming infection or hemorrhage into vital organs.

The International Aplastic Anemia Study Group distinguishes severe and moderate forms of aplastic anemia according to the degree of bone marrow aplasia. Severe disease is characterized by two or more of the following criteria: neutrophil count <500 per mm^3, platelet count <20 000 per mm^3, and reticulocyte count <20 000 per mm^3. Super-severe aplastic anemia is a new form, defined by a neutrophil count <200 per mm^3.

Allogeneic bone marrow transplantation can cure the majority of transplanted patients; current survival rates are 70–90%. Unfortunately, only a minority of patients (25–30%) are eligible for this procedure, either because they lack identical siblings, or because of age restriction.

Immunosuppression can achieve a similar initial response rate. Antithymocyte globulin (ATG) (or antilymphocyte globulin; ALG) is considered the first-line immunosuppressive therapy for aplastic anemia, and is used either alone or in combination with cyclosporin, corticosteroids, androgens or hematopoietic growth factors. ATG and cyclosporin have comparable efficacy; however, combined therapy results in higher and earlier response rates than that achieved with either drug alone. Very high doses of glucocorticoids (prednisone 10–20 mg/kg daily) as single agents may induce response in the occasional patient, but are associated with unacceptably high complication rates. When included in immunosuppressive protocols, they are used at a low dose, as prophylaxis for serum sickness, which is a common side effect of ATG. Hematopoietic growth factors are not beneficial on their own, but can be used in combination with ATG and/or cyclosporin-containing regimens to shorten the period of neutropenia and reduce the frequency of blood-product transfusions. Cyclophosphamide has also been shown to be effective in a small group of patients. Androgens are probably not beneficial in aplastic anemia.

A major limitation of immunosuppressive therapy is that up to 50% of successfully treated patients either relapse or develop a late clonal disorder such as overt myelodysplastic syndrome, paroxysmal nocturnal hemoglobinuria or acute leukemia. Another important drawback to immunosuppressive regimens is that response may take up to 12 weeks; in that period severe and life-threatening infections as well as bleeding complications may occur.

Infection is the leading cause of death in patients with aplastic anemia, and hemorrhage is usually associated with concomitant infection. The pattern of infection in patients treated by bone marrow transplantation is discussed in Part II, Chapter 5. The focus of this chapter is the infections developing in patients with aplastic anemia who do not qualify for bone marrow transplantation and are treated with immunosuppressive agents.

The main source of information is a large study that analyzed the pattern of infection in 150 patients with aplastic anemia who were treated in the Clinical Center of the National Institutes of Health in Bethesda, Maryland, USA, between the years 1978 and 1990 (referred to hereafter as the NIH study). Some 83% of the patients were categorized as having severe aplastic anemia, and the group was followed for a mean of 1.2 years (range from 4 days to 6.6 years). By the end of the study 39% of the patients had died, 62% from infection.

Except for a recently published study describing the significance of fever during ATG treatment, no further studies on the infectious complications in patients with aplastic anemia have been reported since.

I REGARDING THE CLINICAL PRESENTATION AND EVALUATION OF THE PATIENT

1.1 What are the clinically predominant modes of presentation of infection in patients with aplastic anemia?

Fever develops in about two thirds of patients with aplastic anemia at any time from diagnosis, and a specific diagnosis of infection can be made in about 70% of the febrile events. In the NIH study, a lower neutrophil count and the presence of a tunneled central venous catheter (Hickman–Broviac or Port-A-Cath) were associated with a higher likelihood of developing a febrile event.

An etiologic agent can be demonstrated in about two-thirds of infectious events (microbiologically documented infections), and in the other one-third infection is suspected on the basis of clinical presentation (clinically documented infections). Isolation of bacteria or fungi from the bloodstream occurs in about one third of documented infectious episodes.

In about 30% of febrile events no source of infection can be detected. In the NIH study, febrile events without a determined source were significantly associated with ATG treatment and with clinical manifestations of serum sickness.

In a recent study, all 42 patients with aplastic anemia developed fever during the first 2 days of ATG treatment, which lasted for 1–6 (median 2.5) days. Four patients had positive blood cultures with coagulase-negative *Staphylococcus* with no other clinical signs of infection, except fever.

1.2 What are the predominant sites of infection?

The predominant sites of infections in patients with aplastic anemia are the bloodstream (primary bacteremia or fungemia), the respiratory tract, the gastrointestinal tract, the skin and soft tissue, and the urinary tract (Table 2.1).

Bacteria or fungi can be isolated from the bloodstream in about one third of infectious events. A possible portal of entry for bloodstream infection can be defined in only one third of events, the most common source being soft tissue infection, including catheter exit-site infection and cellulitis. Other sources for bloodstream infections are pneumonia, urinary tract infection, intraabdominal and periodontal infections.

Table 2.1 Frequency of the various sites of infection and their etiology in patients with aplastic anemia (data derived from 200 episodes of infections in the NIH study)

	Primary bacteremia	Respiratory tract		Oropharynx	Gastrointestinal tract		Skin and soft tissue	Urinary tract
		Lungs	Sinuses		Abdominal	Perirectal		
Etiology								
CDI	–	29	47	57	40	40	44	9
Fungal	19	42	40	7	–	–	–	–
Bacterial	81	21	13	10	47	60	53	91
Viral	–	–	–	27	7	–	2	–
P. carinii	–	8	–	–	–	–	–	–
Parasitic	–	–	–	–	7	–	–	–
Total (% out out 200 epidosodes	22	19	8	15	8	3	22	6

Site of infection (%)

CDI, clinically documented infection.

Respiratory tract infections account for a further third of infectious events. The most frequently encountered infection is pneumonia, followed by sinusitis, bronchitis and epiglottitis. Concomitant pneumonia and sinusitis are not uncommon.

Another important site of infection is the soft tissue. The major patterns of infection are cellulitis, catheter exit-site infection, paronychia and osteomyelitis. Soft tissue infections tend to recur with discontinuation of antibiotic therapy. Occasionally soft tissue infections may become rapidly progressive and invade subcutaneous tissues or deeper organs.

Any site along the gastrointestinal tract can be involved in infection, including the oral cavity, the esophagus, the colon or the perirectum. Stomatitis, gingivitis and periodontal infection are the most common presentations of oral cavity involvement. Typhlitis, or neutropenic enterocolitis, which was initially described in patients with acute leukemia, can cause severe and life-threatening complications in patients with aplastic anemia. Other intraabdominal infections, such as cholangitis, cholecystitis and diverticulitis, may complicate the course in older patients. Pseudomembranous enterocolitis due to *Clostridium difficile* is the most common cause of nosocomial diarrhea.

Urinary tract infections are not common in patients with aplastic anemia, accounting for about 5% of all infectious events. Primary central nervous system (CNS) infections are rare, and are usually due to opportunistic infections such as *Cryptococcus neoformans*. The CNS may be also involved in disseminated infections, especially due to invasive aspergillosis or candidiasis.

1.3 What are the predominant organisms that contribute (by site)?

In the NIH study, the most common etiologic agents were bacteria (67%), followed by fungi (25%), viruses (7%), *Pneumocystis carinii* (1.5%) and parasites (0.5%).

The majority of bloodstream isolates (BSI) were bacteria, and only 10 were fungi. The predominant bacterial pathogens were Gram-positive bacteria, which accounted for 35% of bloodstream isolates and 70% of nonbacteremic isolates. The most frequently isolated Gram-positive bacteria were coagulase-negative staphylococci, coagulase-positive staphylococci, α-hemolytic streptococci, *Enterococcus* spp., and *Corynebacterium* spp. Gram-negative bacteria accounted for 50% of bacterial bloodstream isolates and 30% of nonbacteremic isolates. The most common Gram-negative bacteria were *Pseudomonas aeruginosa*, *Klebsiella pneumoniae*, *Escherichia coli* and *Acinetobacter* species. Although *P. aeruginosa* has been reported to decrease in frequency in many centers, a wide center-to-center variation exists, and the local pattern should be carefully studied. In the NIH study, *P. aeruginosa* accounted for 11% of bacterial bloodstream isolates, compared with 13% of *K. pneumoniae* and 5% of *E. coli*. Anaerobes were isolated in less than 5% of cases, the most common isolates being *Clostridium* spp.

Fungal BSI consisted only of *Candida* species (*C. albicans* 55%, *C. tropicalis* 33%, *C. lusitaniae* 11%). A switch to non-*albicans* *Candida* species may occur in centers with widespread use of azole antifungal drugs.

A specific pathogen could be documented in more than three-quarters of pulmonary infections. In the NIH study, 60% of the bacteriologically documented cases of pneumonia were due to fungi, 30% due to bacteria and 10% due to *P. carinii*. *Aspergillus* species (*A. fumigatus* 40%, *A. flavus* 33%, *A. nidulans* 7% unidentified *Aspergillus* spp. 20%) accounted for the majority of invasive fungal pneumonia, followed by *Candida* spp. Isolation of more than one *Aspergillus* spp. from respiratory specimens was not uncommon. *P. aeruginosa* was the single most common pathogen associated with bacterial pneumonia, followed by coagulase-negative staphylococci, *Mycobacterium tuberculosis* and coagulase-positive staphylococci. Pneumonia due to multiple pathogens was also observed, usually due to mixed fungal and bacterial pathogens. Occasionally, patients presented with unusual combinations of pathogens, such as *M. tuberculosis*, cytomegalovirus and *P. carinii*, in one.

The majority of sinus infections were also due to fungal pathogens, mainly *Aspergillus* spp., followed by *Candida* and *Fusarium* spp. Bacterial pathogens included *Haemophilus influenzae*, *P. aeruginosa* and coagulase-positive staphylococci.

Soft tissue infections were difficult to document bacteriologically, and in up to 45% no etiologic agent could be defined. The vast majority of infections were caused by bacteria, and a minority by herpesviruses (herpes simplex virus and varicella zoster virus). Gram-positive bacteria (coagulase-positive staphylococci, coagulase-negative staphylococci, α-hemolytic streptococci, *Corynebacterium* spp.) predominated in cutaneous infections, while Gram-negative bacteria (*P. aeruginosa*, *K. pneumoniae*, *E. coli*) were more common in perirectal and perineal infections.

Herpes simplex virus and *Candida* spp. were most commonly associated with infections of the oral cavity, whereas bacterial pathogens were involved in periodontal infections. Intraabdominal infections, such as cholecystitis, cholangitis and typhlitis, were usually caused by Gram-negative bacteria (*K. pneumoniae*, *E. coli*, *Enterobacter cloacae*), *Enterococcus* spp. and anaerobes. Gastroenteritis was frequently hospital acquired and was associated with *C. difficile*.

Urinary tract infections were all due to bacteria, particularly *E. coli* and *K. pneumoniae*.

Fungi alone accounted for 40% of deaths resulting from infection in the NIH study, bacteria for 20%, and concomitant fungi and bacteria for a further 32%. The other deaths due to infection were associated with *P. carinii* pneumonia (one case) or clinically documented cholecystitis (two cases). All patients with invasive pulmonary aspergillosis (IPA) or systemic candidiasis eventually died. The mortality rate was also high for perirectal infection (75%) and *P. aeruginosa* bacteremia (60%).

1.4 How do the organisms vary according to various risk factors?

The depth of neutropenia and failure of the bone marrow to respond to immunosuppressive therapy are the major risk factors for severe and fatal infection in patients with aplastic anemia. In the NIH study, the risk for developing fungal infection was assessed by comparing patients with invasive fungal infection to those with other febrile episodes. Patients with fungal infections differed from the other patients by a lower granulocyte count, both at the start of infection (median 28 versus 44 per mm^3) and when last evaluated (0.5 versus 1182 per mm^3). Similar results were found when episodes resulting in the patient's death were compared to all other episodes (72 versus 285 per mm^3 and 0.4 versus 256 per mm^3, respectively).

P. carinii pneumonia was not affected by the degree of neutropenia, but was significantly associated with the use of cyclosporin therapy.

1.5 How does this differ from other conditions, from center to center, and from country to country?

As in patients with chemotherapy-induced neutropenia or those undergoing bone marrow transplantation, the depth and duration of neutropenia are the major factors that impact on the pattern of infection in patients with aplastic anemia. However, several differences are worth mentioning. The gastrointestinal mucosal barrier is less affected by immunosuppressive therapy than by cytotoxic chemotherapy, which accounts for the significantly lower incidence of gingivostomatitis and esophagitis in patients with aplastic anemia. On the other hand, the duration of neutropenia is expected to last longer in patients with aplastic anemia, and this is an important risk factor for invasive fungal infections. Indeed, there was a high incidence of IPA and *Aspergillus* sinusitis in the NIH study, which resulted in almost unanimously fatal outcome.

A center-to-center variance may be expected in the pattern of isolated bacteria: namely, the relative frequency of Gram-negative versus Gram-positive bacteria, the incidence of *P. aeruginosa* and the frequency of *C. albicans* versus non-*albicans Candida* spp. Similarly, the incidence of β-lactam-resistant staphylococci, vancomycin-resistant enterococci, as well as extended-spectrum β-lactamase-producing and multiresistant Gram-negative bacteria is likely to differ between centers.

Country of origin is likely to affect infection due to endemic pathogens such as *M. tuberculosis*, *Strongyloides stercoralis* or enteric protozoa (*Cryptosporidium*, *Cyclospora* and microsporidia).

1.6 What is the appropriate approach to the initial evaluation and diagnosis of infection in patients with aplastic anemia?

Patients with aplastic anemia may present with infection at admission, and therefore should undergo careful questioning and thorough physical examination to assess the presence of infection both at initial presentation and subsequently when they develop a fever. Neutropenia may mask many of the classic signs and symptoms of infection, and fever may often be the only clue for infection. Pain, on the other hand, can quite reliably direct to the focus of infection (see also Table 2.2).

The oral cavity should be examined for the presence of painful ulcers, white plaques or membranes, periodontal infection, and overt gingivitis or stomatitis. The patient should be questioned about difficulty in swallowing or retrosternal pain, which may indicate esophageal involvement.

The skin should be evaluated for the presence of rash or cellulitis. All parts of the body should be examined, paying special attention to sites such as the perineum, buttocks, axillae and fingernails. Rash may be an extremely important clue to infection. For example, a single or a group of vesicular or crusted lesions is highly suggestive of herpes simplex infection, while dermatomal arrangement suggests varicella zoster. Diffuse vesicular or crusted lesions, which may become hemorrhagic in severely thrombocytopenic patients, are an alarming sign, pointing to the possible diagnosis of disseminated varicella zoster. Lesions with central necrosis may indicate systemic infection with either bacteria (*P. aeruginosa*, *K. pneumoniae* or other Gram-negative species) or a fungal pathogen (*Candida*, *Fusarium*, *Aspergillus*, or even *C. neoformans*). A diffuse rash is more characteristic of *Fusarium* spp. The lesions may vary in size from a few millimeters to a few centimeters, and occur singly or in small numbers. Sometimes they assume the classical appearance of ecthyma gangrenosum, which is more characteristic of *P. aeruginosa* infection. This is a round, indurated nodule which often begins as a vesicle that undergoes hemorrhage, necrosis and ulceration. It is typically surrounded by a rim of erythema and contain little or no pus. In addition, small erythematous papules or papulonodules, which appear singly or diffusely, may be the manifestation of disseminated *Candida* infection.

The skin should be also evaluated for the presence of painful erythema, induration and abscess formation. The fingernails should be evaluated for the presence of paronychia, which can be a source of systemic dissemination for organisms such as *P. aeruginosa*, *Candida* or *Fusarium* spp. Special attention should be devoted to the exit sites of intra-

Table 2.2 Evaluation of infections in patients with aplastic anemia according to the site of infection and the possible etiologic agent

Site of infection	Infectious syndrome (clinical features)	Predominant pathogens*	Workup of infection
Bloodstream	**Bacteremia/fungemia** (fever with or without localizing signs of infection)	**Bacterial** Coag. (−) Staphylococcus P. aeruginosa K. pneumoniae Coag. (+) Staphylococcus Enterococcus spp. E. coli **Fungal** Candida spp. Fusarium spp. (rare) Cryptococcus spp. (rare)	Blood cultures: two sets drawn from separate sites, and at least one set from indwelling central catheters. Fundoscopic examination
Upper respiratory tract (paranasal sinuses, ears, nasopharynx, larynx, trachea)	**Paranasal sinusitis** (rhinorrhea, stuffy nose, ulcerated/necrotic nares lesions, or fever without signs or symptoms)	**Fungal** Aspergillus spp. Candida spp. Fusarium spp. (rare) **Bacterial** P. aeruginosa H. influenzae Coag. (+) Staphylococcus	CT/MRI of the sinuses (may show marked sinus opacification or only mucosal thickening). Specimens for histology and culture: biopsy from the nasal mucosa, aspiration/biopsy (via fiberoptic endoscopy) from the affected sinuses. Blood cultures, fungal serology (antigenemia), (PCR)
Lower respiratory tract	**Bronchopneumonia, pneumonia** (cough, pleuritic chest pain, pleural friction rub, hemoptysis or fever without signs/symptoms)	**Fungal** Aspergillus spp. Candida spp. Mucor spp. Fusarium spp. (rare)	CT/MRI of the chest (more sensitive than plain radiography in the neutropenic patient: may show localized or diffuse alveolar infiltrates). Specimens for histology and culture: expectorated sputum, BAL (± biopsy), OLB, transthoracic needle

Site of infection	Infectious syndrome (clinical features)	Predominant pathogens*	Workup of infection
		Bacterial P.aeruginosa Coag. (+) Staphylococcus K. pneumoniae M. tuberculosis	aspiration/biopsy. Blood cultures, fungal serology (antigenemia), (PCR)
	Pneumonitis (dry cough, exertional dyspnea)	**Pneumocystis carinii** **Viral** Cytomegalovirus	Chest radiography, CT/MRI of the chest (may show diffuse interstitial or patchy infiltrates). Specimens for histology and culture: induced sputum, BAL (± biopsy), OLB, transthoracic needle aspiration/biopsy. Viral serology (antigenemia), PCR
Skin and soft tissue **I Primary infection**	Cellulitis, abscess formation (pain, erythema, swelling and pus if not neutropenic)	**Bacterial** Coag. (+) Staphylococcus Coag. (−) Staphylococcus P.aeruginosa C. jeikeium Group A Streptococcus Enterococcus spp. **Fungal** Candida spp. Mucor spp. (rare)	Specimens for direct examination and culture: pus, discharge, needle aspiration, skin biopsy (histology). Plain radiography may be required to detect gas in tissue; CT/MRI to determine the extent of infection. Blood cultures
	Vesicular rash (local or diffuse, sometimes in dermatomal distribution. May become hemorrhagic or ulcerated)	**Viral** Herpes simplex virus Varicella zoster virus Cytomegalovirus (rare)	Specimens for culture and histology: swab from the bottom of the lesion, needle aspiration, skin biopsy. Tzanck preparation, EIA or DFA for rapid diagnosis
II Secondary infection	Maculopapular rash (diffuse)	**Fungal** Candida spp. Fusarium spp.	Specimens for culture and histology: swab from the bottom of the lesion, needle aspiration, skin biopsy. Blood cultures. Investigation for primary infection

Lesions with central necrosis (local or diffuse)	**Bacterial** P. aeruginosa Klebsiella spp.	As above
	Bacterial P. aeruginosa K. pneumoniae Other Gram-negative organisms **Fungal** Aspergillus spp. Fusarium spp. Mucor spp. (rare) Cryptococcus spp. (rare)	
Vesicular rash (diffuse, may become hemorrhagic or crusted)	**Viral** Varicella zoster virus Cytomegalovirus (rare)	Specimens for culture and histology: swab from the bottom of the lesion, needle aspiration, skin biopsy. Tzanck preparation, EIA or DFA for rapid diagnosis
Gastrointestinal tract		
I Oropharynx		
Stomatitis/mucositis, gingivitis, periodontitis (pain, erythema, ulcers, aphthae, white plaques, sore throat)	**Viral** Herpes simplex virus **Fungal** Candida spp. **Bacterial** K. pneumoniae α-Hemolytic streptococci	Specimens for direct examination and culture: oral/pharyngeal swabs. EIA or DFA for rapid diagnosis. Blood cultures
II Esophagus		
Esophagitis (retrosternal pain, dysphagia)	**Fungal** Candida spp. **Viral** Herpes simplex Cytomegalovirus (rare)	Treatment is mostly empirical in the neutropenic patient. Endoscopy in refractory cases. Specimens for culture and histology: esophageal biopsy
III Lower gastrointestinal tract		
Pseudomembranous colitis (mucous diarrhea, abdominal	**Bacterial** C. difficile	Stool cultures and toxin assay for C. difficile (PCR). Plain abdominal films (may show intestinal dilatation),

Site of infection	Infectious syndrome (clinical features)	Predominant pathogens*	Workup of infection
	tenderness intestinal dilatation)		abdominal US/CT/MRI (may show diffuse thickening of the large intestinal wall). Colonoscopy should be avoided in the neutropenic patient
	Typhlitis (neutropenic enterocolitis) (RUQ pain, vomiting, diarrhea)	**Bacterial** Enterobacter spp. E. coli K. pneumoniae P. aeruginosa Bacteroides spp.	Abdominal US/CT/MRI (may show segmental thickening of the large intestinal wall). Blood cultures
IV Perirectal infection	**Cellulitis, abscess formation** (pain, skin sloughing, inflamed hemorrhoids, abscess formation)	**Bacterial** E. coli Enterococcus spp. P. aeruginosa K. pneumoniae Anaerobes	Blood cultures. Digital rectal examination or rectoscopy should be avoided in the neutropenic patient
Urinary tract	**Urinary tract infection** (dysuria, urgency, frequency, flank pain)	**Bacterial** E. coli K. pneumoniae P. aeruginosa	Midstream urine culture. Blood cultures. Abdominal US/CT (may detect obstruction, abscess formation)
Central nervous system (primary or secondary to disseminated infection)	**Brain lesions, meningitis** (altered mental status, headache, seizures, focal neurologic signs, nuchal rigidity)	**Fungal** Aspergillus spp. Fusarium spp. Mucor spp. C. neoformans	CT/MRI of the brain (may show infarcts or abscess formation). Fungal blood and CSF cultures. Cryptococcal serology (antigenemia) in blood, CSF aspiration/biopsy under stereotactic CT guidance

* Pathogens are arranged according to the order of frequency.

Coag. (−), coagulase negative; Coag. (+), coagulase positive; CT, computed tomography; MRI, magnetic resonance imaging; BAL, bronchoalveolar lavage; OLB, open lung biopsy; PCR, polymerase chain reaction; DFA, direct fluorescent assay; EIA, enzyme immunoassay; US, ultrasonography; RUQ, right upper quadrant; CSF, cerebrospinal fluid.

venous catheters, which should be evaluated for the presence of erythema, tenderness, skin erosion, discharge and swelling. The perirectal area should be evaluated for the presence of skin sloughing, tenderness, inflamed hemorrhoids or overt abscess formation. Routine digital examination is best avoided in the neutropenic patient.

Diagnosis of pneumonia, and particularly invasive fungal pneumonia, is extremely difficult in neutropenic patients, since the usual signs and symptoms may be obtunded by neutropenia. Often, the initial presentation is persistent fever despite broad-spectrum antibacterial or even antifungal therapy. Patients should be questioned about the presence of pleuritic chest pain, which is a common sign in IPA and may antedate radiographic changes by up to 3 weeks. Similarly, pleural friction rub should be looked for during lung examination. Although highly suggestive of IPA, pleural friction rub may occasionally occur with other etiologic agents. Dyspnea and dry cough are common presentations of pneumonia due to *P. carinii*.

A significant advance in the diagnosis of IPA can be attributed to the systematic use computed tomography (CT), which was shown to improve the outcome of patients with IPA through early diagnosis and administration of antifungal therapy. This approach is based on the experience shared by most physicians working in the field, that high-resolution CT (as well as magnetic resonance imaging; MRI) is more sensitive than plain chest radiography for the diagnosis of invasive fungal infections. The finding of a single or multiple areas of nodular infiltrates surrounded by ground-glass attenuation (the halo sign) and pulmonary cavitation (the crescent sign) in the setting of a febrile neutropenic patient is considered highly suggestive of IPA. In addition, any new infiltrate in that setting is also highly suspicious and, in the absence of another etiology, the administration of antifungal therapy is probably required. However, one of the limitations of this approach, as has been shown by several recent studies, is the lack of specificity of the halo and crescent signs. Mucormycosis, embolic infarction, bacterial abscess, organizing pneumonia and fibrosing alveolitis can all assume the radiologic appearance of IPA.

Obtaining respiratory tract cultures for the confirmation of IPA usually requires an invasive procedure, which can result in a high complication rate in patients with aplastic anemia who are severely thrombocytopenic as well as neutropenic. These invasive techniques include bronchoalveolar lavage (BAL), transbronchial biopsy, transthoracic needle aspiration, and open lung biopsy. BAL is least likely to result in significant bleeding, but may have a disappointingly low yield, especially in the presence of localized lung lesions. The major contraindication to BAL is impending respiratory failure. In the majority of patients with IPA, invasive diagnostic procedures can be delayed until bone marrow recovery.

Sputum cultures, especially when repeatedly sampled, may yield *Aspergillus* in about 50% of patients with IPA. Unfortunately, in the majority of patients sputum cultures are not relevant at the time of initial diagnosis, since sputum production usually occurs later in the course of the disease, sometimes after the pulmonary infection has already progressed. Nonetheless, multiple sputum samples for fungal cultures should be attempted whenever available.

Sinus infections may also have a subtle presentation. Patients should be questioned about nasal stuffiness and rhinorrhea, which may be the only clue for invasive fungal sinusitis. With advanced disease facial pain may become a more prominent complaint. The nares should be examined carefully for the presence of necrotic or gray lesions and for areas of hypoesthesia. Periorbital extension of invasive fungal sinusitis may present as periorbital cellulitis, while basal extension may result in upper palate ulceration. CT or MRI is more sensitive than plain sinus radiography, and may reveal either thickening of the nasal mucosa or opacification of the sinus cavity, as well as bony destruction and extension into adjacent tissue. Flexible endoscopy can be used to visualize the involved sinus and to obtain specimens for histologic and bacteriologic studies.

Patients should also be questioned about abdominal pain and the presence of diarrhea. The concomitant appearance of right upper quadrant pain with vomiting and diarrhea is suggestive of neutropenic enterocolitis. It should be stressed that in patients with neutropenia or those receiving immunosuppressive therapy the classic peritoneal signs may be minimal or absent, yet the patient may suffer from a life-threatening intraabdominal infection. When the patient is profoundly neutropenic, any abdominal complaint should be evaluated thoroughly, and should be considered a trigger for initiating broad-spectrum antibacterial therapy, even in the absence of fever.

When infection is suspected on the basis of fever or on clinical grounds, two sets of blood cultures should be obtained. If a tunneled catheter is in place, one set of blood cultures should be obtained via the line. Initial routine cultures should also include throat and urine cultures. In addition, any site of suspected focus of infection should be cultured, and cutaneous lesions should be biopsied. In patients coming from endemic areas, stool should be studied for the presence of parasites such as S. *stercoralis* and enteric protozoa.

Chest radiography should be a routine part of the initial evaluation. In addition, it may be wise to obtain CT (or MRI) images of the lungs and sinuses, the sites most frequently involved in invasive aspergillosis. These imaging studies may help with the early diagnosis of patients who are already infected at presentation, and will also serve as reference for follow-up studies. As mentioned above, a strategy of systematic CT scans allows earlier detection of invasive aspergillosis and has a favorable impact on outcome.

Initial laboratory studies should include blood counts and chemistry, and perhaps estimation of C-reactive protein (CRP) levels. When available, baseline antigen detection assays for *Candida* and *Aspergillus* should be also obtained. In addition, it might be wise to keep a sample of the patient's serum for subsequent comparative polymerase chain reaction (PCR) or serology studies. A purified protein derivative (PPD) skin test should be considered for high-risk patients.

1.7 How should the evaluation be modified according to the severity of the risk?

The severity of neutropenia and its duration are the predominant risk factors for developing invasive fungal infections in patients with aplastic anemia. Fungal infections, and particularly invasive aspergillosis, have the most prominent impact on outcome in this group of patients. Since early diagnosis and early aggressive therapy may increase the chances of survival, the bulk of diagnostic efforts should be focused on the early diagnosis of invasive fungal infections. Although all patients with severe aplastic anemia are at risk, those with a neutrophil count of less than 100 per mm^3 are probably at an increased risk for developing and dying from invasive fungal infections.

Patients who require prolonged (> 1 month) treatment with cyclosporin-containing immunosuppressive regimens may be also at a heightened risk for developing opportunistic infections similar to those in organ transplant patients. They should be monitored carefully for infection with *P. carinii*, cytomegalovirus, *C. neoformans* and intracellular bacteria (*Nocardia*, *Mycobacteria*, nontyphoidal *Salmonella*, *Listeria* and *Legionella* spp.).

1.8 What are the specific evaluation measures? (see also Chapter 2 in Part I)

Evaluation measures according to the site and organism are summarized in Table 2.2.

1.9 What new developments are going to impact on emerging organisms, recognition, evaluation and diagnosis of infection in patients with aplastic anemia?

Immunocompromised hosts, particularly those with severe and protracted neutropenia, provide an excellent niche for the development of fungal pathogens. There are about 200 000 species of fungal pathogens, many of which are ubiquitous in the environment, in food, or even colonizing the skin or gastrointestinal tract. It is only logical to expect that in the compromised host repeated exposure may result in invasion. Indeed, an ever-increasing list of such opportunistic fungal pathogens is being recognized as the cause of invasive and life-threatening infections in neutropenic patients. The most frequently reported infections are due to *Fusarium* spp., *Trichosporon beigelii*, *Malassezia furfur*, *Penicillium marneffei*, *Acremonium* species and dematiaceous fungi (e.g. *Exserohilum*, *Alternaria*, *Curvalaria*, *Bipolaris*). In patients with aplastic anemia, several unusual invasive fungal pathogens have been reported in the literature, including a single case, each, of *Exserohilum rostratum*, *Trichoderma longfibrachitum* (a dermatophyte) and *Fusarium chlamydosporum*. Some of the emerging fungal pathogens may show variable degrees of resistance to the conventional antifungal regimens.

Other epidemiologic trends of fungal infections among cancer and bone marrow transplanted patients may also affect patients with aplastic anemia. These include the shift from *albicans* to non-*albicans Candida* spp. and the emergence of azole resistance among *Candida* spp. Recent reports address the increasing frequency of C. *parapsilosis*, C. *glabrata* and C. *krusei* among cancer and bone marrow transplant patients.

Similarly, the local pattern of drug resistance may impact on nosocomial bacterial infections in patients with aplastic anemia. Of particular importance is the prevalence of β-lactam-resistant staphylococci, vancomycin-resistant *Enterococcus*, extended-spectrum β-lactamase-producing K. *pneumoniae*, carbapenem-resistant P. *aeruginosa* and quinolone-resistant Gram-negative rods. For example, quinolone resistance increased in 1993 to 28% among E. *coli* bloodstream isolates from patients with neutropenic cancer participating in the European Organisation for Research on Treatment of Cancer (EORTC) studies. Other cancer centers have reported on bloodstream infections due to β-lactam-resistant *Enterobacter*, penicillin-resistant *Streptococcus viridans* and *Streptococcus pneumoniae*, as well as vancomycin-resistant enterococci.

The emergence of *Aspergillus* as a predominant etiologic agent in nosocomial pneumonia and a major cause of death was reported not only in patients with aplastic anemia, but also in bone marrow transplant patients and those with hematologic malignancy. This has prompted intensive research efforts at new diagnostic modalities.

The most promising progress in nonculture techniques for the diagnosis of invasive aspergillosis is a commercially available sandwich enzyme-linked immunosorbent assay (ELISA) (Platelia Aspergillus; Sanofi Diagnostics Pasteur, Marnes-La-Coquette, France) which detects galactomannan, a cell wall constituent of *Aspergillus* spp. that is released during growth. A high sensitivity of 67–100% and a specificity of 81–100% were found in patients with hematologic malignancies, especially when sequential serum samples were studied. This antigen assay allows early detection and quantitative measurements (quantitative titers) of the *Aspergillus* load, and can be used for early diagnosis as well as monitoring the response to treatment. The galactomannan antigen can also be detected in cerebrospinal fluid of patients with cerebral aspergillosis. A possible limitation of this assay is a high intralaboratory and interlaboratory variation in antigen titers when measured in different runs.

Another rapidly developing field is pathogen-specific PCR. Small-scale studies have demonstrated high sensitivity in the detection of *Aspergillus* DNA from BAL fluids as well as from patients' sera. False-positive (due to environmental contamination) and false-negative results are still a problem.

2 REGARDING THE RISK FACTORS ACCOMPANYING APLASTIC ANEMIA

2.1 What are the main alterations in host defense mechanisms and what are the appropriate investigations to document them?

The predominant alteration in host defense mechanisms in patients with aplastic anemia is a low neutrophil and monocyte count, which result from bone marrow failure. Since bone marrow recovery in response to immunosuppressive therapy may take up to 12 weeks, the average duration of neutropenia is longer in patients with aplastic anemia than in those with cancer and chemotherapy-induced neutropenia. This is translated into a longer period at risk for severe and fatal infections.

2.2 What are the alterations due to iatrogenic factors?

Following the administration of immunosuppressive therapy, patients with aplastic anemia may develop mild to moderate impairment of cell-mediated immunity. The degree of impairment depends on the intensity and duration of the regimens used. Current treatment regimens contain a combination of ATG, cyclosporin and a short course of low-dose prednisone. ATG is prepared by immunizing horses with human lymphocytes, and has a nonspecifically lympholytic effect. It is mildly immunosuppressive and produces moderate lymphopenia, probably through complement-mediated lysis. Cyclosporin inhibits the release of interleukin-2 from activated T-cells, and consequently decreases T-cell proliferation, as well as the production of lymphokines such as interferon-γ. Glucocorticoids, by affecting the trafficking of peripheral white blood cells, may decrease the number of circulating lymphocytes, monocytes, eosinophils and basophils, and increase the number of neutrophils.

In addition, ATG may cause transient reduction in the number of peripheral granulocytes, and subsequently an increased susceptibility to infection. Glucocorticoids may inhibit the function of leukocytes and tissue macrophages, thereby adding a qualitative component to the already existing quantitative phagocytic disorder in patients with aplastic anemia.

In contrast to cytotoxic chemotherapy in patients with cancer, the currently used immunosuppressive regimens in patients with aplastic anemia lack profound bone marrow toxicity, do not compromise the integrity of the mucosal and endothelial barriers, and do not impair humoral immunity. Suppression of cell-mediated immunity is also milder compared with that in patients receiving an organ transplant.

2.3 What is the influence of environmental factors?

Patients with aplastic anemia are inpatients during the period of maximum immunosuppression, so that their most important exposure is to the hospital environment. Like other groups of hospitalized patients, they may acquire resistant nosocomial pathogens as well as C. *difficile* via the hands of the staff or from the inanimate environmental objects. More importantly, they are exposed to the airborne spores of *Aspergillus*, which is ubiquitous in the hospital environment. In the hospital setting, *Aspergillus* has been cultured from unfiltered air, ventilation systems, fireproofing material, dust arising from renovation and construction work, potted plants, pepper and spices, and even from the hospital water system (shower heads and hot water faucets).

2.4 What are the most significant factors that contribute to the risk of infection in patients with aplastic anemia?

The primary risk of infection in patients with aplastic anemia is the severity and duration of neutropenia, which are influenced by the severity of bone marrow failure and the response to immunosuppressive therapy. Febrile episodes and fungal infections are more likely to develop in patients with a low neutrophil and monocyte count. The majority of patients who die from invasive aspergillosis have no neutrophils at the time of death. ATG treatment may slightly augment this risk by producing a transient decrease in neutrophil count. The most important extrinsic risk for developing invasive aspergillosis is the presence of *Aspergillus* spores in the hospital environment.

Other components of the immunosuppressive regimen, such as cyclosporin and steroids, may also contribute to the risk of infection by altering cell-mediated immunity. They predispose to opportunistic infections such as *P. carinii*, *C. neoformans*, herpesviruses including cytomegalovirus, as well as intracellular bacteria.

2.5 What are the specific or nonspecific measures aimed at minimizing each of these factors?

The strategy of preventing severe and fatal infection in patients with aplastic anemia should be aimed at reducing the neutropenic period on the one hand, and decreasing the exposure to nosocomial pathogens, particularly *Aspergillus* spores, on the other.

Granulocyte colony-stimulating factor (G-CSF) has been shown to have some effect in increasing the neutrophil count in patients with aplastic anemia, but the effect is not lasting when the treatment is used alone. On the other hand, when used as adjuvant therapy with potent immunosuppressive protocols, G-CSF has the potential to reduce the mortality rate and to improve remission rates, as has been shown in recent pilot studies. The combination of G-CSF with erythropoietin β is being currently studied.

In order to decrease exposure to fungal spores, patients with severe aplastic anemia should probably be located in a protected environment, which can be achieved by high-efficacy particulate air (HEPA) filters, directed room airflow, positive room air pressure, well sealed rooms, and a high rate of air exchange in the rooms (see section 4.1 below).

2.6 Are there different levels of risk of infection recognized for patients with aplastic anemia?

Levels of risk for infection have not been studied in patients with aplastic anemia. It may be deduced from the NIH study that a neutrophil count below 100 cells/mm^3 presents an increased risk for invasive aspergillosis. In addition, patients who are slow to respond to the immunosuppressive therapy are at an increased risk for developing and dying from invasive fungal infections.

2.8 What new developments are going to impact on minimizing or suppressing the specific risk factors?

More potent treatment protocols for aplastic anemia causing more rapid and long-lasting restoration of normal hematopoiesis are likely to have the most significant impact on the risk for infection, by reducing the duration of neutropenia. Cyclophosphamide and purine analogs, alone or in combination with cyclosporin, are currently being evaluated.

New growth factors, such as stem cell factor (CSF) and interleukins (IL-3, IL-6 and IL-11), also have the potential to decrease the depth and length of neutropenia. The combination of several growth factors in the treatment of aplastic anemia is intriguing. Small clinical trials with these new agents have so far been disappointing owing to severe systemic toxicity or lack of response. Engineered synthetic growth factors have been synthesized and await clinical evaluation.

3 REGARDING THE SURVEILLANCE OF PATIENTS WITH APLASTIC ANEMIA

3.1 What is the important premorbid information to be gathered?
Before the administration of immunosuppressive therapy, data regarding the country of origin and recent travel history should be collected. This information is required to assess the risk for the reactivation of endemic infections including *M. tuberculosis*, gastrointestinal parasites (e.g. *S. stercoralis*, enteric protozoa) and endemic fungi (e.g. histoplasmosis or coccidioidomycosis). This should be followed by chest radiography, PPD skin test, examination of stool samples and serologic studies, according to the type of exposure.

3.2 What are the surveillance measures to be taken when a patient presents with aplastic anemia?
3.3 What are the other specific measures to be taken when a patient presents with aplastic anemia?
3.4 What development(s) are to be expected for surveillance in patients with aplastic anemia?
The major threat to the lives of patients with aplastic anemia is IPA. Studies regarding the benefit of nasal fungal surveillance cultures in neutropenic patients have yielded conflicting results. Their predictive power probably depends on the circumstances (presence or absence or hospital renovations or an outbreak) and local experience. The value of nasal fungal surveillance cultures has not been evaluated in patients with aplastic anemia. The cost–benefit characteristics of such surveillance should be determined by the individual center.

Nonmicrobiologic surveillance methods for invasive fungal infections include periodic CT (or MRI) of the paranasal sinuses, the chest and the brain as well as antigen detection assays for *Candida* and *Aspergillus*. PCR-based methods for fungal infections, using either a pathogen-specific or universal fungal probes, are promising, but their performance in patients with invasive fungal infections awaits further evaluation. Combining several methods can probably improve the yield.

Prospective screening by one or more method (e.g. CT and serology with or without PCR) can be used to design a preemptive approach to antifungal therapy, thus reducing the need for unnecessary treatment. The optimal time interval for the periodic studies has not yet been elucidated, but undertaking CT once a week and serologic and PCR studies two or three times a week seems a logical approach. This strategy needs to be evaluated in prospective studies.

The utility of environmental control for the prevention of nosocomial infections is another unsolved issue. A recent study by the French Aspergillus Study Group demonstrated a decrease in the number and incidence of invasive nosocomial aspergillosis when periodic monitoring of fungal contamination in the air and surfaces was combined with the monitoring of new cases of IPA and the application of control measures in cases of renovation. In light of the data connecting nosocomial fungal infection with the hospital water supply, there may also be a role for monitoring of the hospital water system.

Studies regarding the absolute or relative utility of the different surveillance methods in patients with aplastic anemia are currently not available, and are a challenge for future research.

4 REGARDING THE PREVENTION OF INFECTIONS IN PATIENTS WITH APLASTIC ANEMIA

4.1 What approaches, if any, to the prevention of infection should be considered in patients with aplastic anemia?

Preventive measures in patients with aplastic anemia have not been studied. Strategies developed for bone marrow transplant patients, including antibacterial and antifungal prophylaxis or protected environment, may also be appropriate for patients with aplastic anemia.

Several antibacterial prophylactic regimens have been studied in febrile neutropenic patients, the most effective ones being trimethoprim sulfamethoxazole (TMP–SMX) and quinolones. Although the current data support the efficacy of these agents in reducing the infectious episodes, particularly those due to Gram-negative bacteria, no survival advantage has been shown. Furthermore, development of resistant Gram-negative bacteria and outbreaks of fatal α-viridans infections are of major concern. Resistance may be even more likely to develop in patients with aplastic anemia who are expected to have a longer duration of neutropenia and of antibacterial therapy. Routine antibacterial prophylaxis should probably not be used in patients with aplastic anemia.

Prospective randomized studies have been able to demonstrate the efficacy of antifungal prophylaxis with fluconazole in reducing invasive candidiasis in patients undergoing bone marrow transplantation, but not for those with acute leukemia or solid tumors. Nonetheless, in the MD Anderson Cancer Center, the use of fluconazole has been associated with an impressive reduction in the incidence of candidemia. However, while fluconazole may have protective effect against candidal infections, it has no known effect against *Aspergillus*, which is of major concern in patients with aplastic anemia. Another concern with wide use of fluconazole treatment is the emergence of non-*albicans* and resistant *Candida* spp. The role of routine fluconazole prophylaxis is questionable in patients with aplastic anemia.

There is no consensus regarding the effectiveness of intranasal or low dose amphotericin B, or of oral itraconazole, as a protective measure against invasive aspergillosis. Studies with itraconazole suspension show some promise, and await confirmation.

Cyclosporin-containing regimens have been shown to increase significantly the risk of *P. carinii* pneumonia. Patients treated with such regimens should probably receive prophylaxis against *P. carinii* pneumonia.

Exposure to fungal spores can be reduced by locating patients with aplastic anemia in a protected environment. The best studied such environment is the room with laminar airflow. This system is highly effective, but is very expensive to install and maintain. HEPA filtered rooms with positive pressure are less costly and have also proved to be effective in preventing nosocomial aspergillosis. Patient stay out of the protected environment should be reduced to a minimum. If a procedure in other areas of the hospital is unavoidable, the route should be planned carefully to avoid areas of construction, and the immediate admission of the patient should be coordinated to minimize waiting time. Although not based on firm data, some authorities suggest that potted plants and shrubs should not be allowed in the immediate vicinity of the patients, and that pepper and other spices should be sterilized before use.

Despite all these measures, the risk of invasive aspergillosis can be reduced but not eliminated. This has been explained by patient's colonization before hospitalization, by occasional breaks in the airflow and by time spent outside the protected room. Recently, the hospital water supply has been suggested as the source of nosocomial aspergillosis and fusariosis. This new route of exposure may be minimized by using boiled or filtered water instead of tap water.

4.2 What are the future challenges and opportunities for reducing the risk of infection?

Future research efforts should be devoted to prevention of invasive fungal infections, and in particularly IPA, which have the most deleterious effect on patients with aplastic anemia. One of the more exciting prospects would be the development of vaccines against *Candida* and *Aspergillus*; however, this is not likely in the near future. Even if such vaccines were available, it is not clear whether the patients would be able to mount a protective immune response, as they will need immunosuppressive therapy.

Future studies should also concentrate on more effective antifungal prophylaxis and strategies to reduce the exposure to fungal spores in the hospital environment.

5 REGARDING THE TREATMENT OF PATIENTS WITH APLASTIC ANEMIA

5.1 What is the role of empirical therapy?

Empirical antibacterial therapy has become the standard of care for the febrile neutropenic patient since the early 1970s. This approach was originally designed for patients with cancer-related neutropenia, and was based on the observations that empirical therapy could reduce the early morbidity and mortality rates associated with undiagnosed and untreated infections. The rationale behind this approach is based on the following arguments:

1 There is a quantitative correlation between the number of circulating granulocytes and the risk of developing infectious complications. The likelihood of severe bacterial and fungal infections significantly increases when the granulocyte count drops below 500/mm^3, and even more so when the count is less than 100/mm^3.
2 Not only does the likelihood of infection increase, but also the severity and rapidity of spread if untreated. This is especially true for Gram-negative bacteria. In the 1960s and the early 1970s, when potent antibiotics were less available, the mortality rate from Gram-negative bacteremia in neutropenic patients was reported to be 70–80%, and even higher in patients presenting with shock. The median length of survival in neutropenic patients with Gram-negative bacteremia was 3–4 days, and one third of patients had died within 24 h. This desperate situation has changed with the availability of more potent antibiotics and the recognition that they should be started as soon as the neutropenic patient became febrile.
3 Delay in therapy further increases mortality.

4   The inflammatory response of the neutropenic patient is muted, and the normal signs and symptoms of infection may be minimal or even absent. Fever remains the cardinal, and sometimes the only, sign of infection.

5   There is no reliable way to predict when fever in the neutropenic patient is due to infection or to other causes. The essence of empirical antibiotic therapy is that fever in the neutropenic patient is considered a sign of infection until proven otherwise.

In December 1997 The Infectious Disease Society of America published revised guidelines for the use of antimicrobial agents in neutropenic patients with unexplained fever in the journal *Clinical Infectious Diseases* (1997; **25**: 551–573).

Many of the above considerations are also true for patients with aplastic anemia, so that many of the guidelines for empirical antibiotic therapy use developed for the high-risk febrile neutropenic patient can be adopted for the neutropenic patient with aplastic anemia. However, several considerations unique to the patient with aplastic anemia do exist. Importantly, in patients with chemotherapy-induced neutropenia the first episode of fever is usually due to a bacterial infection, while fungi are responsible for the secondary febrile events. In patients with aplastic anemia the likelihood of fungal infections at presentation is somewhat higher, and this should be taken into consideration in the initial evaluation (see section 1.6). At the other extreme, patients who develop fever immediately after the administration of ATG may be suffering from the side effect of the drug, rather than an infection. Rigors and other manifestations of serum sickness (arthralgia, myalgia), as well as failure to document a source of infection, also suggest drug toxicity. Other considerations for patients with aplastic anemia are discussed below, and the algorithm for initial evaluation and treatment is presented in Figure 2.1.

Empirical antibiotic therapy should be started with a single oral temperature > 38.5°C, or ≥ 38.0°C over at least 1 h in patients with a neutrophil count of <500/mm³ or <1000/mm³ with a predicted decline of <500/mm³. Considerations for selecting the initial antibacterial regimen should include the patterns of bacterial infections as well as the pattern of resistance to antibacterial therapy in the individual center. Other considerations are the potency of the antibacterial agents in the absence of neutrophils, their toxicity profile as well as known drug allergy or organ dysfunction, which may limit the use of certain antibacterials. In patients with aplastic anemia the potential for interaction between the antibacterial and immunosuppressive agents is an additional consideration.

The empirical regimen may include either a single potent antibacterial agent (monotherapy) or two agents (combination therapy). Monotherapy most commonly includes ceftazidime, cefepime, imipenem or meropenem. Combination therapy usually consists of a β-lactam antibiotic in combination with an aminoglycoside. The β-lactam in the combination is either a ureidopenicillin, with or without a β-lactamase inhibitor (piperacillin, azlocillin, piperacillin–tazobactam), or an antipseudomonal cephalosporin (e.g. ceftazidime, cefepime). Vancomycin should not be routinely incorporated into the initial antibiotic regimen, unless there is a high incidence of β-lactam resistance among Gram-positive organisms (e.g. methicillin-resistant *Staphylococcus aureus* or penicillin-resistant β-hemolytic streptococci) in the individual center, or if there is strong clinical evidence of catheter-related or soft tissue infection.

Considerations for modification of the initial regimen are similar in the patient with aplastic anemia and in those with cancer-related neutropenia. The reasons for modification are usually the subsequent isolation of a resistant organism from the bloodstream or from a site of infection, clinical evidence of infection that is not covered by the empirical regimen, or a progressive infection. Examples are isolation of Gram-negative bacteria

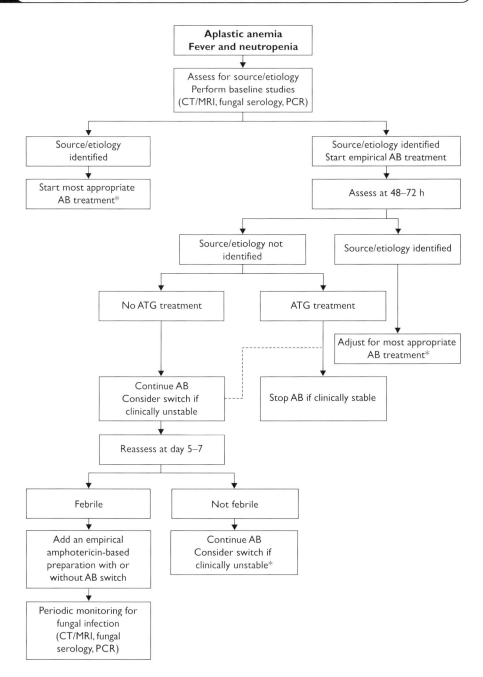

Figure 2.1 Algorithm for the initial evaluation and treatment of the febrile neutropenic patient with aplastic anemia. *If febrile at any time after day 5–7, add an empirical amphotericin-based preparation with or without a switch in the antibiotic treatment, and assess for invasive fungal infection. CT, computed tomography; MRI, magnetic resonance imaging; PCR, polymerase chain reaction; AB, antibiotic; ATG, antithymocyte globulin.

that are resistant to the β-lactam component of the regimen (switch to another β-lactam or a quinolone), β-lactam-resistant Gram-positive cocci (add vancomycin or teicoplanin), evidence of anaerobic bacteria (add metronidazole or clindamycin, if the initial regimen does not provide adequate anaerobic coverage), or evidence of viral or fungal infection (add antivirals or antifungals, respectively). If the initial regimen contained vancomycin and β-lactam-resistant Gram-positive cocci were not documented, vancomycin should be stopped.

The optimal duration of antibacterial treatment has not been studied in patients with aplastic anemia. In the presence of a documented infection, the duration of treatment depends on the nature of infection and its response to antibacterial therapy, as well as the degree of neutropenia and the response of the bone marrow to immunosuppressive therapy. Generally, longer duration of treatment is required in patients with aplastic anemia.

If fever and neutropenia persist beyond 48–72 h without a source of infection, the decision should be made whether to continue the same antibiotic regimen or to switch to another regimen with a broader spectrum. Clinical instability should favor the switch to another regimen. If the patient is being treated with ATG, especially when having other manifestations of serum sickness, there is a high likelihood that the fever is due to ATG treatment rather than infection. If the patient is clinically stable, antibiotic treatment may be discontinued with close monitoring of the patient.

If fever and neutropenia persist beyond days 5–7 of antibiotic treatment, empirical antifungal therapy should be added. Owing to the high incidence of invasive aspergillosis, empirical antifungal therapy in the patient with aplastic anemia should probably consist of an amphotericin-based formulation, rather than fluconazole. A daily dosage of amphotericin deoxycholate (conventional amphotericin B) of 0.6–1.0 mg/kg is probably appropriate. The use of amphotericin deoxycholate is limited by its well-known toxic profile, namely a high incidence of infusion-associated reactions (fever, chills, hypoxic events) and dose-related toxicity (renal toxicity, hypokalemia, anemia). Renal toxicity is a major concern in patients with aplastic anemia who may be receiving concomitant nephrotoxic agents, such as cyclosporin or aminoglycosides. Lipid formulations of amphotericin were developed to improve the therapeutic index of amphotericin deoxycholate.

Three lipid formulations of amphotericin are available commercially: AmBisome, a small unilamellar vesicle formulation; Amphocil/Amphotec (ABCD), a colloidal dispersion; and Abelcet (ABLC), a lipid complex. Two of the preparations have been evaluated as empirical treatment for febrile neutropenic patients. One recent multicenter study compared Amphocil 4 mg/kg daily with amphotericin deoxycholate 0.8 mg/kg daily in a double-blind fashion for the empirical treatment of fever and neutropenia. The vast majority of patients were either bone marrow transplanted or had leukemia. The therapeutic response was comparable between the two groups (50% and 43.2%, respectively); however, infusion-related toxicity was more common in the Amphocil arm. On the other hand, renal toxicity with Amphocil was significantly less frequent compared with that seen with amphotericin deoxycholate, and this was not affected by the concomitant use of cyclosporin or aminoglycosides. Another recently published study compared the empirical use of AmBisome 3 mg/kg daily with amphotericin deoxycholate 0.6 mg/kg daily in febrile neutropenic patients, again in a double-blind fashion. There was a significant reduction in the infusion-related toxicity as well as renal toxicity in the AmBisome arm compared with the amphotericin deoxycholate arm. Furthermore, AmBisome was found to be more protective against the development of systemic fungal infections. On the basis of this study, the US Food and Drug Administration (FDA) approved the use of AmBisome for empirical therapy in febrile neutropenic patients.

The addition of empirical antifungal therapy should be followed by intensive efforts to document the presence of fungal infection if the patient remains persistently febrile and neutropenic. Breakthrough fungal infections are not uncommon in patients with aplastic anemia on empirical antifungal regimens.

5.2 What is the appropriate approach to the patient with aplastic anemia and evidence of infection in various body sites?

The general approach to therapy according to the various sites of infection is similar for chemotherapy-related neutropenic patients and those with aplastic anemia. Empirical therapy should take into consideration the most common pathogens according to site (Table 2.2), as well as the pattern of resistance in the individual center. A high incidence of *P. aeruginosa* infection in patients with aplastic anemia should be remembered when selecting an empirical regimen.

The majority of sinus and pulmonary infections in patients with aplastic anemia are due to fungal pathogens, and particularly *Aspergillus*. Signs and symptoms pointing to the lung or sinuses as a possible site of infection should prompt an intensive search for a fungal pathogen, and empirical therapy should include an antifungal agent.

5.3–5.6 What is the appropriate approach to the patient with aplastic anemia and evidence of a documented bacterial, viral, fungal or parasitic infection?

The principles of pathogen-directed therapy in patients with aplastic anemia are similar to those of other patients with chemotherapy-induced neutropenia (see also Part II, Chapters 4 and 5). The only caveat is that neutropenia is more likely to persist throughout the course of infection, so that a longer duration of antibacterial therapy may be required, and a switch to oral therapy is usually not an option. The following discussion will focus on infections due to *Aspergillus*, which is the predominant cause of morbidity and mortality in patients with aplastic anemia.

The outcome of invasive aspergillosis in patients with aplastic anemia has been extremely disappointing. In the NIH study, 13 of 14 patients with invasive aspergillosis eventually died, and in 12 death could be related directly to the infection. One patient with isolated *Aspergillus* sinusitis, who had also responded to ATG therapy, survived. All patients were treated with variable daily doses of amphotericin deoxycholate (0.5–1.5 mg/kg).

Amphotericin deoxycholate is the gold standard of treatment for invasive aspergillosis. The overall success rate in various groups of patients is around 30%, the range being 0–85%. The higher rates are a single-center experience, describing patients who were diagnosed early and treated with higher doses of amphotericin (1.0–1.5 mg/kg daily). Patients with sinus aspergillosis may have somewhat higher response rates than patients with pulmonary or disseminated aspergillosis. CNS aspergillosis is almost universally fatal.

There is a significant interaction between amphotericin deoxycholate and cyclosporin with regard to renal toxicity. Since cyclosporin is an important component of the current immunosuppressive regimens, the use of amphotericin deoxycholate in patients with aplastic anemia may be problematic. The appropriate dose of amphotericin deoxycholate for the treatment of invasive aspergillosis in patients with severe aplastic anemia is 1.0–1.5 mg/kg daily. Renal toxicity can be reduced by concomitant administration of saline (about 2 liters per day), and the degree of hypokalemia by the administration of amiloride.

The new lipid formulations of amphotericin enable the administration of higher daily doses of amphotericin without increasing renal toxicity. Experience with these formulations as first-line therapy in patients with invasive aspergillosis is limited, since the vast majority of patients have been treated on a compassionate basis, or following amphotericin failure or toxicity. Nonetheless, a recent multicenter randomized study compared AmBisome 5 mg/kg daily with amphotericin deoxycholate 1 mg/kg daily in the treatment of invasive fungal infection. Among patients with suspected or documented pulmonary aspergillosis, 42% of those receiving AmBisome had a complete response compared with only 21% of patients taking amphotericin deoxycholate. Partial and complete response rates were 56% and 50%, respectively. Overall mortality rates were also better in the AmBisome arm (19% versus 38% for amphotericin deoxycholate). Although the results were not statistically significant, the trends are encouraging.

A recent retrospective analysis assessed the efficacy of Amphocil (dose range 2–8 mg/kg daily) in patients with invasive aspergillosis, who participated in clinical trials in six cancer or transplant centers. The response rate (complete and partial) in the Amphocil-treated patients was 49%, compared with 23% in patients treated with amphotericin deoxycholate. The survival rate was also higher in the Amphocil group (50% versus 28%). However, since the study was not prospective or randomized, the authors could not conclude that Amphocil was superior to amphotericin deoxycholate. A third study assessed the efficacy of Abelcet (5 mg/kg) given on an open-label, single-patient basis for emergency use in patients with invasive fungal infection refractory or intolerant to amphotericin deoxycholate. The overall response rate (complete and partial) was 48%: 38% for pulmonary aspergillosis, 30% for disseminated aspergillosis, 64% for sinus aspergillosis and 67% for single-organ extrapulmonary aspergillosis. Finally, summary of the UK data for compassionate use of AmBisome for invasive fungal infections revealed an overall response rate of 59% for patients with aspergillosis and of 80% for those who were not previously treated with amphotericin.

All three lipid formulations of amphotericin have a superior renal toxicity profile compared with the parent drug, even when given at a daily dose of up to five times that of amphotericin deoxycholate. No advantage can be demonstrated as far as hypokalemia is concerned. Infusion-related or immediate toxicity has been shown to be significantly lower with AmBisome compared with amphotericin deoxycholate, even if infused in as short a time as 30–60 min. No advantage in the infusion-related reaction could be demonstrated for the other two lipid formulations. No increased renal toxicity was observed in patients treated concomitantly with AmBisome and cyclosporin, although severe liver toxicity was reported with concomitant Abelcet and cyclosporin use.

In patients with aplastic anemia and invasive aspergillosis who are being treated with cyclosporin, the use of one of the lipid formulations of amphotericin as first-line therapy should be strongly considered. All three available lipid formulations have a comparable decreased risk of renal toxicity, but only AmBisome has demonstrated significantly decreased immediate toxicity. Furthermore, experience accumulated with the use of AmBisome in organ and bone marrow transplant patients treated with cyclosporin has also confirmed its safety and tolerability. The appropriate daily dose of the lipid formulations is 5 mg/kg. Higher doses, up to 8 and 10 mg/kg daily of both Amphocil and AmBisome, are also well tolerated.

Itraconazole has also shown efficacy in the treatment of invasive aspergillosis, although data regarding profoundly neutropenic patients are sparse. In a multicenter open study the overall response rate to itraconazole was 39%. In the USA and several European countries, itraconazole is approved as a second-line therapy for patients with invasive aspergillosis who are intolerant of or refractory to amphotericin deoxycholate. Itraconazole is generally well tolerated and has a favorable toxicity profile. The most frequent side effects are nausea and vomiting (10%), hypokalemia (6%), raised levels of liver transaminases (5%), hypertriglyceridemia (5%), skin rash (2%) and pedal edema. However, the use of itraconazole is limited by its aberrant absorption from the gastro-intestinal tract and by several clinically important interactions with other drugs. Itraconazole inhibition of cytochrome P-450 enzyme systems may result in toxic concentrations of concomitantly administered drugs. This may result in serious cardiac arrhythmias (cisapride, terfenadine) or rhabdomyolysis (lovastatin, simvastatin). Other important interactions are with cyclosporin, tacrolimus, steroids, warfarin, rifampin, digoxin, sulfonylurea compounds, phenytoin, benzodiazepines and protease inhibitors. The interaction with some of these drugs may also result in increased itraconazole metabolism and decreased plasma levels. The levels of both itraconazole and cyclosporin can be monitored to minimize the effect of the drug interaction.

Currently only the oral preparations of itraconazole are approved for clinical use . The recommended itraconazole dose for invasive aspergillosis is 200 mg tid for the first 4 days (loading dose) followed by 200 mg bid. For cerebral aspergillosis a higher dosage (400 mg bid) should be considered. Capsules should be taken with food, but the liquid formulation should be taken without food. An intravenous preparation has been recently approved by the FDA.

In the author's view, itraconazole should probably not be used as first-line therapy for invasive aspergillosis in patients with aplastic anemia. It may be reserved to patients intolerant of amphotericin-based preparations, or as 'follow-up' therapy for those who have responded to initial therapy with an amphotericin-containing regimen and who require prolonged antifungal therapy following bone marrow recovery.

The optimal duration of therapy for invasive aspergillosis is not known. The concept of a 'total dose' of amphotericin has no scientific basis, and is probably meaningless in the era of lipid formulations of amphotericin. Indeed, a daily dose of a lipid formulation may equal a weekly 'total dose' of amphotericin deoxycholate. Early initiation of antifungal treatment and maximally high daily doses of an amphotericin-containing preparation initially may improve the outcome.

In the author's view, patients with aplastic anemia and invasive aspergillosis should be treated with a maximal dose of an amphotericin-containing preparation until the recovery of the neutrophil count and evidence for disease response. These usually occur concurrently in the severely neutropenic patient. After bone marrow recovery, the decision to continue with an amphotericin-based preparation or to switch to oral therapy with itraconazole (follow-up therapy) should take into consideration the site of infection and its extent, as well as the rate of disease response. Six to eight weeks of treatment with an amphotericin-based preparation are usually adequate, although treatment should be individualized.

Several promising new agents are under investigation, including new azoles and echinocandins. The most studied one is voriconazole, a third-generation broad-spectrum triazole which is available in oral and intravenous forms. Voriconazole has shown a good clinical efficacy and was well tolerated in patients with invasive aspergillosis. Multinational randomized comparative trials are currently underway.

The role of surgery in invasive aspergillosis is currently being reevaluated. Until recently surgery was considered useful in the following settings: IPA with hemoptysis (lobectomy), endophthalmitis (vitrectomy), endocarditis (valve replacement) and epidural abscess (drainage). Debridement of sinusitis and osteomyelitis was also found useful in selected patients. The drawback was the risk of perioperative death due to fatal bleeding in patients who were also severely thrombocytopenic. Indeed, in the NIH study, two of three patients undergoing lung resection for IPA died from intrapulmonary hemorrhage in the immediate postoperative period. The third patient died from progressive infection. Advances in surgical technique and perioperative care have probably played a major role in the current favorable results from recent studies. These small non-randomized studies have reported excellent immediate postoperative and long-term survival rate in immunocompromised patients undergoing lung resection for the diagnosis and treatment of IPA. The largest study from the University Hospital of Basel included patients with perioperative profound neutropenia and thrombocytopenia. The 30–day postoperative mortality rate was 11%, and the 3–month survival rate was 77%. Five patients with aplastic anemia and IPA were also included in this study: three of them survived. Of the patients who did not survive, one developed renal aspergillosis following surgery and died from bacterial sepsis at 5 months and the other died from cerebral bleeding at 60 days. A further patient with aplastic anemia and pulmonary mucormycosis also survived. Comparative studies are required to conclude whether surgery offers an additional benefit over early and aggressive medical therapy.

REFERENCES

Antoine GA, Gates RH, Park AO. Invasive aspergillosis in a patient with aplastic anemia receiving amphotericin B. *Head Neck Surg* 1988; **10**: 199–203.

Aquino VM, Norvell JM, Krisher K, Mustafa MM. Fatal disseminated infection due to *Exserohilum rostratum* in a patient with aplastic anemia: case report and review. *Clin Infect Dis* 1995; **20**: 176–178.

Bergen GA, Shelhamer JH. Pulmonary infiltrates in the cancer patient. New approaches to an old problem. *Infect Dis Clin North Am* 1996; **10**: 297–325.

Bretagne S, Marmorat-Khuong A, Kuentz M et al. Serum *Aspergillus* galactomannan antigen testing by sandwich ELISA: practical use in neutropenic patients. *J Infect* 1997; **35**: 7–15.

Burch PA, Karp JE, Merz WG, Kuhlman JE, Fishman EK. Favorable outcome of invasive aspergillosis in patients with acute leukemia. *J Clin Oncol* 1987; **5**: 1985–1993.

Caillot D, Casasnovas O, Bernard A et al. Improved management of invasive pulmonary aspergillosis in neutropenic patients using early thoracic computed tomographic scan and surgery. *J Clin Oncol* 1997; **15**: 139–147.

Collin BA, Ramphal R. Pneumonia in the compromised host including cancer patients and transplant patients. *Infect Dis Clin North Am* 1998; **12**: 781–805.

De Pauw BE. Practical modalities for prevention of fungal infections in cancer patients. *Eur J Clin Microbiol Infect Dis* 1997; **16**: 32–41.

Dearden C, Foukaneli T, Lee P, Gordon-Smith EC, Marsh JC. The incidence and significance of fevers during treatment with antithymocyte globulin for aplastic anaemia. *Br J Haematol* 1998; **103**: 846–848.

Denning DW. Invasive aspergillosis. *Clin Infect Dis* 1998; **26**: 781–803.

Denning DW, Evans EG, Kibbler CC et al. Guidelines for the investigation of invasive fungal infections in haematological malignancy and solid organ transplantation. British Society for Medical Mycology. *Eur J Clin Microbiol Infect Dis* 1997; **16**: 424–436.

Edwards JE Jr, Bodey GP, Bowden RA et al. International Conference for the Development of a Consensus on the Management and Prevention of Severe Candidal Infections. *Clin Infect Dis* 1997; **25**: 43–59.

Groll AH, Piscitelli SC, Walsh TJ. Clinical pharmacology of systemic antifungal agents: a comprehensive review of agents in clinical use, current investigational compounds, and putative targets for antifungal drug development. *Adv Pharmacol* 1998; **44**: 343–499.

Hughes WT, Armstrong D, Bodey GP et al. Guidelines for the use of antimicrobial agents in neutropenic patients with unexplained fever. A statement by the Infectious Disease Society of America. *J Infect Dis* 1997; **25**: 551–573.

Kaiser L, Huguenin T, Lew PD, Chapuis B, Pittet D. Invasive aspergillosis. Clinical features of 35 proven cases at a single institution. *Medicine (Baltimore)* 1998; **77**: 188–194.

Leenders AC, Daenen S, Jansen RL et al. Liposomal amphotericin B compared with amphotericin B deoxycholate in the treatment of documented and suspected neutropenia-associated invasive fungal infections. *Br. J Haematol* 1998; **103**:205–212.

Munoz FM, Demmler GJ, Travis WR et al. *Trichoderma longibrachiatum* infection in a pediatric patient with aplastic anemia. *J Clin Microbiol* 1997; **35**: 499–503.

Osterwalder B, Gratwohl A, Nissen C et al. Invasive pulmonary aspergillosis: a diagnostic and therapeutic problem in patients with severe aplastic anemia. *Schweiz Med Wochenschr* 1985; **115**: 378–380.

Pizzo PA. After empiric therapy: what to do until the granulocyte comes back. *Rev Infect Dis* 1987; **9**: 214–219.

Pizzo PA. Management of fever in patients with cancer and treatment-induced neutropenia. *N Engl J Med* 1993; **328**: 1323–1332.

Pizzo PA. Empirical therapy and prevention of infections in the immunocompromised host. In: Mandell GL, Bennett JE, Dolin R, eds. *Mandell, Douglas and Bennett's Principles and Practice of Infectious Diseases.* 5th edn New York: Churchill Livingstone, 2000:3102–3112.

Reichenberger F, Habicht J, Kaim A et al. Lung resection for invasive pulmonary aspergillosis in neutropenic patients with hematologic diseases. *Am J Respir Crit Care Med* 1998; **158**: 885–890.

Rosenfeld SJ, Kimball J, Vining D, Young NS. Intensive immunosuppression with antithymocyte globulin and cyclosporine as treatment for severe acquired aplastic anemia. *Blood* 1995; **85**: 3058–3065.

Sánchez C, Mauri E, Dalmau D et al. Treatment of cerebral aspergillosis with itraconazole: do high doses improve the prognosis? *Clin Infect Dis* 1995; **21**: 1485–1487.

Segal BH, Walsh TJ, Liu JM, Wilson JD, Kwon-Chung KJ. Invasive infection with *Fusarium chlamydosporum* in a patient with aplastic anemia. *J Clin Microbiol* 1998; **36**: 1772–1776.

Verweij PE, Dompeling EC, Donnelly JP, Schattenberg AV, Meis JF. Serial monitoring of *Aspergillus* antigen in the early diagnosis of invasive aspergillosis. Preliminary investigations with two examples. *Infection* 1997; **25**: 86–89.

Verweij PE, Erjavec Z, Sluiters W et al. Detection of antigen in sera of patients with invasive aspergillosis: intra- and interlaboratory reproducibility. The Dutch Interuniversity Working Party for Invasive Mycoses. *J Clin Microbiol* 1998; **36**: 1612–1616.

Walsh TJ, Hiemenz JW, Seibel NL et al. Amphotericin B lipid complex for invasive fungal infections: analysis of safety and efficacy in 556 cases. *Clin Infect Dis* 1998; **26**: 1383–1396.

Walsh TJ, Finberg RW, Arndt C et al. Liposomal amphotericin B for empirical therapy in patients with persistent fever and neutropenia. National Institute of Allergy and Infectious Diseases Mycoses Study Group. *N Engl J Med* 1999; **340**: 764–771.

Weinberger M. Approach to management of fever and infection in patients with primary bone marrow failure and hemoglobinopathies. *Hematol Oncol Clin North Am* 1993; **7**: 865–885.

Weinberger M, Pizzo PA. The evaluation and management of neutropenic patients with unexplained fever. In: Patrick CC, ed. *Infections in Immunocompromised Infants and Children.* New York: Churchill Livingstone, 1992: 335–356.

Weinberger M, Elattar I, Marshall D et al. Patterns of infection in patients with aplastic anemia and the emergence of *Aspergillus* as a major cause of death. *Medicine (Baltimore)* 1992; **71**: 24–43.

Weinberger M, Hollingsworth H, Feuerstein IM, Young NS, Pizzo PA. Successful surgical management of neutropenic enterocolitis in two patients with severe aplastic anemia. Case reports and review of the literature. *Arch Intern Med* 1993; **153**: 107–113.

White MH, Anaissie EJ, Kusne S et al. Amphotericin B colloidal dispersion vs. amphotericin B as therapy for invasive aspergillosis. *Clin Infect Dis* 1997; **24**: 635–642.

White MH, Bowden RA, Sandler ES et al. Randomized, double-blind clinical trial of amphotericin B colloidal dispersion vs. amphotericin B in the empirical treatment of fever and neutropenia. *Clin Infect Dis* 1998; **27**: 296–302.

Won HJ, Lee KS, Cheon JE et al. Invasive pulmonary aspergillosis: prediction at thin-section CT in patients with neutropenia – a prospective study. *Radiology* 1998; **208**: 777–782.

Wong-Beringer A, Jacobs RA, Guglielmo BJ. Lipid formulations of amphotericin B: clinical efficacy and toxicities. *Clin Infect Dis* 1998; **27**: 603–618.

Yamakami Y, Hashimoto A, Tokimatsu I, Nasu M. PCR detection of DNA specific for *Aspergillus* species in serum of patients with invasive aspergillosis. *J Clin Microbiol* 1996; **34**: 2464–2468.

Young NS, Barrett AJ. The treatment of severe acquired aplastic anemia. *Blood* 1995; **85**: 3367–3377.

Young NS, Maciejewski J. The pathophysiology of acquired aplastic anemia. *N Engl J Med* 1997; **336**: 1365–1372.

Infections in Patients with Solid Tumors

Kenneth V I Rolston

INTRODUCTION

It is well known that patients with cancer develop infection more often than those without cancer. However, such patients do not make up a homogenous group, so that the risk of infection, other major complications, and the overall outcome is different in certain subsets of patients with cancer. The spectrum of infection can differ depending upon the nature of the predisposing factor(s). Patients with hematologic malignancies and those receiving immunosuppressive therapy following bone marrow transplantation often have prolonged granulocytopenia, defects in phagocytosis, and impaired cellular and/or humoral immunity – each associated with a distinct spectrum of infection. In contrast, most patients with solid tumors are not immunosuppressed but are predisposed towards infection as a result of obstructive phenomena (e.g. lung carcinoma; biliary and pancreatic carcinoma), damage to anatomic barriers such as the skin and mucosal surfaces, procedures such as surgery and radiotherapy, central nervous system (CNS) dysfunction, and the use of catheters, shunts, prostheses and other medical devices. Although chemotherapy-induced neutropenia does occur in patients with solid tumors, it is often short lived and does not have the same impact as in patients with hematologic malignancy. This chapter reviews the nature, spectrum, diagnosis and management of infections that occur commonly in, or are unique to, patients with solid tumors.

I REGARDING THE CLINICAL PRESENTATION AND EVALUATION OF THE PATIENT

I.1 What are the clinically predominant modes of presentation of infection in patients with solid tumors?

The frequency of fever or infection depends on the nature and intensity of chemotherapy, the use of antimicrobial (or other) prophylaxis, complexity and duration of surgery, and the presence of other predisposing factors. Consequently, the proportion of clinically and microbiologically documented infections and episodes of unexplained fever differs from institution to institution, depending on the nature of the population being served and local practice patterns. Experience from the National Cancer Institute and from institutions that participate in the International Antimicrobial Therapy Cooperative Group/European Organization for Research and Treatment of Cancer (IATCG/EORTC) trials indicates that the frequency of bacteremia is lower in patients with solid tumors than in those with hematologic malignancies (12% versus 25%), whereas episodes of unexplained fever are more common (65% versus 40–50%).

In contrast, clinically and microbiologically documented infections are documented more often in patients with solid tumors (50–60% versus 40%) and episodes of unexplained fever are less common in these patients (40% versus 60%) at the University of Texas, M D Anderson Cancer Center. This in part may be due to the fact that patients with solid tumors seldom receive prophylactic antibiotics that might render microbiologic cultures negative. Additionally, large bulky tumors that are necrotic, infections related to obstruction (e.g. postobstructive pneumonitis; ascending cholangitis), and the presence of surgical wounds and areas that have been irradiated often provide a clinical and microbiologic focus of infection. Tumor fever is occasionally superimposed upon infection, particularly in patients with large necrotic tumors and those with metastatic lesions in the liver. Tumor fever may be the only cause of fever in approximately 4–8% of patients with a solid tumor (excluding those with Hodgkin disease or lymphoma, who are considered elsewhere).

1.2 What are the predominant sites of infection?

The nature and location of the primary tumor, and the presence and location of metastatic lesions, dictate the predominant sites of infections. Patients with primary tumors of the CNS often have complete or partial loss of the gag reflex and develop a predilection for aspiration resulting in aspiration pneumonia. Neurologic impairment can also lead to urinary tract infection as a result of impaired micturition and urinary retention. Surgical wound infection, epidural and subdural infections, cerebral abscesses, meningitis and shunt-related infections occur following intracranial surgery for tumor resection and the placement of shunts.

Infections of the upper respiratory tract, including sinusitis, pneumonia (including aspiration pneumonia) and local cellulitis following surgical excision and reconstruction, are the most common sites of infection in patients with head and neck tumors. Pulmonary infections such as postobstructive pneumonia, lung abscess, empyema and surgical wound infections are common in patients with carcinoma of the lung. Cellulitis following axillary lymph node dissection is the most common site in patients with breast cancer. Cholangitis with bacteremia, hepatic abscesses and peritonitis are not infrequent in patients with hepatobiliary–pancreatic tumors. Patients with colonic and gynecologic malignancies develop abdominal or pelvic abscesses, occasionally after fistula formation or perforation of a viscus. Ureteral obstruction resulting in urinary tract infection is also fairly common in patients with carcinoma of the cervix, and is caused most often by local extension of tumor, and less often as a result of radiation damage. Osteomyelitis, osteoradionecrosis and infected prostheses with adjacent bone, soft tissue or joint infections predominate in patients with osteosarcoma and other bone neoplasms. Infections related to the presence of foreign medical devices such as vascular access catheters, shunts and prosthetic devices are also encountered quite frequently in patients with solid tumors. The most common sites of infection related to the underlying solid tumor(s) are listed in Table 3.1.

1.3 What are the predominant organisms that contribute (by site)?

Most infections in patients with solid tumors are caused by the normal resident microflora, although acquisition of nosocomial organisms does occur after hospitalization and following antibiotic exposure. Consequently, the distribution of causative organisms usually mirrors the normal flora of that particular site. For instance, surgical wound infections and catheter-related infections are most often caused by organisms colonizing the skin (coagulase-negative staphylococci, *Staphylococcus aureus*, *Streptococcus* spp.,

Table 3.1 Predominant sites of infection in patients with solid tumors

Tumor site	Sites of infection
Central nervous system	Surgical wound infection, epidural abscess, subdural empyema, brain abscess, meningitis and ventriculitis (often shunt related), aspiration pneumonia, urinary tract infection
Head and neck	Surgical wound infection, cellulitis, deep fascial space infections, sinusitis, mastoiditis, retropharyngeal and paravertebral abscess, cavernous (and other) sinus thrombosis, meningitis, brain abscess, aspiration pneumonia, osteomyelitis
Lung	Surgical wound infection, empyema, pneumonia (postobstructive), lung abscess
Esophageal/gastric	Mediastinitis, tracheo-esophageal fistula with pneumonitis, gastric perforation and abscess
Breast	Surgical wound infection, cellulitis/lymphangitis following axillary lymph node dissection, mastitis, breast abscess, bacteremia
Hepatobiliary–pancreatic	Surgical wound infection, ascending cholangitis with or without bacteremia, peritonitis, intraabdominal abscess, hepatic abscess, pancreatic abscess, subdiaphragmatic abscess
Intestinal and pelvic	Surgical wound infection, peritonitis, intraabdominal or pelvic abscess, acute and chronic pyelonephritis, bacteremia, necrotizing fasciitis
Genitourinary	Acute and chronic pyelonephritis with or without bacteremia, prostatitis, catheter/surgery-related urinary infections
Bone	Surgical wound infections, soft tissue infections, osteomyelitis, septic arthritis, infected prosthesis

Corynebacterium jeikeium), although opportunistic pathogens such as *Pseudomonas aeruginosa, Acinetobacter* and *Candida* spp. are not uncommon in a nosocomial setting. Similarly, many respiratory infections are caused by the normal resident oropharyngeal flora (*Streptococcus pneumoniae, Haemophilus influenzae*, mouth anaerobes) with enteric Gram-negative bacilli and *Staphylococcus* spp. gaining predominance in the hospital. Enteric Gram-negative bacilli, intestinal anaerobes and enterococci dominate abdominal and pelvic sites of infection. *Candida* spp. frequently colonize debilitated, hospitalized patients, particularly those who have received broad-spectrum antibacterial therapy. Candiduria and candidemia are not uncommon in this setting, although disseminated candidiasis is uncommon in patients with a solid tumor. Colonization with *Candida* spp., therefore, is not sufficient reason for therapeutic intervention in patients with a solid tumor. Other fungal infections (*Aspergillus, Fusarium*), viral infections [cytomegalovirus (CMV), varicella zoster virus (VZV), Epstein–Barr virus (EBV)] and parasitic infections [toxoplasmosis, *Pneumocystis carinii* pneumonia (PCP), strongyloidiasis] are also quite rare. A breakdown of predominant pathogens by site is provided in Table 3.2.

1.4 How do the organisms vary according to various risk factors?
In patients receiving conventional chemotherapy for solid tumors, the duration of severe neutropenia is short-lived. However, some patients with small cell lung cancer, sarcoma, testicular tumor, breast cancer or other solid tumor do receive intensive chemotherapy

Table 3.2 Evaluation of infections in patients with solid tumors according to the site of infection and the possible etiologic agent

Site of infection	Infectious syndrome (clinical features)	Predominant pathogens	Diagnostic tests
Bloodstream	Bacteremia (fever with or without local signs of infection)	Coagulase-negative staphylococci Staphylococcus aureus Viridans streptococci, Streptococcus spp. Enterococcus spp. (nosocomial outbreaks in some institutions) Gram-negative bacilli (Escherichia coli, Klebsiella pneumoniae, Enterobacter spp., Pseudomonas aeruginosa) Candida spp.	Blood cultures: two sets drawn from separate sites and one set drawn from indwelling intravenous catheter
Intravascular catheter-related infections	Pain, erythema, tenderness, discharge from catheter entry site, occasionally necrotic lesion	Coagulase-negative staphylococci Staphylococcus aureus Corynebacterium jeikeium Bacillus spp. Gram-negative bacilli (especially Pseudomonas spp., Acinetobacter spp., Stenotrophomonas maltophilia) Candida spp., Malassezia furfur, Aspergillus spp. (uncommon) Atypical mycobacteria (M. fortuitum, M. chelonei)	Swab of entry site Culture of catheter Blood cultures (consider drawing blood through each lumen of the catheter)
Oral cavity	Periodontitis Gingivitis Stomatitis/mucositis (aphthae, ulcers) Oral thrush (white plaques)	Viridans streptococci Staphylococcus aureus Aerobic and anaerobic Gram-negative and Gram-positive bacteria Herpes simplexvirus Candida spp.	Swab of lesion Oral wash

Site	Condition (symptoms)	Organisms	Specimen/diagnosis
Throat	Pharyngitis Tonsilitis (sore throat, odynophagia)	*Streptococcus pyogenes* Viruses (rhinovirus, coronavirus, adenovirus, influenza, parainfluenza, herpes simplex) *Chlamydia pneumoniae* *Mycoplasma pneumoniae*	Swab of pharynx Serology
Upper respiratory tract: (ear, nose, sinus, nasopharynx, larynx, trachea)	Otitis externa Otitis media (earache, drainage, irritability)	*Streptococcus pneumoniae* *Streptococcus pyogenes* *Haemophilus influenzae* *Staphylococcus aureus* *Pseudomonas aeruginosa* *Moraxella catarrhalis* *Mycoplasma pneumoniae*	Swab of external auditory canal Tympanocentesis Biopsy (occasionally)
	Sinusitis (tightness of sinus areas, headache, toothache, nasal obstruction, nasal voice)	*Streptococcus pneumoniae* *Haemophilus influenzae* *Streptococcus pyogenes* *Staphylococcus aureus* Gram-negative bacilli (*Escherichia coli*, *Klebsiella pneumoniae*, *Pseudomonas aeruginosa*) Anaerobic bacteria *Moraxella catarrhalis* *Mycoplasma pneumoniae* *Candida* spp. *Aspergillus* spp.	Aspiration of sinus Biopsy (if no improvement after 72–96 h of empirical antibiotic therapy)
	Epiglottitis (sore throat, odynophagia)	*Haemophilus influenzae* *Streptococcus pneumoniae* *Streptococcus pyogenes* *Staphylococcus aureus* *Moraxella catarrhalis* *Mycoplasma pneumoniae* *Candida* spp. (rare)	Culture of supraglottic specimen

Site of infection	Infectious syndrome (clinical features)	Predominant pathogens	Diagnostic tests
	Laryngitis (sore throat, hoarseness, otalgia) Tracheitis (stridor, dyspnea, cough)	Streptococcus pyogenes Haemophilus influenzae Staphylococcus aureus Moraxella catarrhalis	Culture of tracheal secretions
Lower respiratory tract (bronchi, terminal airways, alveoli)	Bronchopneumonia Pneumonia (cough, dyspnea, chest pain, sputum, hemoptysia, pleural effusion)	Gram-negative bacilli (Escherichia coli, Klebsiella pneumoniae, Pseudomonas aeruginosa) Streptococcus pneumoniae Viridans streptococci Staphylococcus aureus Legionella spp. (sporadic outbreaks) Mouth anaerobes (Peptococcus, Peptostreptococcus, Fusobacterium) Mycoplasma pneumoniae Chlamydia pneumoniae Pneumocystis carinii Mycobacteria (M. tuberculosis, atypical mycobacteria) Viruses (influenza, parainfluenza, adenovirus, varicella zoster virus) Candida spp. Histoplasma, Cryptococcus	Chest radiography, CT, MRI Serology Fiberoptic bronchoscopy with bronchoalveolar lavage Transbronchial biopsy Thoracocentesis Open lung biopsy
Skin infection and soft tissue	Cellulitis (pain, erythema, tenderness, necrosis in case of ecthyma gangrenosum)	Primary infections: Coagulase-negative staphylococci Staphylococcus aureus Streptococcus spp. Corynebacterium jeikeium Gram-negative bacilli (Pseudomonas aeruginosa, Escherichia coli, Klebsiella pneumoniae)	Skin swab Aspiration (needle) Skin biopsy (histology and culture)

Site	Clinical presentation	Organisms	Investigations
	Papules, nodules (with or without myalgia and muscle tenderness)	*Enterococcus* spp. (perirectal cellulitis) Anaerobic Gram-negative bacilli (perirectal cellulitis) *Candida* spp. Disseminated infections: *Candida* spp. *Trichosporon* spp. Gram-negative bacilli (*Escherichia coli*, *Pseudomonas aeruginosa*, *Aeromonas hydrophilia*, *Serratia marcescens*)	
	Ulcers, vesicles, hemorrhagic or crusted lesions (isolated or with dermatomal distribution)	Herpes simplex Varicella zoster virus	
	Disseminated vesicles, hemorrhagic or crusted lesions	Varicella zoster virus Herpes simplex	
Gastrointestinal tract:			
Esophagus	Esophagitis (dysphagia, retrosternal pain)	Herpes simplex *Candida* spp., *Aspergillus* spp.	Plain abdominal films Esogastroscopy Colonoscopy Ultrasonography CT, MRI Culture of endoscopic specimens Stool cultures Toxin detection
Small intestine, colon	Enteritis Typhlitis Colitis (nausea, vomiting, bloating, abdominal discomfort, cramp, pain, constipation, diarrhea)	Aerobic and anaerobic Gram-negative bacilli *Clostridium* spp. (typhlitis) *Clostridium difficile* (antibiotic-associated diarrhea) *Strongyloides stercoralis* *Cryptosporidium* Virus (coxsackievirus and rotavirus: sporadic outbreaks)	
Liver Spleen	Hepatitis	Primary viral hepatitis (A, B, C, delta) Other viruses (EBV, CMV, HSV, coxsackievirus, adenovirus) *Toxoplasma gondii* *Candida* spp.	Serology

Site of infection	Infectious syndrome (clinical features)	Predominant pathogens	Diagnostic tests
Biliary tract	Cholecystitis Cholangitis	Aerobic Gram-negative bacilli (*Escherichia coli*, *Klebsiella pneumoniae*, *Proteus* spp., *Enterobacter* spp., *Pseudomonas aeruginosa*) Anaerobic bacilli (*Clostridium* spp., *Bacteroides* spp.) *Enterococcus* spp. *Candida* spp.	Ultrasonography CT, MRI Biopsy (histology and culture)
Urinary tract	Urinary tract infections (dysuria, i.e. frequency, urgency, pain; hematuria; flank pain)	Gram-negative bacilli (*Escherichia coli*, *Klebsiella* spp., *Proteus* spp., *Enterobacter* spp., *Pseudomonas aeruginosa*) *Enterococcus* spp. Coagulase-negative staphylococci (*Staphylococcus saprophyticus*) *Candida* spp. Virus (BK virus, adenovirus)	Culture of urine
Central nervous system	Meningitis Encephalitis (altered mental status, headache, photophobia, seizures, focal neurologic signs, nuchal rigidity) Shunt infections (fever, change in mental status, headache, meningism, raised intracranial pressure; patient may also be asymptomatic)	*Listeria monocytogenes* *Cryptococcus neoformans* *Nocardia asteroides* *Aspergillus* spp., *Candida* spp. Mycobacteria Coagulase-negative staphylococci *Staphylococcus aureus* *Enterococcus* spp. *Corynebacterium* spp. *Propionibacterium* spp. Gram-negative bacilli *Candida* spp. Increased risk of bacterial meningitis due to *Streptococcus pneumoniae*, *Haemophilus influenzae* and *Neisseria meningitidis*	CT, MRI Lumbar puncture Aspiration or biopsy under stereotaxic CT guidance

designed to produce maximal antineoplastic response. In such patients, the duration and severity of neutropenia may approach the levels seen in patients with hematologic malignancy, and result in infections more typically associated with prolonged neutropenia (Gram-positive cocci; enteric Gram-negative bacilli; *Candida* spp.).

The presence and location of prosthetic devices and other foreign materials have a significant effect on the organisms isolated. Although the vast majority of infections associated with central venous catheters are caused by Gram-positive organisms (coagulase-negative staphylococci, *S. aureus*, *C. jeikeium*, *Bacillus* spp.), the overall spectrum of central venous catheter-associated infections is broad and includes Gram-negative bacilli (*P. aeruginosa*, *Acinetobacter* spp. and *Stenotrophomonas maltophilia*, among others). *Candida parapsilosis* and other *Candida* spp. are also associated with line-related infections, particularly in patients with radiation enteritis and others requiring parenteral hyperalimentation. Urinary catheters are associated with infections caused by enteric Gram-negative bacilli, enterococci and *Candida* spp. Ventriculoperitoneal shunts predispose to infections (meningitis and ventriculitis) caused primarily by *Staphylococcus* spp. Interleukin-2 has been associated with an increased frequency of Gram-positive coccal infections.

1.5 How does this differ from other conditions, from center to center, and from country to country?

Most patients with solid tumors are not significantly immunosuppressed, unlike patients with hematologic malignancies, lymphoma, or bone marrow transplant recipients. Consequently, the risk for developing infection is generally not as significant or protracted unless substantial obstruction or other anatomic abnormalities, which cannot be easily reversed, exist. Also, the specific microflora isolated from patients may vary from center to center. For example, the National Cancer Institutes (NCI) has reported a sharp decline in the isolation of *P. aeruginosa* from patients with neutropenic cancer, whereas *P. aeruginosa* remains the second most frequently isolated Gram-negative organism at the University of Texas, M D Anderson Cancer Center. Additionally, Gram-positive organisms are isolated more frequently than Gram-negative organisms at most cancer treatment centers worldwide. However, there are centers at which Gram-negatives still predominate. Disseminated fungal, viral or protozoal infections are distinctly uncommon but should not be overlooked in the diagnostic evaluation of patients with solid tumors. Knowledge of local microflora at specific centers, and of local susceptibility and resistance patterns (which can also differ from center to center, and from country to country) is of vital importance when considering options for initial empirical antibiotic therapy.

1.6 What is the appropriate approach to the initial evaluation and diagnosis of infection in patients with solid tumors?

There is no substitute for a detailed history and thorough physical examination as part of the initial evaluation. Unlike other categories of patients with cancer, a focus of infection can often be identified in patients with solid tumors, and historical information can often lead to the identification of a specific focus. For example, seizure activity might point to an intracranial process, or suggest the presence of aspiration pneumonia. A cough, productive of large amounts of foul-smelling sputum, is consistent with the presence of a lung abscess or postobstructive pneumonitis. The expression of urine or fecal material through the vagina indicates the presence of a vesicovaginal or rectovaginal fistula. During physical examination close attention needs to be focused on the oropharyngeal cavities, the groin and perirectal region, sites where obstruction might occur, surgical wounds, prosthetic devices, irradiated areas, the skin including nail beds and catheter insertion sites, and the paranasal sinuses.

There is nothing special or unique about the initial laboratory evaluation of these patients. Basic evaluation includes chemical analysis of the blood and urine, a complete and differential blood count, tests for hepatic and renal function, and all appropriate microbiologic cultures. Radiographic evaluation of the chest need not be performed on a routine basis but is indicated when primary or metastatic lung disease, or pulmonary symptoms (cough, sputum, hemoptysis, chest pain, dyspnea) are present. Radiographic imaging studies may be particularly useful in evaluating the CNS, paranasal sinuses, pulmonary, abdominal and pelvic foci. Leukocyte-labeled indium scans, bone scans and gallium scans are often done, but seldom provide useful information. Doppler or venous flow studies are useful in the evaluation of deep venous thrombophlebitis that is often not clinically apparent. Serologic studies are generally not very useful unless specific pathogens that elicit a serologic response are suspected.

1.7 How should the evaluation be modified according to the severity of the risk?

A thorough evaluation is warranted regardless of risk. However, the presence of severe neutropenia, septicemia with shock, life-threatening infections such as meningitis, or intestinal perforation require immediate therapeutic intervention, often before a complete evaluation is possible. Procedures such as a lumbar puncture, computed tomography (CT) of the head or abdomen, etc., need to be performed as expeditiously as possible. Close cooperation between radiologic, medical and surgical teams is often necessary since prompt surgical intervention can be critical and life saving.

Conversely, a history of prolonged fever (weeks or months) with few associated symptoms is often indicative of a chronic infection or tumor fever, and can be evaluated at a less hectic pace, often without hospitalization of the patient. The rapidity and extent of the evaluatory process needs to be tailored to the individual patient, as each requires a slightly different approach.

1.8 What are the specific evaluation measures? (see also Chapter 2 in Part I)

Specific evaluation measures depend upon the site and nature of the infection.

Microbiology

Specimens for culture should be collected, if possible before the initiation of antimicrobial therapy, unless the patient's clinical situation dictates otherwise. Two cultures of blood, for bacteria (aerobic and anaerobic) and fungi, should be obtained from all patients. The use of multilumen central venous catheters is commonplace. Since infection may be limited to only one lumen of such catheters, many authorities recommend obtaining blood cultures from each lumen, in addition to a culture from a peripheral vein. Quantitative blood cultures are not always indicated but may increase the yield for specific organisms, and may be useful in differentiating between colonization of catheters versus true catheter-related infections versus bacteremia from other sources. Specimens for culture from other sources including surgical wounds, urine, sputum and cerebrospinal fluid (CSF) should be obtained when clinically indicated. Such specimens should also be examined by Gram staining and appropriate stains for mycobacteria, fungi and other specific pathogens, if suspected clinically. Routine cultures from the urine, stools or rectal swabs, and the oropharynx, are generally not very useful, and are not recommended. They might be indicated for infection control purposes when investigating outbreaks caused by resistant organisms such as vancomycin-resistant *Enterococcus faecium* (VREF), methicillin-resistant *S. aureus* (MRSA), *P. aeruginosa*, multidrug-resistant Gram-negative bacilli (*S. maltophilia*), penicillin-resistant pneumococcus, etc.

In patients with diarrhea, testing for *Clostridium difficile* toxin is often recommended as the first step. If this is negative and the diarrhea is suspected to be of infectious etiology, the stools should be tested for bacteria (e.g. *Aeromonas, Campylobacter, Plesiomonas, Salmonella, Shigella, Yersinia*), protozoa (amoeba, *Cryptosporidium, Giardia*, etc.), viruses (rotavirus, CMV) and mycobacteria (*Mycobacterium avium*-complex, MAC). Urine cultures are indicated if the patient is symptomatic, the urinanalysis is abnormal, a urinary catheter is in place, or surgery involving the urinary tract has been performed. Patients who are neutropenic may be relatively asymptomatic and may not have evidence of pyuria, due to blunting of the inflammatory response. Examination of the CSF, pleural and ascitic fluid should be performed when clinically indicated and specimens should be sent for bacterial and fungal cultures. Pleocytosis may be absent in the presence of neutropenia.

Cutaneous lesions should be biopsied for Gram staining, staining for other specific pathogens (fungi, mycobacteria, protozoa), culture and cytologic examination. Other biopsies (lung, liver, bone, brain, lymph nodes, bone marrow, etc.) should be performed when clinically indicated, and handled in a similar fashion.

Radiographic imaging techniques

Chest radiography does not need to be obtained on a routine basis, but only when signs or symptoms of respiratory tract involvement are present. In patients who are neutropenic, chest radiography may not show evidence of an infiltrate even if clinical evidence of a pulmonary infection is present. Plain radiography of the paranasal sinuses is not helpful. CT should be performed if involvement of the sinuses is suspected. Plain films of the abdomen are also not very useful unless intestinal perforation is suspected. Ultrasonography, radionuclide imaging, CT and magnetic resonance imaging (MRI) are often indicated and used in an attempt to identify a focus of infection.

Routine serologic testing is unhelpful. If specific pathogens that elicit a serologic response are suspected, appropriate serologic testing should be performed. However, such pathogens are not unique to patients with solid tumors. Patients presenting with Kaposi sarcoma, CNS lymphomas or other unusual malignancies should undergo testing for human immunodeficiency virus (HIV) infection.

1.9 What new developments are going to impact on emerging organisms, recognition, evaluation and diagnosis of infection in patients with solid tumors?

The emergence of resistant microorganisms is of considerable concern, but is not unique to patients with solid tumors. Among Gram-positive organisms, vancomycin-resistant enterococci (VRE) are of greatest concern since no effective standard therapy is currently available for the treatment of such infections. VRE now account for 10–20% of enterococcal isolates at some centers. Glycopeptide intermediate *S. aureus* (GISA) and other vancomycin-resistant organisms (*Lactobacillus, Leuconostoc, Pediococcus*) are less commonly isolated, but all appear to be related to increased vancomycin usage (both parenteral and oral). Viridans streptococci and pneumococci are often penicillin resistant and are also of concern when isolated.

Among Gram-negative bacilli, organisms that produce type 1 β-lactamases (*Enterobacter, Citrobacter, Serratia, P. aeruginosa*, etc.), and those that produce extended-spectrum β-lactamases (ESBLs) such as *Klebsiella* spp. and *Escherichia coli*, are of great concern, and can have a big impact on empirical and specific therapeutic regimens. Organisms that produce metallic and nonmetallic enzymes that inactivate carbapenems (e.g. *S. maltophilia, Acinetobacter* spp.) are still relatively infrequent but, with the increased use of the carbapenems for monotherapy, are also of concern. Frequent monitoring for the emergence of multidrug-resistant organisms at individual treatment centers is recommended, since institutional differences are likely.

As previously indicated, some catheter-related infections (particularly those that occur in patients receiving parenteral nutrition) are caused by *Candida parapsilosis* and other *Candida* spp. The emergence of resistant isolates such as *C. krusei, C. lusitaniae, C. rugosa, C. glabrata, C. tropicalis* and occasionally even *C. albicans* has been reported, and should be monitored since standardized antifungal susceptibility testing methods have now been developed and are widely available.

2 REGARDING THE RISK FACTORS ACCOMPANYING SOLID TUMORS

2.1 What are the main alterations in host defense mechanisms and what are the appropriate investigations to document them?

As previously stated, most patients with solid tumors have intact host defense mechanisms, including phagocytosis, cell-mediated immunity (CMI), humoral immunity and the complement cascade. Patients with primary CNS tumors or metastatic lesions in the brain often develop partial loss of the gag reflex, predisposing towards aspiration. Neurologic abnormalities resulting in impaired micturition also occur. Normal anatomic barriers such as the skin and mucosal surfaces can be disrupted by solid tumors originating at these sites (squamous cell carcinoma of skin, melanoma, bronchogenic carcinoma, colonic carcinoma), metastatic lesions from distant primary sites, or rapidly growing tumors which outstrip their blood supply resulting in necrosis and devitalized tissue. Massive infiltration of bone marrow by tumor can occasionally result in myelosuppression, producing pancytopenia.

2.2 What are the alterations due to iatrogenic factors?

The two major effects of cancer chemotherapy on host defense mechanisms are myelosuppression and disruption of normal anatomic barriers, particularly mucosal surfaces. Patients with solid tumors usually have normally functioning granulocytes, and conventional chemotherapy rarely produces severe neutropenia that lasts more than 10 days. The risk of developing infections as a result of the neutropenic state is therefore not as prolonged as in patients with hematologic malignancies, those receiving intensive chemotherapeutic regimens and recipients of bone marrow transplantation. However, several other factors, when associated with neutropenia, substantially increase the risk of infection. Cancer chemotherapy often damages mucosal surfaces, increasing the risk of oropharyngeal, respiratory, gastrointestinal, urinary and bacteremic infections. Agents that are particulary prone to cause mucositis include chlorambucil, cisplatin, cytarabine (Ara-C), doxorubicin (Adriamycin), fluorouracil (5-FU) and methotrexate. Damage to ciliary function in the respiratory tract increases the likelihood of developing pneumonia. Additionally, some chemotherapeutic agents such as methotrexate and vincristine inhibit phagocytosis and the bactericidal activity of granulocytes, producing qualitative impairment in host defense mechanisms. Cytotoxic agents may also produce varying degrees of suppression of CMI. In patients with a solid tumor, however, impaired CMI usually occurs after prolonged corticosteroid administration (e.g. in patients with CNS tumors), and may lead to infections that are more common in that setting (e.g. PCP, mycobacterial infections, fungal infections). A complete and differential blood count and flow cytometric evaluation of lymphocyte subsets (CD4 and CD8 T-lymphocytes) are the two most important methods for the laboratory evaluation of CMI. Lymphocyte subset analysis, however, is seldom useful in general clinical practice. Skin testing for specific recall antigens is another method of evaluating CMI, and is even less useful.

Radiation therapy produces a wide range of undesirable effects including varying degrees of myelosuppression and impairment in cellular and humoral immunity. Radiation damage to the skin causes delayed wound healing and produces favorable conditions for the growth of bacteria by altering the physical and immunologic properties of normal skin and underlying tissues, including the lymphatic system. Radiation also produces damage to respiratory mucosa, resulting in loss of mucociliary function, and to the gastrointestinal mucosa, causing radiation enteritis and other local damage.

Previous antimicrobial usage can influence the spectrum of subsequent infections by selecting resistant organisms. For example, excessive vancomycin usage has been associated with increased isolation rates of VREF and other vancomycin-resistant organisms. The primary drawback of fluoroquinolone prophylaxis is the development of resistant Gram-negative bacilli (*E. coli; P. aeruginosa*, etc.). In general, prophylactic and empirical antimicrobial regimens are used less often and for a shorter duration in patients with solid tumors, than in other, more immunosuppressed, groups. However, local practice patterns do vary and must be considered, along with local susceptibility resistance patterns, when evaluating patients for infection.

A large number of catheters and other foreign devices are used in most oncology practices. The vast majority are used for vascular access or hemodynamic monitoring (peripheral and central venous catheters, arterial lines, Swan–Ganz catheters). The spectrum of infections associated with these devices has been discussed in section 1. Urinary catheters (Foley, suprapubic), shunts and prosthetic devices also increase the frequency of infection.

Surgery, particularly when extensive, results in the breakdown of normal anatomic barriers and in the extravasation of materials and creation of dead spaces that promote the development of infection. Common sites of infection and predominant organisms by site are listed in Tables 3.1 and 3.2.

2.3 What is the influence of environmental factors?

Environmental factors do not have a specific or unique impact on infections in patients with solid tumors. Patients exposed to community outbreaks such as influenza, and those at risk for pneumococcal pneumonia, need to be protected. This is accomplished using standard immunization schedules. Prolonged hospitalization and the frequent use of broad-spectrum antimicrobial agents increases the likelihood of acquisition of multidrug-resistant organisms (VRE, MRSA, resistant Gram-negative bacilli, C. *difficile*). Nosocomial transmission of these organisms is minimized by standard infection control techniques. Routine isolation of patients or the use of protective environments following conventional chemotherapy is not recommended. Foodborne infections are uncommon and the avoidance of fresh fruits and salads, or the use of specialized diets, has not been demonstrated to be of any particular benefit in patients with solid tumors. Reasonable precautions need to be exercised while traveling to endemic areas, but these precautions are usually no different than those recommended by the Centers for Disease Control (CDC) for all travelers.

2.4 What are the most significant factors that contribute to the risk of infection in patients with solid tumors?

Several factors contribute to the risk of infection in patients with solid tumors. The presence of multiple factors in the same patient is not uncommon, and contributes towards increased risk.

Disruption of normal anatomic barriers

Normal anatomic barriers, which include intact skin, oropharyngeal, respiratory, gastrointestinal and genitourinary mucosal surfaces, provide an important defense mechanism against invasion by microorganisms. Disruption of these barriers can be caused by cancer chemotherapy, radiation therapy, surgical procedures, the use of medical devices such as catheters, and the underlying tumor itself, giving rise to infections caused by organisms that form part of the normal flora of these sites, or those that have been nosocomially acquired.

Neutropenia

Neutropenia is most often induced by cancer chemotherapy. Varying degrees of neutropenia can also occur as a result of radiation therapy, and occasionally after extensive infiltration of the marrow by tumor. The degree and duration of chemotherapy-induced neutropenia in patients with solid tumors is generally not as severe or as prolonged as in patients with hematologic malignancies, reducing the period at risk in such patients.

Obstructive phenomena

Obstructive phenomena are quite common in patients with solid tumors and are often associated with infection. For example, bronchogenic carcinoma or metastatic pulmonary lesions can cause partial obstruction of a bronchus leading to postobstructive pneumonia. Biliary tract obstruction in patients with hepatobiliary–pancreatic tumors results in ascending cholangitis. Urethral obstruction in patients with carcinoma of the prostate frequently results in urinary tract infection. Intestinal tumors can cause partial or complete obstruction of the bowel with or without intestinal perforation. In all these situations, mixed or polymicrobial infections are common, and the etiologic agent(s) are usually those that colonize the area of obstruction.

Medical procedures and devices

As previously indicated, medical procedures, surgery, radiation, and the use of catheters and other devices (shunts, prostheses) are often associated with the development of infection. The use of multiple lumen vascular access catheters (e.g. Hickman catheters) has become commonplace. These catheters facilitate the drawing and/or administration of blood or blood products, the administration of chemotherapy or antimicrobial agents, and other supportive medication. Infection is the major complication associated with such catheters. The organisms causing catheter-related infections are listed in Table 3.2. Approximately 80–85% are Gram-positive, with *Staphylococcus* spp. being predominant. Urinary catheters are used frequently when obstruction or urinary incontinence is present. Local involvement of the bladder or ureters with cancer may require the creation of surgical diversions, frequently into ileal or colonic segments. Bacteriuria and acute or chronic pyelonephritis with intestinal microorganisms is a frequent occurrence in these circumstances. The use of CSF shunts is not uncommon in patients with CNS tumors. Symptoms associated with CSF shunt infections depend upon the location of the infection. The most frequent symptoms – headache, mental status changes, nausea and lethargy – usually result when the proximal or CNS end of the shunt is infected. The distal ends of such shunts are generally located in the pleural or peritoneal cavities, giving rise to symptoms of pleuritis or peritonitis when infected. Surgically implanted prosthetic devices are used frequently in patients with osteosarcoma and other bone tumors. Infection is the most common complication associated with these devices, and is most often caused by organisms colonizing the skin.

2.5 What are the specific or nonspecific measures aimed at minimizing each of these factors?

Disruption of normal anatomic barriers can be minimized by limiting the number of invasive procedures performed (e.g. venepuncture), and by using catheters and other medical devices only when absolutely necessary, and not just for the sake of convenience. Meticulous surgical techniques and strict adherence to infection control practices (particularly handwashing) will limit the incidence of postoperative infections and the nosocomial transmission of multidrug-resistant pathogens. Recognizing and dealing with obstructive phenomena early is important. Surgical intervention, radiotherapy and the use of stents can help relieve obstruction and minimize infection. Reduction in the degree and duration of neutropenia is achieved by reducing the intensity of the chemotherapeutic regimen or extending the treatment interval, unless the maintenance of dose intensity for maximal therapeutic response is required. Most patients with solid tumors do not benefit from placement in protected environments, routine reverse isolation, antimicrobial prophylaxis, or the use of filtered water and specialized diets. These measures might be useful in selected situations when intensive chemotherapy is being delivered. The benefits and disadvantages of prolonged corticosteroid administration need to be carefully considered before such therapy is initiated. Patients at risk, particularly those with multiple risk factors, need to be monitored closely, and prompt therapeutic measures need to be instituted when infection develops.

2.6 Are there different levels of risk of infection recognized for patients with solid tumors?

The risk of developing infection, infection-related or other complications, and response to therapy, depends upon a number of factors including, but not limited to, the underlying malignancy, the nature and severity of the impairment in host defense mechanisms, the degree and duration of neutropenia, the presence of comorbidity factors (e.g. renal or respiratory insufficiency; hypotension; seizure activity, thrombocytopenia with bleeding) and the age of the patient. However, the ability of clinicians to predict risk in individual patients, with reasonable accuracy, early in the course of a febrile episode has been limited.

The recent work of Talcott and colleagues has led to the recognition of four well-defined risk groups among febrile neutropenic patients. These researchers initially developed a risk prediction rule in a retrospective study of 261 patients, and subsequently validated this rule in a prospective study of 444 cancer patients with fever and neutropenia. In this model, patients who were considered to be at low risk (morbidity and mortality rates of less than 2%) were generally those with stable or responsive solid tumors, who were hemodynamically stable, and developed fever and neutropenia while receiving conventional antineoplastic therapy in an outpatient setting. However, some patients with hematologic malignancy were also included as low risk in this model. In a pilot study of home antibiotic therapy following early discharge from hospital in low-risk patients conducted by the same group of investigators, there was a high readmission rate (30%) due to persistent fever or the development of complications.

Table 3.3 Risk-based grouping of patients with fever and neutropenia

Risk group	Patient characteristics
High risk	Hematologic malignancy, allogeneic bone marrow transplantation, prolonged neutropenia (> 14 days), multiple comorbidity or risk factors
Moderate risk	Solid tumor with intensive chemotherapy, autologous bone marrow transplant or PBSCT, neutropenia of intermediate duration (> 7 but <14 days)
Low risk	Solid tumor with conventional chemotherapy, short-lived neutropenia (≤ 7 days), no comorbidity, clinically stable

Developed from experience at the University of Texas M D Anderson Cancer Center. Experience at different centers may vary, based on differences in patient populations, clinical practice patterns and other local factors.

PBSCT, Peripheral blood stem cell transplantation.

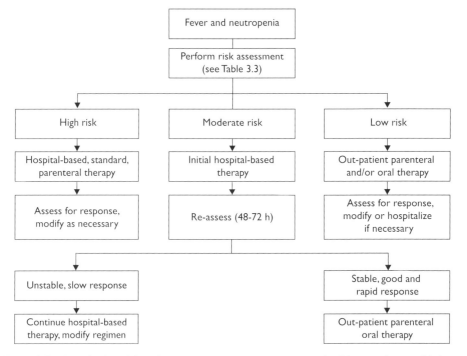

Figure 3.1 Algorithm for risk-based therapy when neutropenic patients with solid tumors become febrile.

The Multinational Association of Supportive Care in Cancer (MASCC) is attempting to refine Talcott's prediction rule in an effort to increase its accuracy, by focusing greater attention on the underlying malignancy (solid tumor versus hematologic malignancy) and the duration of neutropenia (<7 days).

Clinical experience from the University of Texas M D Anderson Cancer Center has led to the recognition of high-, moderate- and low-risk groups among patients with fever and neutropenia (Table 3.3). Treatment algorithms for the management of the various risk groups have been developed (Figure 3.1). It must be emphasized that risk prediction models will never have absolute accuracy, and good clinical judgement must be exercised in all circumstances.

Although a substantial proportion of patients with solid tumors who develop fever are now considered to be at low risk, some are not. Patients receiving highly intensive chemotherapy for certain solid tumors (small cell lung cancer, sarcomas, testicular cancers) resulting in more prolonged neutropenia, those receiving multiple modality therapy (chemotherapy and radiation with or without surgery), elderly patients, those with substantial comorbidity, and those with multiple risk factors (e.g. neutropenia with obstruction or substantial disruption of anatomic barriers) are at much greater risk for the development of infections and/or complications.

2.7 How does the level of risk impact on management?

The level of risk impacts upon several aspects of the management of these patients. Routine surveillance cultures, for example, are not cost-effective or particularly useful. However, such cultures (nares, oropharynx, rectum/stool) are indicated for patients at risk for developing colonization or infection with resistant organisms such as MRSA, VREF and multidrug-resistant Gram-negative bacilli. Identification of patients colonized or infected with these organisms can have a significant impact on prevention of nosocomial transmission and on therapeutic strategies.

Chemoprophylaxis (fluoroquinolones) and other preventive measures, such as the use of hematopoetic growth factors [granulocyte colony-stimulating factor (G-CSF), granulocyte–macrophage colony-stimulating factor (GM-CSF)] or protected environments, are not indicated for low-risk patients. Although practice patterns vary from country to country, and from institution to institution in the same country, seldom can the use of such measures be justified in patients with solid tumors. However, patients at high risk for developing infection due to the presence of multiple predisposing factors need to be monitored carefully, and dealt with at the earliest signs of the development of infection. Some prophylactic measures might be justified in high-risk patients with a solid tumor.

The degree of risk has the greatest impact on the nature and setting in which specific therapeutic measures are administered. High-risk patients with fever and neutropenia need standard, hospital-based, parenteral, broad-spectrum, empirical antibiotic therapy until resolution of infection and/or recovery from neutropenia. In contrast, low-risk neutropenic patients with fever can be treated with parenteral, sequential or oral antibiotic regimens without admitting them to the hospital. An intermediate, or stepdown, approach may be appropriate in moderate-risk patients and consists of initial stabilization in the hospital, followed by early discharge and completion of antibiotic therapy at home (see Figure 3.1). Patients with life-threatening infections need immediate attention, often before a complete evaluation has been performed. This must be conducted in conjunction with the administration of empirical therapy directed at the most likely pathogens in each particular situation (Table 3.2).

2.8 What new developments are going to impact on minimizing or suppressing the specific risk factors?

The hematopoetic growth factors (G-CSF, GM-CSF) have been shown to reduce the severity and duration of neutropenia in patients receiving chemotherapy for various solid tumors including small cell lung cancer, metastatic sarcomas and bladder tumors. These factors are expensive and are not indicated in patients with short-lived neutropenia (<7 days), but their use is justified in patients with prolonged neutropenia. They have also been shown to reduce the incidence and severity of mucositis in patients with solid tumors receiving chemotherapy. Newer molecules such as interleukin-2 (IL-2), IL-15 and the keratinocyte growth factor (KGF) may help in the regeneration of gastrointestinal mucosa, and are being evaluated for their potential role in preventing or reducing the severity and duration of mucositis.

3 REGARDING THE SURVEILLANCE OF PATIENTS WITH SOLID TUMORS

3.1 What is the important premorbid information to be gathered?

As indicated above, most infections in patients with solid tumors are caused by the normal resident microflora or by nosocomially acquired pathogens. However, a history of travel to or residence in areas endemic for specific infections (tuberculosis, endemic mycoses, parasitic diseases) is important, and might help draw attention to them as the patient is being evaluated. Knowledge of previous surgical procedures and implanted prosthetic devices is also an important historic factor in such patients, as it may help identify a specific focus of infection. The prior use of antibiotics and over-the-counter medications can alter the nature and spectrum of subsequent infection, and should be determined when interviewing the patient. Knowledge of immunization history (e.g. pneumococcal vaccine) is also useful.

3.2 What are the surveillance measures to be taken when a patient presents with a solid tumor?

The role of serial microbiologic surveillance cultures in patients with solid tumors has not been established. They can occasionally provide useful information; however, the predictive yield of such cultures tends to be low, and in an era in which cost-effectiveness has gained considerable prominence, they add substantially to the cost of care. Knowledge of local microflora, however, is an important factor when considering the use of surveillance cultures. In institutions where resistant organisms such as VRE, MRSA, *P. aeruginosa*, *S. maltophilia*, *C. krusei*, etc., are relatively common, prior knowledge of colonization with such organisms can help in the choice of appropriate antibiotic therapy when infection develops, and in the prevention of nosocomial transmission of these pathogens from patient to patient. Environmental surveillance is also important in such institutions in order to maintain adequate infection control.

Since patients with solid tumors are not at particular risk of developing disseminated fungal infections (*Candida*, *Aspergillus*) or viral infections (CMV, HSV, VZV, EBV), routine surveillance (microbiologic or serologic) for these pathogens is not helpful. Routine examination of stools to detect the presence of *Strongyloides stercoralis* or other intestinal parasites is also not necessary. Such examination should be performed only in individuals with a history of travel to or residence in an endemic area.

4 REGARDING THE PREVENTION OF INFECTION IN PATIENTS WITH SOLID TUMORS

4.1 What approaches, if any, to the prevention of infection should be considered in patients with solid tumors?

General and specific measures for minimizing the risk factors that predispose toward infection in patients with solid tumors have been outlined in sections 2.5 and 2.8. As indicated previously, routine antibacterial, fungal or viral prophylaxis is not necessary. Recent evidence suggests that when PCP is documented in a patient with a solid tumor, it is generally in the setting of prolonged corticosteroid administration. PCP prophylaxis [trimethoprim–sulfamethoxazole (TMP–SMX) or pentamidine] should be considered, but is not mandatory, in such patients. Appropriate surgical prophylaxis, depending on the nature of the surgical procedure, will help minimize postoperative infections. The use of antibiotic-impregnated catheters, or other specialized catheters, and the meticulous maintenance of these devices, are useful methods for reducing catheter-related infections.

5 REGARDING THE TREATMENT OF PATIENTS WITH SOLID TUMORS

5.1 What is the role of empirical therapy?
Empirical therapy is indicated for the treatment of life-threatening infections, when it is injudicious to wait until a specific etiology has been established. Providing empirical therapy to patients with neutropenia shortly after the onset of fever is standard practice, since the risk of bacteremic infections that can disseminate rapidly without prompt therapy (*P. aeruginosa*, *Enterobacteriaceae*, viridans streptococci) is relatively high in this setting. Emergent management of CNS infections, such as meningitis, ventriculitis and cerebral abscesses, often requires the administration of empirical therapy using drugs that provide coverage against the pathogens commonly isolated from such sites (see Table 3.2). Empirical therapy and prompt surgical intervention are of critical importance in situations such as bowel perforation and spillage of fecal material into the abdominal cavity, situations that are encountered occasionally in patients with intestinal tumors.

Empirical therapy in febrile neutropenic patients generally consists of the administration of parenteral broad-spectrum antibiotics, while monitoring the patient in the hospital. Several choices for initial therapy are available, but specific regimens need to be tailored to local microflora and susceptibility patterns. The choices include combination regimens, with or without vancomycin, and monotherapy.

Initial usage of vancomycin should be considered when the likelihood of infection with resistant Gram-positive organisms (MRSA; viridans streptococci; *C. jeikeium*; coagulase-negative staphylococci) is high. Routine use of this agent should be avoided in order to minimize the emergence of VRE and other glycopeptide-resistant microorganisms. Aminoglycoside β-lactam combinations and double β-lactam combinations have been used worldwide with success rates ranging from 55% to 95%. Broad-spectrum cephalosporins and/or carbapenems are appropriate for empirical monotherapy.

Changes or alterations to the initial regimen are necessary if there is evidence of progressive infection or failure to respond, new clinical developments, or microbiologic data and susceptibility information that indicate the need for a change. Frequent modifications include:

- the addition of vancomycin if not used initially, when Gram-positive coverage needs to be strengthened
- the addition of a second Gram-negative drug (if only one was included in the original regimen), particularly if a Gram-negative infection has been documented and is not responding adequately
- additional anaerobic coverage (metronidazole, clindamycin), especially for infections such as necrotizing gingivitis, neutropenic enterocolitis, perirectal abscesses, or other intraabdominal pelvic sites
- the addition of empirical antifungal agents (fluconazole, itraconazole, amphotericin B)

- surgical intervention (e.g. drainage of a perirectal abscess) or removal of foreign bodies such as infected catheters is occasionally necessary.

Standard therapy for febrile neutropenia in patients with solid tumors does not differ much from that in patients with hematologic malignancies, except that the duration of treatment is generally shorter owing to a shorter period at risk. Recent risk prediction models have enabled clinicians to simplify the therapy of low-risk neutropenic patients, with the use of sequential or oral regimens which enable early discharge from the hospital, or outpatient therapy for the duration of the febrile episode. This 'risk-based' approach to therapy might be more cost-effective and result in improved quality of life for patients and their caregivers than the old 'one size fits all' approach of hospital-based parenteral therapy.

Various parenteral and oral combination regimens have been used in the outpatient setting. Examples include: amikacin plus ceftriaxone, ciprofloxacin plus clindamycin, aztreonam plus clindamycin, ciprofloxacin plus amoxycillin-clavulanate. An algorithm for risk-based therapy is provided in Figure 3.1.

5.2 What is the appropriate approach to the patient with a solid tumor and evidence of infection in various body sites?

The predominant sites of infection in patients with solid tumors and the predominant organisms by site of infection are listed in Table 3.2. Prior to the isolation of specific pathogens, empirical antimicrobial therapy directed at organisms expected to be present at a particular site of infection is warranted. Local (community and hospital) susceptibility/resistance patterns need to be considered when choices for empirical therapy are being made. If specific pathogens are isolated, therapy can be tailored to provide optimal coverage against them. However, patients who are neutropenic should continue to receive broad-spectrum therapy even if a specific organism (Gram-positive, Gram-negative or anaerobic) has been isolated. Bactericidal activity can be critical in neutropenic patients with bacteremic infections, and in those with CNS and cardiovascular infections (meningitis, endocarditis). Adequate tissue penetration is particularly important for infections of the CNS, musculoskeletal infections and lower respiratory tract infections. Although every attempt should be made to treat infections associated with foreign bodies (catheters, shunts, stents, prosthetic devices, etc.) without their removal, it may not be possible to achieve adequate sterilization of the site with antimicrobial therapy alone. Surgical debridement and/or removal of the foreign body may be necessary if adequate medical therapy has been unsuccessful. Surgical debridement is also often necessary in infections such as perirectal abscesses and necrotic soft tissue infections. Unconventional routes of antimicrobial administration (e.g. aerosolization, intrathecal administration) might have to be considered in special circumstances.

5.3 What is the appropriate approach to the patient with a solid tumor and evidence of a bacteremia, with or without site of infection?

Gram-positive bacteremia

Response to standard therapy in patients with a solid tumor who develop Gram-positive bacteremia exceeds 95%. Agents other than vancomycin, to which the specific pathogen is susceptible, are generally appropriate. These include antistaphylococcal penicillins (nafcillin, oxacillin), other β-lactams, macrolides, TMP–SMX, the tetracyclines, clindamycin, and some newer quinolones. The use of bacteriostatic antibiotics in patients with Gram-positive bacteremia should, however, be only a second choice because of the obvious severity of such infections on the one hand, and because of the impaired host defense mechanisms in these patients on the other hand. In this setting, the use of new quinolones might offer advantages over macrolides, tetracyclines and clindamycin.

Vancomycin is indicated when an organism resistant to other antimicrobial agents is isolated (MRSA, MRSE, *S. haemolyticus*, some viridans streptococci, penicillin resistant, *S. pneumoniae*, *C. jeikeium*). Vancomycin may also be necessary in patients allergic to β-lactams or other antimicrobial agents. Occasionally combination regimens that interact synergistically are preferable. Examples include aminoglycoside plus a β-lactam, and vancomycin plus aminoglycoside or rifampicin.

Many Gram-positive bacteremic infections are related to the presence of an indwelling catheter. A large number of these infections can be treated with antimicrobial agents alone, without removal of the catheter. However, persistent bacteremia or fever, significant infection at the catheter entry site, or the isolation of certain microorganisms (*Bacillus* spp., *S. aureus*, *C. jeikeium*) might indicate the need for catheter removal. A prior attempt at saving the catheter by flushing it with urokinase might be indicated in some cases. The duration of therapy is approximately 10–14 days unless evidence of endocarditis, septic thrombophlebitis or other signs of dissemination are present.

Gram-negative bacteremia

A large number of antimicrobial agents with potent activity against commonly isolated Gram-negative bacilli (see Table 3.2) are currently available, and newer agents are being developed and evaluated. The most commonly used agents include extended-spectrum cephalosporins (ceftazidime, cefepime), antipseudomonal penicillins with or without β-lactamase inhibitors (piperacillin–tazobactam, levofloxacin), the carbapenems (imipenem, meropenem), the quinolones (ciprofloxacin, ofloxacin) and the aminoglycosides (gentamicin, tobramycin, amikacin). Agents such as TMP–SMX and rifampicin also have useful activity against many Gram-negative pathogens, although they are seldom used as 'first-line' agents. The aminoglycosides are not appropriate for monotherapy of Gramnegative bacteremia in neutropenic patients, even if in vitro susceptibility of the causative pathogen is demonstrated. This is probably due to multiple factors including a narrow therapeutic index. They are best utilized in combination with other classes of antimicrobial agents, particularly if such combinations are synergistic. Once-daily administration has led to the reduction in aminoglycoside-related toxicity. The choice of specific agents depends upon local susceptibility and resistance patterns.

Unlike Gram-positive bacteremia, the majority of Gram-negative bacteremic infections are not catheter related, even in patients with indwelling CVCs. However, some Gram-negative bacilli are more likely to cause catheter-related infections than others. These include *Acinetobacter* spp., *P. aeruginosa*, *Pseudomonas* spp. and *S. maltophilia*. Quantitative blood cultures might be helpful in identifying such infections, and appropriate management generally includes catheter removal in addition to effective antimicrobial therapy.

There continues to be a debate about the appropriate management of bacteremic infections caused by *P. aeruginosa*. Some authorities recommend the use of combination regimens (preferably synergistic) without exception, in this setting, particularly in patients with severe neutropenia. However, in a large review of *P. aeruginosa* bacteremia in patients with cancer from the M D Anderson Cancer Center, the most critical factors for a favorable therapeutic response were the timing of therapy (i.e. any delay adversely affected outcome) and susceptibility of the organism to the nonaminoglycoside (generally β-lactam) component of the therapeutic regimen. This experience has been confirmed in a follow-up study from the same institution. Although combination therapy may not always be necessary, *P. aeruginosa* is known to be an aggressive pathogen, and is associated with considerable morbidity and mortality. All patients with *P. aeruginosa* infections should be monitored carefully regardless of whether they initially receive monotherapy or combination therapy, and appropriate therapeutic modifications should be made if there is evidence of progressive infection, or lack of response to the initial regimen.

Many empirical regimens contain adequate anaerobic coverage since they include agents such as the carbapenems and piperacillin–tazobactam. However, monotherapy with extended-spectrum cephalosporins, or cephalosporin–aminoglycoside combinations, does not provide adequate anaerobic coverage. In patients receiving such regimens the addition of agents such as metronidazole or clindamycin, or a switch to broad-spectrum agents with anaerobic activity (imipenem, meropenem, piperacillin–tazobactam, levofloxacin) is indicated in patients with necrotizing gingivitis, neutropenic enterocolitis, perirectal abscesses, or other abdominal/pelvic sites of infection. Surgical debridement may be life saving in some anaerobic infections and surgical consultants should be involved in the management of patients with necrotizing anaerobic infections from the onset.

Polymicrobial infections occur commonly when there is tissue involvement. Common examples include pneumonia, neutropenic enterocolitis (typhlitis), perirectal infections, and other skin and skin structure infections. Catheter-associated infections may also be polymicrobial in nature. Gram-positive cocci, Gram-negative aerobic bacilli, and anaerobes are commonly isolated, depending on the site of infection. Occasionally bacterial and fungal and/or viral infections may coexist. The morbidity and mortality rates for many polymicrobial infections have been shown to be greater than those associated with single-organism infections. Appropriate broad-spectrum therapy directed at potential, or documented, pathogens is indicated. Surgical intervention may be vital in some situations (e.g. perirectal abscess, necrotizing fasciitis, and occasionally neutropenic enterocolitis). Removal of infected catheters may be required, in addition to appropriate antimicrobial therapy.

5.4 What is the appropriate approach to the patient with a solid tumor and evidence of a viral infection?

Patients with solid tumors are not at particular risk for developing disseminated viral infections, and there is nothing special or unique about the treatment of viral infections when documented in this patient population. Acyclovir remains the agent of choice for the treatment of infections caused by HSV and VZV. For localized lesions, or when parenteral therapy is no longer necessary, the newer oral agents (famciclovir and valacyclovir) provide greater bioavailability than oral acyclovir. CMV, EBV and human herpesvirus 6 are rarely encountered in patients with a solid tumor.

Community respiratory viruses [influenza, parainfluenza, respiratory syncytial virus (RSV)] have recently been shown to be important causes of morbidity and mortality in bone marrow transplant recipients and in patients with hematologic malignancy. They have not been the subject of extensive study in patients with solid tumors, and in all likelihood do not have the same impact in this setting. Vaccinations, chemoprophylaxis (amantadine, rimantadine) or passive immunization (RSV specific immunoglobulin) should be considered for the appropriate indications. Therapy with agents such as ribavirin is seldom indicated. Two new neuraminidase inhibitors (zanamivir and oseltamivir) were recently approved for the treatment of influenza A and B. Clinical experience with these agents in cancer patients is lacking.

Many patients with a solid tumor develop raised transaminase levels, indicating the presence of hepatitis, but it is often difficult to determine whether the disease is virus or drug induced. The presence of hepatitis may be responsible for substantial delays in the administration of antineoplastic therapy, since it is hazardous to administer hepatotoxic drugs to patients whose liver function is already impaired. Several recent reports have focused on the phenomenon of reactivation of quiescent liver disease due to hepatitis B virus following cytoxic or immunosuppressive therapy. The clinical picture is that of fulminant hepatic failure, which has led to the requirement of liver transplantation in some patients. Hepatitis B virus is also recognized as a major cause of hepatocellular carcinoma in the world today. The risk of developing hepatocellular carcinoma can be as high as 3% per year in hepatitis B surface antigen (HBsAg) carriers, and greater than 12% per year for those with cirrhosis. Consequently, it is recommended that all HBsAg carriers should have regular serial serum α-fetoprotein determinations, and that all carriers with cirrhosis have α-fetoprotein testing and hepatic scanning or ultrasonography for the early detection of hepatocelluar carcinoma. Infection with hepatitis C virus has also been associated with chronic liver disease and hepatocellular carcinoma. Recent data indicate that, in patients with chronic hepatitis C infection, therapy with interferon and ribavirin is effective in inducing virologic and histologic improvement, and should be made available to such patients.

5.5 What is the appropriate approach to the patient with a solid tumor and evidence of a fungal infection?

Fluconazole is effective for the treatment of candidemia caused by susceptible species (i.e. most *Candida* spp., except *C. krusei*). Species other than *C. albicans* might require high doses (800–1200 mg/day) for adequate response to occur. Removal or exchange of offending catheters shortens the duration of candidemia, and hastens response. Amphotericin B is also effective, but its use is limited by substantial toxicity. The lipid formulations of amphotericin B are much less toxic, but much more expensive, and are indicated only when toxicity or refractory infections make the use of amphotericin deoxycholate unrealistic. Fluconazole is also effective for more localized infections (thrush, esophagitis, vaginitis and candiduria). Cryptococcal meningitis is seen occasionally, particularly in patients receiving prolonged corticosteroid therapy. Other disseminated fungal infections are extremely rare in patients with a solid tumor, and their therapy is standard.

5.6 What is the appropriate approach to the patient with a solid tumor and evidence of a parasitic infection?

Parasitic infections (PCP, toxoplasmosis, *S. stercoralis*, *Cryptosporidium*, etc.) are uncommon in patients with solid tumors. Standard therapeutic measures are indicated.

5.7 What is the role of nonantiinfective interventions (including reducing or altering immunosuppression) in the management of established infection?

The hematopoietic growth factors (G-CSF, GM-CSF) have been used not only to prevent infection in high-risk patients but also as adjuncts to antimicrobial therapy for the treatment of established infections in patients with prolonged neutropenia. Some authorities recommend their use in neutropenic patients with disseminated fungal infections and severe bacterial infections that are unresponsive to appropriate antiinfective therapy. A reduction in the duration of neutropenia and a qualitative improvement in granulocyte function are the principles behind the use of hematopoietic growth factors as therapeutic adjuncts. Another approach is the use of hematopoietic growth factors to mobilize granulocytes from normal donors, and to transfuse these granulocytes to neutropenic patients with serious bacterial and fungal infections. These approaches are promising, but their role has not been fully established. Since most patients with a solid tumor do not experience periods of prolonged neutropenia, and are not at risk for disseminated fungal infections, these approaches are less likely to be useful in this specific patient population.

REFERENCES

Elting LS, Bodey GP, Fainstein V. Polymicrobial septicemia in the cancer patient. *Medicine* 1986; **65:** 218–225.

Hughes WT, Armstrong D, Bodey GP et al. Guidelines for the use of antimicrobial agents in neutropenic patients with fever. *Clin Infect Dis* 1997; **25:** 551–573.

Koll BS, Brown AE. The changing epidemiology of infections at cancer hospitals. *Clin Infect Dis* 1993; **17**(Suppl 2): S322– S328.

Ozer H. ASCO Ad Hoc Colony-Stimulating Factor Guidelines Expert Panel: American Society of Clinical Oncology recommendations for the use of hematopoietic colony-stimulating factors: evidence-based, clinical practice guidelines. *J Clin Oncol* 1994; **12:** 2471–2508.

Pizzo PA. Management of fever in patients with cancer and treatment related neutropenia. *N Engl J Med* 1993; **328:** 1322–1332.

Pizzo PA. Fever in immunosuppressed patients. *N Engl J Med* 1999; **341:** 893–900.

Rex JH, Bennett JE, Sugar AM et al. A randomized trial comparing fluconazole with amphotericin B for the treatment of candidemia in patients without neutropenia. *N Engl J Med* 1994; **331:** 1325–1330.

Rolston KVI. New trends in patient management: risk-based therapy for febrile patients with neutropenia. *Clin Infect Dis* 1999; **29:** 515–521.

Rolston KVI, Dholakia N, Rodriguez S, Rubenstein EB. Nature and outcome of febrile episodes in patients with pancreatic and hepatobiliary cancer. *Supportive Care Cancer* 1995; **3:** 414–417.

Rolston KVI, Rubenstein EB, Freifeld A. Early empiric antibiotic therapy for febrile neutropenia patients at low risk. *Infect Dis Clin North Am* 1996; **10:** 223–237.

Talcott JA, Siegel RD, Finberg T et al. Risk assessment in cancer patients with fever and neutropenial a prospective, two-center validation of a prediction rule. *J Clin Oncol* 1992; **10:** 316–322.

Chapter 4

Infections in Patients with Hematologic Malignancies

Michel P Glauser and Thierry Calandra

INTRODUCTION

Hematologic malignancies are quite common forms of cancer, with lymphoma accounting for about 5% of all adult malignancies. Acute myeloid leukemia occurs more often in adults than in children (2.1 versus 0.7 per 100 000 population, respectively), whereas acute lymphoblastic leukemia is found more often in children (boys 2.9 per 100 000 and girls 1.8 per 100 000) than in adults (men 0.6 per 100 000 and women 0.4 per 100 000). Chronic lymphocytic leukemia is especially common in older persons, with an incidence of 10 per 100 000 in individuals older than 70 years compared with 1 per 100 000 in those younger than 50 years.

Chronic granulocytic leukemia occurs in approximately 1 per 100 000 population. In this condition the function of the granulocytes is not clearly impaired, except that neutropenia develops after treatment. However, approximately 10% of patients with CLL have a terminal blast crisis with the clinical features of acute leukemia. The remaining patients develop a slowly progressive leukoerythroblastic picture.

Patients with acute leukemia show failure of normal differentiation and maturation of the leukocytes, with uncontrolled proliferation and failure of bone marrow function, causing neutropenia. The resulting cells tend to be mainly immature precursors. In chronic leukemia there is an inappropriate production of leukocytes in various stages of development and, in addition, humoral immunity is defective in chronic lymphocytic leukemia.

The result of treatment of hematologic malignancies has improved dramatically in recent years. Thus, acute lymphocytic leukemia can be cured in approximately half of adults and in 60–70% of children. Similarly, 70% of patients with Hodgkin disease can be cured by treatment, as can half of those with lymphoma. However, while antineoplastic treatment can cure or produce remission in many patients with hematologic malignancies treatment that targets the normally replicating bone marrow progenitor cells as well as malignant cells increases the risk of infection. The risk is further exacerbated by the disordered number and function of the granulocytes, as well as by cellular and humoral immune disorders resulting from the underlying diseases.

Since patients with hematologic malignancy often suffer from prolonged and sometimes severe granulocytopenia, together with defective granulocyte function, they differ from patients with solid tumors, who are usually less immunosuppressed and who have a shorter duration of chemotherapy-induced neutropenia. Infection in patients with solid tumors is promoted by obstruction of natural passages (bronchial tree, urinary tract, alimentary tract, biliary tract), damage to anatomic barriers, surgery, radiation therapy, surgical shunts and prostheses, and also from neutropenia, but infrequently from immunosuppression. In patients with hematologic malignancy, the risk of infection is related to the low neutrophil count, to alterations in cellular and humoral immunity and, importantly, to changes in mucosal integrity.

The critical factor determining infection in patients with hematologic malignancies is the neutropenia caused by the disease or by antineoplastic treatment. In patients with neutropenia, the likelihood of developing an infection is inversely related to the number of circulating neutrophils, so that the lower the number of neutrophils, the more likely the patient is to develop one or more infections. The risk of infection is increased if the neutrophil count is less than $1000/mm^3$, especially if the number of these white cells is falling rapidly. Severe infection is probable with a neutrophil count of less than $100/mm^3$, especially if such profound neutropenia is prolonged. The probability of developing an infection is also related to the duration of the neutropenia. It has been estimated that, with a neutrophil count of less than $100/mm^3$, 25% of the patients suffer from infections if the low level of neutrophils is maintained for 1 week and all patients become infected if neutropenia of less than $100/mm^3$ lasts for 6 weeks.

I REGARDING THE CLINICAL PRESENTATION AND EVALUATION OF THE PATIENT

1.1 What are the clinically predominant modes of presentation of infection in patients with hematologic malignancies?

Fever
Fever develops in the majority of patients with hematologic malignancies who have disease-related or chemotherapy-induced neutropenia. Although any temperature distinctly above baseline is indicative of fever, fever has been defined by the Consensus Guidelines of the Immunocompromised Host Society (IHS) as a single oral temperature reading greater than 38.5°C (101.3°F) or greater than 38°C (100.4°F) on two or more occasions over a 12-h period or as a single oral temperature reading greater than 38.3°C (100.9°F) or 38°C (100.4°F) during at least 1 h, by a Working Committee of the Infectious Diseases Society of America (IDSA). Temperature should be measured orally or by auditory canal probe.

More than two thirds of febrile episodes are likely to be caused by infection, which may occur with or without focal symptoms or signs. Because of the defect in the inflammatory response, the classic signs of infection such as pain, heat, redness and swelling are often absent in neutropenic patients, so that fever is generally the first and frequently the only sign of infection. Noninfectious etiologies of pyrexia include the underlying malignancy, chemotherapy, transfusion of blood products, and occasionally antimicrobial agents, colony-stimulating factors or allergic reactions. Thus, in neutropenic patients, infection should be considered the cause of fever until proven otherwise. Uncommonly, infection may develop in the absence of fever because of the defective inflammatory response or with certain organisms, such as *Clostridium septicum*.

Classically, infections are classified into three standardized categories:
1 microbiologically documented infections, subdivided into those with and without bloodstream infection
2 clinically documented infections
3 fever of unknown origin (FUO) (synonyms include fever of undetermined origin, unexplained fever or pyrexia of unknown origin).

Table 4.1 Classification of infections in febrile neutropenic patients with hematologic malignancies

Type of infection	No. of febrile episodes (n = 1049)
Microbiologically documented infections (MDI)	326 (31%)
• With bacteremia	301 (29%)
Single organism bacteremia	265
Polymicrobial bacteremia	36
Gram-positive bacteria	235
Coagulase-negative staphylococci	114
Staphylococcus aureus	18
Viridans streptococci	66
Other streptococci	12
Other Gram-positive bacteria	25
Gram-negative bacteria	102
Escherichia coli	47
Pseudomonas spp.	17
Klebsiella spp.	10
Anaerobes	8
Other Gram-negative bacilli	20
• Without bacteremia	25 (2%)
Clinically documented infections (CDI)	260 (25%)
Fever of unknown origin (FUO)	429 (41%)

Data are derived from two consecutive trials of the International Antimicrobial Therapy Cooperative Group of the European Organization for Research and Treatment of Cancer, which included 1049 patients with hematologic malignancies (i.e. acute nonlymphoblastic leukemia, acute lymphoblastic leukemia and chronic myelogenic leukemia with blast crisis) enrolled between August 1991 and June 1994 in 41 cancer centers located in Europe, the United States and the Middle East.

The data presented in Table 4.1 show the frequency of microbiologically documented infection, clinically documented infection and FUO in the 1049 patients with hematologic malignancy enrolled during 1991–1994 in the three most recent trials organized by the International Antimicrobial Therapy Cooperative Group (IATCG) of the European Organization for Research and Treatment of Cancer (EORTC). Although Table 4.1 provides a good estimate of the frequency of each category of infection, it is necessary to remember that the frequency of microbiologically and clinically documented infection may be underestimated as these trials do not include patients with suspected infection but no fever.

Microbiologically documented infection
Microbiologically documented infection includes (1) bloodstream infections, caused predominantly by bacteria (bacteremia) and occasionally by fungi (fungemia), without an identifiable nonhematogenous focus of infection; and (2) microbiologically proven site of infection (e.g. pneumonia, cellulitis, catheter-related infection, urinary tract infection), with or without concomitant bloodstream infection. Microbiologically documented infections account for approximately 25–30% of the episodes of fever in neutropenic patients with hematologic malignancy, most of whom suffer from bacteremia, and the remainder have a microbiologically documented infection without bloodstream infection (Table 4.1). As mentioned previously, the risk of infection is inversely proportional to the

neutrophil count. The development of fever is more likely to be associated with bacteremia when the granulocyte count is less than $100/mm^3$ than when greater than $500/mm^3$.

Clinically documented infection
Clinically documented infection is defined by the presence of a site suggestive of infection (e.g. pneumonia, cellulitis) even though the etiology of the infection has not been documented microbiologically. This category of infection accounts for 20–30% of the febrile episodes occurring in neutropenic patients with hematologic malignancies (Table 4.1).

Fever of unknown origin
FUO refers to a febrile episode that is not accompanied by either clinical or microbiologic evidence of infection. In neutropenic patients, FUO accounts for 40–70% of the episodes of fever (Table 4.1). Although it is difficult to define the exact etiology of fever in the absence of clinically and microbiologically documented evidence of infection, one may retrospectively assume that the fever has probably been of infectious origin if it resolves with antimicrobial therapy. However, the early use of empirical antimicrobial therapy may preclude the possibility of diagnosing or defining an infectious cause for the fever in these neutropenic patients.

1.2 What are the predominant sites of infection?
In 1049 febrile granulocytopenic patients with hematologic malignancies, the origin of infection was localized to the bloodstream (34%), mouth and nasopharynx (22%), the respiratory tract (15%) (upper respiratory tract 1%, lower respiratory tract 13%), skin and soft tissues (13%), the gastrointestinal tract (7%), intravenous catheter sites (5%), the urinary tract (3%) and other sites (2%) (Table 4.2).

Table 4.2 Most common sites of infections in febrile neutropenic patients with hematologic malignancies

	No. of episodes
Total number of febrile episodes	1049
Febrile episodes with an identified site of infection	586
Site of infection	
Bloodstream	200 (34%)
Mouth, tonsil, pharynx	126 (22%)
Respiratory tract	87 (15%)
Upper respiratory tract (nose, sinuses)	8 (1%)
Lower respiratory tract (lung)	79 (13%)
Skin and soft tissue	74 (13%)
Gastrointestinal tract	40 (7%)
Intravenous catheters, phlebitis	31 (5%)
Urinary tract	17 (3%)
Other sites	11 (2%)

Data are derived from two consecutive trials of the International Antimicrobial Therapy Cooperative Group of the European Organization for Research and Treatment of Cancer, which included 1049 patients with hematologic malignancies (i.e. acute nonlymphoblastic leukemia, acute lymphoblastic leukemia and chronic myelogenic leukemia with blast crisis) enrolled between August 1991 and June 1994 in 41 cancer centers located in Europe, the United States and the Middle East.

Mouth and pharynx

Infections of the oral cavity (e.g. mucositis, gingivitis, periodontitis) and pharynx are very common in patients with hematologic malignancies. The frequency and severity of the infections of the oral mucosa are proportional to the degree of mucosal damage (e.g. mucositis) caused by chemotherapy and to the severity of the neutropenia. Since the mucous membranes of the mouth and digestive tract are heavily colonized with microbes, patients with loss of integrity of the mucosal barrier are at high risk of developing both local and disseminated infections, as these lesions are the portal of entry of pathogens causing systemic infections.

Patients with neutropenia and no (or minimal) mucosal damage are at much lower risk of infection. Indeed, patients with acute leukemia often present initially with only mild periodontitis or gingivostomatitis associated with their neutropenia, and possibly altered neutrophil function. In contrast, patients with severe chemotherapy-induced mucositis are at high risk of infection, even in the absence of profound neutropenia. Oral lesions caused by herpes simplex virus (HSV) may mimic chemotherapy-induced mucositis and are also a significant portal of entry for bacterial infections. Because the oral cavity is a frequent source of infection in patients with hematologic malignancies, dental care and removal of all septic foci (e.g. periodontitis, braces) should, whenever possible, precede the initiation of chemotherapy.

Respiratory tract

Infections may involve either the upper or lower respiratory tract. Except for sinusitis, infections of the upper respiratory tract (otitis, epiglottitis, laryngitis and tracheitis) are uncommon in patients with hematologic malignancies. Most lower respiratory tract infections (bronchopneumonia and pneumonia) are primary, but may also be secondary to bloodstream infections. The symptoms indicating pulmonary infection include fever, cough, dyspnea and chest pain. Signs of bronchoalveolar fluid are present in over half of the affected patients and two thirds of these patients have radiographic features – on chest radiography or computed tomography (CT) – of infection. Sputum is seldom found in patients with profound neutropenia (< 100 cells/mm^3), but is usual in patients with higher neutrophil counts (> 1000/mm^3).

Overall, primary pneumonia affected 13% of the neutropenic patients who presented with fever in the IATCG–EORTC trials IX and XI (Table 4.2). Pneumonia was less frequent (3%) among the 650 children aged less than 16 years who were included in these studies. Pneumonia is not as common during the first episode of neutropenia as in subsequent episodes. Moreover, pneumonia occurring during the first episode of neutropenia is more likely to be of bacterial origin, while it is more likely to be fungal in subsequent episodes.

Skin and soft tissue

Cutaneous infections are common in patients with hematologic malignancies. Primary skin and soft tissue infections often result from disruption of the integrity of the cutaneous defense barrier (e.g. needle punctures, intravenous catheters, bone marrow biopsy). Indwelling intravenous catheters, especially those inserted for prolonged periods of time (e.g. Broviac, Hickman, Portacath) are a major source of infection in these patients. Infections most commonly arise at the exit site, but also occasionally affect the tunnelized section of the catheter. Clinical manifestations of cellulitis and catheter-related skin infections include pain, erythema, tenderness, and sometimes necrosis that can be caused by infections due to *Pseudomonas aeruginosa* (e.g. ecthyma gangrenosum), mycobacteria (especially *M. chelonae* and *M. fortuitum*), or to *Aspergillus* or *Mucor* spp.

Disseminated cutaneous infections may reflect septic embolization of the skin secondary to bacteremia, fungemia or viremia. Clinically, the skin lesions are papules or nodules, which may be associated with myalgia and muscle tenderness. Ulcers, vesicles, hemorrhagic or crusted lesions that are either isolated (with or without dermatome distribution) or disseminated are typically associated with herpetic skin infections, but may occasionally be caused by staphylococci or streptococci. A fungal or bacterial (e.g. *Pseudomonas* spp., *Aeromonas* spp.) etiology should be suspected when there are disseminated necrotic skin lesions.

Gastrointestinal tract

The gastrointestinal tract plays an important role in the pathogenesis of infections in neutropenic patients with hematologic malignancies for two reasons. First, it is a major portal of entry of systemic infections when there is chemotherapy-induced mucosal damage and neutropenia, since the endogenous gastrointestinal flora is a large reservoir of microorganisms. Secondly, the gastrointestinal tract itself accounts for 7% of clinically or microbiologically documented infections in febrile neutropenic patients with hematologic malignancies (Table 4.2).

Esophagitis and enterocolitis are the most common gastrointestinal infectious complications occurring in neutropenic patients with hematologic malignancies. Esophagitis presents with retrosternal pain and odynophagia. Symptoms and signs of enterocolitis include nausea, vomiting, bloating, abdominal discomfort, cramps, pain, constipation or diarrhea (often severe in the case of antibiotic-associated colitis).

Typhlitis is a life-threatening necrotizing enterocolitis affecting the cecum. Classically, typhlitis occurs in leukemic patients with a prolonged episode of neutropenia who have been treated with broad-spectrum antibiotics. The clinical manifestations of typhlitis include fever, abdominal pain (initially localized to the lower right abdominal quadrant, but becoming diffuse as the infection progresses), diarrhea and often a profound alteration of the patient's general condition. Bleeding and perforation are the two major complications of typhlitis. Necrotizing fasciitis can also occur, especially with clostridial infection, notably with C. *septicum*, sometimes in the absence of fever.

Viral hepatitis seldom occurs in these patients, but hepatosplenic candidiasis should be suspected in patients with persistent fever (especially at the time of recovery from neutropenia), abdominal pain, hepatosplenomegaly and an elevated alkaline phosphatase level.

1.3 What are the predominant organisms that contribute (by site)?

The majority of infections in granulocytopenic patients with hematologic malignancies are caused by microorganisms of the patient's endogenous flora, usually those that colonize the primary site of infection. Approximately half of the infections are caused by nosocomial pathogens acquired after admission to hospital. Most infections are caused by bacteria (both Gram-positive and Gram-negative species), but fungal infections (*Candida* and *Aspergillus* spp.) and viral infections (HSV and varicella zoster virus (VZV)) also are an important cause of morbidity and mortality in these patients.

In the past decade, most cancer centers have experienced a major change in the etiology of bacterial infections occurring in neutropenic patients. While Gram-negative bacteria were predominant in the 1970s and early 1980s, Gram-positive bacteria have recently increased in frequency, and are now the prevalent pathogens in many institutions. As an example of this change, the percentage of single-agent Gram-positive bacteremia increased from 29% in the first trial (1973–1976) conducted by the

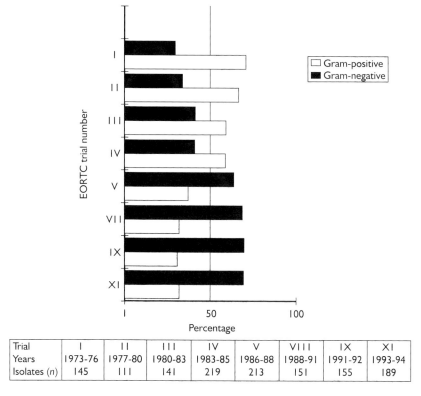

Figure 4.1   Relative incidence of Gram-positive and Gram-negative organisms causing bacteremia in nine EORTC trials from 1973 to 1997.

International Antimicrobial Therapy Project Group of the EORTC to 69% in the 11th trial (1993–1994) of this group (Figure 4.1). Similarly, in a recent study carried out at the National Cancer Institute (Bethesda, Maryland, USA), Gram-positive aerobes accounted for 55% of the primary bloodstream infections.

Fungal infections are a major threat to febrile neutropenic patients. While indwelling intravenous catheters and mucositis are two important portals of entry for fungal infections, the major risk factors include long-lasting and profound neutropenia, the use of broad-spectrum antibiotic agents that alter the endogenous microbial flora and facilitate the proliferation of yeasts and fungi, and the prophylactic use of antifungal agents that may give rise to pathogens with reduced sensitivities to conventional antifungal drugs. Although fungal infections traditionally occur in patients with prolonged neutropenia, they also cause about 5% of the initial episodes of fever.

Bacterial and fungal infections can coexist and the bacterial component may mask the fungal infection. The latter may present as fever after the eradication of the bacterial infection. Disseminated fungal infections have also been demonstrated in 10–40% of autopsies in patients with hematologic malignancies, mainly in patients who have received broad-spectrum antibiotics and corticosteroid treatment.

The fungi that most commonly infect neutropenic patients (85% of patients) include *Candida* spp. (*C. albicans, C. glabrata, C. krusei, C. parapsilosis, C. tropicalis, C. pseudotropicalis*) and *Aspergillus* (*A. flavus* and *A. fumigatus*).

HSV and VZV infections, both primarily acquired or reactivated, are common in patients with leukemia and lymphoma, especially after chemotherapy or treatment with corticosteroids. In contrast to many other immunocompromised patients, especially bone marrow or solid organ transplant recipients, cytomegalovirus (CMV) infections are uncommon in patients with hematologic malignancies, in whom cellular immunity is less altered. In patients with leukemia and lymphoma, the main host defense defect is a lack of neutrophils and anatomic barrier defects.

Although the relative frequencies of the various bacterial pathogens causing infections in patients with hematologic malignancies and neutropenia may vary from center to center, some general observations can be made that apply for most institutions. The predominant pathogens by site of infections are shown in Table 4.3.

Bloodstream infections

About 80–85% of all Gram-positive bacteremias are caused by coagulase-negative staphylococci, viridans streptococci, or *Staphylococcus aureus*. *Enterococcus* spp., *Streptococcus pneumoniae*, *Corynebacterium* spp. and a few species of anaerobes account for most of the remaining 15–20% of Gram-positive bloodstream infections. The striking increase in coagulase-negative staphylococcal infections is related, at least partly, to the extensive use of intravenous catheters, particularly those inserted for prolonged periods of time. Recent reports have shown that viridans streptococci are frequent pathogens in febrile neutropenic patients with acute leukemia or lymphoma. In some institutions today, these organisms comprise the second most common cause of bacteremia and are outnumbered only by coagulase-negative staphylococci.

These streptococcal infections may be severe and present with septic shock or acute respiratory distress syndrome. There are several reasons for the increased frequency of streptococcal bacteremia. Viridans streptococci are normal inhabitants of the mouth, pharynx and gastrointestinal tract. Thus, these infections arise from oral or gastrointestinal mucosa that has been damaged by chemotherapy, especially by treatment with high-dose cytosine arabinoside. Moreover, herpetic ulceration may also represent a portal of entry for streptococcal bacteremia. Another factor predisposing to the streptococcal infections may be the prophylactic use of fluoroquinolone antibiotics. Most of the first-generation quinolones (e.g. ciprofloxacin, norfloxacin, ofloxacin) have limited anti-Gram-positive activity and may not prevent the development of streptococcal infections. However, the frequency of viridans streptococcal infections has also increased in centers not using quinolone prophylaxis, emphasizing that diverse factors may account for the shift in the epidemiology of bacteremia.

Among Gram-negative bacteria, *Escherichia coli*, *P. aeruginosa* and *Klebsiella* spp. are responsible for approximately 80% of the Gram-negative infections in most studies. *Pseudomonas* species are the main cause of life-threatening Gram-negative infections. For reasons that are poorly understood, Gram-negative anaerobes are an uncommon cause of microbiologically documented infections in the neutropenic host. In many centers, the use of quinolones for the prophylaxis of bacterial infections has contributed significantly to the reduction in the incidence of Gram-negative bacteremia in patients with neutropenic cancer.

Intravascular catheter-related infections

Catheter-related infections are caused predominantly by coagulase-negative staphylococci, *S. aureus*, *Candida* spp. and C. *jeikeium*, and less frequently by Gram-negative bacilli.

Table 4.3 Evaluation of infections in patients with hematologic malignancies according to the site of infection and the possible etiologic agent

Site of infection	Infectious syndrome (clinical features)	Predominant pathogens	Diagnostic tests
Bloodstream	Bacteremia (fever ± local signs of infection)	Coagulase-negative staphylococci Staphylococcus aureus Viridans streptococci Enterococcus spp. (nosocomial outbreaks in some institutions) Gram-negative bacilli (Escherichia coli, Klebsiella pneumoniae, Enterobacter spp., Pseudomonas aeruginosa) Candida spp.	Blood culture (two sets drawn from separate sites and at least one set drawn from intravenous catheter)
Intravascular catheter-related infections	Pain, erythema, tenderness, discharge from catheter entry site, occasionally necrosis	Coagulase-negative staphylococci Staphylococcus aureus Corynebacterium jeikeium Candida spp. Gram-negative bacilli	Swab of entry site Culture of catheter tip Blood cultures (consider drawing blood through each lumen of catheter and carrying out quantitative blood cultures)
Oral cavity	Periodontitis Gingivitis, stomatitis/mucositis (aphthae, ulcers) Oral thrush (white plaques)	Viridans streptococci Staphylococcus aureus Aerobic and anaerobic Gram-negative bacilli Aerobic and anaerobic Gram-positive rods Herpes simplex Candida spp.	Swab of lesion Oral wash Direct examination of specimen Culture
Throat	Pharyngitis Tonsilitis (sore throat, odynophagia)	Streptococcus pyogenes Viruses (rhinovirus, coronavirus, adenovirus, influenza, parainfluenza, herpes simplex, Epstein–Barr virus)	Swab of pharynx Serology
Upper respiratory tract	Sinusitis (tightness of sinus areas, headache, toothache, nasal obstruction, nasal voice)	Streptococcus pneumoniae Haemophilus influenzae	Aspiration of sinus Biopsy (if no improvement after

Site of infection	Infectious syndrome (clinical features)	Predominant pathogens	Diagnostic tests
		Streptococcus pyogenes	72–96 h of empirical antibiotic therapy)
		Staphylococcus aureus	
		Gram-negative bacilli (*Escherichia coli*, *Klebsiella pneumoniae*, *Pseudomonas aeruginosa*)	
		Anaerobic bacteria	
		Candida spp.	
		Aspergillus spp., *Mucor* spp., *Rhizopus* spp.	
Lower respiratory tract (bronchi, terminal airways, alveoli)	Bronchopneumonia	Conventional infections:	Chest radiography
	Pneumonia (cough, dyspnea, chest pain, sputum, hemoptysis, pleural effusion)	*Streptococcus pneumoniae*	CT
		Haemophilus influenzae	MRI
		Viridans streptococci	Fiberoptic bronchoscopy with
		Staphylococcus aureus	BAL
		Gram-negative bacilli (*Escherichia coli*,	Transbronchial biopsy
		Klebsiella pneumoniae, *Pseudomonas aeruginosa*,	Thoracocentesis
		Acinetobacter spp.)	Thoracoscopy with biopsy
		Legionella spp. (sporadic outbreaks)	Open lung biopsy
		Viruses (influenza, parainfluenza, varicella zoster)	
		Opportunistic infections:	
		Pneumocystis carinii	
		Aspergillus spp., *Mucor* spp., *Rhizopus* spp.	
		Nocardia asteroides	
		Mycobacterium tuberculosis	
		Atypical mycobacteria	
		Histoplasma capsulatum	
		Cryptococcus neoformans	
Skin infection and soft tissue	Cellulitis (pain, erythema, tenderness, necrosis in case of ecthyma gangrenosum)	Primary infections:	Skin swab
		Coagulase-negative staphylococci	Aspiration (needle)
		Staphylococcus aureus	Skin biopsy (histology and culture)
		Corynebacterium jeikeium	
		Gram-negative bacilli (*Pseudomonas aeruginosa*,	

Clinical manifestation	Organisms	Diagnostic procedures
Papules, nodules (with or without myalgia and muscle tenderness)	*Escherichia coli, Klebsiella pneumoniae*) *Enterococcus* spp. (perirectal cellulitis) Anaerobic Gram-negative bacilli (perirectal cellulitis) *Candida* spp. *Mucor* spp., *Rhizopus* spp., *Absidia* spp. Disseminated infections: *Candida* spp., *Fusarium* spp., *Trichosporon* spp. (less frequent) Gram-negative bacilli (*Escherichia coli, Pseudomonas aeruginosa, Aeromonas hydrophilia, Serratia marcescens*)	
Ulcers, vesicles, hemorrhagic or crusted lesions (isolated or with dermatome distribution)	Herpes simplex Varicella zoster virus Cytomegalovirus	
Disseminated vesicles, hemorrhagic or crusted lesions	Varicella zoster virus Herpes simplex *Staphylococcus aureus* Streptococci	
Skin necrosis	*Aspergillus* spp. *Mucor* spp.	
Gastrointestinal tract		
Esophagus Esophagitis (dysphagia, retrosternal pain)	Herpes simplex *Candida* spp.	Plain abdominal films Esogastroscopy Colonoscopy Ultrasonography CT MRI Culture of endoscopic specimens Stool cultures Toxin detection
Small intestine, colon Enteritis Typhlitis Colitis (nausea, vomiting, bloating, abdominal discomfort, cramp, pain, constipation, diarrhea)	Aerobic and anaerobic Gram-negative bacilli *Clostridium* spp. (typhlitis) *Clostridium difficile* (antibiotic-associated diarrhea) *Strongyloides stercoralis* (uncommon) Rotavirus (children) *Candida* spp.	

Site of infection	Infectious syndrome (clinical features)	Predominant pathogens	Diagnostic tests
Liver and spleen	Hepatosplenic candidiasis (persistent fever, abdominal pain, hepatosplenomegaly, raised alkaline phosphatase levels)		Ultrasonography, CT, MRI, Biopsy (histology and culture)
	Hepatitis	Hepatitis A, B, C and δ viruses	
Urinary tract	Urinary tract infections (dysuria, i.e. frequency, urgency, pain; hematuria; flank pain)	Gram-negative bacilli (*Escherichia coli*, *Klebsiella* spp., *Proteus* spp., *Enterobacter* spp., *Pseudomonas aeruginosa*) *Enterococcus* spp. Coagulase-negative staphylococci (*Staphylococcus saprophyticus*) *Candida* spp.	Urine culture
Central nervous system	Acute meningitis	*Listeria monocytogenes*	CT MRI
	Subacute, chronic meningitis	*Cryptococcus neoformans* *Candida* spp. *Mycobacterium tuberculosis* *Coccidioides immitis* *Histoplasma capsulatum*	Lumbar puncture Aspiration or biopsy under stereotaxic CT guidance
	Focal brain diseases	*Aspergillus* spp. *Mucor* spp. *Nocardia asteroides* *Listeria monocytogenes* *Toxoplasma gondii*	
	Shunt infections (fever, change in mental status, headache, meningism, increase intracranial pressure; patient may also be asymptomatic)	Coagulase-negative staphylococci *Staphylococcus aureus* *Enterococcus* spp. *Corynebacterium* spp. *Propionibacterium* spp.	

Gram-negative bacilli

Candida spp.

Increased risk of bacterial meningitis due to Streptococcus pneumoniae. Neisseria meningitidis.

Haemophilus influenzae

Patients with hematologic malignancies have the same susceptibility to conventional pathogens of the central nervous system (meningitis: Streptococcus pneumoniae, Neisseria meningitidis, Haemophilus influenzae, Gram-negative bacilli; brain abscess: streptococci, Eacteroides spp., Staphylococcus aureus, Enterobacteriaceae) as the general population. Listed above are unique pathogens.

Oropharyngeal infections

The pathogens isolated from oropharyngeal infections in patients with granulocytopenia include bacteria (viridans streptococci, Gram-positive rods, aerobic and anaerobic Gram-negative bacilli and *S. aureus*), viruses (HSV) and yeasts (*Candida*). Mixed infections are common. Oral candidiasis in the granulocytopenic patient often spreads to the esophagus and possibly to the rest of the gastrointestinal tract, which may become a site of invasion and dissemination.

Lower respiratory tract infections

Infections of the lower respiratory tract (e.g. bronchopneumonia and pneumonia) can be subdivided into those caused by conventional pathogens (*S. pneumoniae*, viridans streptococci, *S. aureus*, *E. coli*, *H. influenzae*, *K. pneumoniae*, *P. aeruginosa* and *Legionella* spp.), and those caused by opportunistic pathogens (*Pneumocystis carinii*, *Aspergillus* spp., *Mucor* spp., *Rhizopus* spp., *Nocardia asteroides*, *Mycobacterium tuberculosis*, atypical mycobacteria, *Histoplasma capsulatum* and *Cryptococcus neoformans*).

In a retrospective analysis of 1049 initial febrile episodes in patients with neutropenic cancer enrolled between 1991 and 1994 in two EORTC–IATCG trials, pneumonia was the cause of fever in 79 of 1049 episodes (8%). The infection was clinically documented in two thirds of the patients and microbiologically documented in one third (with bacteremia in 25%). Gram-positive and Gram-negative bacteria accounted for 64% and 29%, respectively, of pneumonias associated with bacteremia. Opportunistic pathogens were isolated in only five of the pneumonias that developed at the beginning of the neutropenic episode. Pneumonia was the cause of approximately 40 episodes of further infection, of which two thirds were documented clinically and one third were documented microbiologically. In contrast to early-onset pneumonias, opportunistic pathogens accounted for the majority (60%) of microbiologically documented late-onset pneumonias: *Aspergillus* spp. (six cases); *P. carinii* (three); *Mucor* spp., *Candida* spp. and CMV (one episode each), confirming the occurrence of these organisms in patients with persistent and profound neutropenia.

Skin and soft tissue infections

Primary cutaneous infections (e.g. cellulitis) are caused by the microorganisms colonizing the skin (*S. aureus*, coagulase-negative staphylococci, streptococci, *Corynebacterium* spp.). *Candida*, *Aspergillus* and *Mucor* spp. also infect needle-puncture lesions, sites of iv catheters, and traumatized skin and soft tissues, resulting in localized infection or septicemia. The skin may also become infected during the course of a bacteremia (staphylococci, streptococci, Enterobacteriaceae and *P. aeruginosa*), fungemia (*Candida*, *Aspergillus* and *Fusarium* spp.), or viremia (HSV, VZV and CMV). Perirectal cellulitis is often a mixed infection caused by Gram-negative bacilli (*P. aeruginosa*, *E. coli*, *K. pneumoniae*), *Enterococcus* spp. and anaerobic Gram-negative bacilli. Necrotic skin lesions are highly suggestive of an infection due to *P. aeruginosa* (ecthyma gangrenosum) or to fungi (*Aspergillus*, *Mucor* or *Rhizopus* spp.).

Central nervous system infections

Infections of the central nervous system (CNS) in patients with hematologic malignancies are uncommon. Patients with hematologic malignancies have the same susceptibility of the CNS to conventional pathogens as the general population. *S. pneumoniae*, *Neisseria meningitidis*, *H. influenzae*, Gram-negative bacilli and *Listeria monocytogenes* are the most frequent causes of acute meningitis. A focal brain lesion may also indicate the development of a brain abscess. Brain abscesses are usually secondary to adjacent infectious lesions (e.g. sinusitis or otitis), pulmonary infection, catheter infections or bacterial endocarditis. The causative organisms are the common aerobic and anaerobic bacteria and *Nocardia* as well as fungal species, especially *Candida* but also *Aspergillus* and *Mucor* spp.

1.4 How do the organisms vary according to various risk factors?

Severity and duration of neutropenia (see also section 2.1)

Severity of neutropenia
Neutrophils are a central component of the host defenses against bacterial and fungal infection. Thus, any alteration either in the function or in the number of neutrophils, as a consequence of hematologic malignancy or cytotoxic therapy, will result in an increased risk of infection. In fact, there is an inverse relationship between the neutrophil count and the incidence of infections, so that as the neutrophil count decreases to less than $500/mm^3$ infections increase markedly, and with neutrophil counts lower than $100/mm^3$ the risk of severe infection (such as bacteremia and bacterial pneumonia) is greatest. On the other hand, with counts greater than $1000/mm^3$ the risk of infection is small. Practically, patients with neutrophil counts lower than $500/mm^3$ are considered to be at increased risk of infection, so that fever in those with a count of less than $500/mm^3$ is considered to reflect ongoing infection and to indicate the need for empirical broad-spectrum antibiotic treatment.

Duration of neutropenia
The duration of neutropenia is also a major determinant of the risk of infection. The longer the duration of neutropenia, the greater the risk of infection (Table 4.4). Neutropenia of $500/mm^3$ or less for 10 days or more, indicating severe and persistent neutropenia, is considered to be a major risk factor for primary infection if there is also a greater likelihood of recurrent or secondary infection despite antibiotic treatment.

Overall, patients have been categorized as being susceptible to a high or a low risk of infectious complications during febrile neutropenia. Patients whose episode of neutropenia lasts less than 7–10 days are assumed to have a lower risk of serious infectious complications than those with longer duration of anticipated neutropenia (more than 10 days). A low risk of infectious complications is confirmed if there is evidence of bone marrow recovery in the form of steadily increasing neutrophil numbers. There appeared to be a low risk (< 1%) of recurrence of fever after empirical treatment of low-risk patients,

Table 4.4 Proportion of patients with cancer developing severe infections with granulocytopenia and the cumulative risk of infection with prolonged granulocytopenia

| | Percentage of severe infections by duration of granulocytopenia (weeks) | | | | | | | |
	1	2	3	4	6	10	12	14
Granulocyte count (per µl)								
< 1000	10	30	45	50	65	70	85	100
< 100	28	50	72	85	100			

Adapted from Bodey et al (1966).

compared with a 38% recurrence rate in patients whose fever recurred if the neutropenia lasted more than 2 weeks. Moreover, 95% of patients with neutropenia for less than 1 week respond to their initial empirical antibiotic regimen without needing a change in the treatment, while two thirds of those with neutropenia for more than 2 weeks may require treatment modification.

Severity of the underlying disease

Although the severity and duration of neutropenia are major determinants of the likelihood of infection, the severity of the underlying disease and its treatment are also important factors in determining the risk of infection. For example, antineoplastic chemotherapy damages mucous membranes, so that the oral and digestive mucosa develops mucositis, which predisposes to infection and invasion. Damage to the mucosa of the upper and lower respiratory tract results in ciliary damage, with predisposition to sinusitis and pneumonia. Injury to the skin by venepuncture, indwelling catheters, bone marrow aspiration and other surgical interventions can also result in infection.

Tubal obstruction by the disease process promotes infection in neutropenic patients. Examples include urinary or biliary tract infections as a consequence of obstruction by neoplastic processes, as well as the development of otitis media as a result of eustachean tube obstruction by malignant involvement of the adenoids. The combination of damage to anatomic barriers or tubal obstruction with neutropenia presents the appropriate conditions for bacterial invasion, dissemination and death.

Preexisting infection may be aggravated by neutropenia. Thus, the periodontal tissues, lungs, colon, perianal tissues and skin are often the sites of infection and foci for bacterial invasion in neutropenic patients.

Table 4.5 Patients at low or high risk for complications during febrile neutropenia

	Low risk	High risk
Neutropenia	Anticipated short duration of neutropenia ($\leq$ 7 days)	Anticipated long duration of neutropenia ($>$ 7 days)
Cancer	Solid tumor, maintenance chemotherapy for leukemia	Leukemia induction, bone marrow transplantation
Mucositis	Absent	Present
Underlying diseases	Absence of comorbid medical conditions	Presence comorbid medical conditions: systemic hypotension, altered mental status, new neurologic changes, respiratory failure, dehydration, abdominal pain, hemorrhage, cardiac compromise or new arrhythmias, catheter tunnel infection/other extensive cellulitis, acute renal or liver failure
Type of infection	Fever of undetermined origin	Bacteremia, pneumonia and other serious documented infections*, age(?)

* Not all of these infections are high risk; for example, a line-related bacteremia caused by coagulase-negative staphylococci, or Gram-negative bacteremia without hemodynamic changes, could potentially be managed in an outpatient setting.

Adapted from Freifeld et al (1997).

The drugs used to treat hematologic malignancies may themselves impair neutrophil function and predispose to infection. These agents can inhibit phagocytosis and neutrophil bactericidal activity.

Patients with a low risk of infectious complications (Table 4.5) are usually not hospital inpatients at the start of the fever, are characterized by an underlying hematologic malignancy that is clinically controlled, and do not suffer from serious comorbidity. Their low neutrophil count is not likely to last more than a few days (<7 days). When these patients develop a fever, the cause of fever often remains unknown.

Conversely, patients with a high risk of infectious complications (Table 4.5) are those with prolonged neutropenia (> 10 days), with comorbid medical conditions including severe mucositis, hemorrhage, dehydration, renal and/or hepatic failure, respiratory and circulatory failure, cardiac failure or neurologic deficits. High-risk patients also include individuals with severe infections such as bacteremia, pneumonia, catheter tunnel infections or cellulitis, especially if hospitalized at the time of onset of the fever, as well as patients whose hematologic malignancies are not controlled by treatment (see Table 4.5).

The categorization of patients as 'low risk' has therapeutic and economic implications. Since few (< 5%) of the patients classified as 'low risk' develop complications, these patients might be selected for outpatient empirical antibiotic therapy, either with intravenously administered antibiotics followed by oral regimens (sequential antibiotic therapy), or wholly with oral antimicrobial therapy. The latter two regimens would involve considerable cost savings compared with hospitalization, if their safety in the context of a home-based schedule could be demonstrated.

1.5 How does this differ from other conditions, from center to center, and from country to country?

Typically, patients with hematologic malignancies (who have not undergone marrow transplantation) differ in several respects from other types of immunosuppressed patients. First, the defective defense against infection results from the abnormally low number of polymorphonuclear leukocytes, which is caused either by the underlying disease or by cytotoxic treatment, so that the majority of infections are caused by bacteria or fungi. Unless the patients have received high doses of steroids or other immunosuppressive drugs, cell-mediated immunity is relatively unaltered so that infections due to intracellular bacteria (e.g. *L. monocytogenes*) or viruses (including the herpes group of viruses, especially CMV) – such as those seen in transplant recipients – are relatively rare. Similarly, virally induced tumors such as those triggered by Epstein–Barr virus (EBV) are exceedingly rare in patients with hematologic malignancies.

Secondly, while the risk of infection is high during the neutropenic episodes, the risk is low when the leukocyte count is normal. The risk of infection persists in patients with profoundly altered cell-mediated immunity, such as that seen in transplant recipients.

Differences from center to center in the same and in different countries have been reported in the relative occurrence and frequency of Gram-positive and Gram-negative bacteria, as well as in the prevalence of *P. aeruginosa* and in the relative frequency of C. *albicans* compared with non-albicans species. Major differences between hospitals have also been observed in the incidence of nosocomial pathogens such as β-lactamase resistant staphylococci, vancomycin-resistant enterococci (VRE) and multiresistant Gram-negative bacteria. Furthermore, as already mentioned, differences may exist in the incidence of environmentally acquired infections such as *Aspergillus* or *Legionella*. Moreover, the country of origin is likely to influence the frequency of infection with pathogens such as *M. tuberculosis* and enteric protozoa such as *Cryptosporidium* and *Cyclospora*.

1.6 What is the appropriate approach to the initial evaluation and diagnosis of infection in patients with hematologic malignancies?

At present, available evaluation techniques do not produce sufficiently rapid results and are not sufficiently sensitive and specific to identify, or exclude, an infective cause for fever in neutropenic patients. Since such infectious episodes may be rapidly fatal, the patients must receive empirical antimicrobial therapy.

For the evaluation of a febrile patient with a hematologic malignancy, it is necessary to establish the risk category of the patient. For this reason, the relationship between the onset of the fever and the first day of the most recent course of cytotoxic therapy should be determined to permit prediction of the approximate duration of the neutropenia.

Granulocytopenic patients in whom infection is suspected require rigorous clinical examination. The mouth should be examined for vesicles and ulcers, and for gingivitis. The mouth and pharynx should also be examined for white patches and pseudomembranes, indicating the possible presence of *Candida*, or for erythema, mucositis, vesicles and ulcerations, indicating the possible presence of HSV infection. The anterior nares should be inspected for signs of congestion, rhinorrhea, crusts, bleeding and ulcers.

The skin often presents the features of a primary infection or lesions secondary to dissemination. Special attention should be paid to evidence of erythema, swelling, tenderness or discharge of the perioral, periungual and perianal skin. The presence of nodules, vesicles, pustules, crusts and ulcers should be recorded and the lesions should be cultured and monitored photographically.

Sites of cutaneous injury (needle punctures, catheter insertion sites, trauma) require special examination for evidence of infection.

Specimens for culture should be obtained during this examination from wherever potential for infection exists. At least two samples of blood should be taken from each patient. Cultures from a peripheral vein should be supplemented by samples from each catheter lumen if an indwelling catheter is present (see section 1.8). Entry sites of catheters should be examined for bacterial, nontuberculous mycobacterial and fungal pathogens.

Oral and pharyngeal lesions can be brushed or biopsied, as can suspected lesions of the paranasal sinuses. All abdominal complaints in neutropenic patients should be thoroughly investigated, with repeated stool cultures, plain radiography of the abdomen and CT, ultrasonography or magnetic resonance imaging (MRI), because of possible necrotizing enterocolitis. Stools from patients with diarrhea should be tested for *Clostridium difficile* toxin and cultured for bacterial species including *Clostridia*, *Salmonella*, *Shigella*, *Campylobacter*, *Aeromonas* and *Yersinia*, and protozoa such as *Cryptosporidium* spp. Care must be taken with diarrheal patients to prevent nosocomial transmission.

Urine cultures are worthwhile, especially if there are urinary symptoms or if the patient has been catheterized. Pyuria may be absent in neutropenic patients with urinary tract infection.

Cerebrospinal fluid (CSF) should be studied only if CNS infection is suspected on clinical grounds. The CSF should be cultured and stained for bacteria and fungi. White blood cells may be absent in neutropenic patients with meningitis. Similarly, if pleural and peritoneal effusions are present, samples should be aspirated, stained and cultured.

Considerable information can be derived from plain radiographs, CT, ultrasonographic or MRI scans of the lungs. In patients with neutropenia, the presence of focal infiltrates, especially cavitating, suggests possible fungal or tuberculous infection or bacterial abscess formation. The diagnosis should be confirmed, if the patient's condition permits, by bronchoalveolar lavage (BAL), transbronchial or transthoracic biopsy, or open lung biopsy. Sputum culture often gives false-positive or false-negative results. In patients with suspected lung infection studied in the EORTC–IATCG trials, microbiologic documentation of the cause of pneumonia was obtained by blood culture in 75%, from sputum culture in 13%, by BAL in 6% and from aspirated pleural fluid in 2%.

Even if the results of all tests are inconclusive, febrile neutropenic patients must receive immediate empirical treatment with broad-spectrum antibiotics.

In conclusion, before starting empirical therapy, each patient should undergo careful physical examination, radiography of the chest, urinalysis, blood cultures and swabbing, aspiration or biopsy of all sites of possible infection.

1.7 How should the evaluation be modified according to the severity of the risk?

Full evaluation may not be possible in patients at greatest risk from severe neutropenia, or from complications such as septicemia with shock, pneumonia, meningitis, or suspected intraabdominal complications such as typhlitis or intestinal perforation. These complications require treatment before extensive investigations are performed.

The estimated duration of the neutropenia can be obtained by relating the onset of the fever to the first day of the last course of chemotherapy. If a short duration of neutropenia is predicted, less extensive investigations are indicated than in patients with more predictably severe and prolonged neutropenia.

Thorough investigation, especially blood cultures, is also indicated in patients with neutropenia who are receiving treatment with high doses of steroids, since this treatment may further obscure the clinical features of infection and inflammation already lessened by the neutropenia.

1.8 What are the specific evaluation measures?

The techniques used for isolating infective pathogens are summarized in Part I, Chapter 2.

Bloodstream

Suspected bloodstream infections require investigation by blood culture. At least two specimens should be sent for culture and the examination should be repeated every 2–3 days, especially if the pyrexia persists. In the presence of an indwelling intravenous device, blood should be taken through each lumen of the catheter, as well as from a peripheral vein at a distal site. When Gram-negative bacteria are isolated, the organisms are causally related to the septicemia. The isolation of Gram-positive organisms, such as *S. epidermidis* or *C. jeikeium*, may be considered significant if cultures from different veins, at different times, are positive, unless the same organism is concomitantly isolated from another infected site. However, culture of *S. aureus*, *S. pneumoniae* and *E. faecalis* usually indicates significant infection. Similarly, isolation of viridans streptococci, such as *S. mitis* in patients with mucositis usually indicates significant infection, as does identification of fungemia.

Culture techniques

To detect bacteremia and fungemia, it is necessary to provide at least two samples of blood during 24 h. Single samples may be falsely negative, or alternatively positive from contamination. About 20–30 ml are required, with appropriately smaller volumes for children. The blood should not be diluted more than 5–10-fold when transferred into broth for culture. Although infections with anaerobes are infrequent, blood should still be incubated under aerobic and anaerobic conditions.

Five-day incubation is sufficient for detecting the majority of pathogens. Longer periods are necessary if infection by *Legionella* or *Brucella* is suspected.

Unfortunately, blood cultures require hours or days of incubation and therefore delay diagnosis, sometimes dangerously. Moreover, some pathogenic microorganisms do not grow in conventional cultures. For these reasons, empirical treatment should be initiated without delay in all neutropenic patients with fever and suspected infection.

Lower respiratory tract

Whenever a lower respiratory tract infection (LRTI) is suspected, it is necessary to carry out careful physical examination, including auscultation of the chest for the presence of rales, ronchi, wheezes, adventitious sounds, pleural friction rubs or signs of pleural effusion. However, since there may be no physical signs of a LRTI, radiographic studies are recommended with each febrile episode. Plain radiographs of the lung should be compared with previous films to identify focal and diffuse parenchymal changes. Further detection of changes involves CT or MRI of the thorax. Sputum should be examined microscopically and by culture but specimens of pulmonary secretions are best obtained by BAL. The absence of neutrophils on microscopic examination does not exclude pneumonia, since neutrophils are visible in only 10% of sputum samples from neutropenic patients with pneumonia. Focal or diffuse lesions require aspiration for culture and histologic examination. The samples can be obtained by BAL, transbronchial or transthoracic needle biopsy or by open lung biopsy if the condition of the patient permits. Serologic studies and polymerase chain reaction (PCR) analyses for viral, fungal and protozoal organisms may be clinically indicated.

Oropharynx

Specimens of smears and brushings from oral, gingival or pharyngeal lesions should be examined by direct staining and culture for bacteria, fungi and viruses. Ulcers, plaques, etc., may require biopsy with histologic studies. Serologic examination for viral infection may be indicated.

Paranasal sinuses

Brushings and endoscopically aspirated samples of secretions should be obtained and examined microscopically and by culture. The sinuses should be studied by CT or MRI for mucosal thickening, obliteration of the sinus lumen and bony erosions.

Skin and soft tissue

Discharge from skin lesions should be examined by staining and by culture for bacteria and fungi. Closed lesions may require needle aspiration or biopsy for histologic samples and material for culture. Serologic studies can help to identify viral pathogens.

Digestive tract

If esophageal symptoms (retrosternal discomfort, pain or dysphagia) are present, endoscopy should be considered, even in neutropenic patients. If there is concomitant thrombocytopenia, the procedure should be performed after platelet transfusion. If endoscopy is possible, samples of secretions and brushings should be cultured for bacteria, fungi and herpesviruses, and examined histologically.

In the presence of diarrhea, stools should be cultured. Special attention should be paid to the possibility of infection with C. *difficile*, by culture and by toxin assay. In neutropenic patients with diarrhea, sigmoidoscopy and colonoscopy are often contraindicated. If the development of typhlitis is suspected, ultrasonography, CT or MRI may show thickening of cecal and ascending colonic mucosa.

Perianal lesions with pain, induration, discharge and bleeding indicate the development of cellulitis. Smears and culture of discharge should be used to identify pathogens.

Liver
In addition to laboratory investigations, ultrasonographic examination and/or radiographic scans (CT, MRI) may show hepatic enlargement with or without focal lesions. These investigations are particularly useful when suspecting hepatosplenic candidiasis.

Urinary tract
Midstream specimens of urine, or of catheter drainage, should be cultured. Radiographic scans may show obstructing lesions or focal renal enlargement.

Cardiovascular system
Bloodstream infection may be associated with, or be the consequence of, endocarditis. The vegetations are demonstrable by transthoracic or transesophageal ultrasonography or CT/MRI.

Septic thrombophlebitis may be the consequence of indwelling catheters and give rise to severe bloodstream infections. The extent of the venous involvement can often be demonstrated by scan or Doppler ultrasonographic examination.

Skeletal system
When osteomyelitis is present, plain radiography and CT or MRI often show the focal lesions. Further information can be derived from technetium (^{99m}Tc) bone scans. The presence of focal suppuration may be demonstrable by use of ^{111}In-labeled white blood cell scans. Suspected septic arthritis, resulting from septicemia, must be confirmed by aspiration, with Gram staining and culture of the aspirate.

Central nervous system
Features of meningitis or focal or diffuse encephalitis require CT or MRI of the brain. Focal lesions may have to be biopsied. If intracranial pressure permits, CSF should be examined by culture, microscopy and serologic investigation.

1.9 What new developments are going to impact on emerging organisms, recognition, evaluation and diagnosis of infection in patients with hematologic malignancies?
The standard use of increasingly broad-spectrum antibiotics may result in the progressive prevalence of resistant bacteria and fungi and the increasing occurrence of infections by opportunistic pathogens.

Emergence of resistant organisms appears to have marked local differences in pattern, depending in part on local antibiotic-prescribing regimens. More and more centers are reporting the presence of β-lactam- and, recently, vancomycin-resistant staphylococci, vancomycin-resistant enterococci, extended-spectrum β-lactamase-producing K. *pneumoniae* and E. *coli* and quinolone-resistant Gram-negative bacteria, such as E. *coli*. The frequent isolation of multidrug-resistant viridans streptococci and *S. pneumoniae* also presents major therapeutic problems, as do organisms producing enzymes that inactivate carbapenems (e.g. *P. aeruginosa*, *Stenotrophomonas maltophilia* and *Acinetobacter* spp.). Among viral infections, CMV and some of the recently identified organisms such as human herpesvirus–6 (HHV-6), HHV-7 and HHV-8 are likely to be recognized as pathogens causing morbidity in neutropenic patients.

The presence of neutropenia also presents an opportunity for the establishment of infection by one of the ubiquitous fungal species in the internal or external environment. Often, these fungal infections are with normally uncommon species including *Fusarium* spp., *Acremonium* spp., *Malassezia furfur* and dematiaceous fungi, or with common species that have become resistant to antifungal agents (such as azoles) including *Candida* spp. Infections with the latter sometimes originate in catheters and include fungi such as C. *parapsilosis*, C. *krusei*, C. *glabrata* and C. *tropicalis*.

The new diagnostic techniques described in Part I, Chapter 2, section 2.1 promise to improve the sensitivity and speed of diagnosis. Two areas that are particularly promising include enzyme-linked immunoabsorbent assays, using antigens from pathogens such as those involved in invasive aspergillosis. This assay, which detects cell wall constituents, released during growth, is sensitive and specific and permits early detection of *Aspergillus* infections and can also be used to monitor treatment. The other very promising technique involves pathogen-specific PCR. This technique is proving valuable in the early diagnosis of, for example, CMV infection. Positive test results before or during treatment are an indication for prophylactic therapy.

The indication for and implications of new imaging techniques in the diagnosis and assessment of the impact of infections in neutropenic patients are provided in Part I, Chapter 2, section 2.2.

2 REGARDING THE RISK FACTORS ACCOMPANYING HEMATOLOGIC MALIGNANCIES

2.1 What are the main alteration in host defense mechanisms and what are the appropriate investigations to document them?

The clinical presentation of infection in patients with hematologic malignancies depends, in part, on whether the infection is associated with granulocytopenia or reflects defects of the anatomic barriers or of cell-mediated or humoral immunity.

Anatomic barriers

Infection in immunocompromised patients is often iatrogenic, due to injury of skin and respiratory or alimentary mucosa. In addition to generalized breaches of the cutaneous mucosal barrier, focal intervention with urethral, nasogastric and intravenous indwelling catheters, bone marrow aspiration, endoscopy and surgery can disrupt anatomic barriers and result in disseminated infections.

Infections are also likely if there is obstruction of tubal organs or ducts. For example, obstruction of the eustachian tubes by adenoids involved in hematologic malignancies may result in otitis media, while biliary tract obstruction by lymph nodes may result in ascending cholangitis.

The infecting organisms tend to be those that colonize locally but which become pathogenic with breaks in the mucosal or cutaneous barriers, with ciliary dysfunction or with tubal obstruction. The combination of anatomic damage and absence of granulocytes permits rapid progression of local invasion and dissemination.

Phagocytes (see also section 1.4)

Granulocytopenia is found especially in patients with acute leukemia and after treatment with myelosuppressive drugs or irradiation. Thus, patients with nonlymphocytic leukemia who have remission-inducing treatment usually have a neutrophil count of less than $100/mm^3$ for 15–20 days, as have patients undergoing bone marrow transplantation. For comparison, the neutropenia produced during treatment of solid tumors usually lasts for less than 10 days.

If neutropenia lasts less than 7 days, the risk of infection is low and 95% of patients respond to the initial choice of empirical treatment without the need for modifications. On the other hand, patients with neutropenia for more than 14 days are at high risk of infection and often suffer recurrence of primary infection or of secondary infections. Persistence of neutropenia may also reflect refractoriness to antineoplastic treatment.

Granulocytopenia predisposes to infection especially when associated with other factors, such as mucosal damage from antineoplastic drugs or skin damage from needles or intravenous catheters, as well as tubal obstruction (e.g. adenoidal involvement in malignancy giving rise to otitis media). In addition to the quantitative abnormalities of the granulocytes in patients with hematologic malignancies, these patients also often have qualitative abnormalities of leukocyte function, especially after treatment with corticosteroids, antineoplastic drugs and irradiation. Decreased macrophage function also interferes with the immune response because these cells, when activated, are the source of cytokines. Cytokines exert multiple biologic effects and play a critical role in host defenses against infections by activating both the innate and adaptive limbs of the immune system. Activated macrophages also represent a defense against intracellular organisms.

Immunoglobulins and complement

Humoral immunity is primarily mediated by B-cell lymphocytes and is abnormal in chronic lymphatic leukemia, Hodgkin disease and multiple myeloma. There is usually an inability to produce antigen-specific neutralizing antibodies against pathogenic organisms in untreated patients with these diseases. Patients with defective humoral immunity and defective antibody production suffer from increased susceptibility to pyogenic infection, even if they are not neutropenic. Patients are also susceptible to infection with encapsulated bacteria, such as S. pneumoniae, H. influenzae and N. meningitidis (see Part I, Chapter 1, Table 1.2).

In patients who do not have circulating opsonizing antibodies to encapsulated bacteria, the activity of all phagocytic cells is impaired. Thus, in patients with multiple myeloma, there is an increased risk of infection with S. pneumoniae or H. influenzae as a result of defective production of polyclonal immunoglobulins. Patients with chronic lymphatic leukemia also often have hypogammaglobulinemia and suffer from infections by these organisms.

Cell-mediated immunity

In patients with leukemia without neutropenia, altered cell-mediated immunity secondary to the underlying disease or to drugs such as antineoplastic chemotherapy or corticosteroids, can predispose to infection. In some conditions (e.g. Hodgkin disease) cellular immune dysfunction is associated with the disease. In these diseases, and especially after specific immunosuppressive treatment, for example to keep acute leukemia in remission or after bone marrow transplantation, there is defective function of the T lymphocytes or of the mononuclear phagocyte system, which results in increased susceptibility to infection. The intensity and duration of the immunosuppressive therapy determine the frequency of infection. Similarly, patients (especially children) who have undergone splenectomy are predisposed to infections by encapsulated bacteria such as S.

pneumoniae or *H. influenzae*. If fever or other features of infection occur in these patients, immediate treatment becomes necessary.

The pathogens that infect patients with impaired cell-mediated immunity are listed in (see Part I, Chapter 1, section 1.2). There is increase in viral (HSV, VZV, EBV, CMV) and fungal infection (*Candida*, disseminated cryptococcosis), and infection by intracellularly replicating bacteria (e.g. *Legionella* or *Salmonella* spp.).

After irradiation of patients with Hodgkin disease, approximately one quarter develop VZV infection. In children with acute leukemias receiving maintenance chemotherapy, approximately 20% become infected with *P. carinii*. In patients with non-Hodgkin lymphoma receiving cytotoxic therapy, *M. avium* infection may occur, while patients with hairy cell leukemia tend to suffer from infection with *M. kansasii*. In these patients, *L. monocytogenes* and *C. neoformans* can also be isolated from blood cultures.

2.2 What are the alterations due to iatrogenic factors?

Chemotherapy
In patients with hematologic malignancies chemotherapy affects host defenses in two major ways.

Alteration of function and integrity of mucosal surfaces
Chemotherapy alters the function (ciliary function in the respiratory tract, motility in the digestive tract) and the integrity of the mucosal surfaces that normally prevent the resident microbial flora from invading the underlying tissues. In addition, daily patient care and indwelling catheters (e.g. venapuncture), provide further tissue and bloodstream access to microorganisms.

Depletion or alteration of cells responsible for host defenses
Chemotherapy depletes and/or alters the cells responsible for combating these pathogens. Furthermore, chemotherapy and steroids may alter cell-mediated immunity, albeit to a lesser degree than in transplant patients. These changes may reactivate latent infections due to intracellular pathogens (e.g. *P. carinii*, *M. tuberculosis*, herpesviruses), or may render patients more susceptible to such infections (*L. pneumophila*, *Candida* spp.).

Antimicrobials
The extensive use in these patients of antimicrobials (both antibacterial and antifungal agents) contributes to the selection of resistant organisms. For example, the increased incidence of streptococcal bacteremia in patients receiving ciprofloxacin prophylaxis may result from the selection of these relatively ciprofloxacin-resistant species. Similarly, fluconazole prophylaxis may select for *C. krusei* or *C. glabrata* colonization and dissemination. In addition, broad-spectrum β-lactam antibiotics may suppress the 'colonization-resistance' (against pathogens) attributable to the normal anaerobic flora, so permitting overgrowth and eventual invasion by both Gram-negative (*E. coli*, and other Enterobacteriaceae, *P. aeruginosa*) and Gram-positive organisms, or by *Candida* spp.

2.3 What is the influence of environmental factors?

Community
While most infections in neutropenic patients are derived from the patient's endogenous flora, viruses that cause respiratory infection or VZV infection may be transmitted by ill

family members or visitors (or hospital staff). Dust and air contaminated by *Aspergillus* spores (e.g. from nearby construction sites) are major sources of infection by this fungus in immunocompromised patients.

Hospital

Hospital-acquired pathogens are derived from the air through ventilation systems and air conditioning. Pathogens are also transmitted in hospital by food and water. Infusion equipment may provide the source of infection, as may intravenous solutions, blood products, catheter and drainage tubes, endoscopes and pressure tapes.

However, human vectors are the most important source of nosocomial infection, with pathogens transmitted by hospital personnel and visitors, but also by water, food, flowers and soap. The organisms most commonly involved include Enterobacteriaceae, *Pseudomonas* spp. and staphylococci.

It has been estimated that within 1 day of admission to the hospital, approximately one half of the endogenous flora of skin and gut of neutropenic patients becomes altered, with aerobic Gram-negative organisms replacing the usual aerobic Gram-positive and anaerobic bacteria. The hospital-acquired flora also includes coagulase-negative staphylococci which have become resistant to β-lactam antibiotics (and therefore require vancomycin for treatment). α-Hemolytic streptococci have also become ubiquitous, with *S. mitis* and *S. sanguis* most common. Vancomycin-resistant and aminoglycoside-resistant strains, refractory to antibiotics, are common causes of nosocomial infections affecting neutropenic patients in some centers.

Enterococci (*E. faecalis*, *E. faecium*) have recently appeared as virulent, difficult to treat, nosocomial pathogens, having acquired antibiotic resistance by transfer of plasmids.

Anaerobes are responsible for about 5% of bloodstream infections and also contribute to the mixed infections in the mouth and perianal areas of neutropenic patients. The dominant organisms involved in these infections include clostridial species (e.g. *C. perfringens*, *C. septicum* and *C. tertium*). Some of these strains are resistant to clindamycin and metronidazole. Nosocomial infection with *C. difficile* (resulting in necrotizing enterocolitis) has become a significant risk in some centers.

In immunocompromised patients with prolonged neutropenia who have received broad-spectrum antibiotics, hospital-acquired fungal infections are common. Fungi found in these patients include *Candida* and *Aspergillus* spp., although *Mucor* spp., *Phycomycetes* and *C. neoformans* may also be found, the latter especially in patients with lymphoma.

Water and food

Food and water can transmit infections to neutropenic patients. Water, directly from the tap, in the form of ice, or aerosolized by vaporizers, humidifiers or from showers can also transmit organisms pathogenic to neutropenic patients. Pathogens can also be found in sink drains, toilets, showerheads and baths. The principal waterborne pathogens include Enterobacteriaceae, *Pseudomonas* spp. and *Klebsiella* spp., as well as cryptosporidiosis from contaminated water, and possibly *Aspergillus*, as recently reported. Moreover, *Legionella* may contaminate the hot water systems and can be responsible for significant morbidity and mortality in hospitals, particularly in immunocompromised patients.

Foods that may transmit pathogens include dairy products, fresh fruit and vegetables, and uncooked or unprocessed meat. Organisms transmitted in this manner may include Enterobacteriaceae, *Pseudomonas* spp., *Klebsiella* spp., *Listeria* spp., staphylococci, streptococci, *Salmonella* spp., *Campylobacter* and *Toxoplasma gondii* in western Europe. While food presents little risk to immunocompromised patients when satisfactorily handled and prepared, infections may be also be derived from the ingestion of large amounts of naturopathic preparations which can contain fungal species.

Region or country
During the past three or four decades there have been marked changes in the types of microorganisms infecting neutropenic patients. In the 1940s and 1950s, before the widespread use of antibiotics, *S. aureus* was the pathogen most frequently isolated from neutropenic patients. After the β-lactamase-resistant antistaphylococcal antibiotics became available, Gram-negative organisms (*P. aeruginosa*, *E. coli*, *Klebsiella* spp.) became predominant. Subsequently, during the past decade, the incidence of *P. aeruginosa* infections has decreased, to be replaced by infections with Gram-negative bacteria resistant to multiple antibiotics (e.g. *Klebsiella* spp., *Enterobacter* spp., *Serratia*). In addition, Gram-positive cocci (*S. aureus*, viridans group streptococci, coagulase-negative staphylococci) have been frequently found. Indeed, during the decades from 1970 to 1990, there has been a 50-fold increase in viridans streptococcal septicemia in neutropenic patients, now accounting for approximately 40% of all bacteremias in some cancer centers. It seems that the risk of streptococcal infections is increased by the use of antacids or gastric secretory inhibitors, and by prophylaxis with fluoroquinolones. These streptococci are similar to the strains found in the normal oropharynx, but may have acquired resistance to penicillin.

2.4 What are the most significant factors that contribute to the risk of infection in patients with hematologic malignancies
Refer to section 2.2.

2.5 What are the specific or nonspecific measures aimed at minimizing each of these factors?

Nonspecific measures
Measures to prevent infection play an important part in lessening the risk of infection for neutropenic patients. Thus, it is important to reduce the acquisition of pathogenic flora by avoiding factors responsible for nosocomial infection. Special emphasis should be placed on careful handwashing. Effective handwashing can lessen or stop transmission of many community and hospital-acquired infections. Education of patients, family members and staff is essential. Contact with staff or visitors with overt respiratory or cutaneous infections must be avoided. The patient should receive a well-cooked, low microbial diet and have a safe water supply. Ice should not be consumed, unless prepared from a safe water supply. For patients with severe neutropenia, air filtration may be desirable in settings where *Aspergillus* infections are observed with a high incidence. When a total protective environment is required, clean air is provided by means of constant positive-pressure air flow. In addition, it is sometimes necessary to employ an intensive regimen to disinfect the patients, including oral non-absorbable antibiotics, antibiotic ointments and sprays, and provision of a low microbial diet.

    Extreme care should be taken with the insertion and management of vascular access catheters, in performing bone marrow aspiration, and in the siting and management of urethral and nasogastric catheters and tubes. These devices should be used only if essential and not for the convenience of healthcare staff. It is also important to ensure that blood and infusion products are free from infectious agents.

Specific measures
Attempts have been made to suppress colonization by pathogens using prophylactic antimicrobial therapy. Thus, fluoroquinolones have been administered long term to prevent (or preempt) infection with Gram-negative aerobes; penicillin has been used to prevent infection by streptococci; trimethoprim–sulfamethoxazole (TMP–SMX) has been given to prevent infection with *P. carinii*; fluconazole has been employed in an attempt to prevent infection with *Candida* spp.; while acyclovir has been used for HSV prophylaxis, especially in seropositive patients (see section 4.1).

2.6 Are there different levels of risk of infection recognized for patients with hematologic malignancies?
Refer to section 1.4.

2.7 How does the level of risk impact on management?
Clearly, different levels of risk have been recognized in patients with hematologic malignancies, and these impact on management (see section 1.4).

Surveillance measures
While it is widely recognized that routine surveillance cultures are not cost-effective (see section 3.2), they may be indicated in some patients at high risk and likely to be colonized with highly resistant organisms [methicillin-resistant *S. aureus* (MRSA), VRE, multidrug-resistant Gram-negative bacilli], or in institutions with a high incidence of *Aspergillus* infections, where preventive measures may be considered suitable for patients with positive nasal swabs.

Serologic testing for herpesviruses continues to provide valuable information. Indeed, patients with positive serology findings, who are at risk from developing mucositis and neutropenia, are candidates for acyclovir prophylaxis (see section 4.1). In addition, routine serial blood cultures are recommended in some centers for patients receiving high-dose corticosteroid treatment because fever and other features of infection may be suppressed. Repeat chest radiography may identify early asymptomatic infection with *Aspergillus* or *P. carinii*.

Preventive measures
If possible, prevention of infection is always better than the cure. Indeed, acyclovir prophylaxis is used in HSV seropositive patients to prevent reactivation during antineoplastic treatment or in otherwise immunosuppressed patients to prevent the development of mucositis and thereby to lessen the chance of bacterial and fungal superinfection. Prophylaxis of VZV is usually contraindicated because the risk of disseminated disease is low, except in patients with severe immunosuppression or recurrent zoster. However, if a seronegative (or clinically naive) immunocompromised individual is exposed to someone with varicella zoster immune globulin (VZIG) should be administered within 48–72 h.

Chemoprophylaxis with TMP–SMX to prevent *P. carinii* pneumonia and with fluoroquinolones to prevent bacterial infections has been used extensively. While such measures are certainly not recommended in low-risk patients, their use might benefit high-risk patients (see section 4.1), but the overall benefit is questionable in view of the great risk of promoting the development of bacterial resistance. Indeed, the IDSA does not recommend the routine use of fluoroquinolones for prophylaxis against bacterial infection.

High-risk patients with profound and long-lasting episodes of neutropenia are also candidates for prophylactic treatment with growth factors (see section 4.1).

Therapeutic measures
The level of risk has its major impact on therapeutic measures (see section 5.1). Indeed, it may soon be possible to manage low-risk patients suspected of suffering from infection in an outpatient setting, with oral antibiotics. Until then a somewhat more cautious approach involves hospitalization of these patients and starting treatment with parenteral antibiotics until a response is obtained, with subsequent discharge of the patient while continuing treatment with oral antibiotics. However, to date, there is no validation of the safety of home therapy for these patients. On the other hand, high-risk patients need hospitalization and broad-spectrum parenteral antibiotics, which often have to be continued (even if there is clinical response to treatment) until recovery in neutrophil numbers.

2.8 What new developments are going to impact on minimizing or suppressing the specific risk factors?

Growth factors and neutropenia
The use of growth factors in patients with hematologic malignancies has not been studied as extensively as in patients with solid tumors, partly out of fear that these agents may promote the proliferation of malignant cells. One of the most controversial issues concerning their use relates to their cost-effectiveness and whether they have any real impact on the morbidity and mortality from infection. Underlying their use is the hope that growth factors may significantly lessen the duration and severity of neutropenia, thus reducing the risks for neutropenic patients and permitting simplification of the anti-infection strategies (see section 4.1). The most recent recommendation from an advisory panel appointed by the American Society of Clinical Oncology (ASCO) even further limits the appropriate use of hematopoietic colony-stimulating factor.

Growth factors and thrombocytopenia
Several growth factors and cytokines have been shown in vitro and in vivo to stimulate platelet production by bone marrow precursors, and their use in patients has given promising results, although indications are not yet fully established. However, the use of granulocyte–macrophage colony-stimulating factor (GM-CSF) has been associated with the development of thrombocytopenia in certain patient populations.

Growth factors and mucositis
Several growth factors [e.g. keratinocyte growth factor (KGF)] and cytokines [e.g. interleukin-2 (IL-2), IL-15] have potent stimulatory activity on mucosal regenerating capacity and are being studied for clinical use. It seems possible that, if successful, their use may profoundly impact on the management of patients with hematologic malignancies.

Predictive markers of infection
At present, one of the key questions in the management of a suspected infection in a neutropenic patient with a hematologic malignancy is to define the level of risk in that patient, so as to provide the best possible coverage for the infection. Thus, 'risk scores' have been proposed, and many studies are underway with the aim of predicting more accurately which patients are likely to have severe or mild infections. However, this approach is likely to remain unsatisfactory in any given patient because the 'risk scores' will always be derived from observations in large cohorts of patients.

An alternative approach is to define so-called 'surrogate markers' which can predict more accurately which patient is particularly at risk. This possibility is being investigated by measuring levels of cytokines such as IL-6, or tumor necrosis factor (TNF), and pro-hormones such as procalcitonin.

In addition, in the future, genomic microbiologic methods may permit the detection of minute quantities of pathogens. However, such techniques will probably always be of only limited use for predicting infection because of the difficulty in differentiating the 'innocent bystander' from the 'true disease-causing pathogen'.

3 REGARDING THE SURVEILLANCE OF PATIENTS WITH HEMATOLOGIC MALIGNANCIES

3.2 What are the surveillance measures to be taken when a patient presents with hematologic malignancy? (see also section 2.7)

The clinical benefits of surveillance cultures have been questioned, and they are now considered to be of only limited use because no single organism found at a given site is consistently predictive, either of the course of an infection in neutropenic patients or of the likelihood of a focal or disseminated infective process. For example, multiple organisms, all potential pathogens in a neutropenic patient, are often identified on surveillance culture, while the actual pathogen responsible for a focal or systemic infection is not isolated. Alternatively, it is not uncommon that the detailed results of surveillance cultures become available only after the results of blood culture. For these reasons, the initial management of pyrexia in a neutropenic patient involves empirical treatment with a broad-spectrum antibiotic, whatever the results of surveillance cultures.

In contrast to surveillance cultures, which are not recommended, a detailed knowledge of the hospital epidemiology with respect to nosocomial antimicrobial-resistant organisms such as MRSA, VRE, extended-spectrum β-lactamase-producing Gram-negative bacteria, C. *krusei* or C. *glabrata* is mandatory so that adequate antimicrobial coverage can be offered to neutropenic patients in such units.

It is critical that a patient, when first presenting with a hematologic malignancy, should be investigated thoroughly to evaluate the risk of infection, such as:

- History of travel to, or residence in, an endemic area (for tuberculosis, endemic mycoses, parasitoses such as, for example, leishmaniasis or *Strongyloides*).
- Previous operative procedures and implantation of prosthetic devices
- Immunization history (and use of repeated vaccines, if necessary, such as pneumococcal vaccine before splenectomy)
- Extensive serologic testing for latent viral infections such as HSV, VZV, CMV (and perhaps in the future HHV-6 and HHV-8), as well as parasitic infections (*T. gondii*).

It is necessary to emphasize that serologic and/or other immunologic tests aimed at measuring an immunologic response to an actual or recent infection are unlikely to be of much help because of the profound intrinsic or iatrogenic immune suppression in patients with hematologic malignances.

4 REGARDING THE PREVENTION OF INFECTION IN PATIENTS WITH HEMATOLOGIC MALIGNANCIES

4.1 What approaches, if any, to the prevention of infection should be considered in patients with hematologic malignancies?

Before starting chemotherapy, serologic tests are required to determine whether a patient with hematologic malignancy has been exposed to HSV, VZV or CMV infection.

Since antineoplastic treatment may reactivate this type of infection, acyclovir prophylaxis is recommended for HSV seropositive individuals who are going to receive treatment that is likely to produce mucositis. Acyclovir is recommended in a dose of 250 mg/m^2 twice daily orally or intravenously. Alternatively, oral valacyclovir can be used. Prophylaxis or preemptive treatment to prevent reactivation of VZV infection requires high-dose acyclovir. In patients who are seronegative for CMV infection, blood products should be screened and only seronegative blood should be used whenever feasible.

In some centers, it is recommended that patients who are granulocytopenic or whose treatment is likely to produce granulocytopenia and who are receiving high-dose corticosteroids should have blood taken repeatedly for serial blood cultures, even in the absence of fever, since these patients may not develop fever even if they suffer from bacteremia.

Considerable controversy still pervades the topic of prophylactic antibacterial antibiotics. Oral nonabsorbable antibiotics have been used in an attempt to achieve alimentary decontamination, since the gut is the source of many of the infections in granulocytopenic patients. However, the use of antibiotics such as vancomycin, gentamicin, polymixin B, nystatin or colistin is associated with many problems. These antibiotics are nonpalatable and poorly tolerated (especially when antineoplastic therapy causes emesis), so that there is poor compliance. Moreover, use of these antibiotics for prophylaxis permits the development of bacterial resistance to, for example, vancomycin, so that prophylaxis with these antibiotics should now be abandoned.

Alternatively, attempts have been made to decontaminate 'selectively' the alimentary tract, using antibiotics such as TMP–SMX to retain the anaerobic flora and thereby to preserve the 'colonization resistance' against aerobic bacteria and fungi. Unfortunately, the efficacy of this type of treatment has not been defined because, although initial results showed decreased infections in granulocytopenic patients, follow-up results have been contradictory. Moreover, TMP–SMX may prolong the duration of the granulocytopenia and may also be followed by the emergence of resistant organisms.

Fluoroquinolones, such as ciprofloxacin, have been used for prophylaxis and may delay the onset of fever in neutropenic patients. Fluoroquinolones reduce the rate of Gram-negative bacteremia, probably at the expense of breakthrough infection by Gram-positive cocci. The emergence of fluoroquinolone-resistant bacteria has also been reported. The use of 'extended-spectrum' fluoroquinolones with extensive activity against Gram-positive bacteria has not been thoroughly evaluated and compared, for instance, with growth factors or placebo. At present, quinolone prophylaxis should be reserved for patients at high risk of developing Gram-negative bacteremia. Other clinicians consider that the use of quinolones for prophylaxis should be discouraged and avoided.

Patients in whom surveillance cultures show heavy colonization with *Candida* may benefit from prophylactic fluconazole. Such treatment (400 mg daily) has been shown to prevent infection with *C. albicans* and *C. tropicalis* in allogenic bone marrow transplant patients, but does not prevent infection with *C. krusei*, and has uncertain activity against *C. glabrata*. The use of prophylactic fluconazole in patients with hematologic malignancies not undergoing bone marrow transplantation is controversial. Indeed, even prophylaxis with ketoconazole, amphotericin B or fluconazole has not resulted in a definite decrease of invasive fungal disease. Moreover, in some centers there has been a shift to infection by more resistant fungal organisms, so that prophylactic antifungal treatment may eradicate *C. albicans* but permits overgrowth and invasion by *Aspergillus*, *C. krusei* and *C. glabrata*. In centers where *P. carinii* is prevalent, prophylactic treatment with TMP–SMX has been extremely useful in reducing the incidence of this infection.

Hematopoietic colony-stimulating factors

During the last decade, the use of CSFs has had a significant impact on the management of patients with cancer. The CSFs have been given to reduce the complications associated with chemotherapy-induced neutropenia. Recommendations for the use of CSFs were published in 1994 by the American Society for Clinical Oncology, and updated in 1996, 1997 and 2000.

Several studies have examined the role of granulocyte colony-stimulating factor (G-CSF, filgrastim) and GM-CSF in the treatment of patients with hematologic malignancies. Three main goals have been pursued: (1) to accelerate hematopoietic recovery and prevent the development of infectious complications; (2) to exert a priming effect and sensitize leukemic cells to the effect of chemotherapy; and (3) to induce differentiation of the leukemic cells.

Overall, the results of the clinical trials conducted in patients with acute myeloid leukemia have been fairly homogenous and have shown that treatment with G-CSF or GM-CSF either concomitantly with or shortly after chemotherapy, moderately shortens the duration of neutropenia. A reduction of the infectious complications of neutropenia, which resulted in reduced antibiotic use and duration of hospitalization, was noted in some, but not all, of these studies. CSFs were found significantly to increase neutrophil counts without leukemogenic effect in neutropenic patients with myelodysplastic syndromes. Intermittent administration of CSFs might be a therapeutic option in patients with profound neutropenia and recurrent infection.

At the present time, there are no data to support the prophylactic use of CSFs in afebrile neutropenic patients. Moreover, the available data do not support the routine adjunctive use of G-CSF or GM-CSF therapy in febrile neutropenic patients. Overall response rates and long-term outcome of patients with acute myeloid leukemia were not affected by the use of G-CSF or GM-CSF, reflecting the lack of beneficial (i.e. priming effect) or detrimental (i.e. stimulation of leukemic clones) effects. Yet, high-risk patients with profound, long-lasting neutropenia and severe infections, such as persistent Gram-negative bacteremia (with or without shock) and pneumonia, or patients with fungal infections (systemic candidiasis or aspergillosis) may occasionally benefit from the administration of CSFs, even though there also is no definitive evidence to support their use under such conditions.

However, it is worth emphasizing that G-CSF and GM-CSF have been coincidentally found to reduce the severity and duration of mucositis in patients with advanced head and neck cancer, sarcoma, or allogeneic bone marrow transplantation, and in children undergoing stem cell transplantation. This action represents another mechanism by which these agents may decrease the incidence of infection. The capacity of other growth factors (KGF) or 'cytoprotective' agents (amifostine, glutamine, sucralfate) either to prevent or to reduce the severity of mucositis is under investigation.

Intravenous immunoglobulins do not benefit neutropenic patients but may help patients with antibody deficiencies, such as patients with chronic lymphatic leukemia or multiple myeloma.

4.2 What are the future challenges and opportunities for reducing the risk of infection?

Refer to sections 2.8 and 4.1 regarding hematopoietic CSFs.

One of the greatest challenges in the management of granulocytopenic patients is the prevention and treatment of infection by *Aspergillus*. It is essential to develop diagnostic techniques for the identification of individuals at risk from this type of fungal infection, since there is at present no satisfactory treatment.

Techniques are required that will permit less generalized use of antibiotics, in order to decrease the development of antibiotic resistance, as well as decreasing the risk of super-infection by antibiotic-selected bacteria and fungi.

It is also necessary to develop more powerful broad-spectrum antibiotics that are active orally and which can be used for ambulant outpatient therapy, thus avoiding the need for hospitalization and the risk of nosocomial infection.

5 REGARDING THE TREATMENT OF PATIENTS WITH HEMATOLOGIC MALIGNANCIES

5.1 What is the role of empirical therapy?

High-risk patients

In high-risk patients with severe prolonged granulocytopenia, the institution of empirical therapy is indicated as an emergency at the first sign of fever or other suspicion of infection. Indeed, before the concept of empirical therapy was developed, infection – with or without hemorrhage – was the cause of death in 50–80% of neutropenic patients with leukemia and in approximately 50% of those with malignant lymphoma. The institution of empirical treatment is mandatory because currently available diagnostic techniques do not yield diagnoses that are sufficiently rapid, or sufficiently sensitive and specific, for identifying or excluding the microbiologic cause of the fever which may, if untreated, be rapidly fatal. Empirical treatment must be based on consideration of the most likely infecting pathogens, taking into account local epidemiologic factors. This is in contrast to antimicrobial treatment of nonneutropenic patients with defective cell-mediated immunity, for whom immediate empiric antibiotic therapy is necessary only if the patient has undergone splenectomy. Otherwise, the specific etiologic infecting agent should be aggressively sought before starting treatment.

In determining whether or not empirical therapy is required for patients with postulated neutropenia, it is necessary to determine the rate at which the granulocyte count is expected to decrease to less than $100/mm^3$, as well as the presence or absence of disrupted mucosal barriers. Undoubtedly, patients will benefit from empirical treatment if the neutrophil count decreases rapidly and/or if there is mucosal or cutaneous damage.

The nature of the empirical treatment is also determined by the duration of the neutropenia and by the severity of the infection and the incidence of complications. If the neutropenia is likely to last longer than 10 days, the risk of infections and complications increases proportionally (see section 1.9). If the neutropenia lasts less than 7–10 days, the risk to the patient is low and the outcome is usually uncomplicated (Figure 4.2).

In high-risk patients, empirical antibiotic therapy, whether combination therapy or monotherapy, should be given parenterally. At least 3 days of empirical treatment are necessary to assess the efficacy of the initial therapy (Figure 4.3). If a specific causal organism is identified during the first 3 days, the treatment can be changed accordingly

Low-risk patients

In low-risk patients, with a short duration of neutropenia and no mucosal or cutaneous damage, there may be no need for aggressive intravenous antibiotic combination regimens (Figure 4.2). Several alternative cheaper and more convenient (to both the patient and healthcare staff) dosing schedules have been used. Two recent reports demonstrate the safety of such orally administered antibiotics compared with parenteral agents, although their safety in the home setting remains to be validated (Table 4.6).

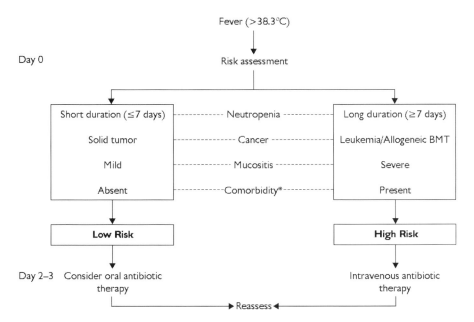

Figure 4.2 Risk assessment in neutropenic patients. *See Table 4.5.

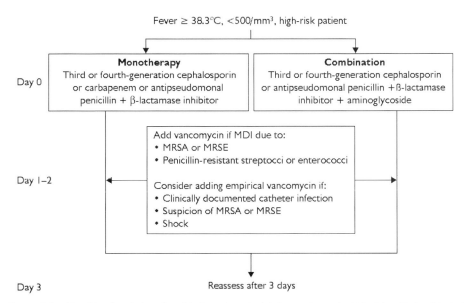

Figure 4.3 Algorithm for choice of antibiotic regimen in febrile, neutropenic, high-risk patients. Adapted from Hughes et al (1997).

Thus, in low-risk neutropenic patients without a clinical focus of infection, monotherapy can be given to the patients provided they are monitored for response, for the development of secondary infection, for the emergence of resistant organisms and for adverse reactions. Such treatment requires good compliance and careful supervision. Oral treatment can be used only if patients are able to swallow tablets and have an intact aliment-

Table 4.6 Antibiotic dosing regimens for low-risk neutropenic patients

Regimen	Details
Monotherapy	Extended-spectrum intravenous antibiotic agents such as third- or fourth-generation cephalosporins or carbapenems, which can be administered on an outpatient basis
Combination therapy	Single daily dosing with an intravenous combination, such as ceftriaxone plus amikacin
Sequential intravenous to oral therapy or initial oral therapy*	Broad-spectrum antibiotic combinations, such as a fluoroquinolone (e.g. ciprofloxacin) plus a β-lactam (e.g. amoxycillin–clavulanate)

* Two recent reports have demonstrated the efficacy and safety of such orally administered antibiotics in comparison with parenteral agents.

ary tract. These patients must not take antacids since divalent cations interfere with antibiotic absorption.

What considerations should direct the choice of antimicrobials?

There has been much discussion regarding the components of antibiotic regimens for the empirical treatment of febrile neutropenic patients. Approximately 80% of the pathogens isolated in febrile episodes in granulocytopenic patients are bacteria. The initial infection is usually caused by either Gram-positive or Gram-negative bacteria, or both, so that the empirical regimen must be broad spectrum, attaining high bactericidal levels in blood and tissues, must be nontoxic and simple to use. Following the widespread use of effective empirical treatment, the overall survival rate of febrile neutropenic patients has been greater than 90%.

For more than two decades, the combination of two or more antibiotics has been described as the 'gold standard' of empirical antibiotic therapy (Table 4.7). The most commonly used combination included an aminoglycoside plus a β-lactam. For example, a popular treatment combination has included the aminoglycoside amikacin and a cephalosporin (ceftazidime). Recently, it has been shown that the combination of piperacillin plus tazobactam and amikacin is also effective, as is the combination of a fourth-generation cephalosporin (cefepime and cefpirome) and an aminoglycoside. The disadvantage of such treatment regimens is that the combination of antibiotics may give rise to toxicologic problems, especially as aminoglycosides are nephrotoxic and ototoxic, and therefore require monitoring of serum levels. Moreover, the preparation and administration of multidrug regimens present technical problems. With the recent increase in Gram-positive coccal and because, in many centers, S. aureus and S. epidermidis infections have become methicillin resistant, vancomycin has increasingly been added to empirical combination antibiotic regimens (see Figure 4.3). Moreover, infections with enterococci and α-hemolytic streptococci have recently increased in frequency, thus rendering the empirical use of vancomycin common in some institutions. However, when these conditions are not present, empirical vancomycin should not be employed.

In an effort to simplify the empirical antibiotic regimens, use has been made of monotherapy with third- and fourth-generation cephalosporins, as well as with carbapenems and most recently with antipseudomonal penicillin and β-lactamase inhibitor (Table 4.7). These antibiotics provide sufficient antibacterial cover to make them suitable for use as monotherapy. There have been many comparisons between single antibiotics and combination regimens. Overall, it has been concluded that monotherapy with modern broad-spectrum antibiotics is often as effective as combination treatment, pro-

Table 4.7 Choices of empirical antibiotic therapy for febrile neutropenic high-risk patients

Regimen	Details
Monotherapy	Third- or fourth-generation cephalosporins
	Carbapenems
	Antipseudomonal carboxypenicillins or ureidopenicillins + β-lactamase inhibitor
Two-drug regimens without a glycopeptide	Third- or fourth-generation cephalosporins + aminoglycoside
	Carbapenem + aminoglycoside
	Antipseudomonal carboxypenicillins or ureidopenicillins (±β-lactamase inhibitor) + aminoglycoside
	Monobactam + aminoglycoside
Two- or three-drug regimens with a glycopeptide	Third- or fourth-generation cephalosporins + glycopeptide ± aminoglycoside
	Antipseudomonal carboxypenicillins or ureidopenicillins (±β-lactamase inhibitor) + glycopeptide ± aminoglycoside
	Carbapenem + glycopeptide ± aminoglycoside
	Monobactam + glycopeptide ± aminoglycoside

vided that patients with documented infection receive additional therapy when the clinical response is not satisfactory, or when culture results dictate.

Therapeutic modifications of the choice of empirical treatment for neutropenic patients include addition of vancomycin if there is a suspected infection involving methicillin-resistant Gram-positive bacteria, or an aminoglycoside plus a carbapenem for Gram-negative resistant organisms. If there is severe mucositis, some recommend the addition of vancomycin. The presence of esophagitis may necessitate the use of acyclovir for HSV infection. Evidence of a pulmonary infiltrate is an indication for the empirical use of an antifungal drug such as amphotericin B. Similarly, TMP–SMX should be given if *P. carinii* infection is suspected.

Azoles have been used prophylactically to prevent candidiasis in severely immunocompromised patients. Fluconazole (400 mg daily) has been shown to prevent infection due to C. *albicans* and C. *tropicalis* but not to C. *krusei* or C. *glabrata*.

Therapeutic modifications upon receiving culture results *(Figure 4.3)*
If cultures grew methicillin-resistant staphylococci, vancomycin should be added to the empirical antibiotic regimen. Similarly, additional vancomycin is necessary if cultures grow penicillin-resistant streptococci, C. *jeikeium* or enterococci. Even though in some centers with a high prevalence of the latter organisms, vancomycin is added to the initial empirical treatment, the glycopeptide antibiotics are best used when pathogen-directed rather than empirically. If Gram-negative bacteria resistant to the β-lactam component of a combination are isolated, the β-lactam should be changed, or exchanged for a new extended-spectrum fluoroquinolone.

What considerations should modulate empirical treatment? *(Figure 4.4)*

Patients with resolution of fever
In patients with negative culture results (i.e. with FUO), it is not usually necessary to continue broad-spectrum antibiotic regimens for longer than 7 days if the patient has

become rapidly afebrile and the neutrophil count has returned to normal levels. Longer courses of antimicrobial therapy may result in superinfection by resistant or opportunistic organisms. However, if profound neutropenia persists, some clinicians elect to discontinue antibiotic therapy in afebrile and clinically stable patients, while others prefer to continue treatment with broad-spectrum antibiotics until recovery of neutrophil numbers. Otherwise, the fever may recur, eventually accompanied by shock. Indeed, nearly half of the patients whose neutropenia persists but whose temperature has resolved with 7 days of antibiotic therapy become febrile again within 3 days of stopping treatment.

Patients who remain febrile after 3 days of treatment
At least 3 days of empirical treatment are necessary to assess the efficacy of the initial therapy.

Clinically stable patients
If the patient is clinically stable but remains febrile after this period of treatment, and if a specific causal organism has been identified, the treatment should be continued, or changed, as appropriate. In this respect, it is important to keep in mind that it has been repeatedly shown in clinical trials that even with appropriate antimicrobial therapy resolution of the fever may take 5–7 days. Thus, persistence of fever for 3 days does not necessarily mean that treatment is ineffective.

Considerable controversy surrounds the optimal management of a patient with FUO, whose clinical condition is stable but who is still febrile after 3 days of empirical treatment. Many clinicians would consider adding empirical vancomycin or teicoplanin in view of a possible occult and resistant staphylococcal infection. In hospitals where there is a high incidence of *Aspergillus* infections, it is usual to add amphotericin B at this time or between days 4 and 7 if the fever persists. However, if the patient remains stable and is not deteriorating, empirical treatment should be continued unchanged for at least two more days since, in at least 50% of patients with FUO, it takes more than 3 days for the fever to resolve. The addition of amphotericin B should be considered after 5–7 days of the initial empirical treatment and after repeated clinical examination and radiography plus CT of the chest and abdomen, especially if there are symptoms suggestive of pulmonary or abdominal infections. An hepatic ultrasonographic examination is indicated to rule out hepatosplenic candidiasis at the time of resolution of neutropenia if the patient remains or becomes febrile. With respect to the addition of vancomycin, its use should be guided by the results of the cultures performed at the onset of fever and not on the basis solely of the persistence of fever.

A fungal cause for the persistent FUO must be considered, especially since fungal infections showing no antemortem evidence have been found in 10–40% of patients who died with prolonged neutropenia. Empirical antifungal therapy is therefore considered desirable for patients with persistent (4–7 days) pyrexia despite treatment with broad-spectrum antibiotics or who have fever and pulmonary lesions, in whom invasive investigations are not possible. In these patients, intravenous amphotericin B should be added to the therapeutic regimen. Alternatively, fluconazole can be used if infection with *Aspergillus* is uncommon locally.

It is worth emphasizing that the optimal time for the addition of either vancomycin or amphotericin B to the treatment of patients who are clinically stable but who remain febrile after 3 days of empirical therapy is still being intensively studied.

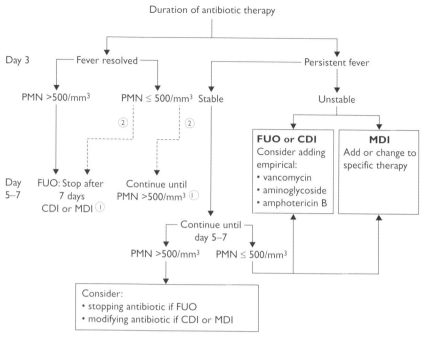

Ⓘ Longer durations of antibiotic therapy may be required for patients with CDI or MDI

② Some investigators elect to stop antibiotic therapy (and to reinstate empirical treatment if fever relapses), whereas others prefer to continue until bone marrow recovery

Figure 4.4 Algorithm for modulation and duration of antibiotic treatment of febrile patients with neutropenia. Adapted from Hughes et al (1997).

Patients in whom the clinical condition is deteriorating

If the patient remains febrile after 3 days of treatment, and the clinical condition is deteriorating, continuing treatment depends on whether or not the patient has developed a clinically obvious focus of infection. If the focus of infection has been found, attempts should be made to identify the causative pathogen by culture or biopsy. The treatment should then be modified accordingly and continued until resolution of the fever and of the neutropenia. If there is no obvious site of infection, the patient must undergo a further thorough clinical examination, including chest radiography and CT, as well as repeat blood cultures. A change in the antibiotic regimen should be considered, such as adding vancomycin, amphotericin B or an aminoglycoside. It is also necessary to keep in mind the possibility that an unusual pathogen (such as *M. tuberculosis*) is responsible for the fever.

5.2 What is the appropriate approach to the patient with hematologic malignancy and evidence of:

For each site, refer to Table 4.3 for a discussion of organisms.

Upper respiratory tract infection?

Sinusitis

Sinusitis occurs especially in patients with obstructing lesions (e.g. lymphomas) and/or if there is mucosal damage due to antineoplastic treatment in patients with leukemia. In neutropenic patients, the main infecting organisms are S. pneumoniae, H. influenzae and Moraxella catarrhalis, as well as P. aeruginosa and anaerobes. If the infection does not improve within 72 h of the start of broad-spectrum empirical antibiotic therapy aimed at covering the above-mentioned organisms, endoscopic sampling, aspiration of sinus contents or biopsy of the sinus mucosa is required for diagnosis. Indeed, fungal infection with Aspergillus or Mucoraceae may occur and progress rapidly to produce facial swelling. Symptoms may be minimal. CT of the sinuses may show bony erosion if there is fungal infection, with subsequent bony necrosis and invasion, leading to cerebral involvement. Treatment involves debridement and high-dose intravenous amphotericin B.

Otitis media and externa

Infection of the middle and outer ear is usually attributable to S. pneumoniae and H. influenzae, which require treatment with broad-spectrum antibiotics. In neutropenic patients, P. aeruginosa may give rise to malignant otitis externa by colonizing and invading the external auditory meatus, with spread to the petrous bone. Aggressive antipseudomonal treatment is necessary for these patients.

Teeth and gingiva

Gingival inflammation and ulceration, as well as periodontal lesions, are common in patients with acute leukemia or in other hematologic malignancies, when patients have received antineoplastic therapy. Moreover, HSV infection may produce mucositis. Patients who are seropositive for HSV before treatment have a 70–80% chance of reactivation during the treatment of leukemia. These patients should be treated prophylactically, either with valacyclovir or famciclovir orally if they can swallow, or with intravenous acyclovir during the severe mucositis.

Oral ulceration after chemotherapy usually results in colonization by endogenous aerobic and anaerobic flora, with local infection and invasion giving rise to septicemia in neutropenic patients. Mucositis and gingivitis occur in up to 85% of leukemic patients. In adults, preexistent periodontal disease is exacerbated by neutropenia. Expert dental care before chemotherapy, as well as intensive oral hygienic measures during neutropenia, is necessary. The organisms most often responsible for infection include S. aureus, C. albicans, P. aeruginosa and streptococci. Necrotic gingivitis caused by anaerobes requires treatment with clindamycin or metronidazole. To control oral thrush, antifungal oral preparations should be used, including fluconazole if the infection is severe.

Lower respiratory tract infection?

Patchy or localized infiltration

Patchy or localized infiltration of the lungs in neutropenic patients may reflect infection by Gram-negative or Gram-positive organisms, as well as viruses, fungi and parasites. The bacteria that produce pneumonitis include especially P. aeruginosa, Klebsiella spp. and Enterobacter spp. In patients with prolonged neutropenia, fungal infection of the lungs is likely. Initially, broad-spectrum antibiotics should be used for 2–3 days to treat patients with pulmonary infiltrates. If the condition improves, treatment should be continued. If the patient deteriorates, diagnosis is necessary with BAL samples obtained bronchoscopically. Biopsies can be performed only if the patient's condition permits (e.g. if there is no thrombocytopenia).

Diffuse pulmonary infiltrates

Diffuse pulmonary infiltrates tend to be caused by bacteria such as *Legionella*, *Mycoplasma*, *Chlamydia* and mycobacteria. Infections due to *Nocardia* present as multiple or confluent nodular lesions rather than diffuse infiltrates, which often become cavitary. Fungi such as *Candida*, *Cryptococcus* and *Histoplasma* also give diffuse pulmonary infiltrates, as do parasites such as *P. carinii* and *T. gondii*. Diffuse viral infection of the lungs is common. The organisms concerned include respiratory syncytial virus (RSV), adenoviruses, HSV, VZV and CMV. If empirical treatment with broad-spectrum antibiotics and TMP–SMX does not result in improvement, histologic diagnosis becomes necessary.

P. carinii can produce patchy or diffuse pneumonia. The diagnosis is made by finding cysts or trophozoites in bronchial aspirate or histologic samples. Patients with suspected *P. carinii* infection should be treated empirically with TMP–SMX.

Viral infections of the lungs are common, with CMV infection particularly prevalent in neutropenic patients with concomitant depressed cellular immunity (i.e. after bone marrow transplantation) (see Chapter 5). The virus can be found in the pharynx, urine and blood of infected patients, as well as in samples obtained by BAL. Treatment involves use of ganciclovir and intravenous immune globulin. Probably, the most common causes of viral infections in patients with hematologic malignancies are community-acquired respiratory viruses such as influenza, parainfluenza and RSV. Other pulmonary viral infections, including HSV and VZV, can occur and may be treated prophylactically and curatively with intravenous acyclovir.

New or progressive pulmonary infiltrates

Fungal pneumonia should be suspected in neutropenic patients who develop new or progressive pulmonary infiltrates while receiving broad-spectrum antibiotic treatment. If the granulocyte count is rising, the patients will do well without change in therapy. However, in many hospitals, *Aspergillus* is ubiquitous in the environment and pulmonary infection with the fungus is common. Many of the patients are also infected with *P. aeruginosa*. Standard treatment is high-dose amphotericin B but itraconazole may also be useful.

Digestive tract infections?

Esophagitis in neutropenic patients is common, especially in patients receiving long-term treatment with antibiotics. Viral, bacterial and fungal organisms may cause esophagitis, especially HSV and *Candida*. The diagnosis is made by means of mucosal brushings or biopsies and treatment is initially empirical.

Patients with severe prolonged neutropenia are at risk of developing perirectal cellulitis, especially if there are preexisting hemorrhoids, mucositis and fissures or if the patient has undergone sigmoidoscopy or colonoscopy. Aerobic Gram-negative organisms (*P. aeruginosa*, *K. pneumonia*, *E. coli*), enterococci or anaerobes are usually responsible for the infection. Antibiotic cover should include clindamycin or metronidazole, in addition to broad-spectrum antibiotics.

Abdominal infection may be primary, or secondary to complications of the malignancy (such as obstruction of the gut or biliary tract). Typhlitis (cecal cellulitis) can develop in neutropenic patients, especially acute leukemic patients after intensive antineoplastic chemotherapy and treatment with broad-spectrum antibiotics. The causal organisms are Gram-negative, especially *P. aeruginosa*. Treatment should be targeted against the Gram-negative bacteria and anaerobes. Neutropenic patients may also develop clostridial peritonitis that disseminates to the bloodstream. In these patients, infection by C. *perfringens* or C. *septicum* may occur in the absence of fever. C. *tertium* infection is less fulminant. These infections are treated with broad-spectrum antibiotic regimens, including vancomycin.

Antibiotic-associated colitis may occur after treatment with any antibacterial agent, but is more frequently associated with clindamycin, ampicillin and broad-spectrum β-lactams. Nosocomial infection with C. *difficile* is often the cause. Treatment involves administration of vancomycin or metronidazole. Since the disease may be nosocomially transmitted, enteric barrier nursing is required.

Genitourinary tract infection?

Medication (e.g. vincristine) and local therapeutic intervention (e.g. catheterization) may predispose to infection, especially with aerobic Gram-negative bacilli (*E. coli*, *Klebsiella* spp., *Proteus* spp., *P. aeruginosa*) and enterococci. In neutropenic patients, a colony count greater than 10^3 per ml of a single organism is diagnostic of infection if the patient is symptomatic, and a count above 10^5 per ml indicates infection even if the patient is not symptomatic. The infecting organisms are either bacterial or fungal. If there is repeated isolation of C. *albicans*, C. *tropicalis* or C. *glabrata* in a patient who is febrile, systemic amphotericin B should be started.

Cardiovascular system infection?

Patients are at risk of cardiovascular infection if there are dental abscesses, intravenous drug abuse or congenital heart disease. Endovascular disease may also result from indwelling venous catheters, especially from infection with Gram-positive bacteria, *P. aeruginosa* and fungi. Diagnosis is made by multiple blood cultures. Treatment should be directed at the specific pathogens and continued for 4–6 weeks or more.

Musculoskeletal infection?

In neutropenic patients, pyomyositis, especially of the psoas muscles, is usually caused by S. *aureus* or Gram-negative organisms. Crepitus may indicate clostridial infection. S. *pyogenes* may produce necrotizing fasciitis, which requires immediate debridement and antibiotic treatment. Septic arthritis or osteomyelitis may be secondary to disseminated Gram-positive or Gram-negative bacteria or fungi.

Skin infection?

The integrity of the skin is frequently disrupted by diagnostic interventions and surgery, as well as chemotherapy. As a result, local infections by bacteria or fungi are common and, in neutropenic patients, often result in disseminated disease. The exit site of indwelling catheters is a common focus of infection, usually by staphylococcal species, Gram-negative bacteria or fungi and may lead to septicemia or fungemia. Reactivation of HSV or VZV is common, for example occurring in 35–50% of patients with Hodgkin disease.

Central nervous system infection?

Meningitis may occur in patients with impairment of cell-mediated immunity and involves organisms such as *L. monocytogenes* and C. *neoformans*. The organisms, or their antigens, are found in the CSF. *L. monocytogenes* infection occurs especially in patients with defective T-cell-mediated immune function. Encephalitis may be caused by viral organisms such as HSV. Diagnosis is made by testing the CSF for PCR patterns characteristic of the virus. MRI may show mass lesions caused by *T. gondii*, as well as encephalitis. The infection may be newly acquired or reactivated by antineoplastic treatment. Focal lesions may also represent brain abscesses, originating from contiguous infected foci (sinuses, ears and teeth) or from endocarditis or pulmonary infections. The causative organisms are aerobic or anaerobic bacteria or fungi.

Foreign bodies in place?

Infection of catheter entry sites and catheter tunnels is common and usually caused by *S. aureus*, coagulase-negative staphylococci, viridans streptococci, *Pseudomonas* spp. and *Candida*. Atypical *Mycobacterium* species may also be found. Catheter removal is often unnecessary but may become necessary if there is tunnel infection, if the catheter is blocked, if there are septic emboli, if there is an *S. aureus* infection that does not respond to treatment, or if the infection is caused by atypical mycobacteria, *Bacillus* spp., *P. aeruginosa*, *C. jeikeium* or *Candida*.

5.3 What is the appropriate approach to the patient with hematologic malignancy and evidence of bacteremia, with or without site of infection?

Bacteremia

Approximately 10–30% of febrile neutropenic patients suffer from bacteremia at the time of presentation (see section 1.2 and Table 4.2). Gram-positive and Gram-negative bacteria are equally commonly responsible for the bacteremia. The Gram-positive bacteria comprise especially *S. aureus*, coagulase-negative staphylococci, streptococcal species (including viridans and enterococci), *Corynebacterium* spp. and *Bacillus* spp. The Gram-negative organisms include *E. coli*, *K. pneumoniae*, *E. cloacae* and, less commonly, *P. aeruginosa*, *S. maltophilia*, *S. marcescens* and *Citrobacter* spp.

Catheter-associated bacteremia

Catheter-associated bacteremia is relatively common and attributable mainly to coagulase-negative staphylococci, *S. aureus* and *Candida*, as well as *Bacillus* and *Corynebacterium* spp. Approximately 80% of catheter infections are attributable to coagulase-negative staphylococci, which can be treated without removal of the catheter. Treatment should include at least 10 days of vancomycin, infused through the catheter. If the cultures remain positive 48 h after the appropriate treatment, the catheter should be removed. Gram-negative infection with *E. coli*, *Klebsiella* or *P. aeruginosa* suggests an alimentary cause or fecal contamination. The infection may be polymicrobial if there is unsatisfactory catheter care.

Gram-positive bacteremia

The risk from Gram-positive infections may be covered by using a broad-spectrum antibiotic empirically, without the initial use of vancomycin, except in clinical environments where methicillin-resistant staphylococci are predominant. If infection is identified, vancomycin is usually needed for the treatment of methicillin-resistant coagulase-negative staphylococci. A localized infected focus in the skin should receive topical treatment. Instead of vancomycin it may be possible to use antistaphylococcal penicillins (nafcillin, oxacillin) if the organisms are sensitive. Vancomycin is used especially with resistant organisms [MRSA, methicillin-resistant *S. epidermidis* (MRSE), enterococci, viridans streptococci, penicillin-resistant *S. pneumoniae*, *C. jeikeium*], and if the patient is allergic to β-lactams. The duration of treatment should be not less than 2 weeks, with longer periods for patients suffering from endocarditis or septic thrombophlebitis.

Gram-negative bacteremia

For patients with confirmed Gram-negative bacteremia who remain neutropenic for prolonged periods, combined treatment (β-lactam plus aminoglycoside) is necessary. If the duration of neutropenia is short, monotherapy with a third-generation cephalosporin or a carbapenem may be used. We recommend that combination therapy be used in high-risk patients. If patients are allergic to β-lactams, a regimen including a fluroroquinolone plus an aminoglycoside can be used therapeutically, except for infections with *P. aeruginosa*. Indeed, most authorities recommend a combination of a β-lactam plus aminoglycoside for treatment of documented *P. aeruginosa* infections, although monotherapy with a β-lactam alone has been shown to be successful in some circumstances.

Anaerobic infection

Anaerobic infections are uncommon in neutropenic patients with hematologic malignancies and involve mainly the sinuses or the digestive tract. Anaerobes cause necrotizing gingivitis, enterocolitis and perirectal abscesses, and are found in intraabdominal septic foci. Treatment involves the use of clindamycin or metronidazole. Therapy with cephalosporins or cephalosporin and aminoglycoside combinations may not provide sufficient anaerobic cover, but require addition of metronidazole or clindamycin, or of amoxycillin–clavulanate, ticarcillin–clavulanate or piperacillin–tazobactam.

Mixed or polymicrobial bacteremia

Polymicrobial infections are common in neutropenic patients, especially in patients with pneumonia, typhlitis, perirectal infections and skin infections. Catheter infections may also be polymicrobial. Polymicrobial infections are caused by Gram-positive, Gram-negative and anaerobic bacteria, while in the lungs polymicrobial infections are often community-acquired viral infections together with bacterial or fungal infections.

5.4 What is the appropriate approach to the patient with hematologic malignancy and evidence of a viral infection?

Herpesviruses

HSV and VZV infections require treatment with acyclovir. Prolonged treatment may be necessary in immunocompromised patients who tend to relapse when treatment is stopped. Prophylactic acyclovir therapy may also be worthwhile in seropositive patients with hematologic malignancies who are going to receive aggressive antineoplastic treatment and are likely to develop mucositis. Repeated or prolonged treatment with acyclovir may infrequently result in HSV resistance to the drug. Under these circumstances, patients should be treated with foscarnet 40 mg/kg iv tid.

Disseminated VZV infection is treated with acyclovir 500 mg/m^2 iv tid. If the lesions of VZV are localized, oral treatment with acyclovir may be sufficient.

Respiratory viruses

Community-acquired viral infections such as influenza, parainfluenza, RSV and adenoviruses are a significant cause of infection during the winter season in patients with hematologic malignancies. The diagnosis is difficult since invasive measures are required to obtain appropriate samples for culture, and specific treatment cannot be instituted unless there is a strong diagnostic suspicion. This is a topic that requires more study in order to improve the management of neutropenic cancer patients, both by developing simpler diagnostic procedures and in terms of treatment.

CMV pneumonia is rare in patients with hematologic malignancies not undergoing bone marrow transplantation. The infection should be treated with ganciclovir 5 mg/kg bid plus high doses of immunoglobulin (500 mg/kg on alternate days) for 10–14 days if the diagnosis is established. Foscarnet 60 mg tid can be used to treat patients with good renal function or patients infected with ganciclovir-resistant CMV.

Hepatitis
Hepatitis B virus (HBV) and hepatitis C virus (HCV) infections are especially dangerous for patients treated with antineoplastic chemotherapy because of potential added liver toxicity. Moreover, such treatment may reactivate latent viral infection and lead to acute hepatitis. It is not known whether interferon plus ribavirin, which has recently been shown to be active in HCV-infected individuals, has a therapeutic role in patients with hematologic malignancies undergoing intensive chemotherapy.

5.5 What is the appropriate approach to the patient with hematologic malignancy and evidence of a fungal infection?
Three themes that are relevant for the management of fungal infections in patients with hematologic malignancies are discussed here: (1) empirical therapy for suspected fungal infections; (2) prevention and treatment of candidiasis; and (3) management of aspergillosis.

Empirical therapy for suspected fungal infections
Invasive fungal infections are a major cause of morbidity and mortality in neutropenic cancer patients. Unfortunately, early diagnosis is difficult, as there are no tests that can reliably establish a diagnosis of invasive fungal infections in these high-risk patients. Fever not responsive to broad-spectrum antibacterial therapy is frequently the only sign of fungal infection. The most common fungal pathogens are *Candida* and *Aspergillus* spp. *Phycomycetes*, *Fusarium* spp., *Pseudallescheria boydii*, *Cryptococcus* spp. and *Trichosporon* spp. are isolated less frequently.

The aim of empirical antifungal therapy is to treat occult fungal infections at an early stage of the disease. There is a consensus among investigators that empirical antifungal therapy is appropriate for neutropenic patients with malignant hematologic disorders who remain febrile after 4–7 days of treatment with broad-spectrum antibiotics and in whom nonfungal causes of fever have been excluded. Only two studies have tested the validity of this concept. In a study by Pizzo et al, which included 50 patients with persistent fever despite 7 days of antibacterial therapy with cefalotin, carbenicillin and gentamicin, amphotericin B was found to reduce the time to fever defervescence and the incidence of fungal infections, but not the overall mortality rate. In a multicenter study conducted by the International Antimicrobial Therapy Cooperative Group of the EORTC, 132 patients with neutropenic cancer who remained febrile after 4 days of empirical antibiotic therapy were randomized to receive empirical amphotericin B 0.6 mg/kg daily or no antifungal treatment. Amphotericin B improved the clinical state of the patients and reduced the incidence of fungal infections and the mortality from fungal infections, but not the overall mortality rate. Patients who benefited most from antifungal therapy were those who (1) had not previously received antifungal therapy; (2) were severely neutropenic; (3) had a clinical documentation of infection; and (4) were older than 15 years of age.

Recently, Walsh et al reported that liposomal amphotericin 3 mg/kg daily was as effective as conventional amphotericin B 0.6 mg/kg daily for empirical therapy of cancer patients with fever and neutropenia who had remained febrile despite receiving broad-spectrum antibiotics for 5 days (resolution of fever, 58% versus 58%; survival, 93% versus 90%). Treatment with liposomal amphotericin B was associated with fewer break-through fungal infections (3.2% versus 7.8%, $P = 0.009$), including candidemia, less infusion-related fever (17% versus 44%, $P < 0.001$) and less nephrotoxicity (19% versus 34%, $P < 0.001$).

Fluconazole has also been used for antifungal therapy. In a pilot study that included 112 febrile neutropenic cancer patients, fluconazole was found to be equivalent to amphotericin B in terms of fever resolution and survival.

However, many questions remain to be answered. What is the most appropriate timing for the initiation of empirical antifungal therapy? No study has examined whether it is better to start empirical antifungal therapy after 3 or 4 days than after 5–7 days of persistent fever during treatment with broad-spectrum antibiotics. The potential advantage of an earlier start must be balanced against the risk of exposing many patients to a substantial risk of unnecessary toxicity or the development of antifungal drug resistance.

What is the most appropriate antifungal regimen? Treatment options include a triazole, such as fluconazole or itraconazole, conventional amphotericin B or a lipid formulation of amphotericin B. None of these treatment regimens has been shown to be superior to the others. Newer agents such as voriconazole or the echinocandins will soon be tested.

What is the optimal dose and duration of empirical antifungal therapy? Therapy should be continued until resolution of fever, disappearance of all signs of infection (if initially present) and until recovery of neutrophil numbers. Studies are currently in progress to address some of these issues. Until the results of these ongoing clinical trials become available, amphotericin B remains the drug of choice for the empirical therapy of suspected fungal infections in persistently febrile neutropenic patients with leukemia or lymphoma. The use of a lipid formulation should be reserved for patients in whom toxicity cannot be prevented by standard preventive measures. Although fluconazole is often widely used in antifungal prophylaxis, it is devoid of activity against *Aspergillus*, which precludes its use as empirical antifungal therapy in febrile neutropenic patients. Similarly, the lack of an intravenous formulation of itraconazole and the fact that the absorption of itraconazole is variable, as well as the paucity of clinical data about its efficacy, preclude its use for empirical antifungal therapy.

Prevention and treatment of candidiasis

Candida spp. are the most common cause of invasive fungal infections in patients with hematologic malignancies. The recent advent of potent and well-tolerated antifungal agents provides an opportunity to prevent these life-threatening infections. Earlier prophylactic studies with oral polyenes (nystatin and amphotericin B) or older miconazoles (miconazole, clotrimazole and ketoconazole) have shown that these agents reduce the frequency of superficial infections caused by C. *albicans*, but not of systemic fungal infections. More recent studies have focused on the use of the newer azoles, fluconazole and itraconazole. In a double-blind placebo-controlled prophylactic study of patients undergoing chemotherapy for acute leukemia, fluconazole (400 mg given orally or intravenously) was shown to prevent colonization and superficial infections by *Candida* spp. other than C. *krusei*. But fluconazole failed to prevent invasive fungal infections, did not reduce the use of amphotericin B and did not decrease the mortality rate. In a small placebo-controlled study of patients with hematologic malignancies, fluconazole reduced the number of febrile days and prevented oropharyngeal candidiasis, but not deep-seated mycoses, and also did not affect prognosis. Other studies have shown that oral or intravenous fluconazole is as effective as oral or intravenous amphotericin B for prophylaxis of fungal infection in leukemic patients. However, the relatively small benefit associated with the use of fluconazole must be balanced against the risk of selecting fluconazole-resistant *Candida* strains, such as *C. krusei* or *C. glabrata*.

Very few studies have examined the role of low-dose amphotericin B in the prophylaxis of *Candida* infections in these patients. There are limited data on the use of itraconazole for antifungal prophylaxis, but large clinical trials are currently in progress. Overall, the utility of fluconazole, itraconazole or amphotericin B for the prophylaxis of fungal infections in patients with hematologic malignancies remains controversial. Local epidemiologic data are essential to determine whether or not to use antifungal prophylaxis, so that strategies may vary from center to center.

While the use of antifungal prophylaxis is debatable, there is general agreement that all neutropenic patients with candidemia should be treated promptly. Several important factors must be taken into account when selecting an antifungal agent for the treatment of patients with candidemia, including the epidemiology of fungal infections within the institution, whether or not the patient has received previous antifungal prophylaxis, the current status of the patient, as well as the severity and anticipated duration of neutropenia. Amphotericin B remains the treatment of choice for critically ill patients, patients with evidence of disseminated candidiasis, patients who have received prophylaxis with azoles, and patients in whom fungemia is suspected to be caused by a non-albicans *Candida* strain such as *C. krusei* or *C. glabrata*. Combined treatment with 5-fluorocytosine and amphotericin B should be considered for patients who fail to respond to amphotericin B alone or in whom infection has relapsed after amphotericin B monotherapy. An intravenous formulation of 5-fluorocytosine is available in Europe but not in the USA. The serum levels of 5-fluorocytosine should be monitored, as bone marrow suppression is of particular concern in patients who have received chemotherapy. Fluconazole is an alternative to amphotericin B in stable patients with uncomplicated candidemia who have not been treated prophylactically with azoles. The recommended dose of amphotericin B is 0.7–1.5 mg/kg daily and that of fluconazole is 400–800 mg/day, but no dose-finding studies with amphotericin B or fluconazole have been performed in this patient population. Treatment should be continued until resolution of all signs of infection and until recovery of neutrophil numbers, and for at least 2 weeks after the last positive blood cultures.

It remains highly controversial whether or not to remove all indwelling intravenous catheters in patients with candidemia. The results of several studies indicate that exchanging the intravenous catheter may shorten the time needed to clear the bloodstream and may also affect the patient's prognosis. It is necessary to change intravenous catheters in neutropenic patients with candidemia if the catheter is thought to be the source of infection. The problem is more difficult in patients with surgically implanted catheters. Under such circumstances, most clinicians may first try to sterilize the catheter with appropriate antifungal therapy. However, the catheter should certainly be removed if the tunnelized section of catheter is infected or if blood cultures remain positive despite appropriate antifungal therapy.

Another unresolved issue is the utility of the colony-stimulating factors [G-CSF, GM-CSF or macrophage colony-stimulating factor (M-CSF)] in patients with candidiasis. At present, there are no data to suggest that this adjunctive therapy improves the morbidity or mortality rates associated with invasive candidiasis in patients with hematologic malignancies. However, despite the lack of data, investigators may choose to use these agents in critically ill and profoundly neutropenic patients with disseminated candidiasis with the aim of accelerating neutrophil recovery and also improving neutrophil function.

Management of aspergillosis

Amphotericin B is the principal drug used for treating invasive aspergillosis. Approximately one third of infected patients can be treated successfully, especially using high doses, up to 1.5 mg/kg daily of conventional amphotericin B or 10 mg/kg daily of liposomal amphotericin B. The greatest therapeutic success has been achieved with aspergillosis of the paranasal sinuses.

The new lipid formulations of amphotericin B permit the administration of higher doses of the drug without increasing renal toxicity. In a recent study, the use of AmBisome 5 mg/kg daily cured twice as many patients (42% versus 21%) with invasive aspergillosis as did amphotericin B 1 mg/kg daily. Similar results were achieved using Amphocil. In the UK, the overall response to AmBisome of patients with aspergillosis was approximately 60%, with a success rate of 80% in patients who had not previously received amphotericin B. Even though these lipid formulations of amphotericin B show less renal toxicity, there is no difference in the development of hypokalemia. The liposomal formulation amphotericin B is indicated especially if cyclosporin is being used, to decrease the renal toxicity of the amphotericin B–cyclosporin combination. The recommended daily dose of AmBisome is 5–10 mg/kg. Patients should be treated with maximal doses of amphotericin B as early as possible until there is evidence that the aspergillosis has disappeared and that the neutrophil count has returned to normal. Six to eight weeks of treatment is usually sufficient, but each patient must be judged individually.

Alternatively, itraconazole has been used to treat invasive aspergillosis, as second-line therapy when patients are intolerant or resistant to amphotericin B therapy. The drug is not well absorbed and has important interactions with hepatic P-450 enzymes, resulting in cardiac arrhythmias (when used with cisapride or terfenadine) or rhabdomyolysis (when given with some statins). There are also interactions with many other drugs, including cyclosporin, warfarin, digoxin or phenytoin. The plasma levels of itraconazole may be lowered by some of these interactions, but circulating concentrations can be monitored. At present, itraconazole is mainly available for oral use (loading dose 200 mg tid for 4 days, followed by 200 mg bid). Higher doses are required for CNS infections. New antifungal drugs, such as voriconazole, are becoming available and are at present the subject of clinical trials.

Recent advances in surgical and postoperative techniques have reestablished the use of surgical resection of localized *Aspergillus* infection, if the patient's clinical condition and platelet count permit.

5.6 What is the appropriate approach to the patient with hematologic malignancy and evidence of a parasitic infection?

Pneumocystis carinii

P. carinii infection usually affects the lungs in immunocompromised patients. The disease is usually preventable if the patient at risk is treated with prophylactic TMP–SMX.

This combination is also used for the treatment of acute pulmonary infection with the organism. Treatment involves administration of TMP–SMX (TMP 20 mg/kg, SMX 100 mg/kg) daily in three or four divided doses, for 14 days. In some patients, adverse reactions (especially nephrotoxicity and sometimes bone marrow damage) necessitates discontinuation of the TMP–SMX therapy. Patients can then be treated with intravenous pentamidine or dapsone.

Toxoplasma gondii

Reactivation of quiescent infection with *T. gondii* is best treated with a sulfonamide plus pyrimethamine. Prophylaxis with TMP–SMX is recommended if patients are seropositive before chemotherapy.

Other parasitic infestations

Other parasitic infestations are rare but evidence should be sought in patients who have visited endemic regions. These infestations should be eradicated before starting treatment associated with neutropenia.

REFERENCES

American Society of Clinical Oncology. Recommendations for the use of hematopoietic colony-stimulating factors: evidence-based, clinical practice guidelines. *J Clin Oncol* 1994; **12**: 2471–2508.

American Society of Clinical Oncology. Update of recommendations for the use of hematopoietic colony-stimulating factors: evidence-based clinical practice guidelines. *J Clin Oncol* 1996; **14**: 1957–1960.

Bodey GP, Buckley M, Sathe YS et al. Quantitative relationships between circulating leukocytes and infection in patients with acute leukemia. *Ann Intern Med* 1966; **61**: 328.

Edwards JE Jr, Bodey GP, Bowden RA et al. International Conference for the Development of a Consensus on the Management and Prevention of Severe Candidal Infections. *Clin Infect Dis* 1997; **25**: 43–59.

Finberg RW, Talcott JA. Fever and neutropenia. How to use a new treatment strategy. *N Engl J Med* 1999; **341**: 362–363.

Freifeld AG, Pizzo PA, Walsh TJ. Infections in the cancer patient. In: DeVita VE Jr, Hellman S, Rosenberg SA, eds. *Cancer Principles and Practice of Oncology*, 5th edn. Philadelphia: Lippincott-Raven, 1997: 2659–2704.

Freifeld A, Marchigiani D, Walsh T et al. A double-blind comparison of empirical oral and intravenous antibiotic therapy for low-risk febrile patients with neutropenia during cancer chemotherapy. *N Engl J Med* 1999; **341**: 305–311.

Glauser M, Boogaerts M, Cordonnier C, Palmblad J, Martino P. Empiric therapy of bacterial infections in severe neutropenia. *Clin Microbiol Infect* 1997; **3**(Suppl 1): S77–S86.

Hughes WT, Armstrong D, Bodey GP et al. 1997 Guidelines for the use of antimicrobial agents in neutropenic patients with unexplained fever. *Clin Infect Dis* 1997; **25**: 551–573.

Kern WV, Cometta A, De Bock R et al. Oral versus intravenous empirical antimicrobial therapy for fever in patients with granulocytopenia who are receiving cancer chemotherapy. International Antimicrobial Therapy Cooperative Group of the European Organization for Research and Treatment of Cancer. *N Engl J Med* 1999; **341**: 312–318.

Viscoli C. The evolution of the empirical management of fever and neutropenia in cancer patients. *J Antimicrob Chemother* 1998; **41**(Suppl D): 65–80.

Walsh TJ, Finberg RW, Arndt C et al. Liposomal amphotericin B for empirical therapy in patients with persistent fever and neutropenia. National Institute of Allergy and Infectious Diseases Mycoses Study Group. *N Engl J Med* 1999; **340**: 764–771.

Warnock DW. Fungal infections in neutropenia: current problems and chemotherapeutic control. *J Antimicrob Chemother* 1998; **41** (Suppl D): 95–105.

Wood MJ. Viral infections in neutropenia – current problems and chemotherapeutic control. *J Antimicrob Chemother* 1998; **41**(Suppl D): 81–93.

Chapter 5

Infections in Blood and Bone Marrow Transplant Patients: Allogeneic and Autologous Transplantation

Raleigh A Bowden

INTRODUCTION

Infection in patients undergoing blood/bone marrow transplantation (BMT) continues to be one of the most common posttransplant complications. Patients having BMT differ from other immunocompromised hosts in that their risk for infection is quite predictable and temporally circumscribed, especially in those who undergo autologous transplantation or when graft-versus-host disease (GVHD) is not a major problem. The infectious risk period has a very specific time of onset, beginning at the time of irradiation and/or chemotherapy conditioning therapy for transplantation. This risk continues until recovery of a functional immune system which begins at engraftment, and which is substantially improved around day 100 after transplant, and is virtually 'normal' by about 18 months after the transplantation. GVHD is the major feature that determines the duration of risk and distinguishes the risks and timing of infection after allogeneic transplant from the risks and patterns observed after autologous transplant.

One of the most significant advances in the technology of stem cell transplantation has been the introduction of sources of stem cells other than the bone marrow. Increasingly, peripheral blood is being used as the source of stem cells for both allogeneic and autologous transplantation because of its ease of acquisition and association, in general, with earlier engraftment. Another source of stem cells being actively investigated is cord blood, which has the advantage of allowing for the expansion of the pool of donors for unrelated stem cell transplantation. These alternative sources of stem cells yield stem cell products that can deliver up to a log more cells to the recipient than bone marrow harvests. The trade-off has been the concomitant increase in the risk of GVHD in some cases compared with marrow as a stem cell source. The implication for a change in the timing and severity of various infectious syndromes with alternative sources of stem cells has not been fully appreciated to date. Infectious patterns will likely reflect those seen with the more traditional bone marrow stem cell source.

The spectrum of infectious diseases has changed dramatically over the past two decades with the introduction of more effective infection prevention strategies. In some cases, such as with trimethoprim–sulfamethoxazole (TMP–SMX) prophylaxis for *Pneumocystis carinii* infection, the incidence has dropped dramatically such that this organism is rarely in the differential diagnosis of fever or pulmonary infiltrates when patients who receive TMP–SMX. For other infections, such as cytomegalovirus (CMV), the use of early antiviral prophylaxis has reduced the incidence of early CMV disease and its associated mortality and has shifted the onset to the time when prophylaxis is discontinued approximately 100 days after transplantation

While the spectrum of infections has changed with the institution of various infectious prophylaxis regimens, our approach to the management of the febrile patient and the treatment of patients with established infection after BMT has not changed appreciably. One possible exception is that economic pressures have created more scrutiny regarding therapeutic choice, duration of therapy and the traditional requirement that febrile or infected patients need to be managed in the hospital setting. Increasing numbers of strategies are being developed which include the use of antibiotics with longer half-lives and those that can be used effectively in outpatient management. Further, many centers now manage the 'low-risk' febrile patient in the outpatient setting as long as the patient is thoroughly evaluated, clinically stable and has close follow-up.

This chapter will present a practical approach to developing (1) a differential diagnosis based on the risk factors by time after transplant, (2) a diagnostic evaluation and (3) suggestions for institution of therapy, either empirical or therapy directed at specific infections. In addition, while much of the information described here will apply to the allogeneic setting, this is because most of the reported literature is in reference to these patients. While diagnosis and treatment studies have not as clearly defined strategies for management of infection in the autologous setting, every effort will be made throughout the chapter to highlight the similarities and differences between these two groups of patients.

1 REGARDING THE CLINICAL PRESENTATION AND EVALUATION OF THE PATIENT

1.1 What are the clinically predominant modes of presentation of infection in patients undergoing BMT?

Table 5.1 provides a comprehensive list of the sites, clinical features, predominant organisms and recommendations for evaluation at each site observed after both allogeneic and autologous transplantation. Fever is most often the first sign of infection after BMT. In certain settings, for example with increasing use of high doses of steroids either for GVHD prophylaxis or treatment, or for management of acute conditioning-related toxicity, fever may be absent. Fever of unknown origin (FUO) is quite common in both the BMT and non-BMT cancer settings and accounts for a significant proportion (up to 40%) of 'infectious' syndromes experienced by these patients. While FUO is presumably due to an occult infection and is managed as such with empirical therapy, other noninfectious causes of fever certainly must be considered. The most common noninfectious cause of fever in the allogeneic BMT setting is acute or chronic GVHD.

1.2 What are the predominant sites of infection?

Of the documented infectious syndromes, the etiologies in order of frequency include bacterial or fungal bloodstream infection, pneumonia, skin and/or indwelling catheter infection, and mucosal infection. This applies to infections in both the allogeneic and autologous settings. In general, the major difference between these two transplant types is the frequency of infection, not the site or type of infection, with the incidence of infection being substantially decreased in patients undergoing autologous transplant for many types of infections.

The etiology of pneumonia varies by time after transplantation (see section 1.4 and Figure 5.1). Bacterial pneumonia leads the list, most commonly caused by Gram-negative enteric organisms (e.g. *Klebsiella*, *Escherichia coli* and *Pseudomonas* spp.) during this

Table 5.1 Evaluation of infections in patients undergoing blood and bone marrow transplantation according to the site of infection and the possible etiologic agent

Site of infection	Infectious syndrome (clinical features)	Predominant pathogens	Diagnostic investigations
Bloodstream	Bacteremia (fever with or without local signs of infection)	Coagulase-negative staphylococci Staphylococcus aureus Viridans streptococci Enterococcus spp. (nosocomial outbreaks in some institutions) Gram-negative bacilli (Escherichia coli, Klebsiella pneumoniae, Enterobacter spp., Pseudomonas aeruginosa) Candida spp. Fusarium spp.	Blood cultures: two sets drawn from separate sites and one set drawn from indwelling intravenous catheter
Intravascular catheter-related infections	Pain, erythema, tenderness, discharge from catheter entry site	Coagulase-negative staphylococci Staphylococcus aureus Corynebacterium jeikeium Bacillus spp. Gram-negative bacilli Candida spp., Malassezia furfur, Aspergillus spp. (uncommon) Atypical mycobacteria (M. fortuitum, M. chelonei)	Swab of entry site Culture of catheter Blood cultures (consider drawing blood through each lumen of catheter)
Oral cavity	Periodontitis Gingivitis Stomatitis/mucositis (aphthae, ulcers) Oral thrush (white plaques)	Viridans streptococci Staphylococcus aureus Aerobic and anerobic gram-negative bacilli Gram-positive rods, Herpes simplex Candida spp.	Swab of lesion Oral wash
Throat	Pharyngitis	Streptococcus pyogenes	Swab of pharynx

Site of infection	Infectious syndrome (clinical features)	Predominant pathogens	Diagnostic investigations
	Tonsilitis (sore throat, odynophagia)	Viruses (rhinovirus, coronavirus, adenovirus, influenza, parainfluenza, herpes simplex) Chlamydia pneumoniae Mycoplasma pneumoniae	Serology
Upper respiratory tract (ear, nose, sinus, nasopharynx, larynx, trachea)	Otitis externa Otitis media (earache, drainage, irritability)	Streptococcus pneumoniae Streptococcus pyogenes Haemophilus influenzae Staphylococcus aureus Pseudomonas aeruginosa Moraxella catarrhalis Mycoplasma pneumoniae	Swab of external auditory canal Tympanocentesis
	Sinusitis (tightness of sinus areas, headache, toothache, nasal obstruction, nasal voice)	Streptococcus pneumoniae Haemophilus influenzae Streptococcus pyogenes Staphylococcus aureus Gram-negative bacilli (Escherichia coli, Klebsiella pneumoniae, Pseudomonas aeruginosa) Anaerobic bacteria Moraxella catarrhalis Mycoplasma pneumoniae Aspergillus spp., Mucor spp., Rhizopus spp. Candida spp. Viruses (influenza, parainfluenza, rhinovirus, adenovirus)	Aspiration of sinus Biopsy (if no improvement after 72–96 h of empirical antibiotic therapy)
	Epiglottitis (sore throat, odynophagia)	Haemophilus influenzae Streptococcus pneumoniae Streptococcus pyogenes	Culture of supraglottic specimen

Site	Clinical presentation	Organisms	Investigations
	Laryngitis (sore throat, hoarseness, otalgia) Tracheitis (stridor, dyspnea, cough)	Staphylococcus aureus Moraxella catarrhalis Mycoplasma pneumoniae Viruses (influenza, parainfluenza, rhinovirus, adenovirus, respiratory syncytial virus) Streptococcus pyogenes Haemophilus influenzae Staphylococcus aureus Moraxella catarrhalis	Culture of tracheal secretions
Lower respiratory tract (bronchi, terminal airways, alveoli)	Bronchopneumonia Pneumonia (cough, dyspnea, chest pain, sputum, hemoptysis, pleural effusion)	Gram-negative bacilli (Escherichia coli, Klebsiella pneumoniae, Pseudomonas aeruginosa) Streptococcus pneumoniae Viridans streptococci Staphylococcus aureus Legionella spp. (sporadic outbreaks) Mycoplasma pneumoniae Chlamydia pneumoniae Nocardia asteroides Pneumocystis carinii Mycobacteria (M. tuberculosis, atypical mycobacteria) Viruses (cytomegalovirus, varicella zoster, influenza, adenovirus, respiratory syncytial virus, parainfluenza) Aspergillus spp., Mucor spp., Rhizopus spp. Candida spp. Histoplasma, Cryptococcus	Chest radiography CT, MRI Serology Fiberoptic bronchoscopy with bronchoalveolar lavage Transbronchial biopsy Thoracocentesis Thoracoscopy with biopsy Open lung biopsy
Skin and soft tissue infection	Cellulitis (pain, erythema, tenderness, necrosis in case of ecthyma gangrenosum)	Primary infections: Coagulase-negative staphylococci Staphylococcus aureus	Skin swab Aspiration (needle) Skin biopsy (history and culture)

Site of infection	Infectious syndrome (clinical features)	Predominant pathogens	Diagnostic investigations
		Corynebacterium jeikeium	
		Gram-negative bacilli (Pseudomonas aeruginosa, Escherichia coli, Klebsiella pneumoniae)	
		Enterococcus spp. (perirectal cellulitis)	
		Anaerobic Gram-negative bacilli (perirectal cellulitis)	
		Candida spp.	
		Mucor spp., Rhizopus spp., Absidia spp.	
	Papules, nodules (with or without myalgia and muscle tenderness)	Disseminated infections:	
		Candida spp., Fusarium spp., Alternaria species	
		Gram-negative bacilli (Escherichia coli, Pseudomonas aeruginosa, Aeromonas hydrophilia, Serratia marcescens)	
		Epstein–Barr virus, adenovirus	
	Ulcers, vesicles, hemorrhagic or crusted lesions (isolated or with dermatomal distribution)	Herpes simplex virus	
		Varicella zoster virus	
		Cytomegalovirus	
	Disseminated vesicles, hemorrhagic or crusted lesions	Varicella zoster virus, herpes simplex virus	
		Staphylococcus aureus, group A streptococci	
	Skin necrosis (toes, fingers) secondary to thrombosis of blood vessels	Aspergillus spp., Mucor spp.	
Gastrointestinal tract:			
Esophagus	Esophagitis (dysphagia, retrosternal pain)	Herpes simplex virus	Plain abdominal films
		Candida spp., Aspergillus spp.	Esogastroscopy
		Cytomegalovirus	Colonoscopy
Small intestine, colon	Enteritis	Aerobic and anaerobic Gram-negative bacilli	Ultrasonography

Site of infection	Infectious syndrome	Predominant pathogens	Diagnostic investigations
	Typhlitis Colitis (nausea, vomiting, bloating, abdominal discomfort, cramp, pain, constipation, diarrhea)	Clostridium spp. (typhlitis) Clostridium difficile (antibiotic-associated diarrhea) Strongyloides stercoralis Cryptosporidium Epstein–Barr virus, cytomegalovirus, adenovirus, coxsackie virus and rotavirus (sporadic outbreaks)	CT, MRI Culture of endoscopic specimens Stool cultures Toxin detection
Liver	Hepatitis	Primary viral hepatitis (A, B, C, delta) Other viruses (EBV, CMV, HSV, coxsackievirus, adenovirus) Toxoplasma gondii	Liver biopsy Serology
	Hepatosplenic candidiasis (persistent fever; abdominal pain, hepatosplenomegaly, raised alkaline phosphatase level)	Candida spp.	Ultrasonography CT, MRI Biopsy (histology and culture)
Urinary tract	Urinary tract infections (dysuria, i.e. frequency, urgency, pain; hematuria; flank pain)	Gram-negative bacilli (Escherichia coli, Klebsiella spp., Proteus spp., Enterobacter spp., Pseudomonas aeruginosa) Enterococcus spp. Coagulase-negative staphylococci (Staphylococcus saprophyticus) Candida spp. Virus (BK virus, adenovirus)	Culture of urine
Central nervous system*	Acute meningitis Subacute, chronic meningitis Focal brain diseases	Listeria monocytogenes Cryptococcus neoformans Candida spp. Mycobacterium tuberculosis Coccidioides immitis Histoplasma capsulatum Aspergillus spp.	CT, MRI Lumbar puncture Aspiration or biopsy under stereotaxic CT guidance

(clinical features)

Progressive dementia	Nocardia asteroides
	Listeria monocytogenes
	Toxoplasma gondii
	Viruses (HSV, varicella, cytomegalovirus, EBV, HHV-6, adenovirus, papillomavirus JC)
	JC virus (progressive multifocal leukoencephalopathy)
Shunt infections (fever, change in mental status, headache, meningism, increase intracranial pressure; patient may also be asymptomatic)	Coagulase-negative staphylococci
	Staphylococcus aureus
	Enterococcus spp.
	Corynebacterium spp.
	Propionibacterium spp.
	Gram-negative bacilli
	Candida spp.

* Patients with BMT have the same susceptibility to conventional pathogens of the central nervous system (meningitis: Streptococcus pneumoniae, Neisseria meningitidis, Haemophilus influenzae, Gram-negative bacilli; brain abscess: streptococci, Bacteroides spp., Staphylococcus aureus, Enterobacteriaceae) as the general population. Listed above are unique pathogens.

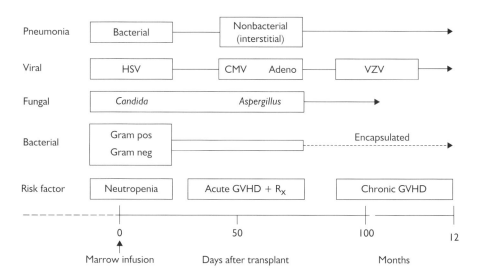

Figure 5.1 Predisposing risk factors and common infections by time after allogeneic transplant. HSV, herpes simplex virus; CMV, cytomegalovirus; VZV, varicella zoster virus; Pos, positive; Neg, negative; GVHD, graft-versus-host disease; R_x, treatment. From Meyers (1985).

period. Pneumonia due to *Pseudomonas* spp. is more common in some centers than others. Pneumonia due to Gram-positive organisms is quite uncommon (including *Streptococcus* spp., *Staphylococcus aureus* and coagulase-negative staphylococci). During the first month after transplantation, aspiration pneumonia is common in patients with significant mucositis and is usually due to Gram-positive mouth flora, including anaerobic species.

CMV is quite uncommon during the first month after transplantation and is more common during the second and third month unless antiviral prophylaxis or preemptive therapy is used. With antiviral prevention, less than 5% of allogeneic transplant patients will develop CMV pneumonia during the first 100 days after transplantation; however, up to 18% of allogeneic BMT patients may develop CMV pneumonia during the first year after transplantation during the period after which antiviral prophylaxis has been discontinued (see section 1.4).

Another group of infections recently appreciated as significant causes of respiratory infection during both the preengraftment as well as postengraftment periods are the community-acquired respiratory viruses, particularly respiratory syncytial virus (RSV), parainfluenza virus and influenza virus. Classically, these infections present with upper respiratory symptoms, with or without sinus symptoms, and often have a fulminant and fatal course despite antiviral therapy.

Fungal pneumonia, most of which is due to *Aspergillus* spp., remains a major challenge in the allogeneic setting. Acquired either before or after transplantation through the inhalation of spores, aspergillosis has two peak times of onset: one peak is during the neutropenic period when both allogeneic and autologous patients are at risk, and the second larger peak occurs during the second and third month after transplantation. Other non-*Aspergillus* molds are also important causes of fungal pneumonia and sinus-related disease, although as a group have occurred with approximately 10% of the frequency of aspergillosis.

Other rarer causes of viral pneumonia include adenovirus, herpes simplex virus (HSV) or varicella zoster virus (VZV), usually seen with other evidence of disseminated viral infection. *Legionella* spp., *Nocardia* spp. and mycobacterial infection (either *Mycobacterium tuberculosis* or one of the rapid growing atypical mycobacterial species) are rare but important causes of bacterial pneumonia. *P. carinii* is generally confined to patients who have not received pre- and post-transplant TMP–SMX due to either allergy or error. Since *P. carinii* pneumonia is an infection seen almost exclusively in the allogeneic setting, the need for prophylaxis with TMP–SMX is controversial in the autologous setting.

The relative frequency of pneumonia may be even higher in the allogeneic and autologous populations of patients since it is often diagnosed clinically in the absence of positive blood cultures, especially for bacterial pneumonia.

There are a number of noninfectious reasons for pulmonary infiltrates, including pulmonary edema, adult respiratory distress syndrome, hemorrhage, atelectasis and idiopathic pneumonia syndrome related to toxicity from the conditioning regimen.

Another, presumably common, site of infection listed in Table 5.1 is paranasal sinuses. Sinusitis is presumably related to the mucosal changes that occur secondarily to conditioning regimens. Again, this holds true for both allogeneic and autologous patients, although many autologous patients receive conditioning that is not associated with the same degree of mucositis seen with many allogeneic conditioning regimens. Few data are available describing the frequency and relative etiologies of infections in the sinuses. It is common for any conditioning therapy that affects the gastrointestinal mucosal lining also to affect the respiratory mucosa, and thickening of sinus linings is a common finding after transplantation. Only more recently have invasive procedures started to be performed, particularly when fungal infection is suspected, and the current literature probably underestimates the frequency of bacterial (including anaerobic infection), respiratory virus infection and fungal infection of the sinuses in the early post-BMT period.

Infections of the urinary, gastrointestinal tracts or the central nervous system (CNS) are quite unusual following BMT, especially during the neutropenic period. Urinary tract infection should be suspected in patients with indwelling catheters or in those with a history of recurrent urinary infection. With the advent of antiviral prophylaxis, recent data have shown that less than 10% of all diarrhea in the early post-BMT period is associated with infection, implying that most of the diarrhea observed is related to the effects of chemotherapy or GVHD on the gastrointestinal lining. CMV or HSV used to be quite common causes of esophagitis or gastrointestinal infection before the routine use of antiviral prophylaxis. Nosocomial infection with *Clostridium difficile* remains a challenging problem in the hospitalized patient on broad-spectrum antibiotic therapy, although many more patients are likely colonized with C. *difficile* than will develop symptoms associated with toxin-positive diarrhea.

1.3 What are the predominant organisms that contribute (by site)?

Table 5.1 outlines the most common types and sites of infection for patients undergoing either autologous or allogeneic transplants.

The most common type of bloodstream infection is caused by bacteria, which account for more than 75% of documented bloodstream infection. The remaining causes of bloodstream infection includes viruses and fungi. While the risk for bacteremia persists as long as the central catheter is in place, the risk of fungemia and viremia is lower for autologous than for allogeneic patients.

CMV has been the most common cause of viral infection after BMT, occurring in up to 70% of CMV-seropositive allogeneic and approximately 40% of seropositive autologous transplant patients before the use of routine antiviral prophylaxis. The risk for CMV pneumonia is approximately 35% in CMV-seropositive patients, compared with 2–7% of autologous patients not receiving antiviral preemptive or prophylactic therapy. Viral blood cultures are now positive for CMV in less than 3% of allogeneic patients during the first 3 months after transplantation, although CMV can be detected more frequently by antigenemia or polymerase chain reaction (PCR) in the earliest stages of viral reactivation. Adenovirus occurs in 5–15% of patients and is more commonly seen after allogeneic transplant. The majority of cases of adenovirus infection are associated with either fever and/or hematuria, with a minority of infections being either asymptomatic or associated with renal, lung or gastrointestinal infection. The mortality rate associated with adenovirus when visceral organs are involved is in excess of 50%. Finally, *Candida* spp. accounted for approximately 10% of bloodstream infections prior to the use of prophylactic fluconazole in the allogeneic transplant setting, occurring substantially less often after autologous transplant. Currently, the incidence of fungemia is approximately 5% for all patients in centers that use prophylaxis and is most often due to non-*albicans Candida*, especially *C. glabrata* and *C. krusei*.

1.4 How do the organisms vary according to various risk factors?

The occurrence of infection is closely associated with predictable risk factors, which have been well defined and vary by time after transplantation. Figure 5.1 describes the three risk periods prior to the era of routine prophylaxis for the most common infections after allogeneic transplantation. In general, patients undergoing T-cell-depleted allogeneic transplantation and allogeneic patients who develop GVHD are at highest risk for infection, while patients undergoing autologous transplantation are at the lowest risk overall.

The three risk periods for infection following allogeneic BMT are (1) the neutropenic period, lasting from the time of conditioning until 2–3 weeks after transplantation; (2) the period from engraftment until approximately day 100 after transplantation; and (3) the 'late' post-BMT period, which extends from day 100 until the end of the first year after transplantation or when GVHD has resolved and its therapy has been discontinued. Patients undergoing autologous transplant share similar risks for infection during the neutropenic period; however, their risk for serious life-threatening infection (e.g. from organisms such as CMV or aspergillosis) is markedly reduced in the post-engraftment period, assuming patients have adequate engraftment.

First risk period (the neutropenic period)

The major organisms causing infection during the neutropenic period include Gram–negative bacterial infection and HSV, the risk for which is augmented by the disruption of the mucosal barrier of the gastrointestinal tract due to conditioning therapy. Gram-positive bacteremia related to intravenous catheters occurs with equal frequency before and after engraftment. VZV, CMV, adenovirus infection and parasitic infections are quite uncommon during the neutropenic period and are more closely related to the presence of GVHD and its therapy during the second 2 months after BMT.

Some centers are experiencing increasing morbidity and mortality rates associated with community-acquired respiratory virus infections. Unlike other viral infections in the BMT setting, the risk for community-acquired respiratory virus infections is almost entirely related to viral exposure rather than engraftment or the presence or absence of GVHD. Fungemia with *Candida* spp. occur in approximately 10–15% of patients, most commonly related to neutropenia, to a disrupted gastrointestinal mucosal barrier from conditioning therapy or GVHD, and to the use of broad-spectrum antibiotics. Approximately one third of posttransplant aspergillosis also occurs during the neutropenic period.

The risk of infection following autologous transplantation is similar to that in patients undergoing allogeneic transplant during the neutropenic period, especially in patients whose conditioning regimens result in severe mucositis. Following engraftment, however, the risk of infections common to the allogeneic setting are low in the autologous setting as long as adequate numbers of neutrophils are maintained. One of the more common infections seen after autologous transplant is Gram-positive bacteremia, especially in the presence of an indwelling intravenous catheter. Infections after day 100 in autologous patients, with the exception of VZV, are quite uncommon.

Second risk period (from engraftment until day 100)

The second risk period affects primarily the allogeneic patient and the most significant risk factors include the presence of GVHD and the use of steroids. Studies have correlated not only an increased frequency of clinically apparent infection (e.g. CMV pneumonia and enteritis) but also a higher mortality rate for patients with GVHD who develop herpesvirus infections, adenovirus or invasive fungal infections.

Before the use of antiviral prophylaxis, CMV was the leading infectious cause of death in the first 100 days, with life-threatening disease occurring in 35% of seropositive patients. The second 2 months after BMT are associated with an increased risk for both adenovirus and *Pneumocystis* infection in patients not receiving prophylaxis. Patients undergoing allogeneic transplantation, particularly those with GVHD and indwelling lines, continue to be at risk for bacteremia and sepsis during this period. The use of T-cell depletion as part of the conditioning regimen delays recovery of antigen-specific T-cells and may prolong the risk period for infections such as CMV beyond 100 days after BMT.

Third risk period ('late' post-BMT period)

Increased risk for infection in the late posttransplant period (more than 100 days after BMT) is almost entirely related to a delay in reconstitution of antigen-specific T cells in patients conditioned with T-cell depletion or in those with chronic GVHD. The exception is VZV infection, whose median time of onset occurs between 4 and 6 months after transplantation. The reasons for this relatively late reactivation pattern have never been fully understood. Both allogeneic and autologous patients are at risk during this late period, although those with chronic GVHD are at highest risk. Other infections that are specific to the late period in high-risk patients include aspergillosis and other molds and infections due to encapsulated bacteria, which are particularly likely to infect the sinopulmonary tree and the middle ear.

As alluded to above, the addition of antiinfective prophylaxis has either significantly reduced the risk of some infections, or in some cases simply delayed their onset until later in the posttransplant course at the time when prophylaxis is discontinued, CMV being the best example. While originally a significant cause of death at the second and third month after transplant, less than 5% of patients now acquire active CMV infection and disease during the first 100 days as long as they are serially monitored and started on prophylactic or preemptive therapy if blood tests prove positive. Because of their inadequate reconstitution of CMV-specific T-cell immunity, allogeneic transplant patients are at continued risk for CMV disease (both pneumonia and gastrointestinal infection) during the late period. In fact, three quarters of all CMV disease in the first year after transplantation now occurs during the late period in up to 18% of seropositive patients undergoing allogeneic transplantation.

1.5 How does this differ from other conditions, from center to center, and from country to country?

In some cases, the types or frequency of infection vary from transplant center to center. For example, aspergillosis occurs rarely in some centers but may occur in up to 15% of patients in other centers. Construction or types of transplant conditioning, including T-cell depletion, have been implicated in these differences. Community-acquired respiratory viruses also appear more common in some centers and are virtually never seen in others.

Endemic infections may also be more common in centers from a particular area. For example, toxoplasmosis is seen more frequently where the endemic rates of infection are high. Likewise, infection with dematiaceous fungi are generally more common in the warmer, southern climates. Rates of infection with *M. tuberculosis* after BMT are also higher in centers located in endemic areas.

1.6 What is the appropriate approach to the initial evaluation and diagnosis of infection in patients undergoing BMT?

Table 5.1 gives an overview as to the specific evaluation approach and diagnostic tools that can be helpful in assessing patients with infection. In general, the best approach to diagnosis of infection in the BMT setting is the use of aggressive diagnostic procedures early in the course of infection or in the highest risk patients to establish the cause. Not only does this facilitate appropriate therapy but also determines the duration of treatment, particularly when it is expensive or is associated with undesirable side effects. This approach is followed for all stem cell transplantation, whether the patient is undergoing autologous, allogeneic or T-cell-depleted transplantation.

The type of diagnostic workup is determined not only by the presenting signs and symptoms of infection, but also by the tune when symptoms present post-transplant. Careful assessment of the pretransplant serologies and the patient's prophylactic antiinfective regimen assists in generating a likely differential diagnosis. For example, a patient who develops pulmonary infiltration just after engraftment but who has received TMP–SMX prophylaxis, and who is known to be CMV seropositive and on ganciclovir preemptive therapy, has a much different differential diagnosis than a patient with new pulmonary nodules on day 80 after transplantation who remains neutropenic with poor engraftment due to GVHD.

In addition to the tests outlined in Table 5.1, the most important approach to the patient with suspected infection in the BMT setting is a careful history of recent changes in symptoms and a meticulous physical examination. The physical examination should focus on sites that are particularly high risk in the BMT patient, including the nasal sinuses, oral and rectal mucosa, the lungs, catheter entry sites and tunnel tracts, and the entire skin surface.

Blood cultures should be obtained in patients with suspected infection. In addition to the usual enteric pathogens, viral blood cultures should also be considered; recognizing that adenovirus can be a cause of persistent fever, and CMV can cause viremia and fever in patients not on antiviral prophylaxis. Blood cultures should be evaluated with a technique sensitive in picking up yeast (either Bac-Tec or isolator methods). Controversy exists as to whether blood cultures should be obtained from both indwelling central venous catheters and a simultaneous venous site, since any positive blood cultures from either site generally warrant treatment, especially in highest risk patients. With rare exception, a single positive blood culture for *Candida* spp. or for coagulase-negative *Staphylococcus* should always be treated.

Chest radiography is also an important part of an infectious workup since many infections reside in the lungs. However, there are no classic radiographic abnormalities pathognomonic for a specific infection, and the best diagnostic evaluation of a radiographic abnormality of the chest involves some sort of invasive diagnostic procedure. Even nodules thought to be classic for aspergillosis can be indistinguishable from the less frequent occurrence of nocardiosis. Patients with a nondiagnostic bronchoalveolar lavage (BAL) result who are particularly high risk or who remain febrile and ill on empirical antiinfective therapy should be considered for a thoracoscopic or open lung biopsy. This may be of particular value in the late posttransplant period in patients with chronic GVHD who are at risk for not only multiple infections, often with unusual organisms, but also for noninfectious chronic lung changes which might be best managed with steroid therapy.

The use of BAL for diagnosis of chest infection can be very sensitive for the diagnosis of pneumonia and is particularly useful in the diagnosis of viral infections (e.g. CMV, community-acquired respiratory viruses) and *Pneumocystis* pneumonia. BAL is less sensitive for fungus. For example, only about 50% of patients with aspergillosis will have their infection identified by BAL. Presence of yeast in the BAL rarely indicate candida pneumonia and most often represent contamination by mouth organisms. BAL is indicated patients who develop a new or a progressive infiltrate on radiography on current antimicrobial therapy. Infection with more than one organism is common, especially after allogeneic transplant. Sputum samples are not reliable and tracheal aspirates or induced sputum samples are rarely performed in the BMT setting. In the critically ill patient whose BAL is nondiagnostic, a thoracoscopic or open biopsy should be considered.

Catheter-related infections are not uncommon. Redness, even with some minimal drainage, that does not extend more than 1 cm from the exit site most often represents local tissue reaction and can be evaluated with a simple Gram stain and culture, with local therapy. Erythema or induration that extend further up the catheter should be evaluated with blood cultures and any purulent material that can be expressed at the entry site. Tender nodules identified on clinical examination of the tunnel tract, particularly in the second or third month after transplantation, should make one highly suspicious of atypical mycobacterial infection. An acid-fast stain of the drainage is critical for early diagnosis. Open debridement both for diagnosis and management of these infections is required.

Lesions involving the skin, mucosa, sinuses or visceral organs highly suspicious of fungal infection should be biopsied. Skin biopsies are easy to perform and should be used early after the appearance of lesions suspicious for any type of infection. All biopsy material in BMT patients should be evaluated histologically, including with special stains for herpesviruses and fungi, and cultured for bacteria, fungi and viruses. Needle biopsies of suspicious visceral lesions, especially in the abdomen, can be helpful but the yield may be only 50%, and often the organism will not grow. However, in such cases, special histologic stains can usually rule in or out fungal infection and assist in the choice of the appropriate type and duration of therapy.

Computed tomography (CT) or magnetic resonance imaging (MRI) can be useful in specific situations to define the extent of infection further. CT is more sensitive than standard radiography in identifying fungal lesions in the lung. The choice of where to scan in search of disseminated fungal disease depends on whether fungus is suspected as the cause of infection. For example, because *Candida* spp. invade through the gastrointestinal tract and then the portal blood system, performing an abdominal CT is appropriate. In contrast, because *Aspergillus* enters the host through the respiratory system and then invades the bloodstream, a chest or head CT is preferred. Both CT and MRI can be useful in defining lesions in the brain in patients who present with CNS symptoms.

1.7 How should the evaluation be modified according to the severity of the risk?
Patients early in the posttransplant course (i.e. prior to engraftment) or those undergoing allogeneic transplant with GVHD on high doses of immunosuppression are at highest risk of infection, and more aggressive diagnostic evaluations should be undertaken in these patients. The major risk for serious infection in autologous BMT patients occurs during the first month. In addition, more frequent culturing may be necessary in some high-risk patients, including those with poor engraftment. An example includes routine blood cultures in patients on high doses of corticosteroids, even in the absence of symptoms, since the use of steroids may interfere with the ability to mount a febrile response or develop local signs and symptoms of infection.

1.8 What are the specific evaluation measures? (see also Chapter 2 in Part I)
Many of the specific measures used for diagnostic evaluation have been listed above. Several comments could be made about the pretransplant evaluation, since this evaluation is aimed at the identification of the patient at high risk for specific infections rather than for specific diagnoses per se. In general, serologic tests are only useful before BMT, when they are used for the identification of patients at high risk for reactivation of previous infection. The typical panel of pre-BMT serologic tests includes tests for CMV, HSV, VZV and *Toxoplasma*. However, following transplant, serologic testing is rarely useful and may be confusing, either because patients do not mount normal antibody responses for months following transplantation or because patients received exogenous antibody from blood products or immunoglobulin. Most BMT centers do not perform Epstein–Barr virus (EBV) serologic testing since most patients are presumed seropositive and the risk of EBV-related lymphoproliferative syndrome, which is much more common after solid organ transplant, is not as clearly implicated in the EBV-seronegative recipient receiving seropositive stem cells. Pretransplant herpesvirus serologies help guide the use of antiviral prophylaxis, and *Toxoplasma* serologies can be helpful in including or excluding toxoplasmosis from the differential diagnosis later after transplant in patients who develop pulmonary or CNS lesions.

Blood cultures should include methodology specific enough to identify yeast, such as the isolator or Bac-Tec systems. Anaerobic cultures should also be set up on bloods even though they are rarely positive. Exudates or drainage should be evaluated with both Gram stains and cultures that include evaluation for fungal species. Acid-fast stains, as mentioned above, may help to identify rapid growing mycobacterial species from catheter drainage material or from lung samples. Tissue obtained for diagnostic purposes should be evaluated for bacteria, fungi, viruses and protozoa as appropriate. Routine surveillance cultures for bacterial or fungi are not considered cost effective.

1.9 What new developments are going to impact on emerging organisms, recognition, evaluation and diagnosis of infection in patients undergoing BMT?
Standard CMV blood and urine cultures have become obsolete with the development of more rapid, early diagnostic tools for CMV. Most centers now test patients weekly for

CMV by either PCR or antigenemia, positive tests are used as a guide for preemptive therapy. Shell vial cultures for the herpesviruses are still quite useful for BAL or tissue specimens when any of the herpesviruses are suspected.

Most infections observed after BMT come from the patient's endogenous flora (e.g. reactivation of viral infection, overgrowth and infection with *Candida* spp., bacteremia from Gram-negative bacterial flora) and are not seasonal. Nasopharyngeal aspirates have recently been added to the diagnostic evaluation in patients who present before or after BMT with upper respiratory symptoms, with increasing appreciation of the morbidity and mortality observed seasonally with community respiratory viral infections. A positive culture in the pretransplant evaluation generally suggests that BMT should be delayed, when possible, until the patient is in the recovery phase of the infection.

Another problematic, although fortunately in most cases not life-threatening, infection has been the rising incidence of C. *difficile* infection. Highly transmissible by the hands or clothing of healthcare workers or patients, C. *difficile* has presented a significant challenge for infection control personnel.

Finally, increasing pressures to control costs have resulted in the elimination of many previously performed tests in the posttransplant setting. Routine surveillance cultures and weekly chest radiography in the lower risk or asymptomatic patient have been eliminated in many centers. This puts increasing importance on the use of ongoing history and physical examination and clinical judgement as a way of guiding the choice of the most appropriate diagnostic tests.

2 REGARDING THE RISK FACTORS ACCOMPANYING BMT

2.1 What are the main alterations in host defense mechanisms and what are the appropriate investigations to document them?

Chapter 1, Part II, outlines in some detail the general factors associated with host defense abnormalities in the immunocompromised host, many of which apply to the BMT patient. In the allogeneic BMT setting, the most significant host defense defects appear to be associated with (a) abnormal anatomic barriers during mucositis related to conditioning therapy or GVHD, and to increased portals of entry due to indwelling intravenous catheters; (b) the number of neutrophils (i.e. their absence during neutropenia) or abnormal neutrophil function during the postengraftment period, particularly in patients on steroids; and (c) abnormal T-cell function. Patients undergoing autologous transplant experience similar defects although, with the exception of neutropenia, they occur with either less severity or a shorter duration than that seen after allogeneic transplant. The role of complement and antibody in host defense in the BMT setting is less clear, since the profound defects in phagocytic and T-cell immunity tend to overshadow the presence or importance of humoral defects.

2.2 What are the alterations due to iatrogenic factors?

Table 5.2 describes the postallogeneic BMT timeline and relates the most common host defense defects to iatrogenic and noniatrogenic factors that contribute to each in this setting. In a sense, all the defects observed after BMT can be considered to be iatrogenic and a result of (1) giving lethal doses of radiation and chemotherapy, followed by (2) transplantation of donor stem cells in their varying degrees of human leukocyte antigen (HLA) mismatch, leading to (3) GVHD, itself immunosuppressive, then (4) requiring

Table 5.2 Alterations in host defense after bone marrow transplantation due to both iatrogenic and noniatrogenic factors

Host defense defect	Iatrogenic factors	Noniatrogenic factors
Neutropenia	Chemotherapy	
	Irradiation	
	Other drugs	
Acute GVHD	Steroids	GVHD
T-cell dysfunction	Anti-T-cell antibody	
Monocyte–macrophage dysfunction	Conditioning therapy	
Chronic GVHD	Steroids	GVHD
		CMV

GVHD, graft-versus-host disease; CMV, cytomegalovirus.

immunosuppressive therapy to treat GVHD. Possibly only CMV infection, which is known to have inherent immunosuppressive effects, can be considered noniatrogenic since patients generally develop this infection as a result of endogenous reactivation. The exception is the CMV-seronegative recipient who acquires CMV from either donor stem cells or from blood product, the latter of which is now preventable with either CMV-seronegative or leukocyte-depleted blood products.

2.3 What is the influence of environmental factors?
Environmental factors play a major role in the risk of certain types of infections in the BMT setting. Exposure from the community, from infected hospital healthcare workers, from food and from environmental factors inherent to the geographic origin of the patient or location of the transplant center all play some role. While most post-BMT infection comes from patients' endogenous flora, viruses that cause respiratory infection or, less commonly, primary VZV infection transmitted from ill family members or healthcare staff can pose a serious threat to patients in the post-BMT period. Dust, and in particular air contaminated with *Aspergillus* spores, is thought to be the major source of aspergillosis after BMT. Food is rarely a source of serious infection and sterile food no longer plays a role in the care of the BMT patient, except in the unusual situation when the patient is in laminar air flow isolation. Careful washing of fresh produce and avoiding nonregulated sources of drinking water may limit the rare source of infections associated with food. Some infections are more common in certain parts of the country or world and a careful travel history may suggest an increased risk to opportunistic pathogens from an endemic region (e.g. coccidioidomycoses or tuberculosis in patients who reside in a region endemic for these infections).

2.4 What are the most significant factors that contribute to the risk of infection in patients undergoing BMT?
In general, the majority of posttransplant infection comes from the endogenous micro-bial flora in the patient. This is particularly true of Gram-negative infection, which is common during the early post-BMT neutropenic period, or during active flares of gas-trointestinal mainfestations of GVHD. The other major infectious risk that comes from within the patient is the common reactivation of various herpesviruses. In patients not receiving any form of antiviral prophylaxis, for example, 70–80% of CMV-seropositive

allogeneic BMT patients (approximately 40% of autologous patients) will develop CMV infection (peak incidence 2–3 months posttransplant). Autologous and allogeneic patients are at similar risks for HSV and VZV. Approximately 80% of HSV-seropositive patients will develop a positive HSV culture, with a peak incidence 1–3 weeks post-transplantation, and 28–40% of VZV-seropositive patients will develop zoster or disseminated VZV infection, with a peak incidence 4–6 months posttransplant.

Exposure from the community and the environment plays an ancillary role in altering the frequency and severity of infection. Significant risks from the community include seasonal transmission of community-acquired respiratory viruses from infected family members or healthcare workers and VZV transmission from exposure of a person with primary VZV to the rare VZV-seronegative recipient. Other significant community exposures include resistant nosocomial bacterial infections e.g. vancomycin-resistant enterococci (VRE) and C. *difficile*.

The region or part of the country or world can also influence the risk for certain infections following BMT. The regional influence on risk of dematiaceous fungal infections, for example, is demonstrated by the increase in infection in the southeastern United States compared with the incidence in more northern transplant centers where it is rarely seen unless the patient travels to those centers already colonized with the organism. In contrast to the infectious risk observed in solid organ transplant patients or patients with human immunodeficiency virus (HIV) infection where *Cryptococcus* is a frequent cause of infection, it is rarely seen after BMT. Perhaps two exceptions include the risks for *M. tuberculosis* and toxoplasmosis after BMT, which are known to be higher in patients who come from endemic areas (e.g. Central and South America, southern Europe and the Mediterranean for *M. tuberculosis*, and western Europe for toxoplasmosis).

Food, if handled with routinely clean precautions, poses little risk to BMT patients, even those most severely compromised, despite common dogma that such patients need sterile or restricted diets. There are simply few data to support this. The same can be said of potted plants or flowers. While most centers restrict such items from patients' rooms, it could be argued that the *Aspergillus* spores in the air patients breathe pose a much higher risk of serious infection than a potted begonia plant. Exceptions, of course, exist and the following are several examples. It is known that immunocompromised patients who ingest large quantities of naturopathic medications containing mold species can develop serious and unusual infections. Outbreaks of cryptosporidiosis have been reported in transplant patients who ingested contaminated water. Other contaminated food products can lead to serious infection in BMT patients as well as normal hosts. Recent data have suggested that molds can also be acquired from contaminated water supplies if ingested in high enough quantities.

2.5 What are the specific or nonspecific measures aimed at minimizing each of these factors?

Because the risk period for patients undergoing autologous transplant is generally shorter than for allogeneic transplant, strategies to minimize risk will need to be extended for the allogeneic transplant patient, especially those with GVHD.

Perhaps the most important measure is the simplest, although not necessarily the easiest to ensure, and that is simple handwashing and keeping sick people away from patients. Handwashing can be quite effective in disrupting the transmission of most community-acquired infections (e.g. community-acquired respiratory viral infections, VRE, C. *difficile*). For these and other nosocomial infections, including VZV, education of family members and healthcare staff, and isolation of the infected patient, is the secondary key to controlling transmission, since, despite best efforts, handwashing is not always performed. Education regarding the use of caution with naturopathic medication during the most intense periods of immunosuppression and use of commonsense precautions in preparation of foods can also avoid most risks from dietary intake.

More difficult are attempts to reduce risks from a patient's own endogenous flora and protection of the patient from infectious molds transmitted through inhalation of airborne spores. A careful history and focused workup pretransplant and during the period of highest immunocompromise after transplantation is the most rationale approach to reduction of risk factors. There are currently no proven ways to ensure absolute protection from exposure to the molds, including *Aspergillus* spp. Neither the use of masks, low-dose amphotericin B or other systemic antifungals, inhalation therapy of antifungals, or routine microbiologic surveillance has been shown unequivocally to be effective. Laminar air flow isolation has been shown to reduce infection due to aspergillosis, although it is very expensive and benefits patients only as long as they remain in isolation for the entire risk period. With pressure to decrease the length of inpatient care, laminar air flow isolation becomes increasingly impractical and most centers have abandoned its use. For those centers who still have operational laminar air flow units, patients with an inordinately long period of neutropenia could be considered for transplant in these rooms. Most centers agree that the use of high-efficiency particulate air (HEPA) filtration is indicated for stem cell transplant patients as long as they remain in the hospital. Again, the use of HEPA filtered air makes more sense in patients who are at increased risk for aspergillosis who will be confined to their rooms for the period of highest risk after BMT.

Testing for *M. tuberculosis* in high-risk patients and initiating therapy prior to transplantation has become standard practice to reduce this rather unusual post-BMT complication, and appears to be effective in anecdotal reports.

3 REGARDING THE SURVEILLANCE OF PATIENTS UNDERGOING BMT

3.2 What are the surveillance measures to be taken in a patient undergoing BMT?

Routine surveillance for both allogeneic as well as autologous transplant patients has played less of a role in recent years as better and more specific ways have been developed to detect infection early. Further, as cost pressures in the healthcare delivery system have increased, there has been elimination of routine microbiologic procedures that, in any event, have a questionable or relatively low yield. One important change has been the elimination of routine body surface cultures both for bacteria and fungi in most centers.

Some forms of surveillance continue to be justified in the asymptomatic patients and include the following. Pretransplant evaluation for both autologous as well as allogeneic patients continues to include serologic testing of all patients for the herpesviruses (see section 1.8) and in some centers for other organisms such as *Toxoplasma*. Cultures of blood and other tissues should be performed before transplantation for patients with obvious exposures or signs and symptoms of active infection. Posttransplant surveillance currently is limited in most centers to routine weekly screening of blood (by viral blood culture, antigenemia or PCR) in CMV-seropositive patients, which identifies patients who might benefit from preemptive antiviral therapy. In addition, routine blood cultures are sometimes performed in allogeneic patients on high doses of steroids because they may not mount a febrile response even in the face of bacteremia or sepsis. Some workers advocate weekly chest radiography to identify early infection, especially aspergillosis, which may present in an otherwise asymptomatic patient. Apart from these examples, most other forms of routine surveillance are no longer used in either the allogeneic or autologous settings.

4 REGARDING THE PREVENTION OF INFECTION IN PATIENTS UNDERGOING BMT

4.1 What approaches, if any, to the prevention of infection should be considered in patients undergoing BMT?

In general, prevention of infection after BMT is more successful than is treatment once infection is already established, especially for infections associated with the highest mortality rates. There have been a number of successful controlled studies published in recent years that have resulted in changes in our approach to the prevention of infection after BMT and in significant improvements in survival.

Perhaps the most significant advance in the past two decades has been the prevention of herpesvirus infections. Acyclovir prophylaxis in the HSV-seropositive patient continues to be routine after allogeneic transplant and is commonly used after autologous transplant in patients receiving conditioning therapy which induces severe mucositis. Acyclovir prophylaxis, given at a dose of 250 mg/m^2 twice daily either orally or intravenously from the onset of conditioning until engraftment in allogeneic patients, has substantially reduced the incidence and severe morbidity of HSV infection early post-BMT. Most centers also give acyclovir prophylaxis to autologous patients when their conditioning regimens are known to result in severe mucositis. Acyclovir alternatives such as valacyclovir may offer a more convenient dosing schedule because they deliver higher doses of active acyclovir orally than do doses of the parent compound. Severe HSV mucositis is rarely seen following an era when more than 70% of HSV-seropositive patients had symptomatic HSV disease in the mouth or esophagus. Figure 5.2 shows the relative reduction in the incidence of HSV-positive cultures by week after transplantation since the routine institution of acyclovir prophylaxis during the first few weeks after transplantation.

Prophylaxis or preemptive ganciclovir (or alternatively foscarnet) has also become routine in the CMV-seropositive allogeneic BMT patient and the seronegative patient with a seropositive donor, but is not used routinely in the autologous setting where the risk of serious CMV disease is substantially lower than in the allogeneic setting. Preemptive therapy is considered 'prophylactic' in that it prevents clinical disease in patients who have DNA or protein evidence of early viral reactivation. Figure 5.3 shows the change in frequency and timing of CMV infection since the routine use of ganciclovir for prevention of CMV infection in allogeneic patients.

Prophylaxis of VZV, which can be successfully achieved with acyclovir or related compounds, is more controversial because the risk period is so long (i.e. continues until the end of the first year after transplantation) and the morbidity is relatively low (84% of patients will have localized zoster). High-risk patients, such as those with severe GVHD, who are early post-BMT or who have experienced recurrent zoster may benefit from routine prophylaxis. There are still patients who die from VZV infection; this occurs most often when the diagnosis is delayed or the patient is started on subtherapeutic doses of acyclovir.

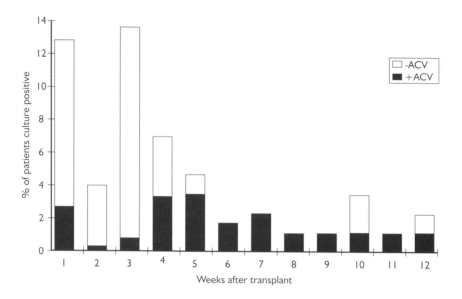

Figure 5.2 Incidence of herpes simplex virus infection with (filled bars) and without (open bars) acyclovir (ACV) prophylaxis, by first positive culture after marrow transplant. From Bowden (1999).

The other infection that is routinely approached prophylactically in the allogeneic setting is candidiasis. Fluconazole, 400 mg daily until engraftment or day 75 after BMT, has been shown in two randomized controlled studies of allogeneic BMT patients successfully to prevent the two major causes of candidiasis, C. *albicans* and C. *tropicalis*.

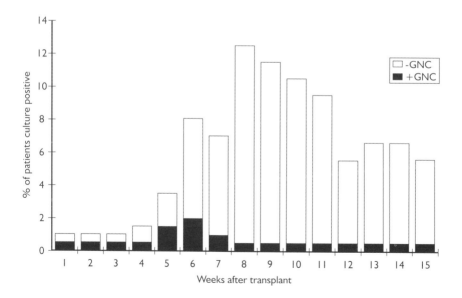

Figure 5.3 Incidence of cytomegalovirus infection with (filled bars) and without (open bars) ganciclovir (GNC) prophylaxis, by first positive culture after marrow transplant. From Bowden (1999).

Unfortunately, it does not prevent mold infections or *C. krusei* and has variable activity against *C. glabrata*, making some question whether the cost is justified in all patients. Because autologous patients are at substantially less risk for candidiasis, fluconazole prophylaxis is not indicated in these patients.

4.2 What are the future challenges and opportunities for reducing the risk of infection?

The most pressing future challenge in infectious disease after BMT is the need to develop effective strategies for prevention of mold infection, and specifically aspergillosis, which is now the leading infectious cause of death after allogeneic transplantation. The development of such a strategy has been difficult to date because of the lack of early diagnostic tests to identify patients at highest risk for development of life-threatening infection. This has been compounded by the lack of availability of effective and safe antifungal agents with activity against *Aspergillus* spp. and the difficulty in conducting adequately powered controlled studies in such a relatively infrequent, though deadly, infection.

Other challenges include the need to focus preventive therapy on those who need it most. When the risk of infection is high (e.g. the incidence of CMV is 70–80% in CMV-seropositive patients), the use of prophylaxis in all patients is more cost effective than when the incidence is low. For example, when the incidence of aspergillosis is 10–15% (and few high-risk indicators are available to date to identify which 10–15% will become infected among all patients), prophylaxis for all patients may be too costly or toxic to justify. Another example includes the use of universal fluconazole prophylaxis when only 5–10% of patients will be infected with susceptible *Candida* spp. Finally, efforts to limit the unnecessary use of prophylactic antibiotics are becoming critical as increases in resistant bacterial species as well as an increase in nosocomial infection with *C. difficile* are being observed. Despite the long-standing dogma to continue all antimicrobial therapy once started until engraftment, early discontinuance of empirical antibiotics in low-risk patients may be justified in some cases.

5 REGARDING THE TREATMENT OF PATIENTS UNDERGOING BMT

5.1 What is the role of empirical therapy?

Empirical therapy with broad-spectrum antibiotics continues to be the mainstay of management of the febrile neutropenic patient. This practice continues because of the high risk of death when therapy is initiated after identification of the cause of fever. Choice of empirical therapy is based on the microbiology of the institution, the side-effect profile of the antibiotics being considered, and cost. Coverage of Gram-positive organisms with vancomycin is not thought to be an essential part of initial empirical therapy in most centers. Withholding vancomycin therapy until the Gram-positive organism has been identified in the blood culture has become accepted practice in most centers because of the high likelihood that a Gram-positive organism in blood culture will be coagulase-negative *Staphylococcus* (greater than 90%) and the low morbidity rate associated with this organism. Therapy is generally continued until neutropenia resolves, although recent recommendations suggest that therapy can be discontinued earlier in the low-risk patient who becomes clinically asymptomatic.

Empirically changing antibiotics during the febrile neutropenic period without positive cultures should be avoided. Modifications of therapy should be guided by changes in the clinical examination, changing microbiologic flora and the microbiologic results from diagnostic procedures.

The initiation of amphotericin B for empirical coverage in the allogeneic and/or neutropenic patient who is persistently febrile for 3–7 days on broad-spectrum antibiotics also remains the standard of care. The timing of initiation varies with the perception of risk. The use of fluconazole prophylaxis has complicated the question of when to add broader antifungal coverage during the neutropenic period, since fluconazole covers the most virulent *Candida* pathogens so well. Recent data for patients undergoing BMT, however, suggest that aspergillosis is also a significant risk during this early period and, thus, the addition of amphotericin B in patients on fluconazole should be considered when the risk of aspergillosis is thought to be significant.

The use of empirical therapy outside the febrile neutropenic period requires experience and clinical judgement because in many cases, when fever occurs after engraftment, the patient can be managed with careful sequential examinations, and cultures and antibiotics can be withheld until the cause of the fever is identified. Exceptions to this include the clinically ill, engrafted patient, those with active acute GVHD, those on steroid therapy and other high-risk patients with a more complicated post-BMT course. In such patients, however, empirical therapy may be initiated with the initial evaluation and discontinued when cultures are negative.

5.2 What is the appropriate approach to the patient undergoing BMT and evidence of:

In general, after both allogeneic and autologous transplantation, specific therapy at differing sites of infection should be based on the organism identified at that site. When it is clinically apparent that an infection is present but an organism cannot be identified, therapy is directed at the most likely organism.

Upper respiratory tract infection?

Infection in the upper respiratory tract is usually confined to the oropharynx and sinuses. The etiologies of infection are numerous and include herpesviruses and community-acquired respiratory viruses, yeasts (i.e. *Candida*), and occasionally bacteria or molds. Infections of the teeth and gingiva, external and middle ear, and eye are uncommon but should be obvious on clinical examination when they occur. Patients should have a pre-transplant evaluation of the teeth and periodontal tissues, and any abnormalities that are identified should be treated before transplantation. Infections of the mucosa have become less frequent after transplantation with the routine use of acyclovir and fluconazole for early post-BMT prophylaxis in the allogeneic setting. Patients who develop new findings on clinical or radiologic examination, particularly during the neutropenic period should have a biopsy or aspirate when feasible.

Lower respiratory tract infection?

Lower respiratory tract abnormalities are common after both autologous and allogeneic transplant and can represent either infection (most common) or noninfectious causes, particularly early after transplantation. Examples of noninfectious abnormalities that may be confused with infection include pulmonary edema, hemorrhage, atelectasis and idiopathic pneumonia syndrome related to toxicity from the conditioning regimen. The only way to treat infections of the lower respiratory tract adequately is to establish the diagnosis. BAL should be used whenever needed as the first diagnostic procedure (see section 1.6).

Empirical treatment is problematic when the evaluation for infection is negative. Resolution of radiographic changes may be slow, resulting in questions about duration of therapy and pressure to discontinue toxic or expensive therapy (e.g. amphotericin B or one of the lipid complex amphotericin products), with little data to guide that decision with confidence.

Gastrointestinal, genitourinary, cardiovascular and musculoskeletal infections?

Specific gastrointestinal, urinary tract , cardiovascular and musculoskeletal system infections are uncommon in patients undergoing BMT. Recent data reporting culture results in hundreds of episodes of diarrhea in BMT patients revealed that less than 10% were a result of infection, and the majority of infections were due to viruses for which there is no therapy (e.g. astrovirus, adenovirus). C. *difficile* can be identified by toxin assay and should be treated with alternatives to metronidazole.

Skin infection?

Skin infections, particularly around the intravenous catheter or other foreign body sites, are relatively common after both allogeneic and autologous transplant, and therapy should be directed by Gram stain, culture or punch biopsy. The most common organisms causing skin infection in the early post-BMT period include staphylococcal species. and Gram-negative organisms. After engraftment, invasive fungal infection, Gram-negative and Gram positive infection and VZV become more common. These infections can have atypical presentation, particularly VZV infection, and attempts to establish the diagnosis should be made as early as possible to assist in initiating the most appropriate therapy.

There are differences of opinion as to which documented infections require removal of the catheter when infection has occurred. Some clinicians advocate that all patients with a single positive blood culture with *Candida* or *Pseudomonas* spp. should have the catheter removed immediately, whereas others would treat with antimicrobials and remove the catheter only if defervescence was not observed within 24–48 h or blood cultures continued to be positive on apparent appropriate therapy. Removal of the intravascular catheter is mandatory when atypical *Mycobacteria* spp. are identified. As always, the risk of inadequately treated infection must be weighed against the cost and morbidity of removing and replacing the catheter. Strict criteria may help increase a successful outcome from catheter-related infections. For example, neutropenic patients should meet the following criteria: defervescence within 24–48 h of starting appropriate and full-dose antibiotic treatment, negative blood cultures within 24–48 h of starting therapy and overall clinical improvement in response to therapy. If blood cultures remain positive or the patient remains febrile, replacement of all indwelling lines should be considered. Of interest, the majority of catheter-related infections can be managed with the catheter left in place.

Central nervous system infection?

CNS infections are uncommon during the early posttransplant period and bacterial meningitis is extremely rare at any time after transplantation. Fungi are the most frequent cause of CNS infection, with aspergillosis being the most common, accounting for 55% of CNS infections and usually presenting as a single lesion on CT. *Candida* infection is responsible for 33% of CNS infections, usually presenting with smaller multiple foci or identified only at autopsy on microscopic examination. CNS toxoplasmosis is quite rare in patients undergoing BMT but can occur. CT should be performed in any patient with changing mental status, particularly if focal signs are present on physical examination. Lumbar punctures are rarely helpful; bacterial meningitis is extremely rare and fungal organisms, even when a CNS abscess is present, are rarely identified by lumbar puncture.

5.3 What is the appropriate approach to the patient undergoing BMT and evidence of bacteremia, with or without site of infection?

The use of empirical therapy has been discussed above. The choice of the antibiotic regimen is based on the organism identified. In general, once a bacterial infection is documented in the blood or other tissue site, the antibiotic of choice is continued for a full 2 weeks, which should encompass the time of resolution of neutropenia. There are few published data in the BMT setting to support this duration of therapy; however, the risk of recurrent infection with the same organism appears to be higher when therapy is discontinued earlier.

Most Gram-positive infections can be treated once the diagnosis is established. Although vancomycin should not be used empirically, its use is appropriate when coagulase-negative staphylococci are identified. Other sites commonly associated with bacteremia include the perirectal area, skin or lungs during neutropenia. In addition to appropriate antibiotic therapy, drainage of the localized infected area should be considered.

Despite pressures to minimize therapy due to cost containment, the use of combination therapy, usually with an aminoglycoside, remains the standard treatment for documented Gram-negative infection. Many centers use combination therapy as initial therapy until blood cultures are negative and the patient is afebrile and clinically stable. At that time it might be appropriate to change to a single antibiotic, including one of the oral quinolones, to complete 2 weeks of treatment in the outpatient setting. Specific infections may require use of combination agents for the entire treatment course if the risk for development of resistance to one is high.

The question has recently arisen as to whether every patient with febrile neutropenia or bacteremia needs to be admitted to the hospital. The predictive risk factors for identifying patients who might be safely managed in this setting have been described recently (see Chapter 4). The highest risk for death appears to be in the first 24–48 h of the presentation of signs and symptoms of infection.

The frequency of anaerobic infections has not been well defined in patients undergoing BMT but appears to be extremely uncommon, accounting for less than 2% of infections. When they do occur, the most common site may include the sinuses or the gastrointestinal tract in the patient with a bowel perforation or rectal fistula (both uncommon now) or necrotizing gingivitis, which is still seen during the neutropenic period.

Mixed polymicrobial infections are common and may occur in up to 10% of patients. Polymicrobial bacterial infections were more common in the days when GVHD of the gastrointestinal tract resulted in perforation than they are today with improved therapy for GVHD. Repeated polymicrobial bacterial infection has been associated with iatrogenic infection, for example contamination of multiuse vials of flushing solution for indwelling intravenous catheters. Clusters of infections, particularly in the outpatient setting, should prompt careful evaluation.

Rarely, infections of the intestinal track, such as with *Strongyloides*, will result in polymicrobial infection due to breakdown of the intestinal wall and creation of a portal of entry for intestinal flora.

Polymicrobial infections where CMV or a community-acquired respiratory infection is identified with another organism (e.g. *Aspergillus* spp., *Enterococcus* spp.) are more frequent than mixed bacterial infection. Indeed, recent data have shown that up to 15% of patients with community-acquired respiratory virus pneumonia have a second organism present. Therapy needs to be directed at both causes of infection. Patients undergoing allogeneic transplant may be at higher risk for mixed polymicrobial infection than those undergoing autologous transplant.

Legionella spp., *Nocardia* spp. and *Actinomyces* spp. are among the rare bacterial infections that occur after BMT, but are important because they can sometimes be confused with more common infections, particularly with fungi.

5.4 What is the appropriate approach to the patient undergoing BMT and evidence of a viral infection?

Treatment of the herpesviruses has been well described and its success has had a significant impact on morbidity and mortality rates in the BMT setting. Not all HSV infections need antiviral therapy and, in fact, patients may need some exposure to active infection at the end of acyclovir prophylaxis to ensure an adequate HSV-specific cytotoxic T-lymphocyte response. Repeated treatment of HSV leads to the occurrence of HSV resistance. Treatment of resistant HSV is problematic, although foscarnet, 40 mg/kg iv tid, can be effective for some period of time.

The standard treatment of CMV pneumonia continues to involve the combination of ganciclovir, 5 mg/kg bid, plus high doses of intravenous immunoglobulin at a dose of 500 mg/kg every other day for 10–14 days. Treatment is the same for both autologous and allogeneic patients because, although the incidence of CMV pneumonia may be lower in autologous patients, morbidity and mortality rates do not differ by type of transplant. There are no controlled studies to support this treatment combination. Initial phase I–II studies from several USA centers reported an improved survival rate of 50–70%; however, European reports and more recent reports from the USA have shown poorer survival rates, in the range of 30%. With the routine use of prophylactic or preemptive ganciclovir, patients who now develop CMV pneumonia are either those with neutropenia who could not take the drug or those with GVHD who had ganciclovir therapy discontinued at day 100. Foscarnet 60 mg/kg tid can be used as an alternative to ganciclovir in patients who are neutropenic and who have good renal function, or in patients with ganciclovir-resistant CMV.

Late CMV disease continues to be a significant problem, occurring after day 100 following BMT. Overall, approximately 18% of CMV-seropositive patients will develop either CMV pneumonia or CMV enteritis, with three quarters of disease now occurring in the late period. Combination of ganciclovir and foscarnet has been used, but data to support this regimen in patients undergoing BMT are unavailable.

Treatment of VZV infection has historically involved the use of intravenous acyclovir at a dose of 500 mg/m^2 tid when infection occurred during the first 9 months. Aggressive intravenous therapy has been given early because deaths still occur from this infection in this timeframe. With the availability of better, orally bioavailable formulations of acyclovir, oral treatment in the patient with localized zoster is becoming routine in the BMT setting, although studies specific to this population are not available. Caution should be exercised when treating any patient with disseminated VZV infection or at high risk for dissemination with oral therapy until it has been established that the infection will not disseminate.

The hepatitis viruses B, C and D occur after transplantation and vary in their clinical severity. Hepatitis B virus (HBV) is a relatively common cause of liver dysfunction, but fortunately is usually not fatal. This may be because patients undergoing BMT are relatively more immunosuppressed and an intact immune system is required for the liver damage from HBV seen in other settings. In these settings, HBV often presents at the time immunosuppression is reduced or withdrawn. Because of its mild impact, HBV in the donor or patient is generally not considered a contraindication to BMT. There is no proven therapy available for HBV infection in the BMT setting. Hepatitis C virus (HCV) is a major cause of life-threatening chronic hepatitis late after transplant. Reports vary on the impact of HCV infection early after transplantation from mild liver disease to fatal venoocclusive disease in different series. Treatment of HCV has not been defined in the BMT setting. Stem cell donors with HCV infection should be excluded from consideration due to the high incidence of life-threatening chronic liver disease in the recipient after BMT.

Posttransplant viral infections for which there are no proven treatment recommendations include human herpesvirus types 6 or 7, EBV, adenovirus, enteroviruses and other very rare viruses such as parvovirus B19, JC or BK viruses.

5.5 What is the appropriate approach to the patient undergoing BMT and evidence of a fungal infection?

Mucosal candidiasis has become much less of a problem with the routine use of prophylactic fluconazole. In the absence of fluconazole, mucosal infection can usually be managed by topical clotrimazole or nystatin troches (or suppositories for vaginal infection). Ketoconazole should be avoided since it can lead to an overgrowth of C. *glabrata*. For infections that develop in patients not already on prophylactic fluconazole, 200 mg daily of fluconazole will also be effective. Lower doses should be avoided since they may lead to the development of resistance.

Amphotericin B remains the treatment of choice for documented invasive fungal infections, particularly in the neutropenic or seriously ill BMT patient. All fungemias should be treated, usually with a daily dose of amphotericin B of 0.5 mg/kg, equivalent to a total dose of 1.5 g in a 70 kg adult. Literature to support the dose and duration of amphotericin B for fungal infections is not available; therefore treatment dosage and duration are empirical. Particularly when prophylactic fluconazole is used and breakthrough fungemia occurs, the consensus is that amphotericin B should be used for treatment. There may be a role for fluconazole in the therapy of fungemia later in the posttransplant period when the patient develops a documented infection with a susceptible *Candida* species (e.g. hepatosplenic candidiasis). Historically, C. *albicans* and C. *tropicalis* have been the two most common causes of infection in the BMT setting. Inference from the results of the two large USA randomized studies might suggest that most hepatosplenic candidiasis is in fact due to C. *albicans* and C. *tropicalis* since it is rarely seen in patients who are receiving such prophylaxis. 5-Fluorocytosine is sometimes used in combination with amphotericin B for disseminated candidiasis, keeping the dose at approximately 75 mg/kg to avoid potential marrow toxicity.

Patients who develop candiduria in the presence of a urinary catheter will usually be managed successfully by removal of the catheter. In low-flow urine states, *Candida* spp. may persist, requiring irrigation with an amphotericin B solution.

As mentioned above, the dose or duration of amphotericin B therapy for most fungal infections remain poorly defined. For more severe disseminated infection (e.g. hepatosplenic candidiasis) patients are generally treated until they have received a total dose of 1.5 g. This usually takes about 6 weeks with a daily dose of 0.5 mg/kg. The alternative in stable patients is fluconazole 400 mg/day, although some would advocate higher doses for 6–8 weeks. It is difficult to determine when to stop antifungal therapy when the infection is found on CT in the lungs or other visceral organs because the resolution of changes on the imaging studies lag behind clinical improvement. Some CT changes never fully disappear and are thought to represent residual scar. Some workers recommend that treatment be continued until resolution or stabilization of findings on CT.

Several lipid-complexed drugs have become available around the world and may be used as an alternative to amphotericin B in patients who fail first-line therapy or in those with invasive fungal infections of all types who also have renal dysfunction, such that using standard amphotericin B is not optimal. While it is likely that lipid preparations of amphotericin B would also be successful as first-line therapy, data to date do not demonstrate that outcome is better with any of the preparations. Further, cost is a significant disadvantage in using these preparations routinely; in some instances they can approach ten times the cost of standard amphotericin B. There is no question that they all have excellent renal-sparing advantages. The incidence of infusion-related side effects so commonly seen with amphotericin B varies with the lipid formulation.

Infection with *Aspergillus* spp. and other molds should be managed aggressively with amphotericin B in a daily dosage of 1.0–1.5 mg/kg for a total dose of 2–3 g in adults. Surgical drainage/debridement should be considered in patients with sinus or facial involvement with aspergillosis, and surgical resection may be considered in patients with isolated pulmonary lesions. The oral formulation of itraconazole has improved absorption over the capsular formation but its role in the treatment of aspergillosis has not been established in controlled studies in the BMT setting. Some centers are using itraconazole as maintenance therapy in patients induced with amphotericin B. There are no data demonstrating that itraconazole or any other antifungal has proven synergistic activity in combination with amphotericin B.

The use of growth factors such as granulocyte colony-stimulating factor (G-CSF) or granulocyte–monocyte colony-stimulating factor in conjunction with an antifungal agent remains controversial and costly. Likewise, the use of G-CSF-stimulated granulocyte transfusion has been shown in anecdotal reports to improve survival in patients infected during the neutropenic period. Other descriptive phase I–II data have shown no benefit, particularly for aspergillosis. The use of growth factors or granulocyte transfusions demands carefully controlled study before it is routinely adopted into clinical practice.

Cryptococcal infection is very rare after BMT and, when it occurs, usually presents as fungemia, which should be managed with amphotericin B. Other molds, dematiaceous fungi, endemic mycoses (histoplasmosis, coccidioidomycosis and blastomycosis) are also quite rare and should be managed as described in other hosts.

5.6 What is the appropriate approach to the patient undergoing BMT and evidence of a parasitic infection?

Other infections that occur after BMT also occur in other immunocompromised settings described in this book and are generally managed in a similar fashion. These include *P. carinii*, *M. tuberculosis* and atypical mycobacterial species, and toxoplasmosis. Parasitic infections, with the exception of *P. carinii* (which some consider a fungus) are so rare in the BMT setting that the reader should use more general infectious disease texts to define the best treatment.

Infection with *P. carinii* is generally confined to the lungs and occurs most commonly in patients who have not received prophylactic TMP–SMX, either because of error or allergy. First-line treatment is TMP–SMX 20 mg/kg in divided doses for 2 weeks. As in other types of patients, alternative therapies include pentamidine or dapsone.

REFERENCES

Bowden RA. Respiratory virus infections after marrow transplantation: the Fred Hutchinson Cancer Research Center experience. *Am J Med* 1997; **102** (3A): 27–30.

Bowden RA. Blood and marrow transplantation. In: Armstrong D, Cohen J, eds. *Infectious Diseases*. London: Mosby International, 1999 (in press).

Bowden RA, Slichter S, Sayers M et al. A comparison of filtered leukocyte-reduced and cytomegalovirus seronegative blood products for the prevention of transfusion-associated CMV infection after marrow transplant. *Blood* 1995; **86:** 3598–3603.

Bowden RA, Ljungman P, Paya CV, eds. *Transplant Infections*. Philadelphia, PA: Lippincott-Raven, 1998.

Goodman J, Winston D, Greenfield R et al. A controlled trial of fluconazole to prevent fungal infections in patients undergoing bone marrow transplantation. *N Engl J Med* 1992; **326:** 845–851.

Goodrich J, Boeckh M, Bowden RA. Strategies for prevention of cytomegalovirus disease after marrow transplantation. *Clin Infect Dis* 1994; **19:** 287–298.

Hughes WT, Armstrong D, Bodey GP et al. Guidelines for the use of antimicrobial agents in neutropenic patients with unexplained fever. *Clin Infect Dis* 1997; **25:** 551–573.

Ljungman P, Lonnquist B, Gahrton G, Ringden O, Sundquist V, Wahren B. Clinical and subclinical reactivation of varicella-zoster virus in immunocompromised patients. *J Infect Dis* 1986; **153:** 840–847.

Meyers, J. Infection in recipients of marrow transplants. In: Remington JS, Swartz MN, eds. *Current Clinical Topics in Infectious Diseases*. New York: McGraw-Hill, 1985: 261–292.

Meyers JD, Flournoy N, Thomas ED. Risk factors for cytomegalovirus infection after human marrow transplantation. *J Infect Dis* 1986; **153:** 478–488.

Ochs, L, Shu, X, Miller J et al. Late infections after allogeneic bone marrow transplantation: comparison of incidence in related and unrelated transplant recipients. *Blood* 1995; **86:** 3979–3986.

Riddell S, Watanabe K, Goodrich J, Li C, Agha M, Greenberg P. Restoration of viral immunity in immunodeficient humans by the adoptive transfer of T cell clones. *Science* 1992; **257:** 238–242.

Wald A, Leisenring W, van Burik JA, Bowden RA. Natural history of *Aspergillus* infections in a large cohort of patients undergoing bone marrow transplantation. *J Infect Dis* 1996; **175:** 1459–1466.

Wingard J, Sostrin M, Vriesendorp H. Interstitial pneumonia following autologous bone marrow transplantation. *Transplantation* 1988; **46:** 61–76.

Infections in Patients Receiving Immunosuppressive Therapy for the Treatment of Autoimmune (Rheumatologic) Diseases and Infections Following Splenectomy

Michael C Sneller

I INFECTIONS IN PATIENTS WITH AUTOIMMUNE (RHEUMATOLOGIC) DISEASES RECEIVING IMMUNOSUPPRESSIVE THERAPY

Infection is a major cause of morbidity and mortality in patients with rheumatologic diseases. Failure to recognize an infectious process in these patients often has disastrous consequences. Although certain rheumatologic diseases may be associated with subtle abnormalities of host defense, the dominant risk factor for serious infection is the use of immunosuppressive therapy. The major immunosuppressive agents used in the treatment of these diseases are glucocorticosteroids, low doses of cytotoxic agents (used alone or in combination with glucocorticosteroids) and cyclosporin A.

The recognition and treatment of infections in this patient population are particularly difficult tasks for several reasons:
- the clinical manifestations of infection may be indistinguishable from those of the underlying rheumatologic disease
- the effects of immunosuppressive therapy may diminish the usual manifestations of an infectious process such as fever and localizing signs of inflammation
- the spectrum of potential pathogens is large, making empirical treatment difficult.

I REGARDING THE CLINICAL PRESENTATION AND EVALUATION OF THE PATIENT

I.I What are the clinically predominant modes of presentation of infection in patients with rheumatologic diseases receiving immunosuppressive therapy?

Fever with or without a clinically obvious source is a frequent presenting feature of serious infection in patients receiving immunosuppressive therapy for the treatment of rheumatologic diseases. Fever in this patient population presents a difficult diagnostic problem since the clinical manifestations of an infectious processes may mimic those of the underlying rheumatologic disease, and vice versa. This point is perhaps best illustrated by the occurrence of fever in a patient with systemic lupus erythematosus (SLE). Fever is one of the most common manifestations of active SLE, occurring in over 80% of patients at some time during the course of their illness. In one series of 160 patients with SLE, nearly one third were hospitalized specifically for the evaluation of unexplained fever. Active SLE was found to be the most common cause of fever, accounting for

60% of febrile episodes. However, 23% of febrile episodes were due to documented infections, with bacteremia accounting for nearly half of the infections. Bacteremia in this study was associated with a high mortality rate (33%) and all deaths occurred in patients receiving glucocorticosteroids. An important point to remember when evaluating these patients is that the antipyretic and antiinflammatory properties of glucocorticosteroids can minimize or mask fever and the usual localizing physical findings of serious infections. For example, the usual manifestations of high fever and signs of peritoneal inflammation associated with gastrointestinal perforation may be minimal or absent in a patient receiving glucocorticosteroid therapy.

Pneumonia is one of the most frequent life-threatening infections seen in patients receiving immunosuppressive therapy for the treatment of rheumatologic disease. The immunosuppressed patient with pneumonia may appear acutely ill with fever, purulent sputum, leukocytosis and evidence of consolidation on chest radiography. Alternatively, the patient may initially present with deceptively mild symptoms and radiographic abnormalities due to the antiinflammatory effects of immunosuppressive drugs. The fact that pulmonary manifestations of certain rheumatic diseases may produce many of the same clinical and radiographic abnormalities as pneumonia complicates the evaluation of pulmonary infiltrates in this patient population. In addition, hypersensitivity reactions to certain medications used to treat rheumatic diseases (especially methotrexate) may produce symptoms and radiographic abnormalities indistinguishable from those of pneumonia.

A variety of rheumatologic diseases can involve the central nervous system (CNS) including Wegener granulomatosis, polyarteritis nodosa, Behçet disease and SLE. Patients with these diseases who are receiving immunosuppressive therapy are at increased risk for developing CNS infections, the manifestations of which may be indistinguishable from those of the underlying disease. This is particularly true in SLE where neuropsychiatric manifestations occur in 25–80% of patients. The major CNS clinical syndromes (infectious and noninfectious) likely to be encountered in these patients are acute or chronic meningitis and focal brain lesions.

Individuals with rheumatoid arthritis are especially susceptible to the development of septic arthritis, which may be polyarticular. Patients with long-standing erosive disease are more likely to develop septic arthritis than are those with mild disease. Septic arthritis in these patients may present as a relatively insidious worsening of joint symptoms that to some extent mimics the underlying disease. Thus, any patient with rheumatoid arthritis who develops acutely inflamed joint or joints should be considered to have septic arthritis until proven otherwise.

1.2 What are the predominant sites of infection? (see Table 6.2, pp. 231–233)
Lower respiratory tract infection accounts for 30–50% of major infections in patients receiving immunosuppressive therapy for the treatment of rheumatologic disease. Other frequent sites of infection include the urinary tract, CNS, musculoskeletal system (in patients with rheumatoid arthritis) and bacteremia without an obvious source.

1.3 What are the predominant organisms that contribute (by site)?
- Respiratory tract – bacterial pathogens, such as *Streptococcus pneumoniae*, *Haemophilus influenzae*, *Staphylococcus aureus*, *Legionella* spp. and enteric Gram-negative rods, are the most frequent cause of pneumonia in these patients. Although less frequent than bacterial pneumonia, pulmonary infection with opportunistic pathogens is often associated with a worse clinical outcome. The higher mortality rate of opportunistic pneumonia is often related directly to a delay in diagnosis.

Pneumocystis carinii is the most common cause of opportunistic pulmonary infection in patients with rheumatologic diseases. Other opportunistic pathogens that may cause pneumonia in these patients include fungi (*Aspergillus* spp., *Cryptococcus neoformans*, *Coccidioides immitis* and *Histoplasma capsulatum*), mycobacteria, *Nocardia* spp. and cytomegalovirus (CMV) (rare).

- Urinary tract – enteric Gram-negative rods, *Enterococcus* spp.
- CNS – more common: *C. neoformans*, *Listeria monocytogenes*, *S. pneumoniae*, *H. influenzae*, *N. meningitidis*, *Nocardia* spp; less common: *Mycobacterium tuberculosis*, *C. immitis*, *Strongyloides stercoralis*, *Toxoplasma gondii*, *Aspergillus* spp., JC virus (PML).
- Bone and joint – *S. aureus* (most common), Gram-negative rods.
- Bacteremia without obvious focus – *S. aureus*, enteric Gram-negative rods.

1.4 How do the organisms vary according to various risk factors?

The types of organisms that cause disease in this patient group are to a large degree determined by the intensity of iatrogenic immunosuppression. Bacterial pathogens (such as *S. aureus*, enteric Gram-negative rods) are the most frequent cause of serious infections in patients receiving glucocorticosteroid therapy. In patients receiving very high doses of glucocorticosteroids (> 1 mg/kg prednisone or prednisolone daily) or in those receiving glucocorticosteroids plus a cytotoxic drug, infections with opportunistic pathogens (e.g. *P. carinii*, *L. monocytogenes*, *C. neoformans*) become more frequent. The risk of all types of infection is significantly reduced in patients receiving alternate-day glucocorticosteroid therapy and in those receiving low doses of cytotoxic drugs without glucocorticosteroids (see section 2.2).

1.5 How does this differ from other conditions, from center to center, and from country to country?

The infections that occur in patients treated with glucocorticosteroids with or without the addition of a cytotoxic agent are predominantly those associated with impaired phagocyte function and, to a lesser extent, with suppressed cell-mediated immunity. Thus, the spectrum of pathogens is somewhat similar to that seen in recipients of solid organ transplantation in the 1–6 month posttransplant period.

In countries with a high prevalence of tuberculosis, *M. tuberculosis* may be a more frequently encountered pathogen in this patient population. In addition to tuberculosis, any chronic infection that is endemic to a particular geographic region can potentially emerge during periods of iatrogenic immunosuppression.

1.6 What is the appropriate approach to the initial evaluation and diagnosis of infection in patients with rheumatologic diseases receiving immunosuppressive therapy?

Any clinical manifestation suggestive of infection in a patient on immunosuppressive therapy requires a prompt and thorough evaluation. Such an evaluation should include a thorough history and physical examination, chest radiography, appropriate laboratory studies to assess the activity of the underlying rheumatologic disease, blood cultures, and other cultures as clinically indicated. Any abnormalities detected on the initial evaluation should be pursued aggressively. See section 1.8 for specific details of how to approach specific signs and symptoms.

1.7 How should the evaluation be modified according to the severity of the risk?

Patients receiving higher doses of glucocorticosteroids (> 0.5 mg/kg prednisone daily) or glucocorticosteroids combined with a cytotoxic agent are at the greatest risk for infections. In such patients investigation for infection should be aggressive with early use of invasive procedures, such as lumbar puncture, bronchoscopy and lung biopsy, when clinically indicated to establish a definitive diagnosis (see section 1.8).

1.8 What are the specific evaluation measures? (see also Chapter 2 in Part I)
This section is focused on the clinical approach to specific infectious syndromes commonly encountered in patients with rheumatologic diseases.

Fever
For patients with fever, evaluation should include a thorough history and physical examination, chest radiography, appropriate laboratory studies to assess the activity of the underlying rheumatologic disease, blood cultures and other cultures as clinically indicated. The presence or absence of leukocytosis needs to be interpreted with caution. It should be noted that glucocorticosteroid therapy can cause a neutrophilic leukocytosis, and that cytotoxic drug therapy may impair a patient's ability to mount a neutrophilic leukocytosis in response to infection. In addition, neutrophilic leukocytosis may be a manifestation of certain rheumatologic diseases, such as active Wegener granulomatosis. Thus, both the patient's underlying disease and current drug regimen need to be taken into consideration when evaluating the white blood cell count in a febrile immunosuppressed patient. Although cutaneous lesions in a febrile patient may be a manifestation of the underlying rheumatologic disease, they may also indicate disseminated bacterial, mycobacterial or fungal infection in the immunocompromised host. Thus, cutaneous lesions in a febrile immunosuppressed patient should be biopsied and portions of the sample submitted for histologic examination (including special stains for bacteria, mycobacteria and fungi) and culture for bacteria, mycobacteria and fungi.

Pulmonary infiltrates
The evaluation of pulmonary disease in this patient population starts with a thorough history and physical examination. First, it is important to establish the time course of the illness. Rapidly progressive symptoms developing over several hours or a day suggests an acute bacterial infection. A subacute course progressing over several days to weeks is more suggestive of an opportunistic infection, such as *P. carinii* pneumonia (PCP), or a flare of the underlying rheumatologic disease. Next, a history of exposure to potential pathogens should be carefully sought. Patients should be asked specifically about exposure to tuberculosis, including a history of a positive skin test, household and occupational exposures, and previous residence in endemic areas (e.g. Latin America, sub-Saharan Africa, Southeast Asia, southern and eastern European and Mediterranean countries). A thorough travel and residential history may also provide relevant information about exposure to other potential pathogens such as *H. capsulatum*, which is endemic in the central river valley areas of the United States, and *C. immitis*, which is endemic in the southwest of the United States. Infection with *S. stercoralis* is usually acquired in tropical climates, and immunosuppressed patients have an increased risk for a fulminant hyperinfection syndrome in which pneumonitis is a prominent feature. Exposure to infants and children such as in a daycare setting may increase the risk of pneumonia from varicella and respiratory syncytial virus.

A detailed physical examination is essential and may provide important diagnostic clues. Erythematous necrotic cutaneous lesions raise the possibility of Gram-negative sepsis, in particular *Pseudomonas aeruginosa*. Disseminated histoplasmosis, cryptococcus and nocardiosis may also produce pulmonary infiltrates and cutaneous lesions. Oral mucosal candidiasis is a manifestation of significant immunodeficiency and is consequently associated with an increased risk of opportunistic infections such as PCP. The combination of pulmonary infiltrates and focal neurologic deficits raises the concern of disseminated infection with mycobacteria, fungi (*C. neoformans*, *Aspergillus* spp.) or *Nocardia* spp.

The chest radiograph is an important aspect of the diagnostic workup and must be evaluated in the context of the patient's symptoms, epidemiologic exposures, underlying disease, immunosuppressive therapy, and the presence or absence of leukopenia (see Table 6.1). The usual radiographic appearance of pulmonary infections may be dramatically altered by immunosuppressive therapy. For example, tuberculosis is more likely to cause diffuse lung infiltrates in a miliary pattern among patients receiving immunosuppressive therapy compared with immunocompetent patients. For patients with a suspected pulmonary infection in whom the chest radiograph is negative or inconclusive, a chest computed tomography (CT) scan should be performed. Chest CT can also better define a pulmonary process and help guide further invasive studies such as bronchoscopy or open biopsy.

Based on careful evaluation of the clinical history, physical examination, chest radiographs and laboratory data, a preliminary differential diagnosis can be established. In patients whose clinical presentation is typical of bacterial pneumonia (i.e. acute onset of fever, respiratory symptoms and a localized pulmonary infiltrate) an adequate sputum sample for Gram staining and bacterial culture should be obtained along with blood cultures. The value of sputum analysis for bacterial infection is debatable; however, the abundance of a single organism in an adequate sample (25 neutrophils and fewer than 25 epithelial cells per $100 \times$ field) is suggestive of infection. If a pleural effusion is present, thoracocentesis should be performed. At a minimum, cell count, chemistry (lactate dehydrogenase, protein, glucose, pH), Gram staining and culture should be performed on the pleural fluid.

For immunosuppressed patients with clinical and radiographic features not suggestive of typical bacterial pneumonia, or in a patient not responding to empirical therapy, a more aggressive approach to establishing a definitive diagnosis is indicated. This is particularly true in patients who exhibit diffuse infiltrates, nodules or hilar adenopathy on chest radiography. In these patients expectorated sputum samples are usually not adequate for diagnosis and empirical antimicrobial therapy is not practical because of the large range of possible opportunistic pathogens. The physician must decide which procedures are likely to provide a definitive diagnosis expeditiously and with the lowest morbidity. If available, sputum induction using hypertonic saline may be useful as an initial diagnostic procedure, especially if PCP is suspected. At my institution, the sensitivity of induced sputum examination for PCP in non-human immunodeficiency virus (HIV)-infected patients is approximately 60%. Sputum induction may also be of value in diagnosing tuberculosis.

If sputum analysis is not diagnostic, fiberoptic bronchoscopy with bronchoalveolar lavage (BAL) and, possibly, transbronchial biopsy should be performed. The diagnostic yield for bronchoscopy is highest in patients with diffuse pulmonary infiltrates due to nonbacterial processes such as PCP or pulmonary hemorrhage. The specificity of BAL for invasive fungal pneumonia due to *Aspergillus* or *Candida* spp. is limited, and the isolation of these agents from BAL fluid should be interpreted with caution in patients with rheumatologic diseases. The main risk factor for invasive aspergillosis is prolonged absolute or functional neutropenia, as commonly occurs in association with intensive antineoplastic chemotherapy or in congenital disorders of neutrophil function such as chronic granulomatous disease. In either of these clinical settings the isolation of

Table 6.1 Differential diagnosis of pulmonary infiltrates in patients with rheumatologic diseases receiving immunosuppressive therapy

Radiographic pattern	Infectious causes	Noninfectious causes
Localized infiltrates	Bacterial pneumonia (including *Legionella* spp.)	Wegener granulomatosis
	Mycobacteria spp.	Churg–Strauss syndrome
	Opportunistic fungi	Pulmonary embolus
	Aspergillus spp.	
	Histoplasma capsulatum	
	Coccidioides immitis	
	Cryptococcus neoformans	
	Pneumocystis carinii (uncommon)	
Diffuse infiltrates	*Pneumocystis carinii*	Systemic lupus erythematosus
	Bacterial pneumonia (hematogenous spread)	Rheumatoid arthritis
	Mycoplasma pneumoniae	Microscopic polyangiitis
	Chlamydia spp.	Wegener granulomatosis
	Mycobacteria spp. (miliary pattern)	Churg–Strauss syndrome
	Opportunistic fungi	Scleroderma
	Viral	Sjögren syndrome
	Influenza	Dermatomyositis/polymyositis
	Cytomegalovirus	Pulmonary edema
	Varicella zoster virus (rare)	Drug-induced
		Methotrexate
		Cyclophosphamide (rare)
		Azathioprine (rare)
Nodules or nodular infiltrates	Septic emboli	Wegener granulomatosis
	Staphylococcus aureus	Churg–Strauss syndrome
	Pseudomonas aeruginosa	Rheumatoid arthritis
	Mycobacteria spp.	Lymphoma
	Nocardia spp.	
	Opportunistic fungi	

Aspergillus from respiratory secretions is likely to represent invasive disease and empirical therapy with high-dose amphotericin B is warranted without further diagnostic evaluation. Invasive pulmonary aspergillosis is less common in patients with rheumatologic diseases and, in the absence of prolonged absolute or functional neutropenia, the isolation of *Aspergillus* spp. from BAL or sputum samples may represent colonization. If invasive pulmonary aspergillosis is suspected, strong consideration should be given to performing a lung biopsy to document tissue invasion before embarking on a potentially toxic course of empirical therapy with high-dose amphotericin B. True pneumonia due to *Candida* spp. is extremely unusual even in patients with severe and prolonged immunosuppression. The isolation of *Candida* from respiratory sections almost always represents colonization, and pneumonia due to *Candida* spp. can be diagnosed only by documenting tissue invasion on a lung biopsy specimen.

The isolation of CMV from BAL or sputum samples must also be interpreted with caution. Asymptomatic shedding of CMV in bronchial secretions is common in immunosuppressed patients and, with the exception of bone marrow and solid organ transplant recipients, rarely represents disease. Thus, isolation of CMV from BAL fluid cannot be equated with the presence of CMV pneumonia in patients receiving immunosuppressive therapy for the treatment of rheumatologic diseases. Definitive diagnosis of CMV pneumonia requires (1) a biopsy showing characteristic intranuclear inclusions or positive immunohistochemical staining for CMV antigens combined with tissue necrosis and/or inflammation and (2) the absence of any other pathogen.

The usefulness of bronchoscopy in the evaluation of immunosuppressed patients with localized infiltrates or nodules is variable. Quantitative cultures from BAL fluid or from a protected brush catheter may increase the sensitivity and specificity in the diagnosis of bacterial pneumonia; however, the use of empirical antibiotic therapy may decrease the yield of this procedure. For large (> 2 cm) pulmonary nodules the diagnostic yield of bronchoscopy ranges from 50% to 80%, but for smaller nodules the diagnostic yield is usually less than 15%. If a definitive diagnosis cannot be made on samples obtained by bronchoscopy, then open lung biopsy may be required. Although fine-needle aspiration may occasionally yield a diagnosis in selected patients with peripheral lesions, open biopsy has the highest yield in patients with pulmonary nodules, masses and cavities. In patients with diffuse lung infiltrates, video-assisted thoracoscopy with biopsy may be a less-invasive alternative to full thoracotomy. Open lung biopsy may be associated with significant morbidity and mortality. Thus, when less invasive procedures fail to yield a diagnosis, the physician must weigh the morbidity and mortality of open lung biopsy against that of prolonged and potentially ineffective empirical therapy.

Central nervous system infection

In evaluating patients with rheumatologic diseases for possible CNS infection, the physician is often dealing with opportunistic pathogens that elicit a minimal inflammatory response in patients whose ability to mount such a response is blunted by pharmacologic immunosuppression. Therefore, the usual signs and symptoms of life-threatening CNS infection may be greatly diminished or absent. If the physician waits for manifestations such as meningism, confusion and obtundation to appear before initiating a diagnostic workup, the chance for treating an opportunistic infection successfully is greatly diminished. Hence, the evaluation of suspected CNS infection in this patient population must be initiated based on vastly different criteria than those used in the normal host. A detailed neurologic examination should be performed and repeated frequently to monitor the patient's progress. Each patient should undergo a careful ophthalmologic examination looking for papilledema, signs of retinal and choroid infection (e.g. crypto-coccosis, toxoplasmosis) and proptosis (suggestive of orbital infection or cavernous sinus involvement). The physical examination may also reveal diagnostic clues suggestive of extraneural sites of infection such as cutaneous lesions (e.g. nocardiosis, fungal infection) or stigmata of endocarditis. Indications for brain imaging CT or magnetic resonance imaging (MRI), lumbar puncture, or both, include unexplained headache with or without fever, personality changes, confusion and focal neurologic deficits. The aggressive pursuit of cerebrospinal fluid (CSF) analysis and brain imaging along with the appropriate use of biopsy procedures for focal lesions can result in early diagnosis and successful therapy of life-threatening opportunistic CNS infections.

Other sites
Patients with rheumatoid arthritis who develop acutely inflamed joint(s) should undergo arthrocentesis with cultures of synovial fluid sent for routine, fungal and mycobacterial cultures.

1.9 What new developments are going to impact on emerging organisms, recognition, evaluation and diagnosis of infection in patients with rheumatologic diseases receiving immunosuppressive therapy?
In the past decade penicillin-resistant *S. pneumoniae* has emerged as a significant cause of community-acquired pneumonia. This fact needs to be considered when choosing an empirical antibiotic regimen in patients with rheumatologic diseases who present with suspected community-acquired bacterial pneumonia. As is true in other immunocom-promised patient populations, infections with vancomycin-resistant enterococci and enteric Gram-negative rods that produce extended-spectrum β-lactamases are likely to become more frequent in this patient population. *Cyclospora* is a parasitic pathogen that can cause significant gastroenteritis in both normal and immunocompromised hosts. Recently this parasite has caused several foodborne outbreaks in the United States. Infection with *Cyclospora* is probably under-recognized as it may be missed by routine stool studies. It is important to diagnose this intestinal infection as it can be successfully treated with trimethoprim-sulfamethoxazole (TMP–SMX).

Given that pneumonia is one of the most frequent life-threatening infections in patients with rheumatologic diseases, new diagnostic tests for respiratory pathogens are likely to have the greatest impact on the evaluation of infections in this patient group. Techniques of DNA amplification applied to throat swabs or BAL fluid are currently being developed to detect pathogens such as *M. pneumoniae*, *C. pneumoniae* and *L. pneumophila*.

2 REGARDING THE RISK FACTORS ACCOMPANYING IMMUNOSUPPRESIVE THERAPY IN PATIENTS WITH AUTOIMMUNE (RHEUMATOLOGIC) DISEASES

2.1 What are the main alterations in host defense mechanisms and what are the appropriate investigations to document them?
2.2 What are the alterations due to iatrogenic factors?
Although certain rheumatologic diseases may be associated with subtle abnormalities of host defense, the dominant risk factor for serious infection is the use of immuno-suppressive therapy. The major immunosuppressive agents used to treat patients with rheumatologic or allergic diseases are glucocorticosteroids, low doses of cytotoxic agents (used alone or in combination with glucocorticosteroids) and cyclosporin A. These

immunosuppressive drugs can have profound effects on multiple aspects of host defense mechanisms.

At pharmacologic doses, glucocorticosteroids have both antiinflammatory and immunosuppressive properties which result from the effects of these agents on the distribution and function of lymphocytes, monocytes and neutrophils. The major anti-inflammatory actions of glucocorticosteroids are in large part due to their suppressive effects on neutrophil function. Glucocorticosteroids inhibit neutrophil migration to inflammatory sites, reduce neutrophil adherence to vascular endothelium, reduce the bactericidal activity of neutrophils, and stabilize lysosomal membranes. The latter two effects are observed only at high glucocorticosteroid concentrations and may not be of clinical importance. Glucocorticosteroid therapy produces a neutrophilic leuko-cytosis by accelerating release of mature neutrophils from the bone marrow, and by reducing the egress of neutrophils from the circulation into inflammatory sites. The total white blood cell count may exceed 20 000/mm^3, but band forms and metamye-locytes almost never increase beyond 6% of the total white blood cell count. An excess of these immature neutrophil forms is suggestive of a superimposed infectious process.

The mononuclear phagocytic system is also affected by glucocorticosteroid therapy. In contrast to the effect on neutrophils, glucocorticosteroid administration produces a peripheral blood monocytopenia that persists for 24 h. Glucocorticosteroids impair a number of monocyte functions important to host defense including chemotaxis, bacteri-cidal activity, clearance of antibody-coated red blood cells and production of proinflam-matory cytokines.

Glucocorticosteroids produce profound changes in lymphocyte function and induce a redistribution of lymphocytes out of the circulation. This redistribution predominantly involves T lymphocytes, with CD4 cells affected more than CD8 T-cells. Gluco-corticosteroids also inhibit T-lymphocyte activation, leading to decreased proliferation and lymphokine production. At high doses, glucocorticosteroids are able to inhibit immunoglobulin production by B cells.

In view of the broad immunosuppressive and antiinflammatory effects of glucocorti-costeroids, it is not surprising that treatment with these agents is associated with an increased frequency of infections. The infections that occur in glucocorticosteroid-treated patients are predominantly those associated with impaired phagocyte function and, to a lesser extent, with suppressed cell-mediated immunity. Although there is no doubt that glucocorticosteroid therapy results in an increased susceptibility to infection, the exact magnitude of this problem is difficult to quantify. Experience in patients with rheuma-toid arthritis, SLE and other autoimmune diseases suggests that the incidence of infec-tious complications increases with doses equivalent to prednisone 20–40 mg/day administered for longer than 4–6 weeks. A number of studies have demonstrated that the risk of infection is considerably less with alternate-day glucocorticosteroid therapy, defined as the administration of a short-acting glucocorticosteroid preparation (i.e. pred-nisone, prednisolone or methylprednisolone) once every 48 h in the morning. In one study, no major infections were seen in 70 patients treated with alternate-day glucocorti-costeroids and followed for a total of 170 patient-years. The reduction in infections may be related to the intermittently normal leukocyte kinetics seen in patients receiving this glucocorticosteroid regimen.

Cytotoxic drugs such as cyclophosphamide, azathioprine and methotrexate disrupt host defense through their inhibitory effects on cell proliferation. These drugs can have profound effects on the production and function of both phagocytic cells and lymphocytes. In the treatment of rheumatologic diseases, cytotoxic agents are usually given in doses substantially lower than those used in the treatment of cancer. While low-dose cytotoxic drug therapy does cause immune suppression and mild leukopenia, it usually does not cause disruption of the mucosal barriers as occurs with the higher dose regimens used to treat malignant diseases. Neutropenia is a common toxic effect in patients with rheumatologic diseases who are treated with low-dose cyclophosphamide. The production of neutropenia is not necessary for this drug to have a therapeutic effect in the treatment of these diseases and this toxicity can be avoided by frequently monitoring the white blood cell count and reducing the dose as needed to keep the neutrophil count above 1500 cells/ μl. Other cytotoxic drugs commonly used to treat rheumatic diseases (azathioprine, chlorambucil and low-dose methotrexate) can produce neutropenia, although the risk is less than with cyclophosphamide. As with cyclophosphamide therapy, the white blood cell count should be monitored closely in patients treated with these agents. When combined with daily glucocorticosteroid therapy, treatment with low doses of cytotoxic drugs is associated with the same types of bacterial and opportunistic infections that occur with high-dose glucocorticosteroid therapy. When cytotoxic drugs are given alone or with alternate-day glucocorticosteroids, the incidence of infectious complications is markedly reduced provided neutropenia is avoided.

Cyclosporin A is a potent immunosuppressive agent that inhibits T-cell activation. Cyclosporin A acts as a prodrug, binding to an endogenous intracellular protein known as cyclophilin. The resulting cyclosporin A–cyclophilin complex inhibits the activity of the Ca^{2+}-regulated protein phosphatase, calcineurin, an enzyme required for the transmission of activating signals from the T-cell receptor. The types of infections seen with cyclosporin A therapy are those associated with defective cell-mediated immunity. However, since cyclosporin A is almost always used in combination with other immunosuppressive agents, the true incidence and spectrum of infections with this agent is difficult to determine.

2.3 What is the influence of environmental factors?
Patients receiving immunosuppressive therapy for the treatment of rheumatologic diseases are at increased risk for reactivation of latent infections such as tuberculosis, coccidiomycosis and strongyloidiasis. Patients who have resided in areas of the world where these infections are endemic are at risk for reactivation during periods of immunosuppression.

2.4 What are the most significant factors that contribute to the risk of infection in patients with rheumatologic diseases receiving immunosuppressive therapy?
As described above, the major risk for infection in these patients is the intensity and duration of immunosuppressive therapy. In patients with severe rheumatoid arthritis, abnormal joint architecture which impedes clearance of bacteria may contribute to the increased risk of septic arthritis.

2.5 What are the specific or nonspecific measures aimed at minimizing each of these factors?
The most important measures that can reduce the risk of infection in these patients is to use the minimum amount of immunosuppressive therapy necessary to control the underlying disease and to continually assess the risk of underlying disease versus the risk of the immunosuppressive regimen.

When glucocorticosteroids are used to treat severe manifestations of rheumatologic diseases, such as SLE or systemic vasculitis, it is often necessary to administer a short-acting agent in divided doses. Usually, therapy is initiated with prednisone (or equivalent) 1–2 mg/kg daily in three to four divided doses. This type of divided-dose therapy is a potent antiinflammatory and immunosuppressive regimen that may also be associated with significant glucocorticosteroid toxicity including serious infection. For this reason, it is advisable to convert from divided dose to single daily dose therapy as soon as the desired therapeutic effect has been achieved. The single daily glucocorticosteroid dose can then be gradually tapered until the lowest dose necessary to control disease activity is reached or glucocorticosteroid therapy can be stopped altogether. Tapering of the glucocorticosteroid dose should begin as soon as the disease activity has been controlled or when severe glucocorticosteroid toxicity makes dose reduction necessary. An attempt should be made to taper to an alternate-day regimen whenever possible. When low-dose cytotoxic regimens are employed, the leukocyte count should be monitored frequently and the dose of cytotoxic drug adjusted downward as necessary to keep the neutrophil count above 1500 cells/ μl.

2.6 Are there different levels of risk of infection recognized for patients with rheumatologic diseases receiving immunosuppressive therapy?

Patients at the highest risk of infection are those being treated for more than 4 weeks with daily glucocorticosteroids (at doses greater than 20–40 mg of prednisone) plus a cytotoxic drug. The spectrum of infections seen in such patients includes severe bacterial infections (pneumonia and bacteremia), PCP and other opportunistic infections. Patients receiving a daily glucocorticosteroid dose equivalent to 20 mg or more of prednisone for more than 4 weeks are at increased risk for severe bacterial infections and, to a lesser extent, opportunistic infections. Patients receiving alternate-day glucocorticosteroid therapy equivalent to 60 mg or less of prednisone (or other short-acting glucocorticosteroid preparations) every other day are at minimal risk for major infections, as are those receiving monotherapy with a low dose of a cytotoxic drug (provided neutropenia is avoided). In this later group of patients, cutaneous herpes zoster is the only infection that is likely to occur with increased frequency.

2.7 How does the level of risk impact on management?

As discussed above, patients receiving daily glucocorticosteroids combined with a cytotoxic agent are at the highest risk for opportunistic infection, with PCP being the most commonly encountered opportunistic infection. The incidence of PCP in these patients is approximately 6%, and the mortality rate from the infection may exceed 30%. Thus, it is the author's policy to provide routine PCP prophylaxis for all patients receiving combined therapy with daily glucocorticosteroids and a cytotoxic agent (see section 4.1).

2.8 What new developments are going to impact on minimizing or suppressing the specific risk factors?

Current investigations in the treatment of rheumatologic diseases are focusing on the development of therapeutic agents that more specifically target pathways of the immune response such as antigen processing, cell trafficking and inhibition of specific proinflammatory cytokines. Using these approaches, the pathogenic mechanisms of autoimmunity may be more specifically regulated, allowing for effective treatment without the induction of global immunosuppression and the associated risk of infection.

3 REGARDING THE SURVEILLANCE OF PATIENTS WITH AUTOIMMUNE (RHEUMATOLOGIC) DISEASES RECEIVING IMMUNOSUPPRESSIVE THERAPY

3.2 What are the surveillance measures to be taken when a patient presents with a rheumatologic disease that requires immunosuppressive therapy?

- Purified protein derivative (PPD) determination for individuals with history of exposure to tuberculosis, including a history of a positive skin test, household and occupational exposures, and previous residence in endemic areas. For such individuals, a reaction ≥ 10 mm should be considered positive.
- Stool examination and serology for *S. stercoralis* is mandatory in individuals with a history of travel or residence in endemic area.
- Serologic tests for HIV, hepatitis B and hepatitis C are important, as immunosuppressive therapy may exacerbate chronic infections with these viruses.

3.3 What are the other specific measures to be taken when a patient presents with rheumatologic disease that requires immunosuppressive therapy?

In addition to the surveillance measures listed in section 3.2, a thorough history, physical examination and laboratory evaluation are needed to rule out any concurrently active infectious process that may be exacerbated by immunosuppressive therapy.

3.4 What developments are to be expected for surveillance in patients with rheumatologic disease receiving immunosuppressive therapy?

The development of more accurate immunologic tests that will predict disease severity and risk of relapses for specific rheumatologic diseases will hopefully help identify subgroups of patients who require less intensive immunosuppressive therapy and thus minimize the risk for infectious complications.

4 REGARDING THE PREVENTION OF INFECTION IN PATIENTS WITH AUTOIMMUNE (RHEUMATOLOGIC) DISEASES RECEIVING IMMUNOSUPPRESSIVE THERAPY

4.1 What approaches, if any, to the prevention of infection should be considered in patients with rheumatologic diseases receiving immunosuppressive therapy?

There are two clinical situations in which antimicrobial prophylaxis may be useful in preventing infectious complications of immunosuppressive therapy in patients with rheumatologic diseases. The first is in the patient with a positive tuberculin skin test (PPD) who is about to be started on immunosuppressive therapy. Pharmacologically immunosuppressed patients are highly susceptible to primary and reactivation disease due to *M. tuberculosis*, and the mortality rate from tuberculosis is high in this group of patients. The American Thoracic Society recommends that patients treated with significant doses of glucocorticosteroids (> 15 mg prednisone daily for 2–3 weeks) or 'other forms of immunosuppressive therapy' should receive preventive therapy with isoniazid (300 mg/day for 12 months) if tuberculin skin testing results in an induration of ≥ 10 mm. Before starting isoniazid therapy, it is important to exclude active tuberculosis. A chest radiograph should be obtained and abnormalities including infiltrates, nodules and effusions should be thoroughly evaluated. It should be pointed out that the risk/benefit ratio of isoniazid treatment in patients with rheumatologic diseases has not been evaluated. In patients receiving hepatotoxic medications such as methotrexate, isoniazid

Table 6.2 Evaluation of infections in patients with autoimmune (rheumatologic) diseases and following splenectomy according to the sites of infection and the possible etologic agent

Site of infection	Infectious syndrome (clinical features)	Predominant pathogens	Diagnostic investigations
Bloodstream	Bacteremia (fever with or without local signs of infection)	Staphylococcus aureus Enterococcus spp. (nosocomial outbreaks in some institutions) Gram-negative bacilli (Escherichia coli, Klebsiella pneumoniae, Enterobacter spp., Pseudomonas aeruginosa) Candida spp.	Blood cultures: two sets drawn from separate sites and one set drawn from indwelling intravenous catheter
Upper respiratory tract*	Sinusitis (tightness of sinus areas, headache, toothache, nasal obstruction, nasal voice)	Streptococcus pneumoniae Haemophilus influenzae Streptococcus pyogenes Staphylococcus aureus Anaerobic bacteria Viruses (influenza, parainfluenza, rhinovirus, adenovirus)	Aspiration of sinus Biopsy (if no improvement after 72–96 h of empirical antibiotic therapy)
Lower respiratory tract (bronchi, terminal airways, alveoli)	Bronchopneumonia Pneumonia (cough, dyspnea, chest pain, sputum, hemoptysia, pleural effusion)	Conventional pathogens: Streptococcus pneumoniae Haemophilus influenzae Staphylococcus aureus Gram-negative bacilli (Escherichia coli, Klebsiella pneumoniae, Pseudomonas aeruginosa) Legionella spp. (sporadic outbreaks) Mycoplasma pneumoniae Chlamydia pneumoniae	Chest radiography, CT, MRI Serology Sputum culture Fiberoptic bronchoscopy with bronchoalveolar lavage Transbronchial or transthoracic needle biopsy Thoracocentesis Open lung biopsy

Site of infection	Infectious syndrome (clinical features)	Predominant pathogens	Diagnostic investigations
		Opportunistic pathogens: *Pneumocystis carinii* *Aspergillus* spp., *Mucor* spp., *Rhizopus* spp., *Fusarium* spp. *Cryptococcus neoformans* *Histoplasma capsulatum, Coccidioides immitis* (endemic areas) Mycobacteria (*Mycobacterium tuberculosis*, atypical mycobacteria) *Nocardia asteroides* Cytomegalovirus†	
Central nervous system	Meningitis Encephalitis (altered mental status, headache, photophobia, seizures, focal neurologic signs, nuchal rigidity)	More common: *Cryptococcus neoformans* *Listeria monocytogenes* *Streptococcus pneumoniae* *Haemophilus influenzae* *Neisseria meningitidis* *Nocardia asteroides* Less common: *Mycobacterium tuberculosis* *Coccidioides immitis* *Strongyloides stercoralis* *Toxoplasma gondii* *Aspergillus* spp. JC virus (PML)	CT, MRI Lumbar puncture Aspiration or biopsy under stereotaxic CT guidance
Urinary tract	Urinary tract infections, dysuria (i.e. frequency, urgency, pain;	Gram-negative bacilli (*Escherichia coli, Klebsiella* spp., *Proteus* spp., *Enterobacter*	Culture of urine Ultrasonography, CT

	hematuria; flank pain)	spp., *Pseudomonas aeruginosa*) *Enterococcus* spp. Coagulase-negative staphylococci (*Staphylococcus saprophyticus*) *Candida* spp.	(if suspicion of renal abscess)
Bone and joint	Arthritis Osteomyelitis	*Staphylococcus aureus* *Haemophilus influenzae* (children < 5 years) Streptococci Gram-negative bacilli (*Escherichia coli*, *Klebsiella pneumoniae*, *Enterobacter* spp., *Pseudomonas aeruginosa*) *Candida* spp.	Radiographic studies Radionuclide imaging Ultrasonography CT, MRI Examination of synovial fluid (biochemistry, cellularity, culture) Culture of aspiration or biopsy specimen

* Pathogens responsible for upper respiratory infections are similar to those seen in the general population. Patients with Wegener granulomatosis have increased susceptibility to sinusitis and middle ear infections due to *Staphylococcus aureus* (see text for details). Non-infectious sinusitis is a frequent manifestation of Wegener granulomatosis (see section 5.2, p. 235)

† Cytomegalovirus is a rare cause of lower respiratory tract infection in this patient population (see text for details).

therapy may be associated with additive toxicity that outweighs the potential benefits of preventive therapy.

The second situation in which antimicrobial prophylaxis may be useful is in the prevention of PCP in patients at risk for this infection. As discussed in section 2.7, patients receiving daily glucocorticosteroids combined with a cytotoxic agent are at significant risk for developing PCP. Based on this fact and the documented efficacy of PCP prophylaxis in patients with leukemia and HIV infection, it is the author's policy to provide routine PCP prophylaxis to all patients receiving combined therapy with daily glucocorticosteroids and a cytotoxic agent. The author's preferred prophylaxis regimen for adults consists of trimethoprim 160 mg combined with sulfamethoxazole 800 mg given three times a week. For patients with sulfa allergy, monthly inhaled pentamidine, dapsone (100 mg/day) or atovaquone (1500 mg/day) can be used as an alternative regimen. Prophylaxis should be continued at least until the glucocorticosteroid dosage can be converted from a daily to an alternate-day schedule.

Primary varicella zoster virus (VZV) infection can be very severe in immunocompromised patients. Thus, postexposure prophylaxis of immunocompromised susceptible individuals is usually indicated. Persons not known to be seropositive for VZV and without a previous history of chickenpox should be considered susceptible; however, it should be noted that the majority (71–93%) of adults in the United States who have negative or uncertain histories are in fact seropositive. If the VZV serologic status of a potentially susceptible individual can be determined within 48 h of exposure, the results can be used to determine whether postexposure prophylaxis is necessary. If rapid serologic testing is not available, susceptible individuals should receive varicella zoster immune globulin (VZIG), which is effective at lowering attack rates among immunocompromised persons if administered no later than 96 h after exposure.

The prevention of infection by vaccination is always desirable. However, patients receiving immunosuppressive therapy respond poorly to vaccination, thus severely limiting the utility of this approach. For example, a large case-controlled study of the efficacy of polyvalent pneumococcal polysaccharide vaccine found the vaccine had little to no protective efficacy in immunocompromised patients. Although antibody responses are poor and clinical evidence of efficacy lacking, it is still reasonable to provide pneumococcal and influenza vaccination to patients with rheumatic diseases who are receiving immunosuppressive therapy.

4.2 What are the future challenges and opportunities for reducing the risk of infection?

See sections 2.8 and 3.4.

5 REGARDING THE TREATMENT OF INFECTIONS IN PATIENTS WITH AUTOIMMUNE (RHEUMATOLOGIC) DISEASES RECEIVING IMMUNOSUPPRESSIVE THERAPY

5.1 What is the role of empirical therapy?

Empirical antibiotic therapy is appropriate in the febrile immunosuppressed patient who appears toxic or develops hemodynamic instability, and should be initiated after appropriate cultures have been obtained. The antibiotic regimen should include agents with activity against *S. aureus* and enteric Gram-negative bacteria as these are the organisms most frequently isolated from blood cultures of patients who are receiving immunosuppressive therapy for the treatment of rheumatologic diseases. Patients receiving cytotoxic therapy who present with fever and neutropenia (absolute neutrophil count <500 cells/

μl) should receive an antibiotic with activity against *P. aeruginosa*. Patients started on empirical therapy should be monitored frequently and the antibiotic regimen adjusted based on clinical response and culture results. Patients responding to empirical therapy should generally be treated for at least 5–7 days after clinical signs of infection resolve.

5.2 What is the appropriate approach to the patient with rheumatologic diseases and evidence of:

Upper respiratory tract infection?

With the exception of patients with Wegener granulomatosis (see below), the pathogens responsible for most upper respiratory tract infections in this group of patients are similar to those seen in the normal population (*S. pneumoniae, H. influenzae*). Initial antibiotic therapy should be directed against these pathogens. Immunosuppressed patients with mastoid, sphenoid, posterior ethmoid, or frontal sinusitis should be managed in consultation with a otorhinolaryngologist as infection in these locations may spread to involve the orbit or CNS. Patients with signs of intracranial or orbital extension require immediate surgical drainage of the involved sinus.

Patients with Wegener granulomatosis are particularly susceptible to sinusitis and middle ear infections. Noninfectious sinusitis is a very common manifestation of Wegener granulomatosis, occurring in approximately 90% of patients, and is a source of significant morbidity. The inflammatory sinus disease often results in permanent damage to the mucosal surfaces that disrupts normal sinus anatomy and drainage. As a result, these patients are very susceptible to colonization and infection with bacterial pathogens, especially *S. aureus*. Such infections can mimic active Wegener granulomatosis and may trigger local and possibly systemic flares of disease. Empirical therapy for sinusitis in patients with Wegener granulomatosis should include an agent with good activity against *S. aureus*. Invasive fungal infections due to *Aspergillus* spp. or the agents of mucormycosis are uncommon in patients receiving immunosuppressive therapy for treatment of rheumatic diseases. However, the possibility of invasive fungal infection should considered in any patient with progressive sinusitis unresponsive to antibiotic therapy.

Lower respiratory tract infection?

In patients whose clinical presentation is typical of bacterial pneumonia (i.e. acute onset of fever, respiratory symptoms and a localized pulmonary infiltrate) it is appropriate to institute empirical antibiotic therapy after obtaining sputum and blood cultures. The empirical regimen used to treat suspected bacterial pneumonia in patients with a rheumatic disease should be directed at the most likely pathogens, which include the common agents of community-acquired pneumonia (*S. pneumoniae, H. influenzae*), *S. aureus*, *Legionella* spp. and enteric Gram-negative bacteria. A third-generation cephalosporin with antistaphylococcal coverage (e.g. ceftriaxone, cefotaxime or cefepime) combined with a macrolide (clarithromycin or azithromycin), or monotherapy with one of the newer quinolones (levofloxacin) are reasonable choices. Empirical coverage for *P. aeruginosa* and other Gram-negative bacteria that are typically widely resistant to antibiotics (e.g. *Enterobacter* and *Acinetobacter* spp.) is usually not necessary in patients with suspected community-acquired pneumonia. However, in severely ill patients or in those with nosocomial pneumonia, the empirical antibiotic regimen should include agents with activity against these pathogens. It is also essential that neutropenic patients with pneumonia receive empirical antibiotics with activity against *P. aeruginosa*.

The approach for patients with clinical and radiographic features not suggestive of typical bacterial pneumonia, or those not responding to empirical therapy, is discussed in section 1.8. In a patient with diffuse infiltrates, hypoxemia or other clinical features suggestive of PCP, empirical treatment with TMP-SMX (or pentamidine) should be instituted while the diagnostic workup is being organized.

Gastrointestinal infection?

Stool cultures for enteric pathogens as well as a thorough stool examination for protozoal pathogens (including *Cryptosporidium*, *Microsporidia* and *Cyclospora*) should be performed on all immunosuppressed patients with gastroenteritis. Patients with gastroenteritis and systemic signs of infection should also have blood cultures performed. All patients should be treated with agents appropriate to the specific pathogen isolated. For patients with suspected bacterial gastroenteritis, empirical treatment with ciprofloxacin or other quinolone is appropriate until stool culture results are available.

Genitourinary tract infection?

Patients with upper urinary tract infection who are being treated with high-dose daily glucocorticosteroids or daily glucocorticosteroids plus a cytotoxic drug should probably be treated for at least 14–21 days; otherwise, the management of urinary tract infections in patients with rheumatologic diseases is the same as in the normal population. For patients who are acutely ill, empirical therapy with a quinolone, third-or fourth-generation cephalosporin, or aminoglycoside should be considered.

Cardiovascular system infection?

The management of patients with rheumatologic diseases and endocarditis is the same as for otherwise normal patients who develop this infection.

Musculoskeletal infection?

Empirical therapy for suspected septic arthritis should include agents with good activity against *S. aureus* (nafcillin, first-generation cephalosporin or vancomycin for patients allergic to penicillin). Adequate drainage (by either needle aspiration or surgical debridement) of the septic joint is critical to controlling the infection and minimizing further damage to the joint.

Skin infection?

The approach to patients with rheumatologic diseases who develop a skin infection is the same as for otherwise normal individuals with the exception that longer courses of antibiotics may be necessary in patients receiving high daily doses of glucocorticosteroids.

Central nervous system infection?

The initial diagnostic approach to CNS infections is outlined in section 1.8. In patients with meningitis, initial empirical therapy should always include agents with activity against *L. monocytogenes* (ampicillin or TMP–SMX).

Patients with cryptococcal meningitis should be treated with amphotericin B (deoxycholate) at a daily dose of 0.6–0.7 mg/kg. 5-Fluorocytosine can be added if the patient is not predisposed to neutropenia or thrombocytopenia because of the underlying disease (i.e. SLE) or its treatment. In patients with normal renal function, the dose of 5-fluorocytosine is 25–37.5 mg/kg every 6 h. 5-Fluorocytosine doses must be reduced in the setting of renal insufficiency. The best way to prevent hematologic toxicity from 5-fluorocytosine is to monitor serum levels frequently and maintain levels between 50 and 100 μg/ml. There are only limited data on the efficacy of various lipid formulations of amphotericin B in the treatment of cryptococcal meningitis. The use of these agents should be restricted to patients who either cannot tolerate or do not respond to therapy with amphotericin B deoxycholate. In the United States, AmBisome is the only lipid amphotericin formulation approved for the treatment of cryptococcal meningitis in this setting. The duration of amphotericin therapy is based on the results of weekly CSF cultures. In general, patients should be treated until cultures have remained negative for at least four consecutive weeks. Approximately 50–70% of non-HIV-infected patients with cryptococcal meningitis can be cured with this amphotericin B regimen. However, all patients must be followed closely for relapse after therapy is stopped. The chances of relapse are much greater in patients who must remain on immunosuppressive therapy, especially if the glucocorticosteroid dose of prednisone is greater than 5–10 mg/day or 20 mg every other day. Thus, every attempt should be made to lower the glucocorticosteroid dose to the absolute minimum necessary to control the underlying rheumatologic disease. Following completion of the above amphotericin B regimen, chronic maintenance therapy with fluconazole (400 mg/day in adults for 6–12 months) may have a role in preventing relapse, especially in patients who must remain on immunosuppressive therapy. Initial monotherapy with fluconazole has not been studied adequately in the treatment of non-HIV immunosuppressed patients with cryptococcal meningitis.

Foreign body in place?
The approach to patients with rheumatologic diseases who develop an infection with a foreign body in place is the same as for otherwise normal individuals who develop such infections.

5.3 What is the appropriate approach to the patient with a rheumatologic disease and evidence of bacteremia, with or without site of infection?
In general, the approach to treating bacteremia in this patient group is the same as in otherwise normal individuals with the exception that longer courses (at least 2 weeks) of antibiotics should be considered in patients receiving daily glucocorticosteroids or combined therapy with a cytotoxic agent and glucocorticosteroids. When bacteremia with anaerobic Gram-negative organisms is discovered in patients receiving daily glucocorticosteroids, appropriate radiographic studies should be done to exclude an intraabdominal focus of infection even in the absence of localizing abdominal findings. The same is true for patients with polymicrobial bacteremia due to intestinal organisms. In addition, the strongyloides hyperinfection syndrome is a rare cause of polymicrobial bacteremia in immunocompromised patients. Individuals who have resided in an area where strongyloides is endemic and develop polymicrobial bacteremia with enteric organisms should have stool samples carefully examined for S. stercoralis.

5.4 What is the appropriate approach to the patient with a rheumatologic disease and evidence of a viral infection?

Herpes viruses
Patients receiving immunosuppressive therapy who develop acute infection with VZV or herpes simplex virus (HSV) are usually treated with either intravenous acyclovir, valacyclovir or famciclovir depending on degree of immunosuppression and severity of manifestations. Highly immunosuppressed individuals with cutaneous or extracutaneous disseminated VZV or HSV infections should be treated with intravenous acyclovir. Chronic suppressive therapy with oral acyclovir, valacyclovir or famciclovir can be used

for individuals with frequently recurring HSV or zoster. CMV is frequently shed from respiratory secretions of immunosuppressed patients in the absence of CMV disease, and CMV pneumonia is uncommon in patients receiving immunosuppressive therapy for the treatment of rheumatologic diseases. Thus, isolation of CMV from respiratory secretions in the absence of other evidence for CMV disease should not be treated (see section 1.8).

Respiratory viruses
The approach is the same as that in otherwise normal individuals with the exception that patients receiving immunosuppressive therapy may be more susceptible to bacterial superinfection and should evaluated for this complication (see section 1.8).

Enteroviruses
The approach is the same as in otherwise normal individuals.

Hepatitis
The approach is the same as in otherwise normal individuals with the exception that the use of methotrexate should be avoided in patients with chronic hepatitis B or C because of the potential hepatotoxicity of this drug.

5.5 What is the appropriate approach to the patient with a rheumatologic disease and evidence of a fungal infection?

Candida
The approach is the same as in other patients who develop candidemia.

Aspergillus
Disseminated aspergillosis is highly unusual with the immunosuppressive regimens used to treat rheumatologic diseases. However, if this should occur, the approach would be the same as in other patients who develop disseminated infection with *Aspergillus* spp.

Cryptococcus
Therapy for patients with coexistent cryptococcal meningitis is described in section 5.2. Patients with isolated cryptococcal fungemia most often require treatment with amphotericin B with or without flucytosine, as described in section 5.2. There are no guidelines for the use of fluconazole in this situation. However, chronic maintenance therapy with fluconazole should be considered in patients who clear their infection with amphotericin B but require continued immunosuppressive therapy.

Mucor
Disseminated infection with one of the etiologic agents of mucormycosis is unusual with the immunosuppressive regimens used to treat rheumatologic diseases. However, if this should occur, the approach would be the same as that in other patients who develop evidence of fungemia with the agents of mucormycosis.

5.6 What is the appropriate approach to the patient with a rheumatologic disease and evidence of a parasitic infection?

Pneumocystis carinii
The antimicrobial treatment of PCP in this patient population is the same as for other patients with this infection. The drug of choice for treating PCP is TMP–SMX. Patients

with severe PCP [arterial partial pressure of oxygen (PaO_2) < 70 mmHg] and a history of severe sulfa allergy (exfoliative dermatitis, anaphylaxis, severe hepatitis) should be treated with intravenous pentamidine 4 mg/kg daily. Patients with significant sulfa allergy and mild to moderate PCP (PaO_2 > 70 mmHg) can be treated with clindamycin 450–600 mg every 8 h combined with primaquine 15 mg/day or dapsone 100 mg/day plus trimethoprim 5 mg/kg three times daily. For all the above regimens the duration of therapy is 21 days. Following 21 days of therapy, it is the author's practice to maintain patients on secondary PCP prophylaxis until all immunosuppressive therapy is discontinued. His preferred regimen for secondary prophylaxis is the same as for primary PCP prophylaxis (see section 4.1).

Patients who develop severe PCP while receiving daily glucocorticosteroids at a daily dose of prednisone less than 1 mg/kg should probably have the glucocorticosteroid dose transiently increased to prevent the deterioration in respiratory function that frequently occurs following the institution of anti-*Pneumocystis* therapy. The glucocorticosteroid regimen that has been used successfully in HIV-infected adult patients with severe PCP consists of prednisone 40 mg twice a day for 5 days, followed by 40 mg once a day for 5 days, followed by 20 mg once a day for 11 days. In patients who develop severe PCP while being treated with high doses of glucocorticosteroids (> 1 mg/kg of prednisone daily), it is the author's practice not to increase the glucocorticosteroid dose further.

Toxoplasma gondii
Clinical toxoplasmosis is unusual in this patient population. The approach to treating acute toxoplasmosis including encephalitis would be the same as for other immunodeficient patients. Initial therapy should be with pyrimethamine combined with either sulfadiazine or clindamycin, and the intensity of immunosuppressive therapy should also be reduced, if possible. Treatment should be continued for at least 4–6 weeks after resolution of all signs and symptoms. Long-term maintenance antitoxoplasmosis therapy may be indicated for patients who must remain on high levels of immunosuppressive therapy.

Strongyloides stercoralis
Uncomplicated gastrointestinal infections are treated with thiabendazole 50 mg/kg daily for 2–3 days or ivermectin 200 μg/kg daily for 2–3 days. Ivermectin is probably the drug of choice as it is equally effective and better tolerated than thiabendazole. Disseminated disease in the immunosuppressed patient is treated with the same drug regimens but the duration therapy is 5–7 days. Repeated courses of therapy may be necessary in chronically immunosuppressed patients. Disseminated disease in the immunosuppressed patient is often associated with bacterial superinfection of the lungs, CNS or abdomen which requires specific antimicrobial therapy.

Cryptosporidia, Isospora, Cyclospora
Trimethoprim 160 mg–sulfamethoxazole 800 mg bid or tid for 10 days is the treatment of choice for *Isospora* and *Cyclospora* infections. In immunosuppressed patients the duration of treatment for both infections should be increased to 21–28 days. There is no proven efficacious therapy for *Cryptosporidium parvum* infection.

5.7 What is the role of non-antiinfective interventions (including reducing or altering immunosuppression) in the management of established infection?
When patients with rheumatologic diseases develop a serious infection, the most important nonantiinfective intervention is reducing the level of pharmacologic immunosuppres-

sion. In some situations, the potential morbidity and mortality of a serious intercurrent infection will be greater than that associated with the underlying disease. Thus, the infectious diseases specialist and the rheumatologist need to balance carefully the risks of exacerbating the underlying rheumatologic disease against the risks of the intercurrent infection and, whenever possible, to reduce the intensity of immunosuppressive therapy.

II INFECTIONS FOLLOWING SPLENECTOMY

The spleen has at least two major roles in host defense. First, it serves as a source for antibody production. Secondly, the anatomy of the spleen is such that it serves as a filter capable of removing bacteria from the bloodstream through its mononuclear phagocytic cells. The spleen is particularly efficient at clearing nonopsonized bacteria. Although surgical removal of the spleen is not clearly associated with an increased susceptibility to infection, certain infections can be much more severe in splenectomized individuals. The only clinical syndromes that clearly occur more frequently following splenectomy are severe hemolysis due to infection with *Babesia* spp. and the syndrome of overwhelming sepsis due *S. pneumoniae* and other encapsulated bacteria. Despite the large amount of published literature on this subject, there are insufficient data available to determine the true incidence, pathogenesis and exact risk factors for either syndrome.

I REGARDING THE CLINICAL PRESENTATION AND EVALUATION OF THE PATIENT

1.1 What are the clinically predominant modes of presentation of infection following splenectomy?

Overwhelming postsplenectomy sepsis usually presents with a brief prodrome of fever and nonspecific complaints (headache, malaise, nausea, vomiting, diarrhea, chills and abdominal pain) followed by a rapidly evolving picture of septic shock, which is often accompanied by disseminated intravascular coagulation. Mortality rates for overwhelming postsplenectomy sepsis range from 50% to 75%, with death usually occurring within 48 h.

Babesiosis is an infection by a malaria-like protozoa (*Babesia*) which parasitizes erythrocytes. Most infections in normal hosts are asymptomatic. However, babesiosis in splenectomized individuals may be associated with fever, severe hemolysis and hemoglobinuria.

1.2 What are the predominant sites of infection? (see Table 6.2)

Up to 50% of patients with fulminant postsplenectomy sepsis have no clinically obvious localized focus of infection. Pneumonia and meningitis are the most frequent localized sites of infection in patients with postsplenectomy sepsis.

1.3 What are the predominant organisms that contribute (by site)?

S. pneumoniae is the major pathogen responsible for postsplenectomy sepsis, accounting for 50–90% of cases. *H. influenzae* is the second most common cause. Less common pathogens include *Escherichia coli*, *S. aureus*, *N. meningitidis*, group B streptococcus and *Capnocytophaga canimorsus* (which has been associated with postsplenectomy sepsis following dog bites). See section 1.5 for organisms causing babesiosis.

1.5 How does this differ from other conditions, from center to center, and from country to country?

The few cases of babesiosis reported in Europe have occurred in splenectomized individuals and involved bovine *Babesia* (*B. divergens* or *B. bovis*). The European cases presented with fever and fulminant hemolytic disease that was usually fatal. *Babesia* infection in the United States is usually due to the rodent strain of *Babesia* (*B. microti*). In contrast to the European experience, only about 30% of the symptomatic cases of babesiosis in the United States have occurred in asplenic individuals, and the disease is clinically milder with few fatalities.

1.6 What is the appropriate approach to the initial evaluation and diagnosis of infection in splenectomized patients?

Initial diagnosis of postsplenectomy sepsis must rely on a high index of suspicion in a febrile splenectomized patient. The most rapid diagnostic test is examination of peripheral blood smear and buffy coat for the presence of bacteria. Blood cultures should be drawn and are usually positive within 24 h. However, this diagnostic workup should never delay institution of empirical antibiotic therapy. Babesiosis is usually diagnosed by microscopic examination of Giemsa- or Wright-stained thin and thick blood smears.

1.7 How should the evaluation be modified according to the severity of the risk?

All patients who have undergone splenectomy are at risk and should undergo the same evaluation.

1.8 What are the specific evaluation measures?

See section 1.6 and Chapter 2 in Part I.

1.9 What new developments are going to impact on emerging organisms, recognition, evaluation and diagnosis of infection in splenectomized patients?

In the past decade penicillin-resistant *S. pneumoniae* has emerged as a significant cause of community-acquired pneumonia and bacteremia. This fact needs to be considered when choosing an empirical antibiotic regimen in patients with suspected postsplenectomy sepsis (see section 5.1).

Polymerase chain reaction (PCR) based assays for babesiosis are being developed.

2 REGARDING THE RISK FACTORS FOLLOWING SPLENECTOMY

2.1 What are the main alterations in host defense mechanisms and what are the appropriate investigations to document them?

See section 2.2.

2.2 What are the alterations due to iatrogenic factors?

The main alteration of host defense is the loss of splenic immunologic function. Probably the most important role of the spleen in host defense is in the phagocytosis and clearance of nonopsonized particles. The anatomy of the spleen is such that it serves as a filter capable of removing bacteria from the bloodstream through its mononuclear phagocytic cells. By virtue of this ability, the spleen is of critical importance to the individual challenged with infection by an encapsulated bacteria to which he or she has no protective antibody.

The spleen also serves as a source for antibody production. Splenectomy has been associated with a decrease in serum immunoglobulin (Ig) M levels, but serum levels of IgG and IgA are not reduced. There is no evidence to suggest that type-specific or total antipneumococcal immunoglobulin levels are reduced by splenectomy. In addition, there is no convincing evidence that splenectomy per se affects the ability to respond to pneumococcal or other polysaccharide vaccines.

Finally, splenectomy is associated with a decrease in the levels of certain factors responsible for opsonization, such as tuftsin and properdin. It has been hypothesized that individuals without a spleen are unable to synthesize normal levels of these factors, leading to defective phagocytosis of encapsulated bacteria.

2.3 What is the influence of environmental factors?

As mentioned above, individuals without a spleen may develop symptomatic disease following infection with the malaria-like protozoa *Babesia*. Infection with *Babesia* has been rarely reported in Europe and Russia. However, infection with *B. microti* is not rare in the coastal and island areas of the eastern United States, where the infection is transmitted from the animal reservoir to humans via a tick vector. Most infections in the United States occur between April and October.

2.4 What are the most significant factors that contribute to the risk of infection in splenectomized patients?

Splenectomy is the most significant.

2.5 What are the specific or nonspecific measures aimed at minimizing this factor?

Where possible, techniques such as splenic artery embolization, splenic repair or partial splenectomy should be substituted for splenectomy in patients with splenic trauma.

2.6 Are there different levels of risk of infection recognized for splenectomized patients?

The majority of cases of overwhelming postsplenectomy sepsis occur in the first 2 years following splenectomy. However, the risk of overwhelming sepsis is lifelong, with cases reported to occur as long as 40 years after splenectomy. Children under 15 years of age have a greater overall risk of overwhelming postsplenectomy sepsis than adults. Presumably this is because adults have had previous exposure to the encapsulated organisms and have preexisting humoral immunity which compensates for the lack of a spleen. The nature the underlying disease also appears to influence the risk of overwhelming postsplenectomy sepsis. Individuals undergoing splenectomy for hematologic or lymphoproliferative diseases have a greater risk than those undergoing splenectomy for traumatic rupture.

2.7 How does the level of risk impact on management?

All asplenic individuals with suspected bacterial sepsis or babesiosis should be managed in the same way.

2.8 What new developments are going to impact on minimizing or suppressing the specific risk factors?

The recent development of protein-conjugated pneumococcal vaccines which are more immunogenic (especially in young children) may afford greater protection for splenectomized individuals than current polysaccharide vaccines.

3 REGARDING THE SURVEILLANCE OF PATIENTS FOLLOWING SPLENECTOMY

3.2 What are the surveillance measures to be taken in splenectomized patients?
None is recommended.

3.3 What are the other specific measures to be taken in a splenectomized patient?
See section 4.1.

3.4 What development(s) are to be expected for surveillance in splenectomized patients?
No particular developments are expected.

4 REGARDING THE PREVENTION OF INFECTION IN SPLENECTOMIZED PATIENTS

4.1 What approaches, if any, to the prevention of infection should be considered in splenectomized patients?
Immunization is one approach to preventing overwhelming sepsis following splenectomy. Vaccines against the major pathogens of this syndrome (*S. pneumoniae, H. influenzae* type B, *N. meningitidis*) are available and should be used in asplenic patients. There is no convincing evidence that asplenic individuals respond less well to these vaccines. Thus, it is not imperative to vaccinate before splenectomy. However, patients treated with cytotoxic chemotherapy respond less well to polysaccharide vaccines (regardless of whether they are asplenic). Thus, if possible, vaccination should be performed before the initiation of chemotherapy. Vaccination does not provide complete protection for asplenic patients and there are multiple documented cases of failure related to infection with both vaccine and nonvaccine strains of *S. pneumoniae*. Chemoprophylaxis against *S. pneumoniae* (which causes 50–90% of infections) is advocated by many experts, especially for children. A single daily dose of amoxycillin or penicillin has been the traditional regimen. However, there are several problems with this approach. This regimen will not protect against the penicillin-resistant strains of *S. pneumoniae* that are being encountered with increasing frequency. Likewise, the emergence of *S. pneumoniae* strains resistant to sulfamethoxazole and macrolides compromises the efficacy of chemoprophylaxis with these agents. In addition to antibiotic resistance, studies have demonstrated poor patient compliance with long-term prophylactic antibiotic regimens. One approach is to give the asplenic patient a supply of antipneumococcal antibiotics to take if they develop a febrile illness and cannot be evaluated immediately by a physician.

4.2 What are the future challenges and opportunities for reducing the risk of infection?
- To develop medical and surgical alternatives to splenectomy.
- To develop more immunogenic vaccines against all serotypes of *S. pneumoniae*.

5 REGARDING THE TREATMENT OF INFECTIONS IN SPLENECTOMIZED PATIENTS

5.1 What is the role of empirical therapy?

Early intervention in the form of appropriate antibiotic therapy is critical to preventing death in patients with overwhelming postsplenectomy sepsis. Empirical antibiotic therapy should be strongly considered in all asplenic patients presenting with fever. When possible, blood cultures should be obtained before instituting antibiotic therapy. However, obtaining cultures or waiting for culture results should never delay institution of empirical antibiotic therapy.

Currently, most experts recommend initiation of broad-spectrum empirical therapy with agents active against *S. pneumoniae*, *H. influenzae* and *N. meningitidis*. Local antibiotic resistance patterns of *S. pneumoniae* need to be considered when selecting an empirical regimen. In areas of the world where strains of *S. pneumoniae* with high-level penicillin resistance (minimum inhibitory concentration > 2.0 μg/ml) are rare, ceftriaxone, cefotaxime or ampicillin plus a β-lactamase inhibitor can still be used as initial empirical therapy. If meningitis is present, ceftriaxone, cefotaxime or meropenem should be used. In areas where high-level penicillin-resistant *S. pneumoniae* are a concern, vancomycin should be included in the empirical regimen. The newer quinolones (gatifloxacin and levofloxacin) also have good in-vitro activity against penicillin-resistant *S. pneumoniae* and may be appropriate as initial therapy in adults without meningitis. Once the results of blood cultures are available, therapy can be adjusted as indicated by susceptibility testing.

5.3 What is the appropriate approach to the splenectomized patient with evidence of bacteremia, with or without site of infection?

For Gram-positive bacteremia, Gram-negative bacteremia and bacteremia with a defined primary site of infection, see section 5.1. Anaerobic infection and mixed or polymicrobial bacteremia are not applicable here.

5.4 What is the appropriate approach to the splenectomized patient with evidence of a viral infection?

Neither herpes viruses, respiratory viruses, enteroviruses nor hepatitis are applicable here.

5.5 What is the appropriate approach to the splenectomized patient with evidence of a fungal infection?

Not applicable.

5.6 What is the appropriate approach to the splenectomized patient with evidence of a parasitic infection?

P. carinii, *T. gondii*, *S. stercoralis*, *Cryptosporidia*, *Isospora* and *Cyclospora* are not applicable here. Severe babesiosis in the asplenic host is treated with a combination of clindamycin (20 mg/kg daily in children; 300–600 mg every 6 h in adults) and quinine (25 mg/kg daily in children; 650 mg every 6–8 h in adults).

5.7 What is the role of non-antiinfective interventions (including reducing or altering immunosuppression) in the management of established infection?

In patients with overwhelming postsplenectomy sepsis, aggressive volume expansion is often necessary. Therapy with vasopressors (for severe hypotension) and heparin (for severe disseminated intravascular coagulation) may be needed in selected cases. Exchange transfusions (to lower levels of parasitemia) may be appropriate in selected patients with babesiosis and severe hemolysis.

REFERENCES

Dale DC, Fauci AS, Wolff SM. Alternate-day prednisone. Leukocyte kinetics and susceptibility to infections. *N Engl J Med* 1974; **291:** 1154–1158.

Hellmann DB, Petri M, Whiting-O'Keefe Q. Fatal infections in systemic lupus erythematosus: the role of opportunistic infections. *Medicine (Baltimore)* 1987; **66:** 341–348.

Lynch A, Kapel R. Overwhelming postsplenectomy infection. *Infect Dis Clin North Am* 1996; **10:** 696–707.

Ognibene FP, Shelhamer JH, Hoffman GS et al. *Pneumocystis carinii* pneumonia: a major complication of immunosuppressive therapy in patients with Wegener's granulomatosis. *Am J Respir Crit Care Med* 1995; **151:** 795–799.

Segal B, Sneller M. Infectious complications of immunosuppressive therapy in patients with rheumatic diseases. *Rheum Dis Clin North Am* 1997; **23:** 219–237.

Shelhamer J, Gill V, Quin T et al. The laboratory evaluation of opportunistic pulmonary infections. *Ann Intern Med* 1996; **124:** 585–599.

Stahl NI, Klippel JH, Decker JL. Fever in systemic lupus erythematosus. *Am J Med* 1979; **67:** 935–940.

Stuck AE, Minder CE, Frey FJ. Risk of infectious complications in patients taking glucocorticosteroids. *Rev Infect Dis* 1989; **11:** 954–963.

Chapter 7.0 | Infection in Solid Organ Transplant: An Introduction

Robert H Rubin and Eric Rosenberg

INTRODUCTION

The past two decades have featured major advances in the development and deployment of immunosuppressive drugs in the management of organ transplant recipients. The advent of cyclosporin, tacrolimus, mycophenolate mofetil and a variety of therapeutic monoclonal antibodies has revolutionized organ transplantation, permitting the development of heart, liver, lung, pancreas and small bowel transplantation (in addition to kidney transplantation) as practical approaches to the treatment of endstage organ dysfunction. One-year success rates better than 90% are now commonplace for the heart, kidney and liver (with the results of lung, pancreas and small bowel transplantation steadily improving). Indeed, infection, rather than acute allograft rejection, represents the greatest clinical challenge for many of these patients, and the prevention and treatment of such infections is of central importance in the care of the transplant recipient. In this chapter, general principles of transplant infectious diseases will be presented; in subsequent chapters, the details of these infections in the different forms of clinical transplantation will be discussed.

1 REGARDING THE CLINICAL PRESENTATION AND EVALUATION OF THE PATIENT

1.1 What are the clinically predominant modes of presentation of infection in solid organ transplant patients?
1.2 What are the predominant sites of infection?

The primary forms and sites of infection that occur in the transplant patient can be divided into seven categories.

Infection related to the transplant operation and perioperative care

As in any patient, immunosuppressed or not, who undergoes significant surgery, such as a transplant operation, the most common forms of infection occurring in the first few weeks posttransplant are those related to the operation and postoperative management: wound and allograft infection, pneumonia, drainage catheter-related infection (most commonly urinary tract infection related to a bladder catheter) and vascular access. Vascular access, particularly central venous and long lines, are important causes of bacteremia in these patients and should be avoided whenever possible. The etiologies of these infections, the bacterial and candidal species involved, are the same as in the general population, although the incidence and potential impact are greater in transplant patients. The difference in incidence of this form of infection among the organ transplant populations is largely due to the degree of complexity in the various operations, and is greatest with liver, lung and small bowel transplants, and least with kidney and heart.

Systemic viral infections

The most common form of infection observed in transplant patients is that caused by systemic viruses, particularly cytomegalovirus (CMV), human herpesvirus–6 (HHV–6) and Epstein–Barr virus (EBV). Both systemic effects (most commonly, a mononucleosis-like syndrome) and local organ dysfunction such as pneumonia, focal gastrointestinal infection, hepatitis and central nervous system (CNS) syndromes (aseptic meningitis and encephalitis) can be caused by these agents, although the systemic effects are usually dominant. Of particular note, the allograft itself (as opposed to a native organ) is particularly susceptible to invasion with these agents. For example, in the case of CMV, hepatitis is a clinical problem almost exclusively in liver recipients, pneumonia is most common in lung recipients, and myocarditis is recognized only in heart recipients.

Respiratory tract infections

Community-acquired viral infections remain a significant problem for transplant recipients, with a far higher rate of resulting pneumonia as a consequence of such infections. Conventional bacterial infection of the lungs, usually following viral infection or an aspirational episode, is the most common form of serious infection encountered. Typically, the rate of superinfection (especially if intubation is required) and the incidence of bacteremia are higher in these patients than in the general population with the same forms of infection.

Less common, although a continuing concern, is opportunistic infection of the lungs with such pathogens as *Pneumocystis carinii*, *Aspergillus fumigatus*, *Nocardia asteroides*, *Cryptococcus neoformans* and *Legionella* spp. If no prophylaxis is given, the rate of *Pneumocystis* infection exceeds 15% in the first year posttransplant. Opportunistic pulmonary infection occurs in transplant patients under two conditions: when the net state of immunosuppression is unduly high or when exposure to the pathogen, either within the community or within the hospital, is great enough.

Gastrointestinal tract infections

Gastrointestinal infections in the transplant patient can be divided into three general categories: diverticulitis, which has a relatively high rate of perforation and abscess formation, and usually requires surgical resection (see section 5.2) plus antibiotic therapy; febrile gastroenteritis, caused by the ingestion of pathogens in food and, less commonly, water; and viral infection of the liver and/or gut. CMV can infect the entire gut, from esophagus to anus, producing a variety of clinical effects: impaired gastric motility, gastrointestinal bleeding, diarrhea and perforation are the most notable. CMV involvement of the gut can occur as part of a more generalized syndrome (fever, pneumonia, etc.) or be the only consequence of CMV replication. Similarly, EBV-associated posttransplant lymphoproliferative disease (PTLD) can involve the gut (causing bleeding, obstruction, perforation or intussception) either as the only manifestation of PTLD or as part of a more generalized process.

Dermatologic infections

The skin is an important site of infection in the transplant patient. On the one hand, damage to the skin can provide a portal of entry for both conventional and opportunistic pathogens, which can then disseminate. Any chronic skin disease, such as eczema or psoriasis, can be a source of bacteremia following transplantation. An important guideline is to control such skin disease prior to transplantation, using whatever therapy is needed. For example, a moderate dose of cyclosporin (4–5 mg/kg daily) is quite effective in the treatment of a number of chronic dermatologic conditions, and the risk of immunosuppression is far less than the benefits of such therapy for the future transplant patient.

On the other hand, the skin can be a site of metastatic infection. Thus, in 20–30% of patients with fungal and nocardial infection, skin lesions may be the first manifestation of disseminated infection that brings a patient to medical attention. Because of the impaired inflammatory response of these immunosuppressed patients, the morphology of skin lesions may be atypical, and early biopsy for histologic examination and culture is of critical importance in the management of transplant recipients.

Central nervous system infections

The transplant patient remains susceptible to the same community-acquired infections affecting the CNS as the general population. However, certain CNS syndromes are particularly common in these patients (Table 7.0.1), predominantly with etiologies different from those occurring in the general population.

Table 7.0.1 Clinical syndromes due to central nervous system infection

Syndrome	Common etiologies in transplantation*
Acute meningitis	*Listeria monocytogenes*
Acute–chronic meningitis	*Cryptococcus neoformans*
	(*Mycobacterium tuberculosis, Coccidioides immitis, Histoplasma capsulatum*)
Focal brain infection	*Aspergillus fumigatus, Nocardia asteroides* (*Listeria monocytogenes, Toxoplasma gondii*)
Progressive dementia	Progressive multifocal leukoencephalopathy (due primarily to the BK virus)

* Less common causes are shown in parentheses. Together, *L. monocytogenes*, *C. neoformans* and *A. fumigatus* account for more than three-fourths of the CNS infections occurring in organ transplant patients.

Urinary tract infections

Urinary tract infection (UTI) is the single most common cause of bacterial infection in renal transplant patients, occurring in 30–50% of patients not receiving prophylaxis during the first 6 months posttransplant. A similarly high rate is found in pancreatic allograft recipients in whom a bladder anastomosis is employed (as opposed to an enteric one) for drainage of exocrine secretions. In other transplant groups, the incidence of UTI is not increased by immunosuppression (although the severity of an episode might be increased). In these patients, risk factors for UTI include urinary tract instrumentation, prostatic disease, poor bladder function – the same risk factors for UTI that occur in the general community.

1.3 What are the predominant organisms that contribute (by site?)

The microorganisms causing infection in the transplant patient can be divided into five general categories: conventional bacteria, viruses, opportunistic bacterial infection, fungal infection and parasitic infection.

Conventional bacteria

These are the most common causes of infection in transplant patients, with the pathogenesis and microbial etiology being quite similar to that observed in the general population: Gram-positive organisms are the most common causes of skin and wound infection; *Escherichia coli*, enterococci and *Pseudomonas aeruginosa* are the most common causes of urinary tract infection; and *Streptococcus pneumoniae* and other upper respiratory flora are the most common causes of pulmonary infection. However, because of continuing contact with the hospital environment, there is a far higher incidence of significant infection with relatively antibiotic-resistant Gram-negative bacilli, methicillin-resistant *Staphylococcus aureus* (MRSA), vancomycin-resistant enterococci (VRE) and *Clostridium difficile* than is observed in the general population.

Viruses

There are four groups of viruses that can have a particular impact on the transplant patient.

The herpes group of viruses

The herpes group of viruses (CMV, EBV, herpes simplex virus (HSV) 1 and 2, varicella zoster virus (VZV), HHV-6, HHV-7 and HHV-8) is the most important group of pathogens affecting the organ transplant patient. They are the direct cause of a variety of infectious disease syndromes and they also have a variety of indirect effects; increasing evidence suggests that cytokines, chemokines and growth factors elaborated in response to replication of these viruses can have three indirect effects:

1. contribute to the net state of immunosuppression
2. play a role in the occurrence of allograft injury
3. play a role in the pathogenesis of certain forms of malignancy (EBV and HHV-8 are essential to the occurrence of posttransplant lymphoproliferative disease and Kaposi sarcoma, respectively; CMV increases the risk of EBV-associated lymphoproliferative disease by a factor of 7–10).

Two characteristics make the herpes group of viruses such effective pathogens in the transplant patient: (1) latency, meaning that infection occurs for life, with viral reactivation occurring in response to the elaboration of proinflammatory cytokines, most notably tumor necrosis factor; and (2) the key host defense (i.e. virus-specific, major histocompatibility complex (MHC)-restricted, cytotoxic T-cells) is the aspect of host defense that is most inhibited by posttransplant immunosuppressive therapy.

Hepatitis viruses

Both hepatitis B virus (HBV) and hepatitis C virus (HCV) are common in transplant patients. Because of the effects of immunosuppressive therapy, these viruses have an accelerated course in transplant patients when compared with the general population. At present, HBV infection is more easily prevented and/or controlled. An effective vaccine is available that is most useful before the initiation of immunosuppression, and the screening of both organ and blood donors is an effective barrier to transmission. In addition, the advent of lamivudine therapy, with or without hyperimmune globulin, has been a major advance in the control of this infection. In contrast, there is no HCV vaccine on the horizon, and therapy with interferon, with or without ribavirin, is effective in the long term in a minority of transplant patients. Prevention remains the best strategy.

Community-acquired respiratory viruses

These viruses, particularly influenza, parainfluenza, adenoviruses and respiratory syncytial virus (RSV) are important pathogens in the transplant patient. The most effective strategy for combating them is avoidance, as neither immunization (in the case of influenza) nor antiviral therapy is sufficiently effective in the management of these infections.

Papovaviruses

A variety of clinical syndromes can be caused by these viruses in transplant patients: warts and squamous cell carcinomas of the skin, as caused by papillomaviruses; progressive multifocal leukoencephalopathy, due to BK virus; and renal dysfunction, due to tubulointerstitial infection of the kidney by BK virus. The driving force behind these clinical effects of these viruses is the intensity and nature of the immunosuppressive therapy being administered.

Opportunistic bacteria

Three forms of opportunistic bacterial infection occur in the transplant patient:

1 mycobacterial infection, especially with *Mycobacterium tuberculosis*, but also including a relatively high incidence of atypical mycobacterial infection
2 nocardial infection, especially that due to *N. asteroides*
3 listeriosis, caused by *Listeria monocytogenes*, which can cause a febrile gastroenteritis syndrome in the transplant patient as well as bacteremia, but whose most common effect is CNS infection. The most common CNS syndrome produced by *Listeria* is acute meningitis, although focal brain disease can occur, including a brainstem syndrome that may resemble poliomyelitis.

Fungi

Fungal infections in transplant patients can be divided into two general categories: those due to the geographically restricted systemic mycoses (blastomycosis, coccidioidomycosis and histoplasmosis) and those due to opportunistic pathogens, most notably *Candida* spp. (the most frequent cause of fungal infection in these patients), *Aspergillus* spp., most notably *A. fumigatus; C. neoformans;* and, uncommonly, the Mucoraceae. The common theme for all these infections is dissemination, and metastatic infection is the rule, whether the portal of entry is the lungs, the skin or contaminated vascular access lines.

P. carinii, formerly categorized as a protozoan, merits special attention. Without prophylaxis, the incidence of *Pneumocystis* pneumonia in organ transplant recipients approaches 15% at many centers. Low-dose trimethoprim–sulfamethoxazole (TMP–SMX) prophylaxis (e.g. one single-strength tablet per day) essentially eliminates this infection from allograft recipients. Atovaquone, dapsone or monthly pentamidine can be substituted in individuals intolerant of TMP–SMX, although these alternative regimens are not as effective.

Parasites

The major concern here is *Strongyloides stercoralis*. Because of the unique autoinfection potential of this pathogen, asymptomatic gastrointestinal carriage may persist for decades after acquisition. With the initiation of immunosuppressive therapy, two syndromes can develop: (1) hemorrhagic enterocolitis and/or pneumonia, essentially an accentuation of the usual effects of *Strongyloides* in the general population; and (2) disseminated tissue infection, often accompanied by Gram-negative infection of the CNS or bloodstream due to gut flora that have traveled with the invading parasite.

Less commonly, recurrent Chagas disease may be an issue for transplant patients from endemic areas.

1.4 How do the organisms vary according to various risk factors? (see also section 2)
The risk of infection in the transplant patient is determined largely by the interaction between two factors: the patient's net state of immunosuppression (Table 7.0.2) and the nature of the epidemiologic exposures encountered by the patient (Table 7.0.3). Indeed,

Table 7.0.2 Determinants of the net state of immunosuppression

- Host defense defects associated with the underlying condition
- Dose, duration and temporal sequence of immunosuppressive drugs
- Presence of leukopenia
- Presence of such technical and anatomic problems as devitalized tissue, undrained fluid collections, compromise of the integrity of the mucocutaneous barrier, and the requirement for indwelling foreign bodies
- Such metabolic abnormalities as protein-calorie malnutrition, uremia and, perhaps, hyperglycemia
- Infection with immunomodulating viruses (cytomegalovirus, Epstein–Barr virus, the hepatitis viruses and/or human immunodeficiency virus)

Table 7.0.3 Epidemiologic exposures of importance in the solid organ transplant recipient

Infections related to community exposures

Systemic mycotic infections in certain geographic areas
    a. *Histoplasma capsulatum*
    b. *Coccidioides immitis*
    c. *Blastomyces dermatitidis*

Respiratory infections circulating in the community
    a. *Mycobacterium tuberculosis*
    b. Influenza
    c. Adenoviruses
    d. Parainfluenza
    e. Respiratory syncytial virus
    f. *Legionella* spp.

Infections acquired by the ingestion of contaminated food or water
    a. *Salmonella* spp.
    b. *Listeria monocytogenes*
    c. *Campylobacter jejunii*
    d. *Strongyloides stercoralis*

Community-acquired opportunistic infection resulting from ubiquitous saprophytes in the environment
    a. *Cryptococcus neoformans*
    b. *Aspergillus* spp.
    c. *Nocardia asteroides*
    d. *Pneumocystis carinii*

Infections related to excessive nosocomial hazard
    a. *Aspergillus* spp.
    b. *Legionella* spp.
    c. *Pseudomonas aeruginosa* and other Gram-negative bacilli
    d. Methicillin-resistant *Staphylococcus aureus*
    e. Vancomycin-resistant enterococci
    f. Azole-resistant *Candida* spp.
    g. *Clostridium difficile*

the relationship between these two factors is a semiquantitative one: if the exposure is great enough, even minimally immunosuppressed individuals may develop life-threatening infection; conversely, if the net state of immunosuppression is great enough, even minimal exposure to normally commensal organisms can be a problem.

Age
Although not considered to play a major role, the age of an individual at the time of transplantation may add to the cumulative risk of infection. The greatest risk of infectious complications related to age occurs in children. Many infections occurring in the transplant recipient result from reactivation of a latent infection, with the possibility of at least partial control by preexisting immunity. However, in immunosuppressed children, risk occurs during primary infection when new immune responses should be generated but are blunted due to immunosuppression. Therefore, primary infection with EBV, CMV and VZV may be particularly severe, as the defect is in generating primary immunity rather then mobilizing existing memory responses. Both primary EBV and CMV infection in the child can be caused by the reactivation of latent virus in the allograft (the donor being seropositive), or due to intimate contact in the community. In contrast, primary VZV infection is always acquired in the community, often with school exposures. Other infections that may be more severe in younger transplant recipients are those due to community-acquired respiratory viruses. In particular, RSV tends to cause a more serious, overwhelming pneumonia in children than in adults. In general, elderly transplant patients are at greater risk from infection because of their general debility, preexisting structural or functional requirements, and, perhaps, a greater level of attenuation of immune function than exists for younger adult patients.

Timetable of infection
A useful way of approaching the transplant patient is to recognize that with standardized immunosuppressive programs there is a stereotypical pattern of when different infections occur in the posttransplant course; that is, there is a general timetable that reflects an integration of the risk factors that occur in the transplant patient. Such a timetable (Table 7.0.4) can be useful in three different ways: (1) in the differential diagnosis of the individual patient who presents with an infectious disease syndrome; (2) in the development and deployment of cost-effective antimicrobial strategies; and (3) as a guide to infection control measures, as exceptions to the timetable usually denote an unusual environmental hazard (often within the hospital) that requires correction. It is convenient to divide the posttransplant course of the transplant patient into three time periods.

First month posttransplant
In this time period, there are three causes of infection:
1 infection present in the recipient before transplant, perhaps exacerbated by surgery and anesthesia
2 infection conveyed with the allograft
3 postoperative bacterial and candidal infection of the surgical wound, vascular access, lungs and drainage catheters.
More than 95% of the infections occurring in this time period are of this last type, with the incidence being determined by the skill of the surgical team and the complexity of the surgery. It is notable that at a time when the highest daily doses of immunosuppression are employed, opportunistic infection does not occur unless an unusually intense

Table 7.0.4 Timetable of infection following solid organ transplantation

First month posttransplant
- Progressive infection in the recipient that was not eradicated before transplantation and has now been exacerbated by surgery and immunosuppression (uncommon)
- Infection of the allograft (rare)
- Bacterial and candidal infection of the wound, lungs, urinary tract or vascular access, related to technical mishaps in surgical and postoperative care (> 95% of infections)

One to six months posttransplant
- Viral infection: cytomegalovirus, Epstein–Barr virus in particular (common)
- Opportunistic infection: *Pneumocystis carinii, Listeria monocytogenes, Aspergillus* infection (uncommon, particularly with prophylaxis)

The late period, more than 6 months posttransplant
Three groups of patients:
1 80% of patients with good results (minimal immunosuppression, good allograft function) – community-acquired respiratory viruses, urinary tract infection
2 10% of patients with chronic hepatitis – progressive liver disease, hepatocellular carcinoma
3 10% of patients with poor allograft function and a history of excessive immunosuppression – highest risk of opportunistic infection: *Pneumocystis carinii, Listeria monocytogenes, Cryptococcus neoformans, Nocardia asteroides, Aspergillus* spp.

exposure occurs. This emphasizes that it is not the daily dose of immunosuppressive drugs that is important; rather, it is the sustained effect, the 'area under the curve'. Preventive strategies are based on perioperative antibiotics and impeccable technical management.

One to six months posttransplant
In this time period, there are two major classes of infection: (1) the most important agents of infection are the immunomodulating viruses (CMV, EBV, HHV-6 and the hepatitis viruses); the combination of sustained immunosuppression and infection with one or more of these viruses makes it possible for (2) such opportunistic infections as *P. carinii, L. monocytogenes* and *A. fumigatus* to occur without a particularly intense exposure. Preventive strategies, then, have three components: (1) antiviral, (2) low-dose TMP–SMX (or equivalent), which effectively eliminates the risk of *Pneumocystis* and *Listeria* (as well as *Nocardia*), and (3) environmental protection during this period of high immunosuppression.

Late period, more than 6 months posttransplant
More than 6 months posttransplant, patients can be divided into three categories in terms of infection risk: (1) the 80% of patients who have had a good result from transplantation, and whose major risk is from community-acquired respiratory infection; (2) 10% of patients with chronic viral infection, particularly with HBV and HCV, which in the absence of effective antiviral treatment will progress inexorably; and (3) the 10% of patients with poorly functioning allografts, most of whom have received excessive amounts of immunosuppression, and many of whom have chronic viral infection. This last group is at highest risk for opportunistic infection with *Pneumocystis, Listeria, Cryptococcus* and other pathogens, and should be considered for chronic TMP–SMX and fluconazole prophylaxis, as well as protection from environmental pathogens.

Technical and anatomic problems

Any technical error that leads to undrained fluid collections (e.g. hematoma, urine collection due to a leak, or a lymphocele) or the creation of devitalized tissue can lead to potentially life-threatening infection. In addition, appropriate care and early removal of vascular access devices, drainage catheters and the endotracheal tube (with adequate protection of the airway postextubation) will decrease the risk of infection.

Nature of immunosuppression

The components, the dose, the duration and the temporal sequence in which immuno-suppressive agents are deployed are the driving forces behind the occurrence of infection posttransplant (Table 7.0.2). In terms of infection risk, most of the thrust of the past three decades has been the development of steroid-sparing regimens. In addition, the specific effects of the different components must be taken into consideration. For example, whereas cyclosporin and tacrolimus have no ability to reactivate CMV from latency, antilymphocyte antibodies are quite potent because of the release of proinflammatory cytokines in response to their administration; in contrast, cyclosporin and tacrolimus are quite potent at amplifying the extent and consequences of CMV and other herpesvirus infection once active viral replication is present, whereas the antilymphocyte antibodies are far less potent in this regard. Thus, the entire regimen must be considered.

Antimicrobial preventive strategies (see section 4.1)

There are two aspects of antimicrobial preventive strategies that are particularly important in the transplant patient. First, the intensity of the antimicrobial strategy prescribed must be closely linked to the intensity of the immunosuppressive program that is required. The so-called 'therapeutic prescription' then, has two components: an immunosuppressive program to prevent and treat rejection, and an antimicrobial one to make it safe. Secondly, in patients with technical or anatomic problems, antimicrobial therapy will delay infection, not prevent it, with antimicrobial resistant infection being the price paid if the anatomic problem is not corrected. Thus, the optimal patient management strategy is to link antimicrobial regimens to correction of the anatomic problem that was critical to the development of the infection in the first place

1.5 How does this differ from other conditions, from center to center, and from country to country?

Three major factors help to explain differences in the occurrence of particular infections among transplant patients transplanted at different transplant centers:

1 The nature of the population being served, and the incidence of active and/or latent infection present in both the donor and recipient. For example, the incidence of dormant tuberculosis or latent CMV infection capable of being reactivated posttransplant is very different in different patient populations, with pediatric patients drawn from middle-class environments having the lowest risk, and older adults from lower socio-economic groups having the highest risk.

2 Environmental exposures to pathogens both within the hospital and the general community can be widely different. Thus, the occurrence of invasive aspergillosis in a hospital undergoing extensive construction or legionellosis in one in which the potable water supply is contaminated is far more common than in transplant patients cared for

at centers free from these problems. Similarly, the endemic mycoses occur only among transplant recipients with recent or remote exposure to the geographic areas where such infections are found.

3 Therapeutic protocols, both immunosuppressive and antimicrobial, at different transplant centers may vary. Thus, some centers utilize far more antilymphocyte antibody therapy, resulting in a greater risk of herpesvirus infection; while the use of TMP–SMX prophylaxis and/or antiviral prophylaxis will greatly decrease the incidence of a wide variety of infections.

1.6 What is the appropriate approach to the initial evaluation and diagnosis of infection in solid organ transplant patients?
1.7 How should the evaluation be modified according to the severity of the risk?
1.8 What are the specific evaluation measures? (see also Chapter 2 in Part I)

The key question to be asked in the initial evaluation of a transplant patient with a clinical syndrome possibly due to microbial invasion is whether the patient represents a therapeutic emergency or a diagnostic dilemma. Therapeutic emergencies require immediate initiation of broad-spectrum antimicrobial therapy after full culturing has occurred. Examples of possible therapeutic emergencies include the patient with signs of possible sepsis (e.g. hyperthermia with rigors, hypothermia, hypotension, acidosis, unexplained tachypnea), the patient with an acute abdomen, the patient with respiratory distress, and the patient with fever and neurologic compromise or evidence of meningism. Patients who are more subacutely ill merit a full diagnostic workup, including biopsy of suspicious lesions, before the initiation of therapy. All patients with unexplained fevers merit chest radiography, urinalysis and urine culture, blood culture, complete blood count and routine chemistries. Abnormalities on physical examination (e.g. skin lesions, abdominal findings, abnormalities of the surgical wound, chest consolidations) require radiologic and/or biopsy assessment. Lesions on chest radiography usually merit fuller characterization by computed tomography (CT) and an aggressive diagnostic approach (focal lesions by percutaneous biopsy, diffuse disease by bronchoscopy with bronchoalveolar lavage with or without transbronchial biopsy). Skin lesions merit biopsy for histologic examination and culture. A neurologic workup is indicated for unexplained headaches, change in mental status or the presence of meningeal signs. Such an evaluation includes a careful neurologic examination, CT or magnetic resonance imaging (MRI) of the brain, and lumbar puncture. Finally, an evaluation of the possibility of CMV viremia by antigenemia or polymerase chain reaction (PCR) assay is appropriate, particularly in the time period 1–6 months posttransplant.

1.9 What new developments are going to impact on emerging organisms, recognition, evaluation and diagnosis in solid organ transplant patients?
(see also section 2.8)

Emerging organisms

Two categories of microbial pathogens merit attention here:

1 antimicrobial-resistant organisms that are being observed increasingly in this patient population (e.g. VRE, MRSA, azole-resistant yeast, highly resistant Gram-negative bacilli and ganciclovir-resistant CMV)

2 newly recognized pathogens whose detection has only now become possible and whose full impact is still being defined (e.g. HHV-6, HHV-7, and HHV-8).

The spread of antibiotic-resistant infection is a problem throughout the hospital, but the transplant patient is at particular risk. Person-to-person spread between patients, from medical personnel to individual patients, and from contaminated hospital environments to patients, with VRE, MRSA, highly resistant *Klebsiella, Serratia, Pseudomonas* and other Gram-negative organisms, as well as azole-resistant *Candida* spp., has been especially important among transplant populations. Typically, gastrointestinal, skin and/or respiratory tract colonization occur first, with invasive infection developing when surgery and vascular access, for example, damage mucocutaneous barriers. Appropriate infection control strategies, including antibiotic usage guidelines, active surveillance, isolation and barrier nursing care, and rigorously enforced handwashing policies, are essential in the limitation of the impact of this growing problem.

The issue of ganciclovir-resistant CMV is a different one, as person-to-person spread of such infection has not been documented. Rather, this represents the selection of resistant clones of actively replicating virus under special circumstances. The selection of resistant CMV occurs most commonly when the following conditions are present: high viral load, as manifested by assays for viremia (e.g. antigenemia assay or quantitative PCR), intensive immunosuppressive therapy, and inadequate dose or duration of intravenous ganciclovir therapy. Particularly important is the recognition that oral ganciclovir, because of its poor bioavailability, is not an adequate substitute for intravenous ganciclovir in the presence of viremia. Oral ganciclovir is of great use prophylactically and to prevent relapse once viremia has been cleared with intravenous therapy; to use it earlier (e.g. when the patient has become asymptomatic but still has measurable viremia) increases greatly the risk of selecting for ganciclovir resistance. Alternative therapies to ganciclovir (e.g. foscarnet) are quite toxic in transplant patients, and this scenario should be avoided.

Over the past two decades, newly discovered pathogens, such as *Legionella* spp., have had a proportionately greater impact on transplant patients once diagnostic techniques were developed that permitted identification of these pathogens. Both for recognized and yet to be identified pathogens, transplant patients can be regarded as 'sentinel chickens' in our hospital and community environments that will reveal any excess traffic in microbes. HHV-6, HHV-7, and HHV-8 are three herpesviruses that are common in transplant patients, but whose impact has been difficult to discern until the recent development of quantitative PCR assays for their presence. With these diagnostic tools, it is now becoming possible to assess both the direct and indirect effects of these viruses. It is likely that dual infection with one of these with CMV will enhance the effects of both viruses, and that antiviral strategies will need to be directed at all the viruses, rather than just one. It is also likely that other heretofore undescribed pathogens will be identified in this patient population.

Diagnosis (see also sections 1.6 and 2.8)

Because of the impaired inflammatory response of these immunosuppressed patients, as well as the range of potential pathogens that might be present, a more aggressive diagnostic approach is necessary than in the general population. In addition to routine cultures, early biopsy, bronchoscopy with bronchoalveolar lavage, CT, and lumbar puncture are indicated in the evaluation of subtle signs of infection. One important point is that serologic studies (the demonstration of circulating antibodies to a particular organism) are relatively insensitive for early infection in these patients; rather, the emphasis is on culture, antigen detection (e.g. cryptococcal antigen) and, increasingly, quantitative PCR.

2 REGARDING THE RISK FACTORS ACCOMPANYING SOLID ORGAN TRANSPLANTATION (see also section 1.4)

2.1 What are the main alterations in host defense mechanisms and what are the appropriate investigations to document them?
2.2 What are the alterations due to iatrogenic factors?
2.3 What is the influence of environmental factors?
2.4 What are the most significant factors that contribute to the risk of infection in solid organ transplant patients?

As previously detailed, there are three major risk factors for infection in the transplant patient:

- the technical skill with which the operation and perioperative care is accomplished
- the epidemiologic exposures the patient encounters
- the patient's net state of immunosuppression.

In recent years, the general technical skill of transplant teams has reached such a high level that major technical problems are uncommon, and are usually the result of a problem with the organ to be transplanted. However, this cornerstone of modern transplantation should never be taken for granted.

The epidemiologic exposures that the transplant patient encounters can be divided into two general categories: those occurring in the community and those occurring within the hospital (see Table 7.0.3). In the hospital, exposure to contaminated water or air (and, occasionally food and medical devices) can take one of two patterns: a non-domiciliary pattern, in which the exposure occurs on the ward where the patient is being cared for; and a nondomiciliary pattern, in which the exposure occurs at such sites in the hospital as the radiology department, operating room, catheterization laboratory or bronchoscopy suite where the patient is taken for an essential procedure. Domiciliary exposures are usually identified relatively easily because of clustering of cases in time and space; in contrast, this may not occur with nondomiciliary exposures, making such environmental hazards far more difficult to identify and correct.

The other major factor determining the risk of infection is a complex function termed the net state of immunosuppression (see Table 7.0.2). The dose, duration and temporal sequence in which immunosuppressive agents are utilized are the major determinants of the net state of immunosuppression, but other factors such as metabolic derangements (particularly protein-calorie malnutrition) and the presence of infection with certain immunomodulating viruses (CMV, EBV, HBV, HCV and human immunodeficiency virus (HIV)) contribute significantly to the net state of immunosuppression.

From these comments, general principles of infection prevention in the organ transplant recipient emerge:

1 Technically impeccable surgery and careful management of endotracheal tubes, vascular access and drainage catheters, as well as protection of mucocutaneous surfaces, are obligatory – the cornerstone of any program for preventing infection in this patient population.
2 Epidemiologic protection, particularly in the hospital environment, is essential, especially at times of maximal immunosuppression. Constant surveillance for hitherto unsuspected environmental hazards is important to monitor the success of epidemiologic protective strategies.
3 Individualized immunosuppression, to limit the extent of host defense depression engendered by antirejection programs, is obligatory.

4 The targeted deployment of antimicrobial agents in conjunction with surgical manipulations and escalations in immunosuppressive therapy, as well as in patients with clinical, laboratory or epidemiologic markers that connote a particularly high risk of
subsequent clinical disease, will prevent many infections.

2.5 What are the specific or nonspecific measures aimed at minimizing each of these factors?

Nonspecific measures

Adequate pretransplant assessment of donor and recipient
Active infection of the bloodstream or the allograft greatly increases the risk of clinically
important infection posttransplant, and potential donors should be carefully evaluated
clinically and microbiologically for these; similarly, all active infection should be eradicated in the recipient before transplantation. HBV and HCV are transmitted efficiently
with allografts from infected donors, and these need to be assessed before harvesting the
organ. In addition, both donor and recipient should be assessed for latent infection with
CMV, EBV, VZV (by serologic assay), and tuberculosis (by skin testing) so that appropriate preventive strategies can be initiated posttransplant (see also section 3.1).

Correction of underlying abnormalities in the recipient
These include nutritional repletion, correction of chronic skin disorders, and evaluation
and correction of anatomic defects. For example, patients with a history of active diverticulitis in the recent past should be considered for pretransplant sigmoid colectomy.

Epidemiologic protection
A continuing assessment of both nosocomial and community environmental hazards is
mandatory. Particular attention to air and potable water quality within the hospital is
important in the avoidance of such infections as aspergillosis and legionellosis. Protection
against person-to-person spread due to standard infection control practices, particularly
handwashing among medical personnel, is essential. A particular emphasis should be
placed on patient education in terms of avoiding travel to high-risk environments, high-
risk foods (e.g. undercooked eggs and poultry products, unpasteurized cheeses) and
high-risk activities (not only drug abuse, high-risk sexual activity and noncompliance to a
medical regimen, but also such common activities as gardening with its inherent risk of
fungal and nocardial infection).

Individualized immunosuppressive programs
Although the general pattern of immunosuppression at most centers is relatively
standardized, constant attention to the possibility of decreasing immunosuppression
is mandatory. When increased doses of immunosuppressive agents are required to
control rejection, this should trigger a reevaluation of antimicrobial preventive
regimens, whose efficacy is often linked to the nature of the immunosuppression being
administered.

Protection of the integrity of mucocutaneous surfaces
Protection of the skin is of particular importance, with a concerted effort necessary to
avoid trauma to the skin, indwelling foreign bodies (at any site, but particularly drainage
catheters, central venous access for prolonged periods, and endotracheal tubes), as well

as protecting the gastrointestinal mucosa against the physical consequences of both severe constipation and diarrhea.

Specific measures

The specific antimicrobial measures needed in the transplant patient represent a combination of both prophylactic and preemptive deployment of antimicrobial drugs. The two general principles are:

1 The nature of the antimicrobial strategy should be closely linked to the nature of the immunosuppressive program (the 'therapeutic prescription' for the transplant patient having two components: an immunosuppressive strategy to prevent and treat rejection, and a closely meshed antimicrobial strategy to make it safe).

2 The higher the risk, the greater the intensity of the antimicrobial program.

Four general areas should be considered in the transplant patient, as described below.

Perioperative antibiotic prophylaxis

A single dose of a first- or second-generation cephalosporin, or equivalent, on call to the operating room will decrease the incidence of significant surgical wound infection in this patient population.

Antibacterial and anti-Pneumocystis prophylaxis

This is best accomplished with low-dose TMP–SMX prophylaxis (e.g. one single-strength tablet at bedtime), which will essentially eradicate urosepsis, *Pneumocystis*, *Nocardia*, *Listeria* and, probably, *Toxoplasma* infection from this population. Appropriate prophylaxis for patients unable to tolerate TMP–SMX is more problematic, with atovaquone or pentamidine plus a fluoroquinolone usually substituted. These alternative regimens are less effective in general, and do not provide coverage for *Nocardia* or *Listeria*.

Antiviral strategies

The primary antiviral effort is in the prevention of CMV disease. The program that we employ (see Table 7.0.5) is a combination of prophylaxis for high-risk patients and preemptive therapy for individuals who develop markers of high risk. Thus, if the donor is seropositive for CMV and the recipient seronegative, the risk of CMV disease is 50–65%, and we therefore advocate prophylaxis with a combination of intravenous (for 5–7 days) followed by oral ganciclovir (for 3–4 months) for all these individuals, who represent approximately 10% of transplant recipients. In contrast, if the recipient is seropositive for CMV prior to transplant and is immunosuppressed with a regimen that does not include an antilymphocyte antibody, then the risk of CMV disease is 10–15% and no anti-CMV prophylaxis is prescribed. Rather, preemptive therapy (intravenous ganciclovir for 10–14 days followed by oral therapy for 4 months) is prescribed when either of two conditions is operative: (1) antilymphocyte therapy with antithymocyte globulin (ATG) or OKT3 is utilized, particularly as antirejection therapy (which is employed in the 15% of individuals with so-called steroid-fast rejection, and which increases the risk of CMV disease to 65–75%); or (2) the patient is being monitored for presymptomatic viremia by antigenemia or quantitative PCR assay, with a positive assay for a significant level of virus triggering preemptive therapy.

VZV merits special attention. VZV-seronegative individuals are at high risk for disseminated primary infection posttransplant, and should receive vaccine, preferably before transplantation, with documentation of seroconversion. In the absence of

Table 7.0.5 Cytomegalovirus prevention strategies employed at the Massachusetts General Hospital for solid organ transplant patients*

High-risk patients

Donor seropositive, recipient seronegative:
- Intravenous ganciclovir 5 mg/kg daily for 7 days, followed by
- Oral ganciclovir 1 g tid for 4 months

Recipient seropositive, treated with antilymphocyte antibody therapy:
- Intravenous ganciclovir 5 mg/kg daily during antilymphocyte antibody therapy, followed by
- Oral ganciclovir 1 g tid for 3 months

Lower-risk patients

Recipient seropositive, no antilymphocyte antibody therapy:
- Oral ganciclovir 1 g tid for 3 months, or
- No therapy, but weekly monitoring by antigenemia assay or quantitative polymerase chain reaction for viremia; when positive, preemptive therapy with intravenous ganciclovir 5 mg/kg twice daily for 2 weeks, followed by oral ganciclovir 1 g tid for 3 months

---

* Ganciclovir dosage is adjusted for renal dysfunction.

seroconversion following vaccine administration, prophylaxis of VZV exposures with zoster immune globulin is mandatory.

Antifungal strategies

Fluconazole prophylaxis is indicated in pancreas–kidney transplant recipients, and should be considered in patients with a poor outcome from transplantation. Preemptive therapy of asymptomatic candidiuria and asymptomatic cryptococcal and coccidioidal infections in the lung, to prevent subsequent serious disease, is indicated. In other circumstances, such as broad-spectrum antibacterial therapy, oral nystatin or clotrimazole is usually quite effective in preventing mucosal infection.

2.8 What new developments are going to impact on minimizing or suppressing the specific risk factors? (see also section 1.9)

There are several evolving areas that will influence the incidence and clinical management of infections in the transplant patient.

New immunosuppressive programs

The driving force in the pathogenesis of infections in this patient population is the nature of the immunosuppressive program employed. Steroid-sparing programs have already had a significant impact; in recent years, the development of increasingly specific reagents targeted at particular components of the immune system has been emphasized. If one were to speculate about the future, the goal is antigen-specific tolerance, which, if achieved, would greatly change the risk for infection over the long term and the need for extended antimicrobial therapies. The concept of a therapeutic prescription remains operative, however, with a close linkage between immunosuppression and antimicrobial deployment.

Emerging pathogens

As previously discussed, transplant patients are a 'leveraged' population in terms of a group of individuals who are likely to feel the brunt of new pathogens, whether these be antimicrobial resistant conventional organisms (e.g. VRE, MRSA, resistant Gram-negatives, azole-resistant yeast) or heretofore undescribed or underappreciated organisms (e.g. HHV-6 and dematiaceous fungi). Constant surveillance of these patients for unique infections remains a necessity.

New diagnostic techniques

Increasingly, noncultural assays for microbial antigens or nucleic acid will become the approach of choice in these immunosuppressed patients, permitting rapid, early and specific diagnosis, and better guidance of therapy.

New antimicrobial therapies

New drugs will be developed, including agents effective against presently resistant species, and improved oral antifungal and antiviral agents. In this group there is a particular need for effective agents, with satisfactory oral bioavailability, against *Aspergillus* infection, herpes group viruses and, particularly, HCV. In addition, new strategies for preemptive therapy will emerge, linked to new generations of diagnostic techniques.

3 REGARDING THE SURVEILLANCE OF SOLID ORGAN TRANSPLANT PATIENTS

3.1 What is the important pretransplant information to be gathered?

Evaluation of the prospective organ donor (see also section 2.5)
Donor evaluation for infection that can be transmitted to the recipient is of critical importance in preventing potentially catastrophic infection. There are two general categories of infection that need to be considered in the donor:
1 active infection that will be conveyed with the allograft
2 latent infection that is at risk for subsequent reactivation in the recipient, and which might influence subsequent antimicrobial strategies.

Active infection
Infection with such viruses as HIV, HBV and HCV is of primary concern, as transmission of these viruses with the allograft has an efficiency approaching 100% if there is active viral replication in the donor. HIV and HBV testing of donor serum is quite efficient in protecting recipients from this risk, provided an appropriate sample is tested (difficulties have occurred when the serum sample in a prospective donor was obtained only after multiple transfusions 'diluted out' the expected result, while the organ transplanted remained fully infectious to the recipient).

More controversial has been how to handle an anti-HCV-positive donor (approximately 5% of the donor pool), since only half of these individuals harbor replicating virus (if present, replicating virus is readily transmitted with the allograft). Because of a shortage of donors and the relatively long time course required for HCV to exert its effects, many centers are utilizing organs from anti-HCV-positive donors. Our policy is to reserve such a practice for individuals with an emergent need for the transplant, highly sensitized patients unlikely to get another allograft in the near future, and older patients; in general, children and young adults do not receive such organs because of their potential for a longer lifespan.

Another active problem is acute infection of a prospective cadaveric donor that is related to the terminal illness or the care of the terminal illness. Active infection that has been inadequately treated in the donor is a major hazard for the recipient. Thus, systemic viral infection and known infection of the organ to be transplanted will rule out the use of the donor or a particular organ. A bigger concern is ongoing bacteremia or candidemia in the donor at the time of organ procurement, which is a major hazard for the integrity of vascular, and other, suture lines. Vascular suture line infection carries a risk of mycotic aneurysm development and catastrophic rupture, so great care is required in evaluating the donor.

Dormant or latent infection
Although rarely a cause for turning down a donor, dormant or latent infection will influence posttransplant antimicrobial approaches. For example, knowing whether or not an individual is seropositive for CMV, EBV and *Toxoplasma* can influence the nature of the antimicrobial program prescribed, as the allograft can carry these infections from the donor. Similarly, potential donors with a history of positive tuberculin tests, or previous active disease with either *M. tuberculosis* or one of the geographically restricted systemic mycoses (e.g. *Blastomyces dermatitidis, Coccidioides immitis* or *Histoplasma capsulatum*) should be carefully evaluated to rule out active disease. If such a donor is utilized, then information regarding the past experience of the donor must be conveyed to the medical team caring for the recipient, as such information may be useful in posttransplant management.

Evaluation of the recipient
The first rule of transplant infectious disease is that, whenever possible, active infection must be eliminated from the recipient before transplantation. In particular, pulmonary, intraperitoneal and bloodstream infection require special attention. Active pulmonary infection has a high rate of superinfection posttransplant, and is far better managed before anesthesia and posttransplant immunosuppression. Intraperitoneal infection carries a hazard for suture lines constructed at the time of kidney, liver, pancreas and small bowel transplantation. Active bloodstream infection with bacterial or candidal species carries at least the same risk of suture line infection, mycotic aneurysm and anastomotic rupture as such infection does in the donor.

Knowledge of both latent infection and chronic infection in the potential recipient will influence both antimicrobial and immunosuppressive strategies posttransplant. Thus, seronegative recipients of organs from CMV- or EBV-positive donors (or, in the case of cardiac transplant patients, *Toxoplasma gondii*) are at higher risk of serious clinical disease, and hence merit more intensive antimicrobial strategies than do seropositive recipients. In the case of VZV-seronegative individuals, immunization prior to transplantation with documentation of seroconversion is warranted. In the absence of such seroconversion, varicella exposures in seronegative individuals require zoster immune globulin prophylaxis.

Chronic HBV or HCV infection in the recipient likewise mandates special attention. Lower-dose immunosuppression protocols are usually employed, particularly the prednisone component, and consideration of antiviral therapies before and after transplantation are predicated on the identification and evaluation of these infections.

An area of continuing controversy is the appropriate approach to tuberculin testing. It is generally agreed that patients awaiting transplant should undergo tuberculin testing, noting that false-negative results may occur as a result of anergy induced by the patient's underlying disease. The question of how to approach a patient with a positive tuberculin test result is a more difficult one, as antituberculous drugs are difficult to manage in the face of cyclosporin- and tacrolimus-based immunosuppression, as well as the approximately 10% incidence of chronic hepatitis in transplant patients. In addition, it is now clear that the incidence of clinical tuberculosis is quite low in transplant patients without other risk factors for tuberculosis. Risk factors include previous history of active tuberculosis, significant abnormalities on chest radiography, protein-calorie malnutrition, other immunosuppressing illnesses and non-Caucasian racial background. Our approach is to follow closely, with 6–monthly chest radiography for 2 years, followed by yearly radiography thereafter, individuals with positive tuberculin tests and no other risk factors. Individuals with risk factors receive 1 year of prophylaxis, preferably with isoniazid, but with the combination of ofloxacin and ethambutol if this is not tolerated.

3.2 What are the surveillance measures to be taken in solid organ transplant patients?
3.3 What are the other specific measures to be taken in solid organ transplant patients?

Constant surveillance of both the individual patient and the entire transplant population is necessary for detection of signs and symptoms indicative of a possible serious infection, especially one that might indicate a particular hazard in the environment. Although the clinician should be constantly aware of a possible cluster of cases due to such a hazard, it is to be hoped that detection of a hazard, especially in the hospital environment, might be accomplished with a single case. The best clue to the presence of an environmental hazard is the occurrence of an infection, particularly an opportunistic infection, at a point in time when the net state of immunosuppression is not normally great enough to allow such an infection to occur without an unusually intense exposure. Two examples of this principle are the occurrence of opportunistic infection in the first month posttransplant or at any time when the timetable suggests that such an infection is a rare event.

3.4 What development(s) are to be expected for surveillance in solid organ transplant patients?

Developments in the surveillance of transplant patients will depend on three major factors: the emergence of new infections; the use of new immunosuppressive programs; and the development and deployment of new surveillance techniques. The 1990s have witnessed not only the emergence of MRSA, VRE, highly resistant Gram-negative bacteria and azole-resistant *Candida* infections, but also the recognition that the transplant patient is at particular risk for these infections. It is likely that this leveraged population will also feel the brunt, in future years, of other emerging infections. Since the driving force for many infections is the program of immunosuppression, the deployment of new immunosuppressive agents will change the infection risk and influence the surveillance strategies that will be necessary. Finally, the development and deployment of quantitative PCR technology for early detection of microbial invasion and replication, as well as gene expression technology to assess host responses, will greatly increase the value and scope of surveillance activities.

4 REGARDING THE PREVENTION OF INFECTION IN SOLID ORGAN TRANSPLANT RECIPIENTS

For details relating to specific organ transplants, see Chapters 7.1 (renal), 7.2 (liver), 7.3 (lung), 7.4 (lung and heart-lung), 7.5 (intestinal) and 7.6 (pancreas).

5 REGARDING THE TREATMENT OF SOLID ORGAN TRANSPLANT PATIENTS

For details relating to specific organ transplants, see Chapters 7.1 (renal), 7.2 (liver), 7.3 (heart), 7.4 (lung and heart-lung), 7.5 (intestinal) and 7.6 (pancreas).

REFERENCES

Hibberd PL, Tolkoff-Rubin NE, Conti D et al. Preemptive ganciclovir therapy to prevent cytomegalovirus disease in cytomegalovirus antibody-positive renal transplant recipients. *Ann Intern Med* 1995; **123**: 18–26.

Pohl C, Green M, Wald ER et al. Respiratory syncytial virus infection in pediatric liver transplant recipients. *J Infect Dis* 1992; **165**: 166–169.

Rubin RH. Infection in organ transplant recipients. In: Rubin RH, Young LS, eds. *Clinical Approach to Infection in the Compromised Host*, 4th edn. New York: Plenum Press (in press).

Rubin RH, Tolkoff-Rubin NE. Minireview: Antimicrobial strategies in the care of organ transplant recipients. *Antimicrob Agents Chemother* 1993; **7**: 619–624.

Snydman D. Infection in organ transplant recipients. *Transplant Infect Dis* 1999; **1**: 21–28.

Infections in Renal Transplant Recipients

Eric Rosenberg and Robert H Rubin

INTRODUCTION

Despite the remarkable progress that has been made in renal transplantation over the past several decades, infection remains a major challenge in patient management. The particular problems to be approached are several: the spectrum of organisms that can infect allograft recipients is extremely broad, including both the infections that affect immunologically normal individuals, as well as opportunistic pathogens that affect only the immunocompromised; and the presentation of infection can be subtle, because of the impaired inflammatory response to microbial invasion, rendering early diagnosis difficult and therapy more complex. Although early diagnosis and therapy are central to the management of clinical infection in these patients, the consequences of infection can be so great that prevention is the first responsibility for the clinician.

1 REGARDING THE CLINICAL PRESENTATION AND EVALUATION OF THE PATIENT

1.1 What are the clinically predominant modes of presentation of infection in renal transplant recipients?

Fever without localizing signs
Fever, not infrequently without localizing signs or symptoms, is the most common finding in renal transplant patients presenting with infection. In addition to infection as a cause of fever, other potential causes need to be considered as well: allograft rejection, posttransplant lymphoproliferative disease (PTLD), pulmonary embolism and drug fevers being the most important causes of noninfectious temperature increases. As a general rule, temperature curves are more hectic in children than in adults with both infectious and noninfectious causes of fever.

Viral infection
Viral infections as a course of unexplained fever occur predominantly in the time period 1–6 months posttransplant (see Table 7.0.4 and section 1.4 in Chapter 7.0); systemic cytomegalovirus (CMV), Epstein–Barr virus (EBV) and human herpesvirus–6 (HHV–6) are the most important causes of fever in this time period. Table 7.0.5 in Chapter 7.0 delineates the anti-CMV strategies employed at the Massachusetts General Hospital to prevent such infections. Two basic principles are embodied: high-risk patients can be

defined, and merit more intense preventive approaches; and the nature of the antiviral program must be linked to the intensity of the immunosuppressive program.

Rejection

Acute rejection as a cause of unexplained fever is most common in the first 4–6 weeks posttransplant. Children are most likely to manifest fever from this cause, often as the first sign of allograft rejection, with the level of fever being roughly proportional to the gravity of the rejection episode. Febrile responses in adults are less common, being seen especially when prednisone therapy is being tapered or eliminated. A negative crossmatch prior to transplantation (the recipient being free of antibodies to donor antigens) and effective immunosuppression are of critical importance in preventing this cause of fever.

OKT3/antithymocyte globulin reaction

Febrile reactions following the administration of these antilymphocyte antibody therapies are to be expected with the first two or three doses of these agents, due to the release of tumor necrosis factor (TNF) and interleukin–1 (IL–1). In general, the height of the temperature response is greater when these agents are employed to treat rejection than when they are used prophylactically as induction therapy. During the course of therapy with these antibodies, an immunologic response to the foreign proteins [murine in the case of OKT3, equine for antithymocyte globulin (ATG)] is common, often inducing a febrile response at the end of a 10–14-day course of therapy. This febrile response usually is a marker for decreased efficacy for this form of antirejection therapy, and the need for alternative immunosuppression. Concomitant administration of pulse doses of steroids (e.g. 500 mg intravenous methylprednisolone in adults) will decrease the febrile response to these therapeutic antibody preparations, as well as increase the immunosuppressive potency of the antirejection regimen.

Bacteremia

When considering bacteremia as a cause of fever, the skin, urinary tract, gastrointestinal tract, and surgical wound are the major portals of entry. Any chronic skin disease, such as eczema or psoriasis, can be a source of bacteremia following transplantation. An important principle is to control such skin disease before transplantation, using whatever therapy is needed. For example, a moderate dose of cyclosporin (4–5 mg/kg daily) is quite effective in the treatment of a number of chronic dermatologic conditions, and the risk of immunosuppression is far less than the benefits of such therapy for the future transplant patient.

Traditionally, the urinary tract has been the most common source of bacteremia in the renal transplant patient. With the advent of improved surgery, early removal of the bladder catheter posttransplant, and antibiotic prophylaxis with trimethoprim–sulfamethoxazole (TMP–SMX) or a fluoroquinolone, urosepsis has been largely eradicated. Indeed, the occurrence of urosepsis in a patient on prophylaxis should suggest an anatomic or functional (e.g. impaired bladder emptying) problem with the urinary tract.

Vascular access, particularly central venous and long lines, are important causes of bacteremia in these patients and should be avoided whenever possible. Thus, although long-term venous access from central catheters and long lines is convenient for the administration of extended courses of antimicrobial agents, the rate of secondary bacteremia (and candidemia) is considerable. Therefore, for as long as possible, repeated placement of short peripheral venous access devices is to be preferred.

The administration of low-dose TMP–SMX prophylaxis not only prevents *Pneumocystis* and nocardial infection, but also has a major effect in terms of preventing urosepsis and *Listeria monocytogenes* bacteremia. Bacteremia from the surgical wound is prevented by the combination of impeccable surgical technique and perioperative antimicrobial prophylaxis (e.g. with a first-generation cephalosporin).

There are two categories of bacteremia from a gastrointestinal source that bear mention: most important is the occurrence of sigmoid diverticulitis, which is usually associated with perforation and abscess formation (and positive blood cultures with bowel flora). In addition, such enteric pathogens as *Salmonella* spp. are a significant problem in these patients, with *Salmonella* gastroenteritis having a high rate of bacteremia and metastatic infection in the transplant population. These infections are best prevented by consideration of a sigmoid colectomy in patients with a history of recent diverticulitis; careful attention to bowel habits following transplantation; and appropriate dietary exposures to avoid the ingestion of enteric pathogens.

Clinically documented infection

Lungs

Pulmonary infection due to conventional bacteria occur in three major clinical settings following renal transplantation: in association with prolonged intubation, following aspiration (especially in association with vomiting), and following viral respiratory infection. These are best prevented by appropriate management of the endotracheal tube (including aggressive weaning from the ventilator after operation); judicious use of antiemetic drugs; and avoidance of exposure to respiratory viruses. Influenza and pneumococcal immunization is recommended, but is most effective before transplantation. Opportunistic pulmonary infection is prevented by limitation of the net state of immunosuppression (see Table 7.0.2 and section 1.4 in Chapter 7.0), avoidance of excessive environmental exposures, especially within the hospital, and (in the case of *Pneumocystis carinii* and nocardial infection) low-dose TMP–SMX prophylaxis.

Central nervous system

Renal transplant recipients share the same risk for conventional infections of the central nervous system (CNS) as the general population, although the initial onset may be more insidious. The most common causes of CNS infection in renal transplant patients, however, are *Listeria monocytogenes, Nocardia asteroides, Aspergillus* spp. and *Cryptococcus neoformans*. The first two of these are well prevented with TMP–SMX prophylaxis, *Aspergillus* by careful monitoring of air quality [with the use of high-efficiency particulate air (HEPA) filters when necessary], and fluconazole prophylaxis for *Cryptococcus*. Fluconazole use is indicated as a preemptive therapy in patients with asymptomatic pulmonary nodules found on biopsy to be due to cryptococcal organisms, and should be considered as prophylaxis for the subgroup of patients who are at particularly high risk for crytococcal infection – the 5–10% of patients who are more than 6 months posttransplant and have had an unsatisfactory result from transplantation (poor allograft function, a history of excessive exposure to immunosuppression, and, often, chronic viral infection due to hepatitis B or C or CMV) (see Table 7.0.4 in Chapter 7.0).

Skin

The skin, with its rich blood supply, is of importance in the infectious disease management of the renal transplant patient in two ways: (1) as a portal of entry, when this primary barrier to infection is compromised by disease or injury; and (2) as a site of metastatic infection when disseminated infection, particularly with fungal species or

Nocardia, is present (approximately 25% of individuals with disseminated infections due to these organisms will present with focal cutaneous lesions, often rather nondescript in appearance). An aggressive biopsy approach of unexplained skin lesions is required to permit early preemptive therapy.

Surgical wound

The leading factor in the occurrence of infection related to the surgical wound is the technical skill and success with which the transplant operation is accomplished. Uncomplicated operations have a rate of wound infection of less than 1%. Perioperative antibiotic prophylaxis (e.g. cefazolin before operation) will reduce the risk further. If reexploration is necessary, if hematomas, urine leaks or lymphoceles develop, then the risk of infection, even with antibiotic prophylaxis, is four to five times as great.

Urinary tract

The surgical and immunologic trauma to which the renal allograft is subjected renders it particularly susceptible to infection, especially in the first 3–4 months posttransplant. The need for the bladder catheter for 1–7 days posttransplant provides an opportunity for introducing bacteria into the urinary tract. Without prophylaxis, the incidence of urinary tract infection (UTI) in the first 4 months posttransplant is approximately 35%, with a rate of pyelonephritis greater than 50% and of bacteremia greater than 10%. TMP–SMX or fluoroquinolone prophylaxis is quite effective in preventing these events (in technically uncomplicated transplants the risk of UTI is less than 5% when such prophylaxis is employed).

In the late period, more than 6 months posttransplant, UTIs occur in three settings:

1 lower tract infection in women and men with prostatic disease (comparable to that observed in the general population)
2 infections due to poor bladder emptying, resulting from diabetic neuropathy or intrinsic bladder disease
3 association with urinary stones (often developing on nonabsorbed suture material).

Prevention is based on optimizing bladder function pharmacologically, removal of stones (and correction of the underlying etiology for the stones), and the appropriate use of TMP–SMX or fluoroquinolone prophylaxis.

Microbiologically documented infection

Urinary tract

The microbial etiology of UTI in transplant patients is similar to that observed in the general population: *Escherichia coli* and the other Enterobacteriaceae, enterococci and *Pseudomonas aeruginosa*. Three factors influence the nature of the organisms infecting the urinary tract: (1) whether the patient is receiving prophylaxis; (2) whether recent instrumentation has occurred; and (3) whether complete bladder emptying or other defect in the structure or function of the urinary tract is present. The first two of these factors will contribute to the occurrence of antibiotic-resistant infection; and the last factor will lead to an increased incidence of infection and a higher incidence of symptomatic pylonephritis. An uncommon form of UTI that merits special mention because of its potential impact on the renal transplant recipient is that due to candidal infection. Particularly in individuals with poor bladder emptying, obstructing fungal balls can develop at the ureterovesical junction, leading to ascending infection, candidal pyelonephritis and, frequently, disseminated infection. It is for this reason that treatment of even asymptomatic candiduria is advocated.

Surgical wound

As in general surgical patients, *Staphylococcus aureus* and *Staphylococcus epidermidis* are the most common microbial causes of surgical wound infection in the renal transplant patient, although there is a higher incidence of Gram-negative and candidal infection than is observed in the general population. These infections are best prevented with technically impeccable surgery, prompt removal of drains and perioperative antibiotic prophylaxis (e.g. a first- or second-generation cephalosporin).

Lungs

Pulmonary infection in the renal transplant patient is best prevented by protecting the airway and by limiting both the net state of immunosuppression and the environmental exposures the patient encounters. In the first month posttransplant, bacterial pneumonias due to normal oral flora or colonizing Gram-negative bacilli are the major causes of pneumonia. These are best prevented by prompt extubation and protection of the airway. In the period 1–6 months posttransplant, CMV plays a role, both as a lung pathogen and, more importantly, as a contributor to the net state of immunosuppression, making possible *P. carinii*, *Aspergillus* and *Nocardia* infection. These opportunistic infections may occur even in the absence of an unusually intense environmental exposure due to the high level of immunosuppression present. These are best prevented with anti-CMV strategies (Table 7.0.5 in Chapter 7.0), low-dose TMP–SMX prophylaxis (or an alternative such as pentamidine or atovaquone in patients who do not tolerate TMP–SMX) and attention to air quality. In the late period, more than 6 months posttransplant, high-risk patients (those with poor graft function and an excessive exposure to immunosuppressive therapy) are most likely to develop an opportunistic infection. They merit lifelong TMP–SMX prophylaxis and consideration of fluconazole prophylaxis (against C. *neoformans* and the geographically restricted systemic mycoses).

Bloodstream infection

Bloodstream infection in the renal transplant patient can be divided into two general categories: (1) those usually due to staphylococcal species but occasionally to *Candida*, stemming from contaminated vascular access sites; and (2) those stemming from invasive infection at other bodily sites, most notably the gastrointestinal tract (*Listeria* and Gram-negative organisms) and the urinary tract (Gram-negative organisms and enterococci). Prevention of these infections requires appropriate vascular access management (avoidance of central lines, frequent changing of lines, etc.), and prompt recognition and therapy of microbial invasion.

Gastrointestinal tract

Infections of the gastrointestinal tract can be divided into two general categories: those due to inherent 'structural' abnormalities, and those due to the acquisition of potential pathogens. In the first category, diverticulitis, with a high rate of perforation, abscess formation and/or free peritonitis, is a significant problem in renal transplant patients. Prevention requires close attention to bowel habits and surgical resection (under antibiotic coverage for the Gram-negatives and bowel anaerobes that are causing disease there) (see also section 5.2). Whereas diverticulitis is common, appendicitis is uncommon in this patient population.

Exogenously acquired infections include *Clostridium difficile* and the community-acquired enteric pathogens – *Listeria*, *Campylobacter* and *Salmonella*. C. *difficile* colonization may occur within the hospital due to person-to-person spread, with active colitis then promoted by the use of antibiotics. Active surveillance for C. *difficile* on transplant wards with infection control precautions to prevent transmission, and the judicious use of antibiotics, are important in preventing this entity. In terms of the enteric pathogens, patient education regarding travel, food handling and limitation of exposure to the enteric pathogens (e.g. avoidance of travel to developing countries, and of undercooked egg and poultry products) is essential. Antibiotic prophylaxis, particularly with TMP–SMX or a fluoroquinolone provides added protection as well, if exposure is likely.

1.2 What are the predominant sites of infection? (see Table 7.1.1)
The predominant sites of infection in renal transplant patients are the urinary tract, lungs and surgical wound in the first month posttransplant, and the lungs, urinary tract and gastrointestinal tract thereafter. Although the skin (following injury of some sort) and CNS can be primary sites of infection, usually they represent sites of dissemination from primary infection in the lung (e.g. with *Nocardia, Cryptococcus* or *Aspergillus*) or gastrointestinal tract (*Listeria*) and vascular access sites (with *S. aureus* or *Candida* spp.).

1.3 What are the predominant organisms that contribute (by site)? (see Table 7.1.1)

Viruses

Herpes group viruses
The human herpes viruses are the most common pathogens affecting the renal transplant patient. This group of viruses includes CMV, EBV, varicella zoster virus (VZV), herpes simplex virus (HSV) 1 and 2, and the recently described human herpesviruses (HHV-6, HHV-7 and HHV-8). These viruses all exhibit latency and cell association, and can exert both direct and indirect effects on the patient. The term latency describes the lifelong presence of the virus following primary infection and the cessation of active viral replication (the laboratory marker for the presence of latent virus being seropositivity). Reactivation of latency appears to be accomplished by the release of such proinflammatory cytokines as TNF, or (in the case of HSV and EBV) in response to lesser stimuli. Three forms of infection are recognized:
• primary infection (which tends to be most virulent)
• reactivation of autologous virus (least apt to be symptomatic)
• superinfection (when a seropositive individual is infected with exogenous virus, often from the allograft)
These viruses are modulated by the intensity of immunosuppression.
    In addition to producing infectious disease syndromes directly (Table 7.1.2), these viruses contribute to patient morbidity by indirect effects: predisposing to opportunistic infection by adding to the net state of immunosuppression; playing a role in the pathogenesis of both allograft injury (CMV and probably HHV-6); and certain malignancies (EBV, essential for the pathogenesis of most cases of posttransplant lymphoproliferative disease, with CMV disease increasing the risk of this process by a factor of 7–10).

Hepatitis viruses
Both hepatitis B and hepatitis C viruses (HBV and HCV) are important pathogens in renal transplant patients. Preexisting infection with these viruses is amplified by immunosuppression posttransplant, and most centers advocate liver biopsy before transplantation to evaluate the suitability of individuals for transplantation (liver function tests are notoriously insensitive in assessing the degree of liver injury and cirrhosis that is present).

Table 7.1.1 Evaluation of infections in renal transplant recipients according to the site of infection and the possible etiologic agent

Site of infection	Infectious syndrome (clinical features)	Predominant pathogens	Diagnostic investigations
Urinary tract	Pyelonephritis (high relapse rate and often associated with bacteremia during first 3 months posttransplant) Cystitis	Gram-negative bacilli (*Escherichia coli*, *Klebsiella* spp., *Proteus* spp., *Enterobacter* spp., *Pseudomonas aeruginosa*) *Enterococcus* spp. *Candida* spp.	Culture of urine Ultrasonography, CT (if suspicion of abscess)
Bloodstream	Bacteremia (fever with or without local signs of infection)	Coagulase-negative staphylococci *Staphylococcus aureus* *Enterococcus* spp. (nosocomial outbreaks in some institutions) Gram-negative bacilli (*Escherichia coli*, *Klebsiella pneumoniae*, *Enterobacter* spp., *Pseudomonas aeruginosa*) *Candida* spp.	Blood cultures: two sets drawn from separate sites and one set drawn from indwelling intravenous catheter
Intravascular catheter-related infections	Pain, erythema, tenderness, discharge from catheter entry site	Coagulase-negative staphylococci *Staphylococcus aureus* *Corynebacterium jeikeium* *Enterococcus* spp. (nosocomial outbreaks in some institutions) *Bacillus* spp. Gram-negative bacilli (especially *Pseudomonas* spp.) *Candida* spp.	Swab of entry site Culture of catheter Blood cultures
Lower respiratory tract (bronchi, terminal airways, alveoli)	Bronchopneumonia Pneumonia (cough, dyspnea, chest pain, sputum, hemoptysia, pleural effusion)	Conventional infections: *Streptococcus pneumoniae* Gram-negative bacilli (*Escherichia coli*, *Klebsiella pneumoniae*, *Pseudomonas aeruginosa*, *Acinetobacter* spp.) *Staphylococcus aureus*	Chest radiography, CT Fiberoptic bronchoscopy with bronchoalveolar lavage Transbronchial biopsy Thoracocentesis

Site of infection	Infectious syndrome (clinical features)	Predominant pathogens	Diagnostic investigations
		Legionella spp. (sporadic outbreaks)	Thoracoscopy with biopsy
		Mycoplasma pneumoniae	Open lung biopsy
		Chlamydia pneumoniae	
		Virus (influenza, parainfluenza, respiratory syncytial virus)	
		Opportunistic infections:	
		Aspergillus spp., Mucor spp., Rhizopus spp.	
		Nocardia asteroides	
		Pneumocystis carinii	
		Mycobacterium tuberculosis	
		Viruses (cytomegalovirus, adenovirus, varicella zoster virus)	
		Histoplasma, Coccidioides	
Central nervous system*	Acute meningitis	Listeria monocytogenes	CT, MRI
	Subacute, chronic meningitis	Cryptococcus neoformans	Lumbar puncture
		Candida spp.	Aspiration or biopsy under
		Mycobacterium tuberculosis	stereotaxic CT guidance
		Coccidioides immitis	
		Histoplasma capsulatum	
	Focal brain diseases	Aspergillus spp.	
		Nocardia asteroides	
		Listeria monocytogenes	
		Toxoplasma gondii	
		Viruses (herpes simplex virus, varicella zoster virus, cytomegalovirus, Epstein–Barr virus, human herpesvirus 6, adenovirus, papillomavirus, JC virus)	
	Progressive dementia	JC virus (progressive multifocal leukoencephalopathy)	
Skin infection and soft tissue	Surgical wound infections	Staphylococcus aureus	Aspiration (needle) or swab of skin exudate
		Coagulase-negative staphylococci	
		Enterococcus spp.	

Clinical finding	Microorganisms	Diagnostic methods
Rash	Gram-negative bacilli (Enterobacteriaceae, *Pseudomonas aeruginosa*), *Candida* spp.	Aspiration (needle) or swab of skin exudate; Skin biopsy (histology and culture); Serology
Cellulitis (pain, erythema, tenderness, necrosis in case of ecthyma gangrenosum)	Primary infections: Coagulase-negative staphylococci, *Staphylococcus aureus*, Gram-negative bacilli (*Pseudomonas aeruginosa*, *Escherichia coli*, *Klebsiella pneumoniae*), *Candida* spp., *Mucor* spp., *Rhizopus* spp., *Absidia* spp., Mycobacteria, Human herpesvirus 6 and 7	
Papules, nodules (with or without myalgia and muscle tenderness)	Disseminated infections: *Candida* spp., *Fusarium* spp., Gram-negative bacilli (*Escherichia coli*, *Pseudomonas aeruginosa*, *Aeromonas hydrophilia*, *Serratia marcescens*)	
Ulcers, vesicles, hemorrhagic or crusted lesions (isolated or with dermatomal distribution)	Herpes simplex virus, Varicella zoster virus, Cytomegalovirus	
Disseminated vesicles, hemorrhagic or crusted lesions	Varicella zoster virus, Herpes simplex virus	
Skin necrosis (toes, fingers) secondary to thrombosis of blood vessels	*Aspergillus* spp., *Mucor* spp.	

Gastrointestinal tract

Esophagus

Clinical finding	Microorganisms	Diagnostic methods
Esophagitis (dysphagia, retrosternal pain)	Herpes simplex virus, *Candida* spp., *Aspergillus* spp., Cytomegalovirus	Esogastroscopy; Culture of endoscopic specimens

Site of infection	Infectious syndrome (clinical features)	Predominant pathogens	Diagnostic investigations
Small intestine, colon	Enteritis, colitis (nausea, vomiting, bloating, abdominal discomfort, cramp, pain, constipation, diarrhea)	*Salmonella* spp., *Campylobacter* spp., *Listeria monocytogenes* (all three are associated with a high rate of bacteremia) *Clostridium difficile* (antibiotic-associated diarrhea) Cytomegalovirus Epstein–Barr virus *Strongyloides stercoralis*	Plain abdominal films Ultrasonography CT or MRI Colonoscopy Culture of endoscopic specimens Stool cultures Toxin detection

*Transplant patients have the same susceptibility to conventional pathogens of the central nervous system (meningitis: *Streptococcus pneumoniae*, *Neisseria meningitidis*, *Haemophilus influenzae*, Gram-negative bacilli; brain abscess: streptococci, *Bacteroides* spp., *Staphylococcus aureus*, Enterobacteriaceae) as the general population. Listed above are unique pathogens.

Table 7.1.2 Infectious disease syndromes associated with herpes group virus infection in the renal transplant recipient*

Virus	Clinical syndrome
Cytomegalovirus	Fever, mononucleosis, focal gastrointestinal disease, pneumonia (hepatitis, encephalitis)
Epstein–Barr virus	Fever, mononucleosis, hepatitis, posttransplant lymphoproliferative disease (encephalitis)
Varicella zoster virus	Primary infection: disseminated visceral disease Reactivation infection: dermatomal zoster
Herpes simplex virus–1	Orolabial disease (esophagitis, bronchopneumonia, disseminated disease, meningoencephalitis)
Herpes simplex virus–2	Anogenital disease (aseptic meningitis, disseminated disease)
Human herpesvirus–6	?CMV-like effects (febrile seizures, encephalitis, pneumonia, exanthema subitum, bone marrow suppression)
Human herpesvirus–7	?
Human herpesvirus–8	Kaposi sarcoma

* Uncommon clinical syndromes are shown in parentheses.

Acquisition of HBV or HCV infection at the time of transplantation has traditionally been a significant problem, as the efficiency of transmission by transplanting an organ from a donor with actively replicating virus is quite high.

HBV is well prevented by checking for the presence of hepatitis B surface antigen (HBsAg) in the donor. Recent studies have shown that the HbsAg-negative, hepatitis B core antibody (HBcAb)-positive individual can be a safe kidney donor (although the livers from such individuals harbor virus that can be transmitted in a significant number of cases). Progression of HBV infection posttransplant is accelerated when compared with the general population, with as many as 50% of transplant patients with HBV infection having endstage liver disease or hepatocellular carcinoma 10 years after transplantation. Although interferon therapy is not particularly effective in these immunosuppressed individuals (and can precipitate rejection), the introduction of lamivudine therapy has been a major advance. Unfortunately, over time, escape mutants resistant to lamivudine tend to emerge, and other new therapies are needed.

Approximately 5% of potential kidney donors are anti-HCV positive, with half of these harboring transmissible virus. In general, the acquisition of HCV infection has, over the first 5 years posttransplant, not been associated with excessive morbidity or mortality, although individual exceptions can occur. At 10 years posttransplant, about 15% of individuals with HCV infection will have endstage liver disease or hepatocellular carcinoma. The transplantation of kidneys from anti-HCV donors should be performed with informed consent and should probably be restricted to older patients, highly sensitized patients, and those who have run out of dialysis access sites. Therapy of HCV infection is in its infancy, with the combination of ribavirin and interferon being the best available at present.

Community-acquired respiratory virus

Community-acquired respiratory viruses remain an important problem in this population, with respiratory syncytial virus (RSV), influenza, parainfluenza and adenoviruses being important pathogens. The rate of pneumonia, due both to the virus itself and to bacterial and fungal superinfection, is considerably higher than that in the general population. Unfortunately, the best approach is avoidance, as both therapy (e.g. ribavirin for RSV) and prevention by influenza vaccine have decreased efficacy in this patient population.

Papovaviruses

Papovavirus replication in renal transplant patients is common. Tubulointerstitial infection of the transplant kidney due to BK virus is being increasingly recognized on renal biopsy (performed because of deteriorating renal function). Documentation of such infection should trigger a marked reduction in immunosuppression, the only known treatment for this entity; in the absence of such a step, progressive loss of allograft function will occur. Uncommonly, BK virus can cause the progressive CNS condition known as progressive multifocal leukoencepholopathy (PML), a dementing illness that has no known treatment.

Conventional bacteria

The causes of bacterial infection in the renal transplant patient are very similar to those in the general population. Skin, soft tissue and wound infections are generally caused by Gram-positive organisms, particularly *S. aureus* and group A streptococci. Bacterial infections of the urinary tract are most commonly caused by the Enterobacteriacae, enterococci and *P. aeruginosa*. *Streptococcus pneumoniae* remains the most common identifiable bacterial cause of pneumonia. Particularly in the more immunosuppressed patients, many of whom have prolonged exposures to the hospital environment, there is an increasing incidence of infection with such antibiotic-resistant organisms as methicillin-resistant *S. aureus* (MRSA), vancomycin-resistant enterococci (VRE) and broadly resistant Gram-negative bacilli. These are nosocomially acquired infections in which colonization, when followed with breaks in integrity in the skin or mucosal surfaces, leads to bacteremia, wound infection and urosepsis. Colonization usually is the result of person-to-person transmission – often on the hands of the medical personnel.

Opportunistic infection

Opportunistic infection in the renal transplant recipient is due to the interaction between two factors: the net state of immunosuppression and the environmental exposures the patient encounters. The relationship between these two factors is a semiquantitative one. Thus, the occurrence of opportunistic infection at a time when the net state of immunosuppression is relatively low (e.g. in the first few weeks posttransplant) is strong evidence of the presence of a significant environmental hazard; conversely, the occurrence of opportunistic infection in the absence of a significant epidemiologic exposure is strong evidence that the patient is overimmunosuppressed (whatever the dose of drugs currently being administered).

Fungi

The most common causes of life-threatening opportunistic fungal infection in the renal transplant recipient are *P. carinii*, *Candida* spp., *Aspergillus* spp. and *C. neoformans*. Unless effective anti-*Pneumocystis* prophylaxis is employed, most transplant centers note an incidence of *Pneumocystis* pneumonia of 10–15%. Mucocutaneous infection due to *Candida* spp. is relatively common, with invasive candidal infection then resulting if there is a break in the integrity of the mucocutaneous surfaces (as with a vascular access device). Once bloodstream infection has occurred, even if the vascular access device is removed, the risk of hematogenous seeding and the development of clinically important metastatic infection is greater than 50% in transplant patients (as opposed to 2–6% in normal hosts). Disseminated infection due to *Aspergillus* or *Cryptococcus* is common, with evidence of macroscopic metastatic disease being found in more than 50% of cases at initial diagnosis. Particularly common are metastases to the skin, brain and lungs.

In addition, progressive pulmonary and/or disseminated infection due to the geographically restricted systemic mycoses (blastomycosis, coccidioidomycosis and histoplasmosis) can occur in this patient population. Three epidemiologic patterns are observed:

1 progressive primary infection with bloodstream dissemination
2 reactivation infection with secondary dissemination
3 superinfection, which occurs when the immunity of a previously infected individual is attenuated by the immunosuppressive therapy and reinfection then develops.

Again, dissemination is common. Presenting complaints in these patients include unexplained fever and/or cough, or signs and symptoms due to sites of metastatic infection (e.g. skin findings with blastomycosis, CNS findings with coccidioidomycosis, and mucocutaneous findings with histoplasmosis).

Bacteria

Nocardia spp. (particularly, but not exclusively, *N. asteroides*) and *L. monocytogenes* are the major causes of opportunistic bacterial infection in the renal transplant patient. Interestingly, both are effectively prevented by low-dose TMP–SMX prophylaxis. Nocardial infection shares several clinical characteristics in common with the opportunistic fungal infections and tuberculosis: a pulmonary portal of entry, where the radiographic picture is usually that of a focal consolidation or a nodule; a high rate of systemic dissemination, particularly to the skin and CNS; and a requirement for extended courses of therapy (a minimum of 4–6 months in the cases of *Nocardia*).

Listeria, in contrast, has a gastrointestinal portal of entry, with a variety of foodstuffs, but particularly dairy products, being the source of the infection. The clinical effects of *Listeria* infection in the transplant patient include a febrile gastroenteritis syndrome, bacteremia with or without endocarditis, and CNS infection. The CNS infection can take a variety of forms: a purulent meningitis, focal infection of the brainstem which can produce a clinical picture akin to bulbar polio, and focal cerebritis.

Parasites

The most important parasitic infection in renal transplant patients is that due to *Strongyloides stercoralis*. This organism, because of its unique autoinoculation cycle, can remain asymptomatically in the gastrointestinal tract of a normal host for decades after initial acquisition. After immunosuppression is begun, two clinical syndromes can result: a hyperinfestation syndrome, which amounts to an exaggeration of the usual effects of this infection, with resulting hemorrhagic pneumonia and/or enterocolitis; and disseminated infection, in which *Strongyloides* organisms leave the confines of the gut and invade other tissues, including the CNS. Often, Gram-negative bacteria from the gut accompany the parasites, resulting in a clinical presentation of Gram-negative sepsis and/or meningitis that is unresponsive to conventional antibacterial therapy. Successful treatment requires therapy with thiobendazole or ivermectin as well as antibiotics. Even with this, the mortality rate from these syndromes posttransplant is greater than 50%. As a result, emphasis is placed on pretransplant screening (ideally, with serology or, alternatively, with duodenal intubation) and preemptive therapy with thiobendazole or ivermectin before the initiation of immunosuppression. Routine stool examination for ova and parasites has a sensitivity of less than 20% for this organism and is not recommended to rule out infection.

T. gondii is an uncommon infection in renal allograft recipients. *T. gondii* is rarely transmitted via the allograft, and clinical reactivation disease is rare, particularly in the face of TMP–SMX prophylaxis.

1.4 How do the organisms vary according to various risk factors?

Technical and anatomic problems
Any technical error that leads to undrained fluid collections (whether these be hematomas, urine collections due to a leak, or a lymphocele) or the creation of devitalized tissue can lead to potentially life-threatening infection. In addition, appropriate care and early removal of vascular access devices, drainage catheters and the endotracheal tube (with adequate protection of the airway postextubation) will decrease the risk of infection.

Nature of immunosuppression
The components, the dose, the duration and the temporal sequence in which immunosuppressive agents are deployed are the driving force behind the occurrence of infection posttransplant. In terms of infection risk, most of the emphasis of the past three decades has been the development of steroid-sparing regimens. In addition, the specific effects of the different components must be taken into consideration. For example, whereas cyclosporin and tacrolimus have no ability to reactivate CMV from latency, antilymphocyte antibodies are quite potent because of the release of proinflammatory cytokines in response to their administration; in contrast, cyclosporin and tacrolimus are quite potent at amplifying the extent and consequences of CMV and other herpesvirus infection once active viral replication is present, whereas the antilymphocyte antibodies are far less potent in this regard. Thus, the entire regimen must be considered.

Antimicrobial preventive strategies
There are two aspects of antimicrobial preventive strategies that are particularly important in the renal transplant patient. First, the intensity of the antimicrobial strategy prescribed must be closely linked to the intensity of the immunosuppressive program that is required. The so-called 'therapeutic prescription' has two components: an immunosuppressive program to prevent and treat rejection, and an antimicrobial one to make it safe. Secondly, in patients with technical or anatomic problems, antimicrobial therapy will delay infection, not prevent it, with the price paid if the anatomic problem is not corrected being antimicrobial resistant infection. Thus, the optimal patient management strategy is to link antimicrobial regimens to correction of the anatomic problem that was critical to the development of the problem in the first place.

Timetable of infection
The three risk factors listed above are integrated into a 'timetable' that defines when different infections occur posttransplant. As delineated in detail in Chapter 7.0 (and as summarized in Table 7.0.4), this timetable can be utilized in three ways:
1 in the differential diagnosis of the transplant patient with an infectious disease syndrome
2 as an infection control tool, as exceptions to the timetable usually connote excessive environmental exposure, particularly within the hospital
3 as a guide for devising cost-effective infection prevention strategies.

1.5 How does this differ from other conditions, from center to center, and from country to country?

Differences among categories of immunocompromised patients

Renal transplant patients differ from other categories of immunocompromised patients in terms of infection risk because of the nature of the underlying conditions being treated and the immunosuppressing drugs being administered. With current immunosuppressive regimens, prolonged neutropenia and damage to mucocutaneous barriers are uncommon in renal transplant recipients. Hence, bacteremia and candidemia are far less common than in other compromised hosts. Instead, in kidney transplant patients the major defects in host defense are in cell-mediated immunity and due to technical or anatomic complications of the transplant operation and postoperative care. As a result, herpesvirus, hepatitis virus and respiratory virus infection, fungal infection and wound-related infections are the particular problems that distinguish transplant patients from other immunocompromised patients.

When comparing the different organ transplant patients, the overall pattern of infection is similar, with the major differences having to do with the frequency of technical complications of the transplant operation. The incidence of this class of infection is highest in liver, lung and heart–lung recipients, and lowest in renal allograft recipients because of the differences in the technical demands of the operation itself and the invasive devices required for the perioperative care of the liver and lung recipients (compared with the minimal need in kidney recipients, and an intermediate need in the heart recipient).

Differences among renal transplant centers

Three major factors help explain differences in the occurrence of particular infections among renal transplant patients transplanted at different transplant centers. Firstly, the nature of the population being served, and the incidence of active and/or latent infection present in both the donor and recipient. For example, the incidence of dormant tuberculosis or latent CMV infection capable of being reactivated posttransplant is very different in different patient populations, with pediatric patients drawn from middle-class environments having the lowest risk, and older adults from lower socioeconomic groups having the highest risk.

Secondly, environmental exposures to pathogens both within the hospital and the general community can be widely different. Thus, the occurrence of invasive aspergillosis in a hospital undergoing extensive construction or legionellosis in one in which the potable water supply is contaminated is far more common than in renal transplant patients cared for at centers free from these problems. Similarly, the endemic mycoses occur only among transplant recipients with recent or remote exposure to the geographic areas where such infections are found.

Thirdly, therapeutic protocols, both immunosuppressive and antimicrobial, at different transplant centers may vary. Thus, some centers utilize far more antilymphocyte antibody therapy, resulting in a greater risk of herpesvirus infection whereas the use of TMP-SMX and/or antiviral prophylaxis will greatly decrease the incidence of a wide variety of infections.

1.6 What is the appropriate approach to the initial evaluation and diagnosis of infection in renal transplant patients?

to

1.9 What new developments are going to impact on emerging organisms, recognition, evaluation and diagnosis of infection in renal transplant patients?

See sections 1.6 to 1.9 in Chapter 7.0, pp. 256–257.

2 REGARDING THE RISK FACTORS IN RENAL TRANSPLANT RECIPIENTS

2.1 What are the main alterations in host defense mechanisms and what are the appropriate investigations to document them?

The dose, duration and temporal sequence in which immunosuppression is deployed are responsible directly or indirectly for the alterations in host defense that are produced. The cornerstone of the immunosuppressive program for the past 30 years has been the development of steroid-sparing regimens that will still prevent rejection. Of all the immunosuppressive agents, steroids have the broadest suppressant effect on host defenses. It is also important to recognize that not only do the different agents directly inhibit a given defense, but also, by modulating the extent of such infections as CMV, EBV, HBV and HCV, the immunosuppressive program can make an even greater contribution to the net state of immunosuppression.

Microbe-specific cell-mediated immunity

The antirejection therapy employed has, as its major impact on host defenses, a suppressing effect on the normal function of both helper and cytotoxic T–lymphocytes. The result is a major defect in cell-mediated immunity (and some depression in the humoral response, particularly to vaccines, as well), thereby increasing the clinical impact of herpes group viruses, the hepatitis viruses, fungi, such bacterial species as *Mycobacteria*, *Nocardia* and *Listeria*, and other intracellular pathogens.

Nonspecific immunity

The two most important aspects of nonspecific immunity affected by the transplant experience are the primary mucocutaneous barriers to infection and an adequate number of functioning granulocytes. The mucocutaneous barriers can be adversely affected in the transplant patient in several ways: the surgical wound and vascular access clearly provide potential portals of entry for microbial invasion; chronic steroid administration will cause thinning of the skin, decreased wound healing and decreased tensile strength of the skin and other tissues; herpetic and candidal mucocutaneous infection can likewise cause breakdown and secondary invasion of these structures. A general tenet of transplant infectious disease is that these mucocutaneous structures should be protected from injury, whether such injury is due to surgery, vascular access devices, maceration under occlusive dressings, water immersion injury or other forms of trauma. Granulocytopenia in transplant patients can be a side effect of mycophenolate- or azathioprine-induced bone marrow toxicity, drug reactions, or a consequence of such viral infections as those caused by CMV or EBV. The incidence and severity of granulocytopenia in renal transplant patients are far less than in other immunocompromised patients who are treated with intensive cytoreductive therapy, and usually responsive to dosage or drug adjustment with or without granulocyte colony-stimulating factor (G-CSF) therapy.

2.2 What are the alterations due to iatrogenic factors?

In addition to the immunosuppressive therapy, the technical skill with which the patient is managed and the epidemiologic factors that have been discussed above, there are other iatrogenic factors that affect the occurrence of infection and which bear emphasis.

Nutrition

Nutritional health is often overlooked in surgical patients, even though it is well documented that adequate nutrition is essential for wound healing and maintenance of effective immunologic function. In particular, protein-calorie malnutrition plays an important role in the pathogenesis of infection in transplant patients, as delineated by the following statistic: there is a 10-fold increase in the incidence of life-threatening infection in transplant patients with serum albumin levels below 2.5 g/l. There are a number of factors that can lead to hypoalbuminemia in renal transplant patients: inadequate dietary intake; loss of albumin with inadequate replacement during peritoneal dialysis; nephrotic syndrome due to recurrent or de novo glomerular disease in the allograft; significant liver disease; and a variety of hypercatabolic states. Nutritional repletion should begin before transplantation, and continue as needed posttransplant.

Drug interactions

Any patient on a highly complex medical regimen is at risk for potential drug interactions that could influence the occurrence of infection. This is particularly true in the transplant patient, where drug interactions with cyclosporin and tacrolimus, the two mainstays of modern immunosuppression, can be quite important. There are three types of drug interaction that antimicrobial agents (and other drugs) can have with cyclosporin and tacrolimus, the first two of which are involved with the key step in the metabolism of these drugs via hepatic cytochrome P-450-linked enzymes: upregulation and downregulation in metabolism, and synergistic nephrotoxicity.

Upregulation in metabolism

Certain drugs (most notably rifampicin, isoniazid and nafcillin among antimicrobial agents) increase the metabolism of cyclosporin and tacrolimus, decreasing blood levels and promoting rejection.

Downregulation in metabolism

Certain drugs, most notably the macrolides (erythromycin, clarithromycin and azithromycin) and the azoles (ketoconazole, itraconazole and fluconazole) among antimicrobial agents, decrease the metabolism of cyclosporin and tacrolimus, increasing blood levels and promoting both overimmunosuppression and nephrotoxicity.

Synergistic nephrotoxicity

The combination of therapeutic drug levels of cyclosporin or tacrolimus with therapeutic levels of such antimicrobial agents as gentamicin, amphotericin, vancomycin and high-dose fluoroquinolones or TMP–SMX will promote synergistic nephrotoxicity. The consequences of these potential interactions is to emphasize infection prevention and to modify antibiotic prescribing practices to avoid aminoglycosides, vancomycin, amphotericin and high-dose fluoroquinolones and TMP–SMX. In addition, close attention to blood levels of cyclosporin and tacrolimus is required when either initiating or ending a course of therapy with one of the antimicrobial agents that modifies their metabolism.

One further drug interaction that merits mention is that between allopurinol and azathioprine, which results in synergistic bone marrow toxicity, neutropenia and increased infection risk. Allopurinol blocks the metabolism of azathioprine, thus increasing its potency at a given dosage level. The drugs can be utilized together, provided the azathioprine dose is decreased by 50–75%.

2.5 What are the specific or nonspecific measures aimed at minimizing each of these factors?
See section 2.5 in Chapter 7.0, pp. 259–261.

2.8 What new developments are going to impact on minimizing or suppressing the specific risk factors?
See section 2.5 and 2.8 in Chapter 7.0, pp. 259–262.

3 REGARDING THE SURVEILLANCE OF RENAL TRANSPLANT RECIPIENTS

3.1 What is the important pretransplant information to be gathered?
See section 3.1 in Chapter 7.0, pp. 262–264.

3.2 What are the surveillance measures to be taken in renal transplant recipients
Constant surveillance of both the individual patient and the entire transplant population is necessary for detection of signs and symptoms indicative of a possible serious infection, particularly one that might indicate a particular hazard in the environment. Although one should be constantly aware of a possible cluster of cases due to such a hazard, it is to be hoped that detection of a hazard, especially in the hospital environment, could be accomplished with a single case. The best clue to the presence of an environmental hazard is the occurrence of an infection, particularly an opportunistic infection, at a point in time when the net state of immunosuppression is not normally great enough to allow such an infection to occur without an unusually intense exposure. Two practical ways of acting on this principle are the occurrence of opportunistic infection in the first month posttransplant or at any time when the timetable suggests that such an infection is a rare event.

3.3 What are the other specific measures to be taken in renal transplant recipients
As emphasized previously, active infection should be eradicated before transplantation, and preexisting hepatitis should be adequately assessed, including in most cases a biopsy. In addition, a variety of serologies (e.g. CMV, EBV, VZV and, if the epidemiologic history is appropriate, *Strongyloides*) that will influence antimicrobial use must be carried out. An area of continuing controversy is the appropriate approach to tuberculin testing.

It is generally agreed that patients awaiting transplantation should undergo tuberculin testing, noting that false-negative results can occur due to uremia-induced anergy. The question of how to approach a positive tuberculin test is a more difficult one, as antituberculous drugs are difficult to manage in the face of cyclosporin- and tacrolimus-based immunosuppression, as well as the approximately 10% incidence of chronic hepatitis in transplant patients. In addition, it is now clear that the incidence of clinical tuberculosis is quite low in transplant patients without other risk factors for tuberculosis. Risk factors include previous history of active tuberculosis, significant abnormalities on chest radiography, protein-calorie malnutrition, other immunosuppressing illnesses and non-Caucasian racial background. The authors' approach is to follow closely, with 6-monthly chest radiography for 2 years, followed by yearly radiography thereafter, individuals with positive tuberculin tests and no other risk factors. Individuals with risk factors receive 1 year of prophylaxis, preferably with isoniazid, but with the combination of ofloxacin and ethambutol if isoniazid is not tolerated.

4 REGARDING THE PREVENTION OF INFECTION IN RENAL TRANSPLANT RECIPIENTS

4.1 What approaches, if any, to the prevention of infection should be considered in renal transplant patients?

Prevention of infection, rather than treatment of clinical infection, should be the primary goal of the clinician in terms of the approach to the transplant patient. In addition to the careful evaluation of the prospective organ donor and of the prospective recipient (see section 3.1 in Chapter 7.0), there are several components to the preventive process (see also section 2.5 in Chapter 7.0).

Antimicrobial use

The basis for antimicrobial preventive strategies in the transplant patient is an evaluation of relative risk. Once the risk is delineated, then focused antimicrobial strategies can be deployed. Two preventive modes of prescribing antimicrobial agents are available: (1) a prophylactic mode and a (2) preemptive mode.

The prophylactic use of antibiotics is employed when a particular infection is sufficiently common and important to justify the administration of a nontoxic regimen to an entire population before an event. Preemptive therapy is defined as administering antimicrobial agents to a subpopulation defined as being at high risk for a clinically important disease on the basis of clinical and epidemiologic characteristics or a laboratory marker.

(1) Prophylactic strategies of value in transplantation include the following:

- Low-dose TMP–SMX (which has largely eliminated the risk of *Pneumocystis*, *Listeria*, *Nocardia* and, probably, *Toxoplasma* infection from transplant patients)
- Perioperative antibacterial prophylaxis
- Antiviral prophylaxis against CMV in patients at risk for primary infection (donor CMV seropositive, and recipient seronegative) since the risk of disease is so high in this group of patients (50–75%).

(2) In contrast, preemptive strategies are reserved for the following subgroups of patients:

- CMV-seropositive patients who are shown to be at high risk because of evidence of asymptomatic viremia (by PCR or antigenemia assays), or because of antirejection therapy with antilymphocyte antibodies, receive preemptive ganciclovir therapy.
- Colonization of the respiratory tract with *Aspergillus* spp. is treated preemptively with antifungal therapy, because of a 50–75% risk of invasive disease. Similarly, even asymptomatic fungal infection of the lung, urinary tract and biliary tree are treated preemptively, because of the risk of systemic spread.

Technical expertise

The presence of anatomic or technical factors related to the surgical procedure and postoperative management (including the endotracheal tube, vascular access, and drainage catheters and devices) will have a major impact on the incidence and gravity of infection. Any intervention that leads to devitalized tissue, compromise in the integrity of mucocutaneous surfaces, undrained fluid collections, and the need for indwelling foreign bodies to correct these abnormalities will eventually lead to infection. The administration of antibiotics in this situation will delay the occurrence of infection, providing a 'window of opportunity' for correcting the abnormality. If, however, this opportunity is not taken, antibiotic-resistant infection will develop. Hence, there are two rules of antimicrobial prophylaxis in transplant patients:

1 Technical skill in accomplishing the transplant operation and perioperative care is the key factor in preventing early posttransplant infection; antibiotic prophylaxis should be regarded as adjunctive.
2 Maximal efficacy in patient care is accomplished when antibiotic therapy is linked with the technical or surgical management of the patient.

Environmental protection

A primary consideration for any transplant program is to ensure that the air the patient breathes, the potable water and food that the patient ingests, and the people encountered are free from contamination with infectious agents. In the hospital, air contaminated with *Aspergillus* spores or Gram-negative bacilli, potable water laden with *Legionella pneumophila*, and individuals harboring such organisms as MRSA, VRE, fluconazole-resistant *Candida* spp. and C. *difficile* pose a great hazard for these immuno-compromised patients. Constant surveillance is necessary to prevent catastrophic nosocomial infections of these types. In addition, community exposures to respiratory viruses, foodborne pathogens (e.g. *Salmonella* and *Campylobacter* spp.), tuberculosis and fungal species should be minimized.

5 REGARDING THE TREATMENT OF RENAL TRANSPLANT RECIPIENTS

5.1 What is the role of empirical therapy?

Unlike the situation in the leukemic patient, there is generally little indication for the empirical initiation of antimicrobial agents in the renal transplant patient with unexplained fever. Two exceptions to this statement should be kept in mind:

• If a frank rigor has occurred in association with the fever, empirical therapy is indicated, aimed at the most likely organisms.
• If significant neutropenia is present, an approach analogous to that employed in the management of neutropenic cancer or bone marrow transplant patients is advocated.

5.2 What is the appropriate approach to renal transplant patients with evidence of:

Upper respiratory tract infection?

Bacterial and most viral infections of the upper respiratory tract in the renal transplant patient are similar in both etiology and management to those observed in the general population. Group A streptococcal pharyngitis merits penicillin or other appropriate therapy, and rhinovirus, influenza and parainfluenza virus infection merits careful follow-up for bacterial superinfection, but little in the way of specific management. RSV infection is a significant problem in transplant patients, adults as well as children, and consideration of aerosolized ribavirin therapy should be given in patients with documented RSV infection, even before RSV pneumonia is evident. Orolabial herpetic infection merits therapy with acyclovir (and is effectively treated with ganciclovir or famciclovir if these are being utilized to treat or prevent other herpes group viral infections). In the face of active HSV infection, intubation of both the respiratory and upper gastrointestinal tract should be avoided in order to prevent herpetic lower respiratory tract and esophageal infection. Fungal infection of the upper respiratory tract is usually well treated with oral nystatin or clotrimazole, with fluconazole as a backup for more resistant infection. *Aspergillus* infection of the sinuses merits systemic therapy with an amphotericin preparation plus surgical drainage.

Table 7.1.3 Differential diagnosis of pneumonia in the renal transplant patient according to radiologic abnormality and the rate of progression*

Chest radiography	Etiology according to the rate of progression	
	Acute	**Subacute or chronic**
Consolidation	Bacterial	Fungal
	Thromboembolic	Nocardial
	Hemorrhage	Tuberculous
	(Pulmonary edema)	(Viral, *Pneumocystis*)
Peribronchovascular	Pulmonary edema	Viral
	Leukoagglutinin reaction	*Mycoplasma*
	(Bacterial)	*Pneumocystis*
Nodular infiltrate	(Bacterial, pulmonary edema)	Fungal
		Nocardial
		Tuberculous
		(*Pneumocystis*)

* An acute illness is one that develops and requires medical attention in less than 24 h; a subacute or chronic process develops over several days to weeks. Note that unusual causes of a process are shown in parentheses.

Lower respiratory tract infection?

Much like the situation in other immunocompromised patients, unless an etiologic diagnosis is obvious from expectorated sputum examination or on clinical grounds, an invasive diagnostic procedure (bronchoscopy with bronchoalveolar lavage, thorascopic biopsy, needle aspiration or open lung biopsy) rather than empirical therapy is indicated in the management of these patients, provided significant coagulopathy is not present. The decision as to which diagnostic procedure should be undertaken is in large part determined by the nature of the chest CT findings: diffuse lung disease is initially approached by bronchoscopy; focal, pleural based cavitary disease by needle aspiration; focal disease without a cavity by transthoracoscopic biopsy; and rapidly progressive disease by open lung biopsy. Therapy is then guided by the results of such an assessment. If specific diagnosis is not possible, then empirical therapy is based upon the epidemiologic history, the expected timetable of infection, and an assessment of the morphology of the chest radiographic findings combined with the mode of presentation of the process (Table 7.1.3).

Gastrointestinal infection?

Diverticulitis is both a common and extremely serious problem in the renal transplant patient, with a high rate of perforation, peritonitis and abscess formation. Unlike the situation in the general population in which antibiotic therapy without surgery will often suffice, the general rule in transplant patients is surgical resection (usually with colostomy construction, with later reconstruction of the continuity of the bowel once the inflammation has subsided) with antimicrobial coverage aimed at Enterobacteriaceae and bowel anaerobes. A variety of antibiotic programs can be utilized for this purpose (e.g. a fluoroquinolone plus metronidazole, ampicillin–sulbactam, piperacillin–tazobactam). Gentamicin is to be avoided in the management of such patients because of toxicity issues.

Febrile gastroenteritis (i.e. fever and diarrhea) is also a common problem in this patient population, with a higher rate of bacteremia than in the general population with similar infection. After culturing such a patient, it is the authors' policy to initiate therapy with ampicillin–sulbactam because of the consequences of both *Salmonella* and *Listeria* bacteremia in this patient population, with discontinuation of antibiotic coverage if the cultures of stool and blood remain negative after 48 h and the patient is clinically improved.

Urinary tract infection?
Infection of the urinary tract in the renal transplant patient is quite common if the patient is not receiving TMP–SMX or fluoroquinolone prophylaxis; it is uncommon in the setting of such prophylaxis. Indeed, symptomatic UTI in a compliant renal allograft recipient receiving prophylaxis suggests a functional or structural abnormality of the urinary tract, and a search for such with ultrasonography and urologic assessment must be considered in this circumstance. Fluoroquinolones or TMP–SMX are the cornerstones of therapy for UTI in these patients, with other drugs being deployed on the basis of antibiotic susceptibility testing. Two weeks of therapy is standard, with a consideration of long-term prophylaxis afterwards. Candidiuria is treated aggressively, even when asymptomatic. If an indwelling bladder catheter is present, topical therapy with bladder irrigation with nystatin or amphotericin is reasonable until the catheter is removed. Then, systemic therapy with fluconazole is the treatment of choice, with initiation of therapy in conjunction with catheter removal. For fluconazole-resistant infection, low dose (5–10 mg) amphotericin plus 5–fluorocytosine therapy is quite effective.

Cardiovascular infection?
The risk of cardiovascular infection in renal transplant patients is similar to that in the general population; that is, seeding of heart valves or blood vessels is not influenced significantly by immunosuppression. Thus, the same factors that lead to these infections in the general population (e.g. underlying structural cardiovascular disease, high-level Gram-positive bacteremia, particularly with *S. aureus*) are operative as well. Both diagnosis and treatment algorithms are likewise the same as in the nonimmunosuppressed patient with endocarditis.

Musculoskeletal infection?
Renal transplant patients are at similar risk to nonimmunosuppressed patients to such processes as bacterial osteomyelitis, necrotizing fasciitis and myonecrosis. Septic arthritis due to superinfection of joints damaged by gout and other metabolic disorders is more common in these patients, with similar management guidelines: specific microbial diagnosis through aspiration of the involved joint with antibiotic therapy guided by these results; therapy of the gout and other metabolic derangements; and adequate drainage, usually repetitively. The particular concern, however, in the transplant patient is opportunistic infection due to such organisms as *N. asteroides, C. neoformans* and other fungal species, and *Mycobacterium* spp. Thus, a bone scan is indicated in the evaluation of a patient with one of these processes to rule out metastatic infection to the musculoskeletal system. In patients with musculoskeletal infection as the primary reason for consultation, biopsy is essential to guide therapy since the diagnostic possibilities are so broad. Blood cultures, biopsies of other sites, and measurement of the serum cryptococcal antigen level may also be of use. For virtually all these processes, therapy for 6 months or longer is usually required.

Skin infection?
Cellulitis in most renal transplant patients is of Gram-positive origin and merits treatment with semisynthetic penicillins or first-generation cephalosporins, as in the general population. Focal skin lesions, particularly those with dermal or subcutaneous induration, must be biopsied to rule out disseminated opportunistic infection. Trivial-appearing skin lesions can be the first manifestation of disseminated cryptococcal, nocardial or other opportunistic infection. It is rare that such lesions do not connote systemic seeding,

and hence 4–6 months of systemic therapy is indicated, rather than just local therapy aimed at the skin.

Central nervous system infection?

Approximately 5% of renal transplant patients will develop CNS infection, with 25–50% of these exhibiting only a febrile headache as evidence for such infection. The majority of the CNS infections represent metastatic infection from the lungs (cryptococcal, *Aspergillus* and nocardial infection) or gastrointestinal tract (*Listeria*). Indications for a neurologic evaluation (CT or MRI of the head, and lumbar puncture) include a febrile headache, decreased level of consciousness, and new onset of seizures. Similarly, a neurologic evaluation should be part of a metastatic workup when one of the above mentioned infections is diagnosed at another site. Viral infections of the CNS (e.g. CMV, HHV-6, EBV and HSV) are uncommon among renal transplant patients, as are conventional forms of bacterial meningitis observed in the community (e.g. pneumococcal and meningococcal meningitis). Therapy is predicated on the specific diagnosis that is made and, not surprisingly, given the pathogens, is usually prolonged.

Intraabdominal infections?

In general, intraabdominal infections in renal transplant patients occur at a similar rate as other postsurgical patients. However, the introduction of immunosuppressive therapy can have several adverse effects on the diagnosis and prognosis of individuals who develop intraabdominal infections, especially secondary to intestinal perforation. The impaired inflammatory response in transplant recipients may result in difficulty and delay in making the correct diagnosis of intraabdominal infection. Classic signs and symptoms of acute peritoneal inflammation including fever, leukocytosis, pain, abdominal tenderness, rebound or guarding are often mild or absent in these patients, delaying the diagnosis of intraabdominal infection. Secondly, the immunosuppressed patient may experience a more rapid dissemination of infection introduced at the time of intestinal perforation and peritoneal soilage because of the impaired ability to wall off an infected area and form an abscess. The often occult nature of intraabdominal infection in these individuals, combined with the potential for rapid systemic spread of infection, should result in a heightened clinical suspicion, prompt initiation of antimicrobial therapy and an attempt to make a rapid diagnosis resulting in surgical repair.

5.3 What is the appropriate approach to the renal transplant patient with evidence of bacteremia, with or without site of infection?

Gram-positive bacteremia

The key to success in treating Gram-positive bacteremia appropriately is rapid identification of the source of infection. Whenever possible, lines or catheters that can serve as both portal of entry and persistent source of bacteremia should be removed. Appropriate antimicrobial therapy should be initiated, based on the most likely source. Any available data from previous cultures should be reviewed and used to help guide therapy while awaiting identification and antibiotic sensitivities of the infecting organisms. In individuals with previous history of colonization or infection with antibiotic-resistant organisms such as methicillin-resistant staphylococci, the presumption should be made that the infecting pathogen has similar antibiotic sensitivities and initial therapy should be with vancomycin. In patients with *S. pneumoniae* pneumonia and bacteremia, empirical therapy must be based on the incidence of penicillin resistance in the community.

Gram-negative bacteremia

A careful evaluation aimed at revealing the source of Gram-negative bacteremia is essential. Antibiotics with a broad Gram-negative spectrum should be initiated without delay. The most notable difference in the approach to empirical therapy in renal transplant patients with Gram-negative bacteremia compared with normal hosts is the strict avoidance of aminoglycoside therapy. The combination of an aminoglycoside, potentially nephrotoxic immunosuppressive therapy and a transplanted kidney can cause irreversible nephrotoxicity. Given the widespread availability of third-generation cephalosporins, extended-spectrum penicillins and fluoroquinolones with excellent Gram-negative activity, it is relatively easy to avoid using an aminoglycoside. In addition to aggressive broad-spectrum therapy, it is essential to search for surgically correctable sources of bacteremia.

Anaerobic bacteremia

Anaerobes are less commonly identified as causes of bacteremia. However, isolation of anaerobic bacteria warrants examination of the gastrointestinal tract and the female genital tract for a potential source. Likewise, identification of an anatomic problem in the gastrointestinal or female genital tract should raise the possibility of anaerobic infection. Metronidazole remains the antibiotic of choice for serious anaerobic infection, but many of the extended-spectrum β-lactams also have excellent anaerobic activity. The use of clindamycin is generally avoided in the transplant patient given the higher risk of C. *difficile* infection in this population.

Polymicrobial bacteremia

Appropriate broad-spectrum antimicrobial therapy targeting organisms identified should be initiated as soon as possible. The most likely source of polymicrobial bacteremia is the gastrointestinal tract, including the biliary system, and studies evaluating both the bowel and biliary system are indicated.

Bacteremia with a defined source

Any identified portal of entry should be evaluated for the possibility of surgical correction to avoid persistent or recurrent entry of organisms. If the identified source is a catheter or other foreign body, it should be removed whenever possible. Therapy should always be tailored on sensitivities of the infecting organism. In general, the most efficacious antibiotic with the narrowest spectrum of activity should be used in cases of bacteremia with a defined source when the identification of the organism and antibiotic sensitivities are known.

5.4 What is the appropriate approach to the renal transplant patient with evidence of a viral infection?

Therapy of viral infection in the transplant patient can be divided into two components: (1) decrease in immunosuppressive therapy, and (2) specific antiviral therapy. The major host defense involved with recovery from the viral infections that occur in the transplant patient is the development of MHC-restricted, virus-specific, cytotoxic T cells. Both cyclosporin and tacrolimus, the mainstays of current immunosuppressive programs, are potent inhibitors of this defense. Therefore, the first step in antiviral therapy is to decrease the dose of immunosuppression being administered, particularly cyclosporin and tacrolimus. In terms of specific antiviral therapy of active infection, there are three major opportunities currently available: therapy of herpes group virus infection, therapy of hepatitis B and therapy of hepatitis C. In terms of active herpes group viral infection, with the exception of mucocutaneous herpes simplex infection and herpes zoster (oral acyclovir for the former and oral fanciclovir for the latter), adequate therapy requires relatively high blood levels of the drug. Until recently, this meant intravenous ganciclovir (for CMV in particular) or intravenous acyclovir (for primary varicella). The advent of valine esters of these drugs (e.g. valacyclovir and valganciclovir) offers the promise of far greater bioavailability and the ability to treat orally rather than parenterally. In the case of hepatitis B, chronic lamivudine therapy is quite useful, although resistance begins to emerge after a year or so. In terms of hepatitis C, the best therapeutic program currently available is the combination of ribavirin and interferon.

5.5 What is the appropriate approach to the renal transplant patient with evidence of a fungal infection?

The key question to be asked in prescribing systemic antifungal therapy to a transplant recipient is whether the patient is a therapeutic emergency or is more subacutely ill. If a therapeutic emergency, conventional amphotericin B remains the drug of choice until the patient is stabilized, at which time a decision can be made regarding the substitution of less toxic therapy (a lipid-containing amphotericin preparation or an azole) for disease eradication. In patients who are less acutely ill, primary therapy with the less toxic drugs is usually initiated. At present, there is relatively little information available on the efficacy of the lipid-containing amphotericin preparations in transplant recipients with serious fungal infections, hence the restriction of their use to patients who have already responded to conventional amphotericin but need more therapy, or those who have suffered unacceptable amphotericin toxicity. Of the azoles, fluconazole has been of great use in the treatment of invasive candidal and cryptococcal infection, although there has been a slow increase in the incidence of infection with fluconazole-resistant *Candida* spp. (primarily in patients with uncorrected anatomic abnormalities who have received extended courses of fluconazole therapy). Itraconazole has found its primary use as 'wrap-up' therapy for *Aspergillus* or *Histoplasma* infection.

Candida infection

Initial therapy is usually with fluconazole (5 mg/kg daily for 2–4 weeks, with dosage adjustment for renal dysfunction). For fluconazole-resistant infection (e.g. that caused by *C. glabrata* and *C. krusei*), amphotericin is employed (0.5–0.75 mg/kg daily of conventional amphotericin versus 2.5–4.0 mg/kg daily of a lipid preparation). In patients with urinary tract candidal infection not responding to fluconazole, 5-fluorocytosin plus low-dose amphotericin (5–10 mg/day) is quite effective.

Aspergillus infection

Conventional amphotericin B (at a daily dose of 1.0–1.5 mg/kg) remains the initial treatment of choice for invasive aspergillosis in transplant patients. If a lipid preparation is substituted, a daily dose of 4.0–7.5 mg/kg is required. Itraconazole is not recommended as primary therapy, but it can be useful to follow a course of amphotericin treatment at a dose of 200–400 mg/day, preferably with monitoring of blood levels. Treatment should be continued until all evidence of disease is gone, a process that normally takes 2–4 months, and a dosage of conventional amphotericin of more than 2 g.

Cryptococcus infection

In most patients, amphotericin and fluconazole are of equal efficacy. Because of the difference in toxicity, fluconazole (usually at a dose of 400 mg/day, with dosage adjustments for renal dysfunction) is the preferred therapy. Therapy should be continued until cryptococcal antigen is cleared from the blood and cerebrospinal fluid.

Mucormycosis
Invasive mucormycosis is an infection that requires surgical excision on an emergent basis, followed by adjunctive high-dose amphotericin therapy (1.25–1.50 mg/kg daily).

Endemic mycoses
Clinical disease due to *Blastomyces dermatitidis*, *Coccidioides immitis* and *Histoplasma capsulatum* usually requires a two-stage approach: initial control with an amphotericin preparation, followed by long-term maintenance therapy with an oral azole (itraconazole for blastomycosis and histoplasmosis; fluconazole for coccidioidomycosis).

5.6 What is the appropriate approach to the renal transplant patient with evidence of a parasitic infection?

Pneumocystis carinii
Infection with *P. carinii* is almost a completely preventable disease with appropriate TMP–SMX prophylaxis. Nevertheless, in some individuals, disease does occur and high-dose TMP–SMX is the drug of choice for treatment of acute infection. TMP–SMX therapy is sometimes limited by adverse reaction to the drug, especially bone marrow toxicity and nephrotoxicity. Second-line therapy of severe disease in patients intolerant to TMP-SMX is intravenous pentamidine, which is also highly efficacious.

Toxoplasma gondii
T. gondii infection is usually caused by reactivation of latent infection and is most effectively treated with the combination of sulfadiazine and pyrimethamine. Toxoplasmosis is not commonly seen in renal transplant patients, perhaps because of the widespread use of TMP–SMX prophylaxis.

Strongyloides stercoralis
The most effective way of avoiding complications of *Strongyloides* is to detect the presence of parasitic infestation before transplantation when the organism causes asymptomatic infection. In individuals with the appropriate epidemiologic history, testing for antibody against *S. stercoralis* should be performed before transplantation. Individuals with evidence of infection with *Strongyloides* should be treated preemptively with thiabendazole or ivermectin. Eradication of this parasite during asymptomatic infection before transplantation is relatively easy but treatment of *Strongyloides* superinfection complicated by Gram-negative polymicrobial bacteremia in immunosuppressed individuals is often difficult and associated with a high mortality rate.

5.7 What is the role of nonantiinfective interventions (including reducing or altering immunosuppression) in the management of established infection?

Management of immunosuppression
Perhaps the most difficult aspect of managing infection in renal transplant patients is in balancing the need for immunosuppression to prevent allograft rejection with the need for immune responses to eradicate opportunistic pathogens. Although most infectious processes can be effectively managed with appropriate antimicrobial therapy, reduction

of immunosuppression is also used to allow a more effective host defense. This strategy is of particular importance in situations where rejection of transplanted kidney is acceptable in an attempt to eradicate life-threatening infection.

Granulocyte colony-stimulating factor (G-CSF)

More recently, immunomodulating therapies have played an increasing role in augmenting host immune responses during periods of heavy immunosuppression. In renal transplant patients, G-CSF is used to increase the number of circulating granulocytes as a bridge to avoid the complications of neutropenia. Although neutropenia is much more common in bone marrow transplant patients, occasionally renal transplant recipients become transiently neutropenic secondary to drug therapy or concurrent infection, and judicious use of G-CSF appears to be beneficial during these infrequent periods.

REFERENCES

Ettinger NA, Trulock EP. Pulmonary considerations in organ transplantation. *Am Rev Respir Dis* 1991; **143:** 386–405, 1991; **144:** 213–223, 433–451.

Fishman JA, Rubin RH. Infection in organ-transplant recipients. *N Engl J Med* 1998; **338:** 1741–1751.

Hadley S, Karchmer AW. Fungal infections in solid organ transplant recipients. *Infect Dis Clin North Am* 1995; **9:** 1045–1074.

Rubin RH. Infectious disease complications of renal transplantation. *Kidney Int* 1993;**44:**221–236.

Rubin RH. Infection in the organ transplant recipient. In: Rubin RH, Young LS, eds. *Clinical Approach to Infection in the Compromised Host*, 3rd edn New York: Plenum, 1994: 629–705.

Rubin RH, Tolkoff-Rubin NE. Antimicrobial strategies in the care of organ transplant recipients. *Antimicrob Agents Chemother* 1993; **37:** 619–624.

Terrault NA, Wright TL, Pereira BJG. Hepatitis C infection in the transplant recipient. *Infect Dis Clin North Am* 1995; **9:** 943–964.

Turgeon N, Fishman JA, Basgoz N et al. Effect of oral acyclovir or ganciclovir therapy after preemptive intravenous ganciclovir therapy to prevent cytomegalovirus disease in cytomegalovirus seropositive renal and liver transplant recipients receiving antilymphocyte antibody therapy. *Transplantation* 1998; **66:** 1780–1786.

Chapter 7.2 | Infections in Liver Transplant Recipients

Peter K Linden

INTRODUCTION

Liver transplantation is associated with a higher rate of posttransplant infection than most other categories of solid organ transplantation. This observation is particularly manifest in the early posttransplant period because of the lingering effects of severely debilitated patients with endstage chronic liver disease or acute liver failure, coupled with the length and intricacy of the transplant surgery which involves multiple vascular, biliary and gastrointestinal manipulations. Despite such obstacles, the 1-year retransplant-free survival rate for 1987–1996 and for 1996 was 81% and 86%, respectively, for liver transplant programs in the United States. This remarkable trend is a result of multiple factors; however, improvements in surgical techniques (venovenous bypass, decreased blood product requirements) and more refined immunosuppression (diminished corticosteroid requirements owing to the use and quantitative titration of cyclosporin and tacrolimus) have been dominant in bringing about higher survival rates. A third dominant factor has been advances in the prevention, early diagnosis and treatment of infection, which has reduced both the overall incidence of infection and infection-associated mortality rate. This review outlines the pathogenesis, clinical presentation and management of infectious complications following orthotopic liver transplantation.

I REGARDING THE CLINICAL PRESENTATION AND EVALUATION OF THE PATIENT

1.1 What are the clinically predominant modes of presentation of infection in liver transplant recipients?

Similar to other solid organ recipients, the etiology and timing of infections seen in a liver transplant recipient conform in part to a 'timetable' concept, detailed in Chapter 7.0 (Table 7.0.4, pp. 254), which partitions the posttransplant course into early (first month), intermediate (1–6 months) and late (> 6 months) periods. The infections most likely to occur in these respective periods for the liver recipient are illustrated in Table 7.2.1.

Early infections are highly dependent upon the effects of pretransplant conditions (colonization with hospital-acquired bacteria, severe malnutrition, recent bacterial peritonitis or aspiration pneumonia), high immunosuppressive burden, and the length and technical complications of the transplant surgery itself. Fever or frank sepsis with or without early localizing symptoms or signs is the most common inciting presentation. The magnitude of the temperature increase does not necessarily correlate with either the likelihood of an infectious source or the severity of infection. Conversely, the absence of

Table 7.2.1 Timetable of infection following liver transplantation

Early period: first month posttransplant

1 Intraabdominal infection due to effects of operation or allograft technical complications:
   - Peritonitis (bacterial or *Candida*)
   - Intrahepatic abscess, infarct
   - Cholangitis
   - Peritoneal collections (i.e. hematoma, abscess)
   - Perforated viscera
2 Hospital-acquired infections:
   - Bacterial pneumonia
   - Catheter infection
   - Urinary tract infection
   - Surgical wound infection
3 Infections related to immunosuppression:
   - Reactivated herpes simplex virus (orolabial, genital or, rarely, visceral disease)
   - *Candida* infection (i.e. stomatitis, esophagitis)
   - *Aspergillus* spp. (increased with nosocomial exposure)

Intermediate period: 1–6 months posttransplant

1 Viral infection:
   - Herpes virus family (CMV, EBV, HHV-6, HHV-7)
   - Viral hepatitides (recurrent hepatitis B or C)
   - Other viruses (adenovirus, polyomavirus)
2 Opportunistic pathogens:
   - *Aspergillus* spp. and other mycelia, *Mycobacterium tuberculosis*, *Pneumocystis carinii*, endemic mycoses, *Cryptococcus neoformans*, *Listeria monocytogenes*
3 Delayed complications of graft function:
   - Intrahepatic abscess (arterial insufficiency)
   - Cholangitis (arterial insufficiency, biliary obstruction or obliteration)

Late period: > 6 months posttransplant

   - Community-acquired infection (UTI, pneumonia)
   - Late allograft complications (cholangitis due to vanishing bile duct syndrome, biliary casts or hepatic arterial thrombosis)
   - Recurrent viral hepatitis B and C
   - Reactivated dormant pathogens (shingles, *Mycobacterium tuberculosis*, endemic mycoses)
   - Other opportunistic pathogens (*Nocardia* spp., *Listeria monocytogenes*, *Pneumocystis carinii*, *Cryptococcus neoformans*, *Aspergillus* spp. (highest risk in recipients with high immunosuppression, chronic rejection)

fever or hypothermia, although less common, may still be compatible with a mild or even life-threatening infection. Liver recipients with a complete or partially open abdominal cavity or those on continuous extracorporeal artificial kidney machines are characteristically hypothermic. Other common nonlocalizing symptoms and signs include an altered sensorium (delirium), unexplained tachypnea or tachycardia, respiratory alkalosis or metabolic acidosis, and oliguria. Early nonlocalizing laboratory abnormalities include leukocytosis or leukopenia with a predominance of immature forms (left shift) in bacterial and fungal infection or a predominance of lymphocytes (right shift) in viral infection.

Noninfectious etiologies that may mimic an infectious presentation include allograft rejection, preservation injury or necrosis, drug- or transfusion-related reactions, and rare episodes of graft-versus-host disease.

1.2 What are the predominant sites of infection?

Infection may also present as a symptom-complex with prominent or subtle localizing findings referable to the abdominal wound or intraabdominal cavity (peritonitis, abscess), the lung (pneumonia, metastatic abscess), skin (rash or discrete lesions), central nervous system (CNS) (encephalopathy or focal neurologic signs), or disseminated syndromes affecting two or more organ systems (candidiasis, invasive aspergillosis, cytomegalovirus (CMV)). Not uncommonly, a positive blood culture is an early finding which only upon further diagnostic workup will reveal the primary source (e.g. hepatobiliary tree or multilumen venous catheter). Finally, an increase in the level of liver enzymes is a sensitive indicator of hepatitis (de novo or reactivated hepatitis B or C, CMV, and other viral hepatitides), biliary outflow obstruction or leakage, or vascular insufficiency of the hepatic allograft.

The liver recipient can manifest infection at a diverse number of anatomic sites; however, intraabdominal foci comprise the majority of serious infections particularly in the first posttransplant month, although late technical allograft complications may occur in the middle or even late posttransplant periods. Intraabdominal infections include diffuse postoperative peritonitis associated with or without a visceral perforation. Localized intraabdominal infections may occur in the free peritoneal space (infected fluid collections due to hematoma, bile collections, ascites) or intraparenchymal (intrahepatic bilomas, infarcts abscesses or cholangitis). Most intraabdominal infection is associated with either a surgical technical complication (e.g. hepatic arterial stenosis or thrombosis, biliary leak, or obstruction), hepatic allograft dysfunction, or risk factors that predispose to postoperative infection (prolonged intraoperative time or high intraoperative transfusion requirement, severe coagulopathy, pretransplant immunosuppression, recent spontaneous bacterial peritonitis and chronic hepatitis C infection).

Bloodstream infection is often the first microbiologically documented site in liver recipients and is usually due to a subsequently documented secondary site. However, less commonly, primary bacteremia may occur without a clear inciting focus.

Liver transplantation surgery is classified as 'clean-contaminated' (planned surgical entry into the gastrointestinal and hepatobiliary tree). Thus, surgical wound infection of the abdominal incision or femoral/axillary venous cutdown sites are not uncommon and may be more frequent in recipients requiring a repeat laparotomy or retransplantation.

Bacterial pneumonia is usually due to aspiration of hospital-acquired microflora in the setting of prolonged mechanical ventilation and/or encephalopathy; however, hematogenous dissemination of extrapulmonary foci may also culminate in lower respiratory tract infection. Other important but less common sites of serious infection include hepatitis (see viral discussion), the CNS (abscesses, meningitis, encephalitis), cutaneous or mucocutaneous infection, gastrointestinal tract, and disseminated syndromes involving multiple sites due to an invasive pathogen. Common sites of infection of variable severity include intravascular access sites, urinary tract, cellulitis and the cranial sinuses.

1.3 What are the predominant organisms that contribute (by site)?

Bacterial organisms are the dominant category of pathogens following liver transplantation, although the fungi and viruses are also very important. Enteric bacteria (*Escherichia coli*, *Klebsiella*, enterococci) are the most common intraabdominal pathogens and are significantly more likely to have multi- or pan-resistance to antibiotics in recipients with previous heavy antibiotic exposure, long length of stay, or repeat transplantation. *Candida* spp. are commonly isolated from the intraperitoneal space or hepatic collections, particularly during or after a course of antibacterial therapy.

The staphylococci (*Staphylococcus aureus* and coagulase-negative staphylococci) are still the dominant bloodstream pathogens, often due to intravascular catheter infection, although bacteremia due to enterococci, Gram-negative enteric bacteria and *Candida* spp. are fairly common.

The microbial etiology of lower respiratory tract infection includes *S. aureus*, facultative Gram-negatives (*E. coli, Klebsiella, Enterobacter* spp.), and strict aerobes (*Pseudomonas aeruginosa, Acinetobacter* spp.). *Aspergillus* spp. and rarely other mycelial pathogens may also cause invasive pulmonary disease. Reactivated or, less commonly, primary pulmonary disease due to *Mycobacterium tuberculosis* is very infrequent, but *M. tuberculosis* is an important pathogen because of its potential for aerosol transmission and ability to disseminate to multiple organs.

The hepatic allograft itself is a common target for several viral pathogens. Recurrence of hepatitis B or C occurs at a high rate, but with variable severity, in recipients with end-stage liver disease due to chronic viral hepatitis. Diagnosis is established by typical histologic findings on liver biopsy (lobular inflammation), the lack of inclusions, coupled with serologic evidence of hepatitis B or C virus replication.

The liver allograft is the most common site of CMV disease in the liver recipient, although the incidence of CMV hepatitis and extrahepatic CMV disease has diminished with preemptive and prophylactic anti-CMV strategies (see section 4).

Gastrointestinal infection includes esophagitis [herpes simplex virus (HSV), CMV, *Candida* spp.], enteritis (CMV, protozoa, parasites) and colitis (*Clostridium difficile*). Community-acquired enteric pathogens (*Campylobacter, Shigella, Salmonella*) do not appear to infect liver recipients at a higher rate than the general population, although the clinical severity may be greater.

Aspergillus remains the dominant cause of focal brain abscesses and may occur as a solitary finding or with concomitant pulmonary, sinus or other visceral infection.

Cryptococcus neoformans is a rare cause of subacute meningitis. Acute meningitis is also uncommon but has a wider differential which includes *Listeria monocytogenes, Streptococcus pneumoniae*, and rarely the Gram-negative bacilli. Encephalitis is a rare condition in liver recipients. Most reported cases have involved a viral pathogen [CMV, varicella zoster virus (VZV), HSV, human herpesvirus-6 (HHV-6), adenovirus, enterovirus, polyomavirus]. Nonviral etiologies include toxoplasmosis, histoplasmosis, coccidioidomycosis, nocardiosis, *Listeria, Mycoplasma* and the rickettsial pathogens.

Organisms most capable of causing disseminated syndromes involving two or more noncontiguous anatomic sites include bacteria (*M. tuberculosis, S. aureus*), fungi (*Aspergillus* spp., *Candida* spp.) and viruses (primary infection due to the herpes virus family).

1.4 How do the organisms vary according to various risk factors?

There are several important associations between the native or iatrogenic risk factors and subsequent infection by specific organisms in the liver recipient. Such risk factors may be critical to direct the type, timing and duration of prophylactic or preemptive chemotherapy following liver transplantation, discussed later in this chapter. Multiple studies have demonstrated a strong risk for *Candida* infection and prolonged transplantation operating time, high red blood cell transfusion requirement, retransplantation with a choledochojejunostomy biliary anastomosis, posttransplant bacterial infection and alcoholic liver disease.

Previous tissue-invasive CMV disease (hepatitis, pneumonitis) increases the risk for serious bacterial infection, fungal disease (yeast and mycelial) and *Pneumocystis carinii* infection in the absence of chemoprophylaxis. Invasive CMV disease is more likely after previous antilymphocyte therapy (OKT3, antilymphocyte globulin), a CMV-seronegative recipient of a CMV-seropositive donor liver, and fulminant hepatitis as the reason for liver transplantation. The incidence of Epstein–Barr virus (EBV)-related posttransplant lymphoproliferative disease (PTLD) ranges from 1% to 4%. The risk is enhanced with the administration of antilymphocyte therapy, 'overimmunosuppression', EBV-seronegative recipients of EBV-seropositive allografts (less than 5% of adult liver recipients).

The pretransplant antigen replicative status of hepatitis B of the recipient is predictive of the likelihood of recurrent hepatitis. Hepatitis B virus (HBV) DNA or hepatitis B e antigen (HBeAg)-positive recipients have a 70–100% chance of developing posttransplant chronic hepatitis B infection of their allograft, which usually culminates in accelerated hepatic failure and death. In contrast, de-novo hepatitis B infection in the patient transplanted for nonhepatitis B infection has a less severe outcome.

Pretransplant colonization with multiresistant bacterial strains such as vancomycin-resistant enterococci (VRE) or methicillin-resistant *S. aureus* (MRSA) appears to increase the incidence of early posttransplant VRE and MRSA infection, respectively.

1.5 How does this differ from other conditions, from center to center, and from country to country?

The incidence, pattern and etiology of infection following liver transplantation differs in some respects from other solid organ categories and may vary significantly when compared with different liver transplant centers and countries. Amongst the major solid organ categories, liver recipients have the highest rates of bacteremia and candidemia. This observation reflects the extensive nature of the surgery, high risk for technical complications and heavy antibiotic selection pressure. In particular, VRE have disproportionately affected the liver recipient population because of high rates of VRE colonization at liver centers and the predilection of the *Enterococcus* to cause hepatobiliary infection.

The overall incidence of CMV disease before the use of prophylactic and preemptive strategies ranged from 30% to 50%, but was as high as 80% in the primary CMV infection subset. Comparably, the incidence and severity are higher than for kidney or heart recipients but CMV infection has a less serious course than for lung recipients. CMV hepatitis is much less common in other solid organ categories versus the liver transplant recipient, in whom it is the most common manifestation of CMV disease.

Although not unique to liver transplantation, recurrence of viral hepatitis (B or C) is certainly most common within this category. Despite replacement of the chronically infected liver, evidence of early posttransplant viral infection is uniformly high; however, histologic and clinical severity is variable.

Differences in the incidence and severity of specific infections may differ amongst liver transplant centers within the United States based upon the type of induction, maintenance and rejection episode immunosuppressive protocol, antiinfective prophylactic or preemptive strategies, acceptable level of candidate risk, and systematic exclusion of viral disease in the liver transplant candidate (HBV, human immunodeficiency virus (HIV) 1) by some programs. Geographic areas with a higher incidence of the endemic mycoses (*Coccidioides immitis* in the southwestern United States, *Histoplasma capsulatum* in the Tennessee and Ohio river valleys) predictably see a higher incidence of reactivated coccidioidomycosis and histoplasmosis, respectively, as many recipients native to these region have had exposure to and thus latent infection with these fungi. Similarly, countries with a higher incidence of tuberculosis, strongyloidiasis, trypanosomiasis and other pathogens in the general population will observe a higher incidence of such disease in the posttransplant period.

1.6 What is the appropriate approach to the initial evaluation and diagnosis of infection in liver transplant recipients?

Evaluation of the liver recipient with possible infection requires a meticulous consideration of the patient's pre- and posttransplant history, physical examination and recent laboratory tests. The time interval since the transplant procedure is also an important guide to the inclusion or exclusion of some pathogens.

Some transplant centers maintain a bedside wallchart which details the chronology of immunosuppression, rejection episodes, CMV serology, previous major infections and technical complications, antiinfective therapies, and hematologic and liver enzyme values, and facilitates the diagnosis.

Unequivocal localizing signs (i.e. abdominal findings, wound drainage or erythema, seizure or other focal neurologic signs, or increased purulence and quantity of sputum) may be present at the onset and allow a more tailored diagnostic scheme than in recipients who manifest only fever and no localizing signs or symptoms. Recipients in the intensive care unit who are encephalopathic, sedated or otherwise unable to communicate symptoms require evaluation despite the absence of signs (esophagitis, intraperitoneal infection).

The pattern of liver enzyme increases may point towards allograft rejection, biliary obstruction or leak, vascular insufficiency or viral hepatitis. For example, a disproportionate increase in the levels of bilirubin and γ-glutamyltranspeptidase (GGT) points to a biliary process (obstruction, cholangitis), while a predominant rise in the hepatocellular enzymes (serum glutamic–oxaloacetic transaminase (SGOT), serum glutamic–pyruvic transaminase (SGPT)) is more indicative of a hepatic vascular insufficiency or a viral hepatitis etiology.

In addition to obtaining appropriate cultures, prompt examination of fluid and tissue specimens with Gram stain and special stains (silver, acid-fast) can help direct the choice of antiinfective therapy. Special virologic studies (CMV pp65, polymerase chain reaction (PCR), shell vial, direct immunofluorescence techniques) may be indicated.

Early evaluation may require radiographic studies such as plain films of the chest or abdomen and computed tomography (CT) of the chest, abdomen or head. Ultrasonography of the hepatic artery is a rapidly available study for the demonstration of hepatic arterial thrombosis leading to cholangitis, hepatic infarction or abscess. Percutaneous or T-tube cholangiography remains the procedure of choice to rule out biliary leak or obstruction. The former procedure is utilized in the absence of a functioning biliary drain (T tube) but does carry the risk of intrahepatic or subcapsular hemorrhage. Antibiotic prophylaxis directed at known or potential biliary pathogens is administered 30 min before the procedure.

In general, gallium- and indium-labeled white blood cell scanning techniques have not proven helpful in the initial evaluation of fever in this population.

1.7 How should the evaluation be modified according to the severity of the risk?

Diagnostic and therapeutic delay for liver recipients with certain rapidly evolving processes are poorly tolerated and may enhance the risk for morbid sequelae. The appearance of frank bile or enteric contents in the abdominal drains, peritoneal signs or rapidly progressive soft tissue infection require urgent surgical exploration. The recipient with an acute neurologic syndrome also has a high risk for rapid deterioration. Thus, recipients with a meningeal presentation should promptly undergo lumbar puncture and immediately receive antimicrobial coverage tailored according to Gram staining of the cerebrospinal fluid and the epidemiologic setting. Focal neurologic signs coupled with objective signs of infection (fever, leukocytosis) require immediate CT of the head. Back pain and sensory or motor dysfunction should prompt magnetic resonance imaging (MRI) of the spinal cord to look for an epidural abscess or vertebral osteomyelitis.

Most viral infections do not require urgent diagnostic and therapeutic interventions. However, recipients seronegative for VZV who present with cutaneous vesicular and/or visceral lesions require high-dose intravenous acyclovir and respiratory/contact isolation measures. Another exception are patients suspected of having HSV encephalitis. High-dose intravenous acyclovir should be started concomitantly with the appropriate diagnostic workup (CT of the head and lumbar puncture for HSV PCR studies).

1.8 What are the specific evaluation measures?
See Table 7.2.2 and Chapter 2 in Part I.

1.9 What new developments are going to impact on emerging organisms, recognition, evaluation and diagnosis of infection in the liver transplant recipient?
Viral diagnostic techniques have become more sophisticated during the past decade and this has affected the prospective management of several conditions following liver transplantation. Early detection of CMV replication in the circulating leukocyte mass using the antigenemia assay (CMV pp65) or PCR technique provides a preemptive window of opportunity for the clinician. Thus, many centers have coupled weekly CMV pp65 or PCR monitoring (during the high-risk 1–6-month period) with preemptive antiviral treatment (intravenous or oral ganciclovir, or high-dose oral acyclovir) to abort progression to organ-invasive disease.

Quantitative detection of hepatitis B viral load by HBV-DNA PCR methods is the most sensitive diagnostic strategy to gauge the benefits of lamivudine induction during the candidate or posttransplant periods in recipients transplanted for chronic hepatitis B infection. Later generation antigen assays for hepatitis C (PCR, reverse transcriptase activity) have increasing utility in the liver recipient population to detect recurrence of hepatitis C viremia in recipients with chronic infection or de-novo infection in recipients with posttransplant allograft dysfunction.

Fungal antigen detection systems for deep-seated *Candida* and *Aspergillus* infection have not shown adequate sensitivity and specificity, although novel detection systems will continue to undergo investigation in the future.

What are the new or emerging organisms?
The greatest immediate concern are established pathogens that have evolved resistance mechanisms to the currently available antiinfective agents. Colonization and infection due to enterococci with high-level resistance to vancomycin and all other conventional antimicrobials have had a more adverse impact on the liver recipient population than on other solid organ transplant categories.

The combination of VRE-selective antibiotic pressure, prolonged length of stay and hepatobiliary or other intraabdominal foci of infection has promoted the emergence of VRE. Many candidates for liver transplantation become colonized with VRE while

Table 7.2.2 Evaluation of infections in liver transplant recipients according to the site of infection and the possible etiologic agent

Site of infection	Infectious syndrome (clinical features)	Predominant pathogens	Diagnostic investigations
Bloodstream	Bacteremia (fever with or without local signs of infection)	Coagulase-negative staphylococci Staphylococcus aureus Enterococcus spp. (nosocomial outbreaks in some institutions) Gram-negative bacilli (Escherichia coli, Klebsiella pneumoniae, Enterobacter spp., Pseudomonas aeruginosa) Candida spp.	Blood cultures (two sets drawn from separate sites and at least one set drawn from intravenous catheter)
Intravascular catheter-related infections	Pain, erythema, tenderness, discharge from catheter entry site	Coagulase-negative staphylococci Staphylococcus aureus Enterococcus spp. (nosocomial outbreaks in some institutions) Gram-negative bacilli Candida spp.	Swab of entry site Culture of catheter tip Blood cultures (consider drawing blood through each lumen of catheter and doing quantitative blood cultures)
Peritoneum and peritoneal space	Peritonitis or infected fluid collection (abscess, hematoma)	Gram-negative bacilli (Enterobacteriaceae, Pseudomonas aeruginosa) Enterococcus spp. Candida spp. Anaerobic bacilli (Clostridium spp., Bacteroides spp.) (uncommon)	Ultrasonography CT or MRI Culture of peritoneal fluid
Hepatobiliary tract:			
Liver	Hepatitis	Viral hepatitis (B, C): reactivation in graft Epstein–Barr virus Cytomegalovirus Herpes simplex Adenovirus	Liver enzymes Biopsy Serology Ultrasonography of hepatic artery

Site	Clinical features	Organisms	Investigations
	Liver abscess	Gram-negative bacilli (Enterobacteriaceae, *Pseudomonas aeruginosa, Acinetobacter* spp.) *Enterococcus* spp. *Candida* spp. *Staphylococcus aureus* Anaerobic bacilli (*Bacteriodes* spp., *Peptostreptococcus*, streptococci, *Fusobacterium*)	Ultrasonography CT or MRI Aspiration under CT guidance for culture
Biliary tract	Cholangitis Biloma	Aerobic Gram-negative bacilli (Enterobacteriaceae, *Pseudomonas aeruginosa*) Anaerobic bacilli (*Bacteroides* spp., *Clostridium* spp.) *Enterococcus* spp. *Candida* spp.	Cholangiography Ultrasonography CT or MRI Culture of biliary drainage fluid
Oral cavity	Stomatitis/mucositis (aphthae, ulcers) Oral thrush (white plaques)	Herpes simplex *Candida* spp.	Direct examination of specimen Culture
Throat	Pharyngitis Tonsilitis (sore throat, odynophagia)	*Streptococcus pyogenes* Epstein–Barr virus Adenovirus, rhinovirus, coronavirus Influenza, parainfluenza	Swab of pharynx for culture Serology
Upper respiratory tract (ear, nose, sinus, nasopharynx, larynx, trachea)	Sinusitis (tightness of sinus areas, headache, toothache, nasal obstruction, nasal voice)	Community-acquired sinusitis: *Streptococcus pneumoniae*, *Haemophilus influenzae*, *Moraxella catarrhalis*, viruses (influenza, parainfluenza, rhinovirus, adenovirus)	Aspiration of sinus Biopsy (if no improvement after 72–96 h of empirical antibiotic therapy)

Site of infection	Infectious syndrome (clinical features)	Predominant pathogens	Diagnostic investigations
		Nosocomial sinusitis:	
		Aerobic/facultative	
		Gram-negative bacilli, *Staphylococcus aureus*	
		Aspergillus spp., *Mucor* spp.,	
		Rhizopus spp.	
		Candida spp.	
Lower respiratory tract (bronchi, terminal airways, alveoli)	Bronchopneumonia	Conventional infections:	Chest radiography, CT, MRI
	Pneumonia (cough, dyspnea, chest pain, sputum, hemoptysia, pleural effusion)	Gram-negative bacilli (*Escherichia coli*,	Serology
		Klebsiella pneumoniae, Pseudomonas	Fiberoptic bronchoscopy with
		aeruginosa, Acinetobacter spp.)	bronchoalveolar lavage
		Staphylococcus aureus	Transbronchial biopsy
		Streptococcus pneumoniae	Thoracocentesis
		Haemophilus influenzae	Thoracoscopy with biopsy
		Legionella spp. (sporadic outbreaks)	Open lung biopsy
		Moraxella catarrhalis (late onset)	
		Mycoplasma pneumoniae (late onset)	
		Chlamydia pneumoniae (late onset)	
		Opportunistic infections:	
		Aspergillus spp.	
		Cytomegalovirus	
		Pneumocystis carinii	
		Nocardia asteroides	
		Mycobacterium tuberculosis	
		Cryptococcus neoformans	
		Adenovirus	
		Herpes simple	

Skin and soft tissue infection	Clinical presentation	Organisms	Diagnosis
	Surgical wound infections	Staphylococcus aureus Coagulase-negative staphylococci Enterococcus spp. Gram-negative bacilli (Enterobacteriaceae, Pseudomonas aeruginosa) Candida spp.	Aspiration (needle) or swab of skin exudate
	Rash Cellulitis (pain, erythema, tenderness, necrosis in case of ecthyma gangrenosum)	Primary infections: Coagulase-negative staphylococci Staphylococcus aureus Gram-negative bacilli (Pseudomonas aeruginosa, Escherichia coli, Klebsiella pneumoniae) Candida spp. Mucor spp., Rhizopus spp., Absidia spp. Human herpesvirus 6	Aspiration (needle) or swab of skin exudate Skin biopsy (histology and culture) Serology
	Papules, nodules (with or without myalgia and muscle tenderness)	Disseminated infections: Candida spp., Fusarium spp. Gram-negative bacilli (Escherichia coli, Pseudomonas aeruginosa, Aeromonas hydrophilia, Serratia marcescens) Epstein–Barr virus Adenovirus	
	Ulcers, vesicles, hemorrhagic or crusted lesions (isolated or with dermatomal distribution)	Herpes simplex Varicella zoster virus Cytomegalovirus	
	Disseminated vesicles, hemorrhagic or crusted lesions	Varicella zoster virus, herpes simplex Staphylococcus aureus, streptococci	
	Skin necrosis (toes, fingers) secondary to thrombosis of blood vessels	Aspergillus spp., Mucor spp.	
	Warts Molluscum contagiosum	Papillomavirus Poxvirus-related virus	Skin biopsy (histology)

Site of infection	Infectious syndrome (clinical features)	Predominant pathogens	Diagnostic investigations
Gastrointestinal tract:			
Esophagus	Esophagitis (dysphagia, retrosternal pain)	Herpes simplex Candida spp. Cytomegalovirus	Esogastroscopy Culture of endoscopic specimens
Small intestine, colon	Enteritis, colitis (nausea, vomiting, bloating, abdominal discomfort, cramp, pain, constipation, diarrhea)	Salmonella spp., Campylobacter spp., Listeria monocytogenes (all three are associated with a high rate of bacteremia) Clostridium difficile (antibiotic-associated diarrhea) Cytomegalovirus Epstein–Barr virus Strongyloides stercoralis	Plain abdominal radiography Ultrasonography CT or MRI Colonoscopy Culture of endoscopic specimens Stool cultures Toxin detection
Urinary tract	Urinary tract infections (dysuria, i.e. frequency, urgency, pain; hematuria; flank pain)	Gram-negative bacilli (Escherichia coli, Klebsiella spp., Proteus spp., Enterobacter spp., Pseudomonas aeruginosa) Enterococcus spp. Coagulase-negative staphylococci Candida spp.	Culture of urine Ultrasonography, CT (if suspicion of renal abscess)
Central nervous system*	Acute meningitis	Listeria monocytogenes	CT, MRI Lumbar puncture Aspiration or biopsy under stereotaxic CT guidance
	Subacute, chronic meningitis	Cryptococcus neoformans Candida spp. Mycobacterium tuberculosis Coccidioides immitis Histoplasma capsulatum	

Focal brain disease	*Aspergillus* spp. and other mycelia (e.g. *Dactylaria* spp. and *Pseudallescheria boydii*)
	Nocardia asteroides
	Listeria monocytogenes
	Toxoplasma gondii
	Viruses (herpes simplex virus, varicella, cytomegalovirus, Epstein–Barr virus, human herpesvirus-6, adenovirus, papillomavirus, JC virus)
Progressive dementia	JC virus (progressive multifocal leukoencephalopathy)

* Transplant patients have the same susceptibility to conventional pathogens of the central nervous system (meningitis: *Streptococcus pneumoniae*, *Neisseria meningitidis*, *Haemophilus influenzae*, Gram-negative bacilli; brain abscess: streptococci, *Bacteroides* spp., *Staphylococcus aureus*, Enterobacteriaceae) as the general population. Listed above are unique pathogens.

hospitalized during the donor search period at VRE-endemic transplant centers. Such patients may develop early posttransplant VRE infection due to the unavailability of effective prophylactic antimicrobial agents. Strategies to reduce VRE cross-transmission (cohorting VRE-colonized patients, use of VRE-dedicated equipment) may reduce but not eliminate the VRE burden at endemic centers. Currently there are several investigational antimicrobials with in-vitro activity against VRE (quinupristin–dalfopristin, linezolid, everninomycin and LY-333328) which are under active clinical investigation for VRE and other serious Gram-positive infections.

Gram-negative bacilli will continue to become even more problematic as the prevalence of species that express chromosomal-mediated β-lactamase or plasmid-mediated extended-spectrum β-lactamase production drastically narrow the spectrum of effective therapeutic agents. Pretransplant colonization with resistant Gram-negative bacilli will affect the choice and efficacy of perioperative prophylaxis.

An increase in azole-resistant *Candida* infection (*Candida krusei, Candida glabrata*) is a looming concern as many centers have increased the use of fluconazole for fungal prophylaxis and therapy.

Ganciclovir resistance amongst exposed strains of CMV remains a rare occurrence in this population compared with those with HIV infection. However, vigilant monitoring for resistant CMV strains is indicated with prolonged or repetitive use of ganciclovir (particularly the oral formulation).

Several pathogens have emerged in the last decade due primarily to improvements in clinical acumen and laboratory diagnostic techniques. HHV-6 has been shown to cause a variable syndrome of fever, leukopenia, hepatitis, CNS derangement and other symptoms in liver recipients, usually during the intermediate posttransplant period (1–6 months). Two phenotypic variants have been described: variant A, which is ganciclovir-susceptible, and variant B, which is susceptible only to foscarnet. A similar symptom complex has also been described with HHV-7. The overall clinical importance of these viruses in liver recipients remains unestablished and requires further investigation.

Parvovirus B19, the etiologic agent of 'fifth disease' and aplastic crisis in patients with sickle cell anemia has been implicated in blood dyscrasias (anemia, leukopenia) associated with fever, and even in extra-marrow invasion in liver recipients. Detection of parvovirus B19 DNA can be performed in blood, bone marrow and other tissues by PCR. γ-Globulin may modify and shorten the course of serious disease, although its therapeutic benefit remains anecdotal.

Improvements in mycologic identification with the use of major reference laboratories is primarily responsible for the increased reports of non-*Aspergillus* mycelial pathogens (*Dactylaria* spp., *Trichosporon begeilii, Pseudallescheria boydii, Fusarium solani, Cladosporium trichoides*, and others). Antifungal susceptibility testing in such species may be critical as some are variably or completely resistant to the azoles and amphotericin B.

2 REGARDING THE RISK FACTORS FOR LIVER TRANSPLANT RECIPIENTS

2.1 What are the main alterations in host defense mechanisms and what are the appropriate investigations to document them?

Host defense mechanisms may be altered due to both native and iatrogenic factors. Certain defects may be carried over from the pretransplant period in the patient with endstage liver disease. Patients with cirrhosis may have dysfunction in splenic antigen processing, humoral responsiveness, and the reticuloendothelial 'filtering' function performed by liver macrophages. Such function is not immediately corrected by successful liver transplantation. Patients with autoimmune liver disease due to various conditions (primary biliary cirrhosis, primary sclerosing cholangitis, autoimmune hepatitis) may be on long-term immunosuppression up to the time of liver transplantation with corticosteroids, methotrexate, azathioprine or cyclosporin A. Such patients thus carry a higher immunosuppressive burden earlier in the posttransplant period. Other conditions such as uremia, diabetes mellitus and malnutrition continue to exert an 'immunosuppressive effect' and potentiate the risk for infection in the posttransplant period.

The main host defense defects are due to surgical manipulations and other breeches of anatomic integrity, and to the immunosuppressive burden of the induction, maintenance and rejection episode therapy which affect neutrophil, cell-mediated and humoral immunity. Compromise of both the de-novo immunologic responses to newly acquired pathogens and the immunologic memory to latent pathogens may occur. Other factors include the immunosuppressive effect of CMV disease and hepatic allograft dysfunction due to ischemic preservation injury, vascular insufficiency, rejection or recurrent viral disease.

Specific prospective evaluation of immunologic impairment is generally not performed but rather is interpreted empirically by experienced clinicians managing the liver recipient. However, baseline determinations of previous exposure (and immunologic response) are important for such pathogens as CMV, VZV, HBV, *M. tuberculosis*, and less common pathogens in special circumstances.

2.2 What are the alterations due to iatrogenic factors?
The effects of surgery and other breaches in anatomic barriers in the perioperative period (intravascular and bladder catheterization, artificial ventilatory support) are all iatrogenic, but necessary, interventions that enhance the risk of infection. Excessive length of transplant surgery, hypothermia, high red cell transfusion requirement, choledochojejunostomy, early retransplantation or repeat laparotomy are all markers of increased postoperative risk for infection.

Iatrogenic immunosuppression (usually corticosteroid-based with parenteral cyclosporin A or tacrolimus with or without azathioprine or mofetil mycophenolate) is usually added to the protocol in the immediate posttransplant period but subsequently tailored to the individual graft tolerance of the recipient, presence of other risk factors (e.g. CMV-negative recipient of a CMV-positive allograft) and toxicity of immunosuppressive agents.

2.3 What is the influence of environmental factors?
The liver recipient, like all solid organ recipients, is exquisitely sensitive to potential pathogens in the nosocomial environment. Cluster outbreaks of aspergillosis are usually traced to poorly confined hospital construction resulting in the airborne dissemination of *Aspergillus* spores which can inoculate the pulmonary tree or even an open wound or abdominal cavity. Other airborne threats may arise from the inanimate environment (other mycelia) or other patients (aerosolized *S. aureus*, *M. tuberculosis*, primary varicella infection). *Legionella* growth within the hospital warm water supply is routinely suppressed by superheating and/or chlorination. Outbreaks of hospital-acquired legionellosis may be traced to water decontamination failure or even aerosolization from nearby hospital construction. Breaches in appropriate contact precautions (handwashing, glove use) remain the

principal route for cross-transmission of multiresistant nosocomial pathogens (VRE, MRSA, Gram-negative bacilli). Contaminated hospital equipment (stethoscopes, blood pressure cuffs, thermometers) are also implicated in cross-transmission of some pathogens.

The community environment presents a more variable and less controllable threat to the liver transplant recipient. Respiratory (influenza virus, pneumococci) and gastrointestinal pathogens (rotavirus, *Salmonella*, viral hepatitides) that affect the general population may present in a more fulminant manner. Close contact with an incubating case of 'chickenpox' in a VZV-seronegative recipient may result in disseminated cutaneous and visceral varicella infection. Regional community pathogens include the endemic fungi (*C. immitis, H. capsulatum, Blastomycoides dermatitidis*), parasites (*Strongyloides stercoralis*), and protozoa (*Toxoplasma gondii, Cryptosporidium*). Other sporadic pathogens such as *C. neoformans* and community-acquired *Legionella* are often not traceable to a specific environmental focus. Diagnostic consideration is altered in recipients who have traveled to, or are natives of, tropical climates where exposure to a more diverse range of pathogens occurs (i.e. malaria, trypanosomiasis, leishmaniasis, schistosomiasis).

2.4 What are the most significant factors that contribute to the risk of infection in liver transplantation?

The dominant risk factors for infection are the length of operation, occurrence of technical complications, dysfunction of the allograft, type and quantity of immunosuppression, and the epidemiologic exposure(s) of the recipient. Extremes of age may contribute to a lesser degree to the risk of infection. The incidental effects and unanticipated complications of the transplant operation are the dominant risk factors for early infection.

The liver transplant procedure requires an extensive and meticulously skilled disruption of the recipient's cutaneous, myofascial, vascular, biliary and gastrointestinal systems to implant the donor liver allograft in contiguity with the recipient's vascular, biliary and gastrointestinal systems. The native liver hepatectomy can be even more difficult in recipients with adhesions due to previous abdominal surgery or spontaneous bacterial peritonitis, severe coagulopathy or morbid obesity.

Reconstruction of the biliary drainage may be either by direct anastomosis of the donor and recipient bile ducts (choledochocholedochostomy) or by implantation of the donor bile duct into a constructed Roux-en-Y limb of the recipient's jejunum (choledochojejunostomy). The latter technique, reserved for discrepancy in the size of the donor and recipient bile ducts or for recipients with established extrahepatic biliary disease (primary sclerosing cholangitis), is associated with higher rates of postoperative infection due to surgical entry into the proximal small bowel.

Two or three intraperitoneal drains (suprahepatic, subhepatic and left subphrenic) are customarily left in place at the conclusion of the operation. Such drains do not necessarily evacuate residual or new fluid collections (bile, hematoma, chyle). Moreover, these drains may eventually be a 'reverse conduit', allowing cutaneous flora to invade the intraperitoneal space in the posttransplant period.

Other routine but unavoidable anatomic breeches in the periliver transplant period include endotracheal intubation, multiple intravascular catheters and a bladder drainage catheter.

Major technical complications invariably culminate in serious intraabdominal infection. Hepatic arterial insufficiency due to stenosis or thrombosis occurs in 5% of liver transplant recipients and presents as bile duct necrosis with cholangitis or biloma formation, hepatic infarcts or abscesses, or fulminant hepatic necrosis. Biliary leakage usually occurs at the surgically fabricated duct-to-duct anastomosis or at the donor duct implant site in recipients with a choledochojejunostomy, and usually presents as intraabdominal sepsis often with bacteremia. Biliary leakage at the T-tube exit site before or after removal of the T tube (in duct-to-duct recipients) may also occur. Other technical complications include bowel perforation, vascular suture breakdown with intraabdominal hemorrhage and obstruction of the biliary drainage.

The quantity and quality of immunosuppression may influence the incidence, severity and type of the pathogens causing infection. Overimmunosuppression or high immunosuppressive requirements which are indicated due to refractory allograft rejection enhance the risk for opportunistic infection by nonselective impairment of the appropriate immune defense against specific organisms.

Corticosteroids impair the immune defenses most broadly, affecting qualitative neutrophil function, T- and B-lymphocyte function, and even wound healing. Bacteria, fungal and, to a lesser extent, early viral pathogens (HSV) are promoted by steroid administration.

Cyclosporin A and tacrolimus both impair the lymphocyte recruitment response arm (sensitized T-helper lymphocyte, cytotoxic T-killer lymphocyte) to latent or newly encountered organisms usually contained by a cell-mediated response.

Antilymphocyte therapy (OKT3, antilymphocyte globulin) significantly enhances the risk for serious CMV disease and EBV-related PTLD. Other important factors include the presence or absence of recipient immunity (CMV, VZV, EBV), harboring latent organisms (*M. tuberculosis*, endemic mycoses), occurrence of CMV disease leading to higher rates of bacterial and fungal superinfection, nosocomial environmental hazards and the burden of invasive interventions (catheterization, repeat surgery) and pretransplant conditions (see sections 2.1 and 3.1).

2.5 What are the specific or nonspecific measures aimed at minimizing each of these factors?

Reducing the major risk factors in the liver recipient includes nonspecific or automated approaches for all patients, and specific interventions aimed at special pathogen(s) or only select patients.

Immunosuppression

Avoidance of empiric overimmunosuppression is best accomplished with liver biopsy-directed management in patients with a liver enzyme elevation pattern consistent with possible rejection. Judicious weaning or discontinuance of all immunosuppression may be possible in recipients with high graft tolerance and/or patients with life-threatening infection.

Quantitative monitoring of blood cyclosporin A or tacrolimus levels to the desired therapeutic range may reduce both the incidence of opportunistic infection and dose-related toxicities (neurotoxicity, nephrotoxicity). Prospectively lowering cyclosporin A or tacrolimus dosage should be considered in patients started on other agents with cytochrome P-450 inhibitory properties (fluconazole, itraconazole, erythromycin) to avoid sudden and undesired increases in blood levels.

Organism exposure

Reliance upon routine decontamination and surveillance of hospital air and water supplies is the principal barrier to nosocomially acquired *Aspergillus* and *Legionella*, respectively. The use of hospital tap water rather than distilled water has become more widely accepted to minimize costs; however, epidemiologic surveillance should be in place to ensure that endemic or epidemic waterborne pathogens have not become a problem. Appropriate contact precautions (handwashing, glove-wearing) are fundamental to reducing cross-transmission of multiresistant organisms. Patient cohorting should be considered in refractory endemic or epidemic situations to minimize the exposure of noncolonized individuals. Respiratory isolation measures (masks, closed doors, negative-pressurized room vented to the outside) should be implemented promptly for patients suspected to have active *M. tuberculosis*, incubating or active primary VZV infection, influenza, and other respiratory-transmitted agents.

Donor and blood product screening for transmissible agents is routinely performed. HIV-1 and HIV-2 positive donors are automatically excluded; however, donors positive for hepatitis B core or hepatitis C antibody may be utilized for desperately ill or elderly candidates or for recipients with chronic hepatitis B or C infection. CMV-seronegative or leukocyte-depleted blood units can be utilized in CMV-seronegative recipients of CMV-seronegative donor allografts to avoid subsequent primary CMV infection. Knowledge of the CMV donor status is also used to guide prophylactic or preemptive anti-CMV strategies (see section 4).

Technical complications and other invasive interventions
Minimizing technical complications ultimately depends upon matching the surgeon's skill level to the anticipated degree of difficulty of the recipient and donor organ. Adequate hemostasis and caval/portal venovenous bypass and antimicrobial wound chemoprophylaxis are important factors to reduce early postoperative wound infection. Recent investigation has shown intraoperative hypothermia to be an important risk factor for postoperative infection. Active warming of the patient during such prolonged surgery may reduce this risk, although this concept remains prospectively unproven. Early removal of intraabdominal drains, unused single- or multi-lumen intravascular devices, and bladder catheters will reduce the chance of infection.

2.6 Are there different levels of risk of infection recognized for liver transplant for recipients?
In general, liver recipients who require life support at the time of transplantation [United Network of Organ Sharing (UNOS) I or UNOS 2A candidate status (hospitalized and on some measure of life support)] experience higher rates of infection due to a variety of incorporated factors (antibiotic and nosocomial exposure, severe debilitation, and more advanced clinical deterioration in organ function). Recipients with hepatocellular disease (Laënnec cirrhosis, chronic viral hepatitis and fulminant hepatic failure) also have higher rates of early infection compared with patients with cholestatic disease (primary biliary cirrhosis or sclerosing cholangitis).

Higher levels of risk are well established for some specific posttransplant pathogens.CMV-seronegative recipients of CMV-seropositive liver allografts have at least a 50–70% chance of developing invasive disease in the preprophylaxis era. CMV-seropositive blood products on the other hand are much less efficient in both transmitting CMV to a seronegative recipient and causing CMV-invasive disease.

Similarly, pediatric and, less commonly, adult recipients who are EBV-H seronegative have the highest rates and severest expression of posttransplant lymphoproliferative disease with receipt of an EBV-positive allograft and, less commonly, EBV-positive blood products. The clinical presentation of EBV-related disease is protean and ranges from a febrile syndrome to lymphatic and/or visceral tumors with either monoclonal or polyclonal cell types. Measures for preventing EBV-related disease, other than avoiding overimmunosuppression, have not shown convincing efficacy. Previous antilymphocyte therapy also enhances the risk for CMV- and EBV-related disease.

Recipients with MRSA or VRE colonization documented by surveillance or clinical site cultures at the time of or shortly after transplantation are at increased risk of developing wound, catheter and bloodstream infection due to these multiresistant organisms. A positive donor culture (blood, liver biopsy) places the recipient at risk for infection within the hepatic allograft, vascular or biliary anastomoses.

Serious *Candida* infection is highly correlated with prolonged operating time, early retransplantation, increased steroid use, hyperglycemia and antecedent bacterial infection requiring broad-spectrum therapy.

The pretransplant replicative status of HBV correlates well with the posttransplant risk of recurrent hepatitis B. Recipients positive only for hepatitis surface antigen have about a 50% incidence of recurrence, whereas those positive for HBeAg or hepatitis DNA polymerase have a 70% and near 100% risk of recurrent infection, respectively.

Interestingly, concomitant infection with hepatitis delta (δ) agent also appears to protect the recipient from recurrent hepatitis B. Hepatitis C has a high uniform rate of early virologic recurrence; however, infection with serotypes Ia and Ib is associated with a more aggressive clinical course than non-Ia/Ib serotypes.

2.7 How does the level of risk impact on management?

Liver recipients estimated to be at high risk for infection due to a specific organism may be managed prospectively to reduce the probability and/or severity of subsequent infection. Most commonly, evidence of increased risk is linked to a prophylactic or preemptive antiinfective agent directed at a category of pathogens or a specific pathogen. The most sophisticated approaches based upon risk strata are antiviral regimens calibrated to CMV donor–recipient pairing and coupled with repetitive determinations of CMV replication [e.g. shell vial assay of the more sensitive antigenemia (pp65) or PCR assays]. Use of antilymphocyte therapy (OKT3, ALG) may be another trigger for anti-CMV preemptive treatment. These schemes are elaborated in section 4.

Antifungal chemoprophylaxis can be directed selectively or further intensified in patients with an aggregate of risk factors (long operating time, repeat laparotomy, repeat transplantation or prolonged antibiotic exposure) using either fluconazole or low-dose amphotericin B (10–20 mg/day) for a finite period. Positive donor cultures can guide the postoperative choice and duration of empirical antibiotics. Isoniazid (INH) prophylaxis is used by some centers in recipients with a positive purified protein derivative (PPD) finding, radiographic evidence of old tuberculosis or a history of inadequate therapy. Some transplant centers do not utilize INH due to the ubiquity of liver enzyme increases in liver recipients, risk of hepatotoxicity and overall low risk of tuberculous disease.

The level of risk may also dictate the chosen duration of otherwise standard chemoprophylaxis. For instance, patients with a high immunosuppressive burden due to chronic rejection or severe CMV disease have an enhanced and more prolonged risk of *P. carinii* infection. Extending trimethoprim–sulfamethoxasole (TMP–SMX) prophylaxis beyond the first posttransplant year may be prudent in such cases. Several preventive strategies which are currently undergoing investigation include hyperimmune CMV globulin for PTLD prevention in EBV-seronegative pediatric recipients, as this formulation also has a high level of anti-EBV antibody. Others include the use of antihepatitis B immunoglobulin with lamivudine to prevent the recurrence of chronic hepatitis B infection and interferon-α with oral ribavirin for prevention of hepatitis C recurrence.

Empirical therapeutic coverage based on the epidemiologic circumstances is prudent in cases where the level of risk is prohibitively high. Such intervention should also be coupled with a reduction in immunosuppression on a case-by-case basis.

2.8 What new developments are going to impact on minimizing or suppressing the specific risk factors?

Recent new immunosuppressive agents have shown greater potency or less toxicity (tacrolimus, mycophenolate), although they have not further diminished the risks of posttransplant infection. Advances in immunosuppression that confine their effect selectively to the host's immunologic attack upon the antigens of the hepatic allograft with less collateral suppression of the normal immune system would significantly reduce many of the opportunistic infections currently observed. A reduction in CMV-induced immunosuppression and bacterial or fungal superinfection should be an extended benefit from reductions in CMV disease with improvements in surveillance and prevention.

Augmenting pretransplant immunity in the 'at-risk' recipient remains an appealing but elusive goal. Sustained protective levels (> 10 IU/ml) of hepatitis B surface antibody are achieved only in the minority of liver recipients receiving recombinant hepatitis B vaccination. Development of an efficacious hepatitis C vaccine would reduce the threat of this highly prevalent pathogen to the new liver recipient. Experimental CMV vaccination in CMV-seronegative recipients has shown some promise in kidney transplantation, but this has not become a commercially available product. Eliminating the risk of primary CMV infection in liver recipients would prove enormously beneficial to this subset, which experiences the most morbid sequelae from CMV.

Novel antimicrobials (quinupristin–dalfopristin, linezolid, everninomycin, LY-333328) with activity against the multiresistant Gram-positive species such as MRSA and VRE are currently available as investigational agents; they should be validated clinically within the next several years and will hopefully fulfill both therapeutic and prophylactic needs. Several emerging antifungal compounds (pneumocandins, voriconazole) appear to have promising activity against *Aspergillus* spp. and other mycelial pathogens. The next decade should see advances in xeno- and genome-hybridized liver transplantation, which will pose important new challenges in the field of posttransplant infection.

3 REGARDING THE SURVEILLANCE OF LIVER TRANSPLANT RECIPIENTS

3.1 What is the important pretransplant information to be gathered?
3.2 What are the surveillance measures to be taken in the liver transplant recipient?

A complete epidemiologic exposure history of the liver recipient must be available to clinicians providing posttransplant care. This should include viral serologies (CMV, EBV, VZV, hepatitis A, B, C, δ), syphilis serology, PPD and anergy panel (*Trichophyton*, mumps, *Candida*), and a current chest film. Further surveillance studies may be indicated based upon the nosocomial and community exposure risks of the patient. Such tests include surveillance cultures for VRE (rectal swab), MRSA (nasal swab), *Aspergillus* spp. (sputum or nasal swab), fungal serology (*H. capsulatum, C. immitis, B. dermatiditis*), serology for *S. stercoralis*, and stool for ova and parasites. Other important historic data should include all significant previous infections (spontaneous bacterial peritonitis, endocarditis, pneumonia), an immunization history (childhood vaccination, Pneumovax, hepatitis A and B, influenza, varicella vaccine), previous surgery or permanently implanted foreign materials (prosthetic valve, vascular grafts, orthopedic appliances), residence or travel to tropical areas or regions with a high prevalence of endemic mycoses, unusual domestic exposures (pets, farm animals), pretransplant immunosuppression, and exposure to or prior treatment for *M. tuberculosis*.

Environmental cultures would be considered only at centers experiencing an incidental outbreak of a nosocomial pathogen spread via airborne routes (*Aspergillus*), hospital water (*Legionella*), or contact with other inanimate objects in the patient care environment (VRE).

3.3 What are the other specific measures to be taken when a patient presents for liver transplantation?

There is no evidence that the routine isolation for all liver transplant recipients reduces the risk of infection or improves outcome. However, certain situations merit special isolation procedures. Respiratory isolation should be implemented for patients with suspected or documented respiratory infections due to agents capable of airborne transmission (*M. tuberculosis*, VZV, influenza virus). Gowns should be worn for the care of patients where there is a chance of body fluid contact and particularly for open draining wound care. Strict adherence to glove-wearing and handwashing with an antiseptic–antibacterial agent for all patient care is imperative to contain cross-transmission of hospital-acquired organisms. Removal and disposal of gloves when leaving the immediate patient care environment is also important. Patients with problematic multi- or pan-resistant organisms (VRE, MRSA, *Pseudomonas, Enterobacter* spp.) should be isolated in private rooms or in endemic situations, cohorted with other colonized or infected patients.

4 REGARDING THE PREVENTION OF INFECTION IN LIVER TRANSPLANT RECIPIENTS

4.1 What approaches, if any, to the prevention of infection should be considered in the liver transplant recipient?

The core principles of prophylaxis routinely administered to the liver recipient are described below.

Surgical wound prophylaxis

A parenteral agent(s) directed at faculative enteric Gram-negative bacilli (*E. coli, Klebsiella*, etc.), enterococci, and methicillin-susceptible staphylococci should be administered for 24–48 h. Commonly used regimens are ampicillin–sulbactam, piperacillin–tazobactam, and cefotaxime plus ampicillin.

Herpes simplex virus

Oral acyclovir at a dose of 400–800 mg three or four times daily effectively suppresses reactivated orolabial, cutaneous and genital HSV infection in the early posttransplant period. This practice is usually implemented even for adult HSV-seronegative recipients who are at risk for primary HSV infection. Some centers elect not to use oral acyclovir and prefer close observation of the patient for lesions consistent with HSV reactivation. Centers that utilize early parenteral or oral ganciclovir for CMV prophylaxis have no need to add oral acyclovir.

Cytomegalovirus

There is a diverse number of approaches, but the optimal regimen has not yet been established. Parenteral ganciclovir either given uniformly to all recipients or targeted at high-risk recipients with virologic evidence of CMV replication (positive CMV pp65 or antigenemia) is now the most prevalent approach. At the University of Pittsburgh we follow the CMV pp65 antigenemia assay on a weekly basis between weeks 2 and 16, and every 2 weeks between weeks 17 and 24. CMV-seropositive recipients receive a 14-day parenteral course of ganciclovir for a pp65 assay with more than 10 positive leukocytes per 200 000 leukocytes, while CMV-seronegative recipients receive a 14–21-day course for one or more positive leukocytes. This approach has yielded a dramatic decrease in the progression to organ-invasive CMV disease in both groups compared with our historic experience.

High-dose oral acyclovir (3200 mg/day) or oral ganciclovir has also been utilized, although gastrointestinal side effects and diminished bioavailability in the liver population may compromise their efficacy. Hyperimmune anti-CMV globulin has not shown protective benefit in liver recipients with primary CMV infection (D+/R–) when given during the first 3 months following transplantation.

Pneumocystis carinii

Oral TMP–SMX started within 1–2 weeks of transplantation (one double-strength tablet three times per week or one single-strength tablet from Monday to Friday) has nearly 100% prophylactic efficacy. The risk of *P. carinii* is highest during the first posttransplant year, although some programs extend the duration of prophylaxis in higher-risk cases (chronic rejection, antilymphocyte therapy). Serendipitous protection against other TMP–SMX-sensitive organisms (*Listeria*, *T. gondii*, *Nocardia*) has been proposed but remains unproven.

Alternative approaches in the sulfa-intolerant individual include aerosolized pentamidine (300 mg per month) or dapsone (50 mg/day). Atovaquone is another prophylactic option; however, there is only very limited experience with this drug at present.

Candida

Most centers in the United States are utilizing some antifungal formulation to prevent superficial (stomatitis, esophagitis) *Candida* infection. Oral mycostatin (nystatin) at a dose of 2–8 million units per day reduces the incidence of superficial candidiasis; however, its prophylactic efficacy against deep-seated infection is debatable. Lower rates of candidiasis have been observed with oral fluconazole (200–400 mg/day) for the first month after transplantation, or low-dose amphotericin B (10–20 mg/day) in high-risk recipients.

Selective bowel decontamination (SBD) has been studied repeatedly in the liver transplant population. The most common regimens have been two agents with aerobic/facultative Gram-negative activity (colistin plus gentamicin or tobramycin) and an enteral antifungal agent (mycostatin or amphotericin B) administered both enterally and as a topical paste to the oropharynx. A reduction in Gram-negative infection has been reported, but a reciprocal increase in Gram-positive colonization and infection was also observed. Currently, most liver transplant centers in the United States do not administer SBD routinely.

Preventive approaches for special circumstances include varicella zoster immune globulin (VZIG) given intramuscularly within 72–92 h of exposure of a VZV-seronegative recipient to an incubating or active case of chickenpox; isoniazid (INH) for 12–18 months in patients with pre- or post-transplant positive PPD reactions, or exposure to an active case of tuberculosis or radiographic evidence of old untreated disease.

4.2 What are the future challenges and opportunities for reducing the risk of infection?

The development of resistance to the current generation of agents remains a potential threat to several effective prophylaxis options. Despite a decade of increased use of ganciclovir, there have been only rare reports of ganciclovir-resistant CMV strains in liver and other solid organ recipients. Oral ganciclovir, due to its limited bioavailability and potential for prolonged usage, may favor the development of resistance. Azole-resistant non-albicans species (C. *krusei*, C. *glabrata*) and even azole-resistant *Candida albicans* have become more prevalent with the systematic overuse of fluconazole.

The worsening liver organ shortage will remain a continuing challenge. A protracted donor search (and a longer hospitalization period) will increase the incidence of candidates who become colonized with the more resistant nosocomial pathogens and cannot receive effective antibacterial prophylaxis at the time of transplantation.

5 REGARDING THE TREATMENT OF LIVER TRANSPLANT RECIPIENTS

5.1 What is the role of empirical therapy?

The major considerations to begin empirical therapy in the liver recipient include a sufficient level of clinical suspicion that an active infection is present and/or concern that any further delay in appropriate therapy places the recipient at a high risk for rapid and significant clinical deterioration. Recipients with septic presentations of intraabdominal, pulmonary or unknown origin should all receive empirical therapy. In cases where empirical therapy is deferred, serial observation of the patient's vital signs and pertinent local findings are critical. In most instances there should be sufficient time to obtain the appropriate cultures before initiating therapy. However, patients with acute meningeal presentations in whom lumbar puncture cannot be performed immediately should receive appropriate antimicrobial coverage for bacterial meningitis.

The choice of antimicrobial(s) is influenced by the posttransplant time period (see Table 7.2.1 and Chapter 7.0, section 1.4), the suspected site(s) of infection and the most likely pathogen(s). Other important factors to weigh include the likelihood of multiresistant bacteria (i.e. methicillin-resistant staphylococci which obligates vancomycin use, imipenem–cilastatin for extended-spectrum β-lactamase Gram-negative bacilli, or coverage with two antipseudomonal agents for suspected *P. aeruginosa*), end-organ toxicities, a history of patient intolerance or noncompliance with *P. carinii* prophylaxis.

Empirical treatment should not be continued in cases where cultures, radiographic studies and other diagnostic interventions effectively rule out an infection. Usually this does not exceed a 3–4-day period. Protracted empirical treatment may further obfuscate the clinical picture, select or induce multiresistant bacteria, and promote bacterial or fungal superinfection. Conversely, empirical therapy may be extended to a definitive course of treatment or modified based upon subsequent microbiologic findings or the clinical trend of the patient.

5.2 What is the appropriate approach to the liver transplant recipient with evidence of:

Upper respiratory tract infection?

Sinusitis

The microbial etiology of sinus infection is highly dependent upon the clinical setting (e.g. community versus nosocomial acquisition, specific radiographic findings). Therapy for nosocomial sinusitis should be guided by the sinus aspirate Gram stain and culture as multiresistant hospital-acquired bacteria are the primary etiology. CT evidence of bone erosion with high-density changes correlate with *Aspergillus* or *Mucor* invasion, for which sinus debridement and high-dose amphotericin B or a lipid formulation of amphotericin B is indicated. Community-acquired sinusitis can usually be treated empirically unless there are unusual features at presentation or the patient fails to respond.

Otitis media

A similar distinction for nosocomial versus community-acquired pathogens based upon the clinical setting is also pertinent to guide the selection of antimicrobial(s). Diagnostic and therapeutic tympanocentesis may be required for patients who fail to respond to well-chosen empirical antimicrobial therapy.

Conjunctivitis

Initial workup should include bacterial, fungal and viral cultures of the conjunctival discharge/sac. Concomitant visual disturbances should prompt a formal ophthamologic evaluation of the anterior and posterior chambers to rule out contiguous spread or metastatic infection to the eye. Bacterial conjunctivitis can be treated with topical therapy (gentamicin, erythromycin, sulfa agents). However, herpetic disease (herpes zoster, herpes simplex) requires systemic therapy with oral or parenteral acyclovir.

Oropharynx

Painful vesicular eruptions consistent with herpes simplex should have a Tzanck preparation stain, direct fluorescent assay and/or viral culture followed by empirical acyclovir therapy. Scrapings of any white-yellow adherent coatings on the tongue or buccal mucosa can be examined by potassium hydroxide or Calcofluor staining to confirm the presence of fungal stomatitis, which should respond to nystatin (as either a 'swish and swallow'; liquid suspension or troches), fluconazole or low-dose amphotericin B.

The presence of exudate with or without tonsillar/adenoid enlargement should be cultured for group A *Streptococcus*, which is managed most effectively with oral penicillin. EBV infection should be considered in patients with unexplained tonsillar or peritonsillar lymphoid enlargement or inflammation. Heterophile antibody (Monospot), quantitative EBV PCR, and biopsy are required to confirm the diagnosis of PTLD. Nonherpetic viral pharyngitis is a diagnosis of exclusion with this presentation.

Teeth and gingiva

Common pyogenic complications of the teeth and gingiva are more likely in recipients whose baseline dentition is poor, and are best managed with appropriate dental or periodontal care. Unusual gingival lesions, however, should undergo culture and biopsy. Gingival hyperplasia due to cyclosporin may be an aggravating factor.

Lower respiratory tract infection?

Initial diagnostic studies should include chest radiography and examination of a respiratory secretion specimen for stains and culture (routine aerobic, *Legionella*, viral and mycobacteria depending on the clinical and epidemiologic circumstances). CT of the chest is more sensitive for lesions in the posterior basilar regions, associated mediastinal disease and pleural collections. Bronchoscopic studies, especially bronchoalveolar lavage (BAL), appear to be more sensitive for the detection of *P. carinii*, mycelia, *M. tuberculosis* and viral infections. BAL should also be performed for patients who fail to respond to a course of empirical therapy, nodular or cavitary lesions, and for inspection of the large airways for mucosal lesions. Transbronchial, CT-guided or open lung biopsies are diagnostic options in patients whose diagnosis cannot be ascertained by less invasive methods. The etiologic pathogens, and thus empirical therapy, are highly dependent upon the posttransplant period, nosocomial or community exposure, and prophylaxis history.

Gastrointestinal infection?

Diagnostic workup may be directed based upon the symptomatology (odynophagia, nausea/vomiting or hematemesis, or diarrhea). Similar to other hosts, C. *difficile* is the major infectious cause of hospital-acquired diarrhea in the liver recipient and is easily detected by tissue culture or enzyme immunoassay. Community-acquired cases and nosocomial cases with a compatible epidemiologic history should undergo workup for the common enteric pathogens (including rotavirus) and ova and parasites if there are risk factors (foreign travel or native from an endemic area, unexplained eosinophilia). Recipients with symptoms referable to the esophagus (odynophagia, dysphagia) or stomach (nausea, vomiting, pain, hematemesis) require endoscopic examination with biopsy and/or culture for *Candida*, HSV and CMV. PTLD may present as an obstructive or hemorrhagic gastrointestinal condition for which upper endoscopy or colonoscopy is diagnostically indicated.

Genitourinary tract infection?

In the early posttransplant period bladder catheterization is the principal inciting factor for urinary tract infection (UTI). Local and/or systemic symptoms are variable. Diagnosis and management rest upon the results and sensitivities of a positive urine culture. Removal of the bladder catheter, if possible, will usually help clear the infecting pathogen. Candiduria is often seen in this setting and can be managed with either a 5-day amphotericin bladder irrigation with (50 mg/day) or a short course of fluconazole. Refractory candidal UTIs may indicate parenchymal kidney disease (fungus ball, hematogenous spread to the kidney) and require radiographic imaging of the upper urinary tract. Less common urinary tract pathogens (polyomavirus, adenovirus, *Cryptococcus*, *M. tuberculosis*, *M. hominis*) should be considered in atypical or treatment-refractory cases.

Cardiovascular infection?

A wide range of organisms may cause cardiovascular infection, usually by metastatic spread to valvular or other cardiac tissues; however, the overall incidence is very low. Patients who require pericardiotomy to complete the hepatic venous anastomosis are at risk for deep postoperative infection extending into the pericardium. Echocardiography (transthoracic or transesophageal), coupled with appropriate blood and tissue cultures, is required for diagnosis and definitive management.

Musculoskeletal infection?

Uncommon but serious cases of osteomyelitis are described in liver recipients, often from hematogenous dissemination (*S. aureus*, *Candida* spp., *Aspergillus*). Medical and surgical management is similar to that in patients with other underlying predisposing factors.

Skin infection?

Superficial surgical wound infections may occur at the abdominal incision site or at the axillary and/or femoral venous cutdown sites. These are manageable by opening the incision, drainage and antibiotic therapy based upon initial Gram staining and cultures. Vesicular or painful lesions should prompt viral culturing techniques for a herpetic (herpes simplex, herpes zoster) etiology. Cellulitis in the late posttransplant period may be treated empirically for staphylococci and streptococci, although patients with toxicity or those not responding to empirical therapy require broader coverage. Hematogenous cutaneous dissemination of yeast, mycelial or other pathogens requires skin biopsy and culture to direct the appropriate management.

Central nervous system infection?

The most common CNS presentations include focal neurologic signs (seizure, paresis), an altered level of consciousness (lethargy, obtundation), or acute (meningismus) or subacute (headache) presentations. CT of the brain is usually the first diagnostic test to screen for discrete lesions, mass effect, demyelination or hemorrhage. However, MRI is a more sensitive technique for smaller cerebral lesions, brainstem or spinal cord involvement. Lumbar puncture, if not contraindicated, has excellent sensitivity for cryptococcal and other meningitides, but is quite insensitive for detecting the etiology of brain abscesses, which are better diagnosed by stereotactic brain biopsy. Therapeutic delay is poorly tolerated so empirical treatment (tailored to the differential diagnosis) is quite important during the diagnostic process. Noninfectious CNS processes that may mimic an infectious cause include tacrolimus- or cyclosporin-induced demyelination syndromes, and aseptic meningitis due to OKT3 administration.

Foreign body in place?

Retained removable foreign devices such as intravascular or urinary tract catheters may be an impediment to curing some common infections such as line-related bacteremia or UTI, respectively. Liver recipients may have had previously implanted permanent prosthetic devices (orthopedic implants, cardiac valves, vascular grafts, pacemaker devices) which become incidentally infected due to hematogenous spread from a distant source. Failure to clear the bloodborne pathogen, relapse after appropriate antimicrobial therapy, or local changes around the device indicate that the foreign body is infected. Management options for such situations are determined on an individual basis and include an extended course of treatment, adding agents for microbicidal or intracellular activity (i.e. rifampicin, gentamicin), or device removal if possible.

Intraabdominal infection?

Serious infections in the abdominal cavity are clustered within the first month posttransplant, although sporadically such infections can arise later. They can be separated into technical complications of the liver allograft (intrahepatic abscess or biloma, cholangitis, or an infected anastomosis) and other incidental complications of the operation itself (peritonitis, intraperitoneal abscess or hematoma, intestinal perforation)

The speed and type of diagnostic evaluation is based upon the clinical severity and specific elements of the presentation, which may direct the workup. Appearance of bile in the abdominal drains represents a leakage of bile from the reconstructed biliary duct until proven otherwise. Confirmation can be performed by either a T-tube or percutaneous cholangiogram, although some may advocate immediate exploratory laparotomy. Prompt surgical revision of the bile duct to a choledochojejunostomy, drainage and antibiotic coverage empirically directed to enteric organisms are the main features of therapy.

Hepatic arterial insufficiency may be due to thrombosis, kinking or stenosis of the reconstructed hepatic artery. This condition may manifest as hepatic infarct or abscess, cholangitis or biloma formation, with or without bacteremia or even candidemia. Fever, raised transaminase values, or unexplained bacteremia are other indicators of this condition. Hepatic arteriography is the 'gold standard' investigation to confirm the problem. CT or ultrasonographically guided drainage of intrahepatic collections coupled with appropriate antiinfective therapy may stabilize the patient. Surgical or fibrinolytic revascularization of the hepatic artery may salvage the allograft but only if performed very early. Otherwise, retransplantation offers the only chance for a definitive cure.

Cholangitis (fever, raised GGT/bilirubin levels) may also be due to biliary outflow obstruction, resulting from stricturing at the biliary anastomosis, an obstructing Silastic stent left in place after a choledochojejunostomy, or biliary sludge/cast syndrome. Bile duct strictures require surgical revision of the biliary duct and antibiotic treatment based empirically or on the results of blood/bile cultures. However, obstruction due to a retained stent or biliary sludge may be successfully managed with endoscopic removal of the stent or percutaneous biliary drainage, respectively.

Evaluation and management of other intraperitoneal infection does not differ significantly from that in other hosts. A high index of suspicion for intraperitoneal infection should be reserved for recipients with prolonged surgical time or previous intraabdominal bleeding, and for retransplanted patients. The clinician needs to be mindful that a muted clinical expression (i.e. loss of peritoneal signs) due to the antiinflammatory effects of immunosuppression may occur in the setting of local or diffuse peritonitis.

5.3 What is the appropriate approach to the liver transplant patient with evidence of bacteremia, with or without site of infection?

Isolation of a bloodborne pathogen should in almost all cases prompt the initiation of antimicrobial therapy. The principal exceptions are asymptomatic patients with late growth (> 48 h) or single bottle growth of coagulase-negative staphylococci. Bacteremia occurring while the patient is already on antimicrobial(s) should lead to consideration that the pathogen(s) are either resistant to the current regimen or that a closed space infection is present which requires a nonantimicrobial intervention (i.e. biliary drainage, abscess or line removal). The species of bloodborne pathogen may be a valuable hint to the primary site of infection. Enteric species (*E. coli*, *Klebsiella*, *Enterobacter* spp. and other facultative Gram-negative bacilli or enterococci) are most commonly associated with an intraabdominal focus, which may or may not be clinically apparent by the time that the bacteremia is documented. A concomitant increase in the levels of hepatocellular (SGOT, SGPT) or biliary duct (GGT, alkaline phosphatase) enzymes may also point to vascular insufficiency or cholangitis, respectively, as the source of the bacteremia (see section 5.2).

Empirical coverage should be guided by the initial morphologic description of the blood isolate(s), local susceptibility patterns, and the suspected primary site of infection. Thus, facultative Gram-negative bacteremia may be covered with either a β-lactam/β-lactamase inhibitor (piperacillin–tazobactam), cefepime, aztreonam, carbapenem or a quinolone. Ceftazidime, due to its potent cephalosporinase induction properties, should be avoided. Gram-negative bacilli that are present only in the aerobic bottles and/or suspicion of nosocomial Gram-negative pneumonia should be covered for *P. aeruginosa* and *Acinetobacter* spp. until final identification and susceptibilities are available. Isolation of anaerobes is usually due to lower gastrointestinal obstruction or perforation, or biliary obstruction, and can be predictably covered with metronidazole or a β-lactam with good

($> 90\%$) coverage of *Bacteroides* spp. Staphylococcal bacteremia is most likely due to an infected intravascular device, pneumonia or surgical wound site.

Vancomycin is still the only effective agent for methicillin-resistant staphylococcal infection (coagulase-negative staphylococci and *S. aureus*); however, methicillin-susceptible *S. aureus* infection may respond more favorably to an antistaphylococcal penicillin (nafcillin, oxacillin). Quinpristin/dalfopristin (Synerid), a recently approved antimicrobial agent with broad Gram-positive activity, has excellent activity against both methicillin-susceptable and methicillin-resistant staphylococci. This agent should provide another treatment option for the vancomycin-allergic or -refractory patient.

5.4–5.6 What is the appropriate approach to the liver transplant recipient with evidence of a viral, fungal or parasitic infection?
See Table 7.2.2 and refer also to Chapters 7.1, 7.3, 7.4, 7.5 and 7.6.

5.7 What is the role of nonantiinfective interventions (including reducing or altering immunosuppression) in the management of established infection?
Surgical or radiologically guided drainage is often the primary adjunct to antiinfective therapy for closed space infection and has been emphasized previously in this chapter.

A reduction in the degree of immunosuppression or selective alteration of the composition of immunosuppression can be implemented in some cases. Enthusiasm for such management, however, has to be balanced by the fact that the likelihood of breakthrough allograft rejection and elective graft removal is not an option as it is with pancreas, kidney and intestinal recipients. Certain infections (CMV, EBV) may clearly benefit from a reduction in cyclosporin or tacrolimus dosage. However, aggressive monoclonal-type PTLD may also require antilymphoma chemotherapy. Since corticosteroids impair all arms of the immune system, a reduction in steroid dosage below the equivalent of 10 mg/day is intuitively appealing for serious bacterial, fungal, mycobacterial and parasitic disease. Even complete withdrawal of immunosuppression in life-threatening infection has been reported by the transplant program at Pittsburgh. Such an approach is more difficult to achieve in the early posttransplant period when graft tolerance is lowest, and in patients with a positive cytotoxic crossmatch, multiple episodes of acute rejection or documented chronic rejection. Clearly, serial liver biopsies are required to monitor these patients for breakthrough allograft rejection.

Immunostimulatory therapies have increasingly attracted interest as an adjunct to conventional treatment for infections that are notoriously difficult to treat. Granulocyte or granulocyte–monocyte colony-stimulating factors have been utilized in *Aspergillus* and other fungal infections, although controlled experience is lacking. These agents are also indicated for posttransplant neutropenia usually due to drug-associated myelosuppression. Interferon-α appears to have a salutary biochemical effect on posttransplant hepatitis C infection and is currently under investigation as a combination regimen with oral ribavirin. Triggering allograft rejection remains a real concern with the use of interferon. Thus, a balanced approach with immunosuppressive therapy needs to be maintained.

Infections in Heart Transplant Recipients

Patricia Muñoz and Emilio Bouza

INTRODUCTION

Heart transplantation has become a viable therapeutic option for patients with advanced heart disease. Approximately 3500 heart transplants are performed each year worldwide. Because of limited availability of organs, criteria for donor acceptance have been liberalized, mainly with respect to donor age, ischemic time and potential infection. Remarkably, the use of infected donors, even with positive blood cultures, has resulted in surprisingly few infectious complications.

The recipient pool has also broadened to include infants less than 6 months of age, adults older than 60 years and carefully selected diabetics, amongst others. Given the shortage of organ donors, several investigators have proposed the use of 'marginal' donors for older recipients.

The number of pediatric transplantations continues to increase, especially transplantations of infants with hypoplastic left heart syndrome and patients with congenital defects. Actuarial survival rates are 85% at 1 month, 72% at 1 year, 64% at 3 years and 60% at 5 years. However, these improved rates are still not equal to the survival of the overall cardiac transplant population, in part because of lower survival rates in neonates. Ventricular dysfunction and rejection, rather than infection, are the leading causes of death. However, rejection and infection are the most frequent complications. Also common are hypertension (39%) and seizures (25%), whereas coronary artery disease (8%) is unusual. Functional results are excellent in the 85% who survive, and only 7% are disabled.

The incidence of infection after a heart transplant is about 45%. Infections are more frequent and severe than those suffered by renal recipients but less than in liver or lung transplantation.

Solid organ transplant recipients share a common immunosuppressive regimen which is associated with a predictable time line of posttransplant infectious complications. Both predominant site of infection and offending microorganism will depend strongly on this chronology.

Infections may be classified into three categories (see also Chapter 7.0, section 1.4): early infections (those occurring during the first month after operation); intermediate infections (from 1–6 months after operation); and late infections (those detected after 6 months):

- Early infections are usually nosocomially acquired and do not differ significantly from the infections in other patients who have undergone heart surgery. Infections transmitted with the allograft and infections previously present in the recipient may also appear at this time.

- From months 1–6, patients suffer infections caused by opportunistic pathogens secondary to the immunosuppressive therapy that must be administered to avoid rejection. Heart transplant recipients are at greatest risk for life-threatening infection in the first 3 months after transplantation.
- After month 6, if chronic rejection is not present, community-acquired infections predominate. However, microorganisms specifically associated with immunosuppression have continued to be responsible for 27% of infections occurring more than 1 year after transplantation in some series. A precipitating event (rejection necessitating bolus therapy, surgery, etc.) may sometimes be identified before the development of a serious late infection.

Overall survival rate for the first year after heart transplantation in adults is 79%. From the second year and subsequently, approximately 4% of patients die each year. Infection is a leading cause of death (30% of early deaths, 45% of deaths between 1 and 3 months and 9.7% thereafter). The operative mortality rate remains at approximately 10% and sepsis is the major contributor to death in patients who survive the operation but die in hospital. In the intermediate period, acute rejection and infection are responsible for a similar proportion of deaths. Later, the most common causes of death are cardiac allograft vasculopathy, malignancy and acute rejection.

I REGARDING THE CLINICAL PRESENTATION AND EVALUATION OF THE PATIENT (Table 7.3.1)

1.1 What are the clinically predominant modes of presentation of infection in heart transplant recipients?

Most common presentation complaints are fever without obvious site of infection and fever with upper or lower respiratory tract manifestations.

Fever without a defined site of infection

Fever is a usual alarm sign in most immunosuppressed patients. Fever with no localizing signs soon after operation may represent a deep wound infection, a secondary bacteremia related to pneumonia, tracheobronchitis, urinary tract or catheter-related infection. If the patient is still intubated and the chest radiograph does not reveal infiltrates, the possibility of a nosocomial bacterial sinusitis should be considered. This infection mainly complicates nasotracheal intubation or nasogastric feeding tube due to irritation of the nasal mucosa, resulting in mucosal edema and obstruction of sinus drainage. Pericardial effusions and mediastinal bleeding should also be considered.

Knowledge of the serologic status of both the recipient and donor is of the utmost importance. For example, the possibility of a primary infection should be suspected immediately if a seronegative recipient receives a heart from a cytomegalovirus (CMV) or *Toxoplasma*-positive donor and the patient is not receiving prophylaxis. Drug fever is another possibility and induction therapy with OKT3 or antithymocyte globulin (ATG) is frequently accompanied by the presence of fever spikes.

Subsequently (after the first month), the initial suspicion in a patient who presents with fever of undetermined origin should focus on possible CMV reactivation, especially if the patient has leukopenia and mild hepatitis. Other infections should also be excluded if CMV is not confirmed.

Rejection may also occasionally be a cause of fever, although this is not common after heart transplantation. Endomyocardial biopsy and standard microbiologic techniques are usually necessary in this setting, but determination of serum procalcitonin level may

Table 7.3.1 Evaluation of infections in heart transplant recipients according to the site of infection and the possible etiologic agent

Site of infection	Infectious syndrome (clinical features)	Predominant pathogens	Diagnostic investigations
Bloodstream	Bacteremia (fever with or without local signs of infection)	Coagulase-negative staphylococci Staphylococcus aureus Streptococcus pneumoniae Enterococcus spp. (nosocomial outbreaks in some institutions) Gram-negative bacilli (Pseudomonas aeruginosa, Escherichia coli, Klebsiella pneumoniae, Salmonella spp.) Listeria monocytogenes Candida spp.	Blood cultures (two or three sets drawn from separate sites)
Intravascular catheter-related infections	Pain, erythema, tenderness, discharge from catheter entry site	Coagulase-negative staphylococci Staphylococcus aureus Bacillus spp. Gram-negative bacilli (especially Pseudomonas spp.) Candida spp., Malassezia furfur, Aspergillus spp., Mucor spp. (uncommon) Atypical mycobacteria (Mycobacterium fortuitum, Mycobacterium chelonae)	Swab of entry site and hub Culture of catheter tip Blood cultures (consider drawing blood through each lumen of catheter and doing quantitative blood cultures)
Heart	Endocarditis Pericarditis	Staphylococcus aureus Enterococcus spp. Gram-negative bacilli Coagulase-negative staphylococci Viridans streptococci Aspergillus spp. Candida spp.	Blood cultures Echocardiography Biopsy Culture of pericardial fluid
	Myocarditis	Toxoplasma gondii Cytomegalovirus	

Site of infection	Infectious syndrome (clinical features)	Predominant pathogens	Diagnostic investigations
Oral cavity	Stomatitis/mucositis (aphthae, ulcers) Oral thrush (white plaques)	Herpes simplex virus *Candida* spp.	Direct examination of sample Culture
Throat	Pharyngitis Tonsilitis (sore throat, odynophagia)	*Streptococcus pyogenes* Epstein–Barr virus Adenovirus, rhinovirus, coronavirus Influenza, parainfluenza Herpes simplex virus	Swab of pharynx Serology ELISA, Fluorescence
Lower respiratory tract (bronchi, terminal airways, alveoli)	Bronchopneumonia Pneumonia (cough, dyspnea, chest pain, sputum, hemoptysia, pleural effusion)	Conventional infections: *Streptococcus pneumoniae* *Haemophilus influenzae* Gram-negative bacilli (*Escherichia coli.* *Klebsiella pneumoniae. Pseudomonas aeruginosa. Acinetobacter* spp.) *Legionella* spp. (sporadic outbreaks) *Moraxella catarrhalis* (late onset) *Mycoplasma pneumoniae* (late onset) *Chlamydia pneumoniae* (late onset) Opportunistic infections: Cytomegalovirus *Aspergillus* spp. *Pneumocystis carinii* *Nocardia asteroides* *Mycobacterium tuberculosis* *Rhodococcus equi* *Cryptococcus neoformans*	Chest X-ray, CT, MRI Serology Fiberoptic bronchoscopy with bronchoalveolar lavage Transbronchial biopsy Thoracocentesis Thoracoscopy with biopsy Open lung biopsy

Skin and soft tissue infection	Surgical wound Mediastinitis Osteomyelitis	*Staphylococcus aureus* Coagulase-negative staphylococci Gram-negative bacilli *Candida* spp. *Aspergillus* spp. *Mycobacterium* spp. *Mycoplasma hominis* *Legionella* spp.	Skin swab Aspiration (needle) Skin biospy (histology and culture) Radiographs sometimes helpful
	Folliculitis Cellulitis (pain, erythema, tenderness, necrosis in case of ecthyma gangrenosum)	Primary infections: Coagulase-negative staphylococci *Staphylococcus aureus* Gram-negative bacilli (*Pseudomonas aeruginosa, Escherichia coli, Klebsiella pneumoniae*) *Candida* spp. *Mucor* spp., *Rhizopus* spp., *Absidia* spp. *Trichophyton* spp., *Microsporum* spp. *Epidermophyton* spp.	
	Papules, nodules (with or without myalgia anc muscle tenderness)	Disseminated infections: *Fusarium* spp. *Aspergillus* spp. Gram-negative bacilli (*Escherichia coli, Pseudomonas aeruginosa, Aeromonas hydrophila, Serratia marcescens*) Epstein–Barr virus, adenovirus	
	Ulcers, vesicles, hemorrhagic or crusted lesions (isolated or with dermatomal distribution)	Herpes simplex virus Varicella zoster virus Cytomegalovirus	
	Disseminated vesicles, hemorrhagic or crusted lesions	Varicella zoster virus, herpes simplex virus *Staphylococcus aureus*, group A streptococci	

Site of infection	Infectious syndrome (clinical features)	Predominant pathogens	Diagnostic investigations
	Skin necrosis (toes, fingers) secondary to thrombosis of blood vessels	Aspergillus spp., Mucor spp.	
	Warts	Papillomavirus	
	Molluscum contagiosum	Poxvirus-related virus	
Urinary tract	Urinary tract infections (dysuria, i.e. frequency, urgency; pain; hematuria; flank pain)	Gram-negative bacilli (Escherichia coli, Klebsiella spp., Proteus spp., Enterobacter spp., Pseudomonas aeruginosa) Enterococcus spp. Staphylococcus aureus Coagulase-negative staphylococci (Staphylococcus saprophyticus) Candida spp.	Culture of urine Ultrasonography, CT (if suspicion of renal abscess)
Gastrointestinal tract:			
Esophagus	Esophagitis (dysphagia, retrosternal pain)	Herpes simplex virus Candida spp., Aspergillus spp. Cytomegalovirus	Plain abdominal films Esophagogastroscopy Colonoscopy
Small intestine, colon	Enteritis Colitis (nausea, vomiting, bloating, abdominal discomfort, cramp, pain, constipation, diarrhea)	Salmonella spp., Campylobacter spp., Listeria monocytogenes (all three are associated with a high rate of bacteremia) Clostridium difficile (antibiotic-associated diarrhea) Cytomegalovirus	Ultrasonography CT-Scan, MR Culture of endoscopicl specimens Stool cultures Toxin detection

Diverticulitis	Strongyloides stercoralis Cryptosporidium	
Liver Spleen Hepatitis	Cytomegalovirus, Herpes simplex Primary viral hepatitis (A, B, C, δ)	Biopsy Serology
Biliary tract Cholecystitis Cholangitis	Aerobic Gram-negative bacilli (Escherichia coli, Klebsiella pneumoniae, Proteus spp., Enterobacter spp., Pseudomonas aeruginosa) Anaerobic bacilli (Clostridium spp., Bacteroides spp.) Enterococcus spp. Candida spp.	Ultrasonography CT, MRI Biopsy (histology and culture)
Central nervous system * Acute meningitis Subacute, chronic meningitis	Listeria monocytogenes Cryptococcus neoformans Candida spp. Mycobacterium tuberculosis Strongyloides stercoralis Coccidioides immitis Histoplasma capsulatum	CT, MRI Lumbar puncture Aspiration or biopsy under stereotaxic CT guidance
Focal brain disease	Aspergillus spp., Mucor spp. Nocardia asteroides Listeria monocytogenes Toxoplasma gondii Viruses (herpes simplex virus, varicella, cytomegalovirus, Epstein–Barr virus, human herpesvirus 6, adenovirus, papillomavirus, JC virus)	
Progressive dementia	JC virus, herpes virus, cytomegalovirus, Epstein–Barr virus (progressive multifocal leukoencephalopathy)	

* Transplant patients have the same susceptibility to convent oral pathogens of the central nervous system (meningitis: Streptococcus pneumoniae, Neisseria meningitidis, Haemophilus influenzae, Gram-negative bacilli; brain abscess: streptococci, Bacteroides spp., Staphylococcus aureus, Enterobacteriaceae) as the general population. Listed above are unique pathogens.

also help in differentiating between rejection and infection. In some series, procalcitonin values over 1 ng/ml were related with nonviral infections, while values over 10 ng/ml were found in patients with systemic infections or in septic patients. Values for patients with rejection did not differ significantly from those of the healthy transplant recipients.

Fever with a clinically documented site of infection

The main clinical characteristics of pneumonias after heart transplantation are fever (86%), cough (63%), costal pain (32%), dyspnea (52%), purulent expectoration (52%) and bloody expectoration (15%). Tachypnea and hypoxia are important clinical clues and correlate with the severity of the infection.

Mucocutaneous infections may have quite different presentations (nodules, papules, vesicles, rashes, erythematous indurated areas and necrosis) and they should never be dismissed as irrelevant in an immunocompromised host. Skin lesions may be primary to the skin or may provide a means to diagnose a systemic infection.

Gastrointestinal symptoms have been present in up to 51% of heart transplant patients in recent series, although only 15% are significant enough to warrant endoscopic, radiologic or surgical procedures. Possible manifestations include gastrointestinal bleeding, diarrhea, abdominal pain, jaundice, nausea or vomiting, odynophagia or dysphagia. Hepatobiliary, peptic ulcer and pancreatic complications are the most prevalent.

Infection of the upper gastrointestinal tract with CMV is a major cause of morbidity in cardiac transplant patients. In one series 53 of 201 heart transplant patients had persistent upper gastrointestinal symptoms (abdominal pain, nausea and vomiting). Of the 53 patients, 16 (30%) had diffuse erythema or ulceration of the gastric mucosa ($n = 14$), esophagus ($n = 1$) and duodenum ($n = 1$) with biopsy results that were positive for CMV on viral cultures. All patients with positive biopsy results were treated with intravenous ganciclovir at a dose of 10 mg/kg daily in two divided doses for a period of 2 weeks. Recurrence developed in six of the 16 patients, and necessitated repeated therapy with ganciclovir. None of the 16 patients died as a result of gastrointestinal CMV infection. Esophageal candidiasis and *Helicobacter* infection are probably underreported in cardiac transplant recipients.

Fever and loose stools most commonly represent antibiotic-associated diarrhea, *Clostridium difficile* infection or CMV disease.

Central nervous system (CNS) manifestations are uncommon. They include acute meningitis, subacute meningitis, meningoencephalitis and focal mass lesions. Brain abscesses occur in 1% of heart transplant recipients.

Ophthalmic complications were detected in 59 (44%) of 133 heart transplant patients in one series. However, fever was not common in this setting. The most frequent problem was lens changes, which is typical of prolonged oral corticosteroid therapy. CMV retinitis was found in only two (3%) of the 59 patients.

Microbiologically documented infections

In the authors' experience, 92% of defined infectious episodes detected in heart transplant recipients can be documented microbiologically. The diagnostic yield is enhanced by a very close collaboration between the microbiology laboratory and the infectious diseases clinicians. The most frequently recovered microorganisms are CMV (33%), herpes virus (20%), bacteria (24%), fungi (9%) and others (6%).

Clinically documented infection

Syndromes most commonly diagnosed on a clinical basis are upper and lower respiratory tract infections. In the authors' experience 29% of the pneumonias and 33% of upper respiratory tract infections had a negative culture. A definite underlying cause is usually established for almost all nosocomial pneumonias in heart transplant patients, but in most series 15–30% of respiratory tract infections elude a microbiologic diagnosis. Prior administration of antimicrobial therapy may impede the diagnosis of the causative microorganism.

Bacteremia

Bacteremia is not uncommon in this population. We detected 26 episodes in 19 of 100 heart transplant patients analyzed. The most common microorganisms were: *Staphylococcus epidermidis, Pseudomonas aeruginosa, Streptococcus aureus, Enterococcus faecalis, Escherichia coli, Klebsiella pneumoniae, Listeria monocytogenes, Salmonella enteritidis* and *Streptococcus pneumoniae.* Some 60% of the episodes occurred in the first 3 months after transplantation and four were catheter-related. Late bacteremias were due to community-acquired infections.

1.2 What are the predominant sites of infection? (see Table 7.3.1)

In the authors' experience, and considering all postoperative periods together, the predominant infectious complications include disseminated (i.e. systemic) syndromes (29%), pneumonia (18%), stomatitis (18%), urinary tract infection (UTI) (12%), catheter-related (7%), gastrointestinal tract (7%), skin and soft tissues (3%) and others (4%). When only severe infections are considered, the frequencies are lung, 28–31%; blood, 26–33%; gastrointestinal tract, 17–18%; UTI, 9–12%; wound, 7–9%; skin 7–8%; endocarditis, 2–6%; CNS, 1%; soft tissue, 1%; pericardium 0.4–1%.

In the first month following transplant, the predominant sites of infection are pneumonia, catheter-related infections, antibiotic-associated diarrhea, stomatitis and surgical site infections. Special attention should be paid to postsurgical mediastinitis (2–9%) (a complication unique to this type of transplantation).

Disseminated infections become predominant in the intermediate period, caused mainly by CMV, although pneumonia is still quite common.

Infective endocarditis is a relatively rare complication of heart transplantation. Most series refer to an incidence of 2–6%. Most of the cases are associated with previous nosocomial infections, mainly venous access devices and wound infections. Interestingly 80% of solid organ transplant patients who developed endocarditis in one series had no previous history of valvular disease.

1.3 What are the predominant organisms that contribute (by site)? (see Table 7.3.1)

Immunosuppressed patients are susceptible to infection by any microorganism; the most common will be highlighted.

Oropharyngeal infections

Most common etiologies are herpes simplex virus (HSV) and *Candida* spp. HSV presents as painful vesicular lesions of the oral mucosa (the lips and face may also be involved). One series reported that children receiving immunosuppression for cardiac transplantation may be at risk for head and neck infections from unusual or unsuspected organisms [82 head and neck infections in 27 (61%) of 44 patients]. There were 26 episodes of sinusitis, 27 of otitis media and 20 episodes of tonsilitis/pharyngitis. Unusual middle-ear pathogens included *Morganella morganii* and *P. aeruginosa*.

Pneumonia

The characteristics of pneumonias in the first year after transplantation have been studied in a multiinstitutional review of 307 heart transplant recipients in Spain. There were 21 cases of pneumonia per 100 heart transplants and 75% of these occurred in the first trimester. Approximately 60% were caused by opportunistic microorganisms, 25% by nosocomial pathogens and 15% by community-acquired bacteria and mycobacteria. The most frequent isolates were CMV (20), *Aspergillus* spp. (13) and *Pneumocystis carinii* (11).

Opportunistic microorganisms

Pneumonia caused by opportunistic organisms in heart transplant patients is often polymicrobial, ranging from 25% to 60% of the cases in various studies, with CMV the most common co-infection. The presence of CMV is generally associated with a poor prognosis, although it is not clear whether it should be treated when detected in association with *P. carinii* pneumonia (PCP). *P. carinii* and *Aspergillus* spp. are less commonly found as coinfections.

CMV is the microorganism that most frequently causes pneumonia after heart transplantation (accounting for approximately one quarter of cases), with an overall incidence of five to eight cases per 100 heart transplants.

Aspergillus is the second cause of pneumonia (16% of isolates; an incidence of 4% in the first year posttransplant) in the authors' study. The overall incidence of invasive aspergillosis in heart transplant patients has decreased in recent years: it was 25% before the cyclosporin A era and decreased to 3–14% after the routine use of cyclosporin. It is the most frequent invasive mycosis affecting heart transplant recipients and is still responsible for significant morbidity and mortality. Aspergillosis should be considered in the differential diagnosis of every lung infection in a heart transplant patient. *Aspergillus fumigatus* predominates, although other species have also been found.

P. carinii is the third cause of pneumonia (13% of isolates) in the authors' study. The incidence was four cases per 100 heart transplants (2–8% in other studies). Prophylactic cotrimoxazole (trimethoprim–sulfamethoxazole) reduces the incidence of PCP to virtually zero. The period of highest risk for PCP is the first 2–6 months posttransplant, when immunosuppressive therapy is more intense. PCP is sometimes concurrent with the tapering of steroids and the recovery of the inflammatory response. The mortality rate associated with PCP in human immunodeficiency virus (HIV)-negative patients is significantly higher than that in HIV-infected patients, reaching 50% in some series. Other factors associated with the poor outcome from PCP include cyclosporin immunosuppression, an older age, the need for mechanical ventilation, low serum albumin concentration and CMV coinfection.

The incidence of *Nocardia* pneumonia (2–13%) has also been reduced significantly since the widespread use of cotrimoxazole prophylaxis. It is usually a late infection that may present as nodular asymptomatic lung infiltrates. CNS and skin involvement must be investigated.

Rhodococcus equi is an opportunistic pathogen that may also cause pneumonia in heart transplant recipients. Infection with *Rhodococcus* presents with nodules, a consolidated alveolar pattern or cavitation.

The incidence of pulmonary tuberculosis in heart transplant recipients in Spain (1%) is 20–25 times higher than that in the general population. *Mycobacterium tuberculosis* infection in nonrenal transplant recipients has been described almost exclusively in Europe and the United States, and the frequency ranges from 1% to 1.4%. In the authors' experience, tuberculosis was diagnosed a median of 76 days after transplantation.

Nontuberculous mycobacteria are an exceptional cause of pneumonia after heart transplantation.

Nosocomial bacteria

Taking all microorganisms together, nosocomial bacteria are the leading cause of pneumonia in the posttransplant period (29% in the authors' series: 6.9 episodes per 100 heart transplants). Gram-negative rods (57%), especially nonfermenting bacteria, predominate (*Acinetobacter baumannii, P. aeruginosa*). Nosocomial pneumonia occurs predominantly in the early posttransplant period. In nosocomial outbreaks, the incidence of *Legionella pneumophila* pneumonia following heart transplantation ranges from 0.5% to 8%.

Community-acquired bacteria

Haemophilus influenzae and *S. pneumoniae* are the most common community-acquired bacteria causing pneumonia following cardiac transplantation. Community-acquired pneumonia occurs particularly during the intermediate and late posttransplant periods. The incidence of pneumococcal pneumonia among heart transplant patients ranges from 2% to 3.6% (one case per 100 heart transplants in the authors' study) and is clearly higher than that in the general population. Accordingly, vaccination is recommended.

Influenza virus, parainfluenza virus, parvovirus B19, respiratory syncytial virus (RSV), HSV, *Mucor* spp. *Toxoplasma gondii*, regional mycoses and *Strongyloides stercoralis* are unusual causes of pneumonia in heart transplant patients.

Late pneumonias

After 6 months posttransplant, community-acquired pathogens (*S. pneumoniae, Moraxella catarrhalis*, respiratory viruses) predominate in patients without chronic rejection. However, *P. carinii, Nocardia asteroides, Cryptococcus neoformans* and even CMV may present late after transplantation. The age of the patients, severity at presentation, speed of evolution, radiologic manifestations, occupation, travel history, animal exposure and many other factors provide useful clues to the microbial etiology of a given case.

Adenovirus pneumonia also has been reported after cardiac transplantation. Chest radiography usually shows bilateral diffuse interstitial infiltrates and occasionally pleural effusions. This complication is associated with a significant mortality rate, which may exceed 60%.

Outcome of pneumonia

Pneumonia is one of the leading causes of death after heart transplantation. Mechanical ventilation is required in 37% and death occurs in 23–31% of the patients. This rate varies widely depending on the etiology, *Aspergillus* pneumonia having the worst prognosis. The mortality rate was 13% for CMV pneumonia and 26% for nosocomial pneumonia (50% among patients receiving ventilatory support).

Disseminated infections

As mentioned above, early after transplantation the most common causes of disseminated infections are catheter-associated bacteremias, pneumonia, wound- or urinary tract-related bacteremias. Gram-positive microorganisms predominate in patients receiving quinolone prophylaxis. However, Gram-negative organisms and *Candida* should also be considered.

Later in the posttransplant period, disseminated infections are usually caused by CMV. Less commonly *Toxoplasma*, other viruses [varicella zoster virus (VZV), human herpesvirus-6 (HHV-6), adenovirus], *M. tuberculosis*, or fungal pathogens may be isolated.

CMV is the most common etiologic agent infecting heart transplant recipients. Without prophylaxis, 30–90% of patients show laboratory evidence of CMV replication and 10–90% have associated clinical manifestations (CMV disease). The likelihood of disease depends on the serologic status of both recipient and donor.

Primary infection [seronegative receptor/seropositive donor (R–/D+)] is symptomatic in a high proportion of cases; the most common source of the virus is the transplanted allograft and, less commonly, blood products. The mortality rate of primary infection ranges from 6% to 28%.

Positive recipients (R+) may suffer either reactivation of their own CMV or an infection by viruses transmitted with the allograft. This latter situation results more commonly in symptomatic infection than reactivation (40% versus 20%). Finally, 10–25% of patients who have suffered CMV disease will have recurrence at a later time period.

EBV commonly infects transplant patients, although it is rarely symptomatic. It may result in posttransplant lymphoproliferative disorder (PTLD), which may affect up to 2% of heart transplant recipients. The presentation varies from local invasion of the allograft to disseminated disease with extranodal or CNS involvement.

Patients with toxoplasmosis have fever, altered mental status, focal neurologic signs, myalgia, myocarditis or lung infiltrates. Organ-transmitted infection in a serologically naive recipient is often associated with acute disease (61%), while reactivation of latent infection is less frequent (7%).

Central nervous system infections

Acute meningitis is usually caused by *L. monocytogenes* and subacute or chronic meningitis by *C. neoformans*. However, other pathogens may present in a similar way (*M. tuberculosis, Histoplasma capsulatum, N. asteroides, S. stercoralis*). Therapy with OKT3 monoclonal antibody has been related to the production of acute aseptic meningitis [cerebrospinal fluid (CSF) pleocytosis with negative cultures, fever and transient cognitive dysfunction].

Focal brain infection (seizures or focal neurologic abnormalities) may be caused by *Listeria, T. gondii* (commonly at 3 months posttransplant), fungi (*Aspergillus, Mucorales*), PTLD or *Nocardia* (at 5 months). Finally, progressive dementia of infectious origin has been related to JC virus, HSV, CMV and Epstein–Barr virus (EBV).

Pyogenic bacterial brain abscess is quite uncommon in this patient population. *Aspergillus* is the principal causative organism, followed by *T. gondii* and *N. asteroides*.

Surgical wound infection, mediastinitis and osteomyelitis

The most common site of osteomyelitis is the sternum, and the predominant cause is bacterial pathogens (Staphylococci, Gram-negative rods). However, *Candida, Mycobacterium* spp., *Legionella, Mycoplasma, Aspergillus* and other nonbacterial etiologies have also been described. Most of these infections occur early after the transplantation procedure (median 9 days), although cases caused by *Nocardia, Mycoplasma* and other uncommon microorganisms may appear later.

Cardiac infections

For infective endocarditis, the etiology of 15 cases described in heart transplant recipients were *S. aureus* (4), *Enterococcus* spp. (2), Gram-negative bacilli (2), coagulase-negative staphylococci (2), viridans streptococci (1), *Aspergillus fumigatus* (1), *Candida* (1) and polymicrobial (2).

Early pericardial complications include aspergillosis and bacterial infections, hemopericardium and rejection. Late complications are more frequently related to epicarditis and the transplant-associated coronary disease (chronic rejection), in which lymphoplasmocytic nodules and a myocardial vasculitis are the predominant histopathologic features.

CMV or *Toxoplasma* causes myocarditis in this population. Other pathogens, such as parvovirus B19, have also been described.

Mucocutaneous infections

Opportunistic viral and fungal infections are the leading causes of skin lesions in heart transplant patients. Bacteria cause 2–25% of dermatologic lesions in transplant patients (folliculitis, wound infection, cellulitis and abscesses).

Among the herpesviruses, HSV, VZV and, less commonly, CMV, cause cutaneous lesions in this population. HSV may cause oral, anogenital or cutaneous lesions (including herpetic whitlow). CMV has been related to localized skin ulcers, maculopapular eruptions, vasculitis, purpura and vesiculobullous lesions. VZV lesions consist of vesicular lesions following a dermatomal distribution. Both VZV disseminated cutaneous infections and spread to organ systems may occur. Papillomavirus infections are also common, and the high tendency toward malignant degeneration should always be considered. Rarely mycobacteria or *Nocardia* may be isolated.

Fungi may cause primary skin lesions. The most common are *Aspergillus* and *Mucor*. Other fungi like *Cryptococcus*, *Coccidioides* or *Histoplasma* may also produce cutaneous manifestations, especially in patients residing in or originating from endemic areas. Finally, dermatophytes may cause extensive lesions in this population.

Gastrointestinal infections

Candida and HSV cause esophagitis. Erosive gastritis and colonic ulcers are usually caused by CMV, which may involve both the upper and lower gastrointestinal tract. The incidence of gastrointestinal CMV infection is 8% in some series, with 37.5% recurrence in spite of prompt therapy. Symptoms may include abdominal pain, fever, diarrhea or hematochezia. The prognosis is good, although it may lead to perforation and even death if unrecognized.

Long-term use of steroid therapy is associated with a high risk of acute colonic diverticulitis (4% in one series) and perforation. Anatomic abnormalities need to be diagnosed and occasionally corrected before transplantation (e.g. pretransplant colectomy for significant diverticular disease or in patients who have developed diverticulitis in the past). However, prophylactic colectomy cannot be performed safely in heart transplant patients with terminal heart failure.

In the authors' experience 17% of heart transplant recipients suffer *C. difficile*-related diarrhea. All patients had received antimicrobials before the episode. Liquid diarrhea was present in all the patients, with a median of 10 movements per day. Other manifestations were abdominal pain (29%), fever (14%) and gastrointestinal bleeding (14%).

Patients exposed to foodborne pathogens (*Salmonella*, *Campylobacter*, *L. monocytogenes*) may develop severe diarrheal disease with a higher incidence of positive blood cultures. It may be promoted by opportunistic infection of the digestive tract.

Urinary tract infections
UTIs are frequent in heart transplant patients. Enterobacteriaceae, enterococci, *Candida* and *S. aureus* are the most common etiologies. The possibility of mycobacterial infection should be investigated in the presence of sterile pyuria.

Ophthalmic infections
As mentioned above, most ocular problems after heart transplantation are of noninfectious origin. However, CMV, *Cryptococcus*, VZV and HSV can cause eye disease in this patient population.

Intraabdominal infections
Pancreatitis is rare after heart transplantation, although cyclosporin, azathioprine, corticosteroid, CMV infection and surgery involving cardiovascular bypass have each been independently associated with an increased risk of acute pancreatitis.

Hepatitis following heart transplantation is usually caused by CMV. However, hepatitis B virus (HBV) and hepatitis C virus (HCV) have also been described (see section 3).

Symptomatic cholelithiasis was described in 6.7% of 90 cases of pediatric heart or heart–lung transplants at one center. Studies concerning the incidence of gallstones in adult kidney and cardiac transplant patients have shown that there is an increased risk associated with cyclosporin, possibly related to raised serum levels and hepatoxicity. Cases of acalculous cholecystitis have also been reported in the cardiac transplant population.

1.4 How do the organisms vary according to various risk factors?
Various risk factors may increase the possibility of infection caused by a particular organism:

State of health before transplantation
Patients in a poor state of health before transplantation (chronic congestive heart failure, intubation, cardiac cachexia) should be evaluated carefully for bacterial infection before the procedure. Bacterial pneumonia and UTI is more common in patients with previous predisposing conditions (chronic obstructive pulmonary disease and prostatic hyperplasia, respectively). Finally, the underlying disease that leads to transplantation may influence later infections. For example, ischemic cardiomyopathy was overrepresented in heart transplant recipients presenting with PCP in the authors' experience (78.5%), while this underlying disease was present in only 25% of their overall heart transplant patient population.

Postsurgical complications
The risk of nosocomial bacterial infections is increased in patients with postsurgical complications, reintervention, bleeding, prolonged mechanical ventilation, intravenous catheters or mechanical circulatory support.

Immunosuppression and serologic status
The drugs, dosage, duration and temporal sequence in which immunosuppressive agents are given will influence the relative incidence of opportunistic infections (see section 2.1).

Cytomegalovirus
Increased immunosuppression or administration of OKT3 or ATG as induction or rescue therapy increases the risk of earlier and more frequent viral infection. Antilymphocyte

antibodies may reactivate CMV from latency due to cytokine release mediated by lymphocyte activation. Cyclosporin and tacrolimus are quite potent at amplifying the extent and consequences of CMV and other herpesvirus infections once active viral replication is present (see Chapter 7.0). However, the serologic status of the recipient and donor is the most important risk factor for CMV infection. Seronegative recipients with positive donors have the highest risk of primary severe disease. Massive transfusions will also increase the risk of CMV disease. Finally, CMV infection per se can increase the risk for other opportunistic infections in the host by depressing cell-mediated immunity.

Transmission of HHV-8 from the graft in renal transplant recipients has been demonstrated recently, and primary infection with this virus is a risk factor for transplantation-associated Kaposi sarcoma. The extent to which such transmission occurs in heart transplant recipients remains to be determined.

Fungi

Increased doses of immunosuppression heightens the risk of invasive aspergillosis. In the authors' experience, a rejection episode occurred in 64% of the patients some time during the 3 months before the episode, and in 26% of cases the rejection episode occurred concomitantly with the episode of invasive aspergillosis. Previous (56%) or concomitant (24%) bacterial infections were also common, most cases in pneumonia, bacteremia or surgical site infections. Almost half of the heart transplant patients had had CMV disease before the aspergillosis (47%), and in 54% of these it was present at the time of the diagnosis. Neutropenia was detected in only 9.7% of patients with invasive aspergillos, reintervention in 22% and allograft dysfunction in 15%. Finally, it has been suggested that toxic levels of cyclosporin A, especially when administered with steroids, may increase the risk of invasive aspergillosis by reducing the fungicidal properties of granulocytes.

Toxoplasma gondii infections are associated with significant morbidity and mortality in heart transplant patients. Organs from a seropositive donor may contain cysts, which may reactivate when the organ is transplanted into an antibody-negative recipient, thus producing a primary infection (see section 4.1 for prophylaxis recommendations).

Environmental exposure

Infections caused by multiresistant microorganisms [methicillin-resistant *S. aureus* (MRSA), vancomycin-resistant enterococci (VRE)] or *L. pneumophila* infection will be more common in centers with epidemic or endemic situations. Residency or travel to endemic areas as well as contact with an infected patient increases the risk of tuberculosis in heart transplant patients (see section 3). Increased environmental contamination is also an important risk factor for invasive aspergillosis, and outbreaks have been related to the contamination of air ducts.

Remote or recent exposure to geographically restricted systemic mycoses (*Blastomyces dermatitidis*, *Coccidioides immitis* and *Histoplasma capsulatum*) increases the risk of infection by these pathogens and should be carefully investigated. In a recent series from Arizona, 4.5% of heart transplant recipients suffered coccidioidomycosis.

Parasites other than toxoplasma are not a common cause of disease in solid organ transplant recipients. Travel to endemic regions and, in the future, xenotransplantation may result in the emergence of unusual parasitic complications in such recipients. It is essential to evaluate transplant candidates with residence or travel history in endemic zones to rule out that they harbor *S. stercoralis*. Human infection with this nematode is endemic in some tropical and warm areas of the world, including parts of Europe and southeastern United States. The clinical presentation of strongyloidiasis is multifaceted and the parasite may persist undetected for decades as a chronic, almost asymptomatic, infection. With immunosuppression, extensive tissue invasion may develop, producing life-threatening systemic syndromes. Patients should be carefully evaluated and treated before the immunosuppression is started.

Antimicrobial preventive strategies
Patients not receiving prophylaxis with cotrimoxazole have a higher risk of PCP, *Listeria* or *Nocardia* infections. The risk for PCP is heightened by the intensity and duration of immunosuppressive therapy. A dose of steroids equivalent to 30–40 mg of prednisone for a median of 8–12 weeks can increase the risk for PCP.

Other factors
With current immunosuppressive regimens, prolonged neutropenia and damage to mucocutaneous barriers are uncommon in organ transplant recipients (see Chapter 7.0).

1.5 How does this differ from other conditions, from center to center, and from country to country?

Differences with other conditions
The complexity of heart transplant surgery and the need of postsurgical mechanical ventilation, transfusions and central venous devices is higher than in renal transplantation but less than in liver transplantation. The rate of nosocomial infections parallels the complexity of surgery and the need for supportive care.

The intensity of immunusuppression differs according to the type of solid organ transplant, and is higher in heart than in kidney recipients.

In heart transplant recipients, as in all thoracic transplantations, both fatal and nonfatal infections involve the lung and are related to the underlying functional and anatomic conditions: chronic congestive heart failure before transplantation, intubation, cardiac cachexia, difficulty in coughing, chest tubes, postoperative atelectasis and microaspiration. This patient population may also suffer postsurgical mediastinitis, a complication unique to thoracic transplants. Heterotopic heart transplantation requires a prosthetic vascular conduit between the donor and the recipient pulmonary artery, which may become infected.

Finally, there is a higher susceptibility to some pathogens in heart transplant patients, some of which may be transmitted with the allograft (e.g. *Toxoplasma*). The risk of primary toxoplasmosis is greater in heart transplant-mismatched patients (more than 50%) than in either liver (20%) or kidney (< 1%) mismatched recipients.

Differences from center to center and country to country
Specific centers and countries may show differences in the incidence of a specific pathogen or complication. The population served and the incidence of latent infections usually account for most of these differences (e.g. tuberculosis or CMV). The intensity of the immunosuppressive regimen and the prophylaxis protocol may also be related to some of these differences in the patterns of infection.

Each center should know its own rate of antimicrobial resistance to guide empirical therapy and the incidence of highly resistant microorganisms like VRE, MRSA or multi-resistant *A. baumanii*. Environmental exposure differs among centers and countries.

Whenever an unexpectedly high incidence of antimicrobial resistance is reported, the possibility of outbreaks or specific nosocomial problems should also be considered (aspergillosis or legionellosis).

1.6 What is the appropriate approach to the initial evaluation and diagnosis of infection in heart transplant recipients?

The following approach is suggested:

a) Establish the severity of the patient's condition (blood pressure, heart and respiratory rate, blood gases, electrocardiogram, time of progression, careful physical examination) and carefully investigate the clinical presentation (symptoms, rate of progression). This will guide the subsequent measures to be taken.

b) Decide whether the management should be in the hospital (emergency room, transplant unit, intensive care unit) or as an outpatient. It should be remembered that most fatal infections occur within the first year following the transplant, a period when rejection must also be considered.

c) Take a careful history including risk factors for infection, such as exposures to animals, children, food or to ill people, the compliance to prophylactic regimens and to immunosuppressive agents, and the history of previous infections, surgical and non-surgical complications. Serologic data from donor and recipient should always be recorded (see section 3.1), as well as the history of travel or hobbies.

d) In most cases a careful diagnostic workup is necessary (oriented by the findings of the history and physical examination). Such workup usually includes:

- Imaging studies (chest radiography and others as clinically indicated).
- Obtaining samples for microbologic workup (blood, urine, respiratory samples, wound, etc). In addition to the search for bacteria, specific mycobacterial and fungal cultures should also be ordered. Polymicrobial infections should always be sought. Whenever necessary, direct examination of the samples, performed by an expert microbiologist adequately informed about the clinical situation, may reveal useful information. Antigen detection tests may also be performed (*Cryptococcus*, *Legionella*, group A streptococci).
- Viral investigation through cultures and other techniques is a routine in solid organ transplant patients at least in the first year [CMV antigenemia and when available more sophisticated techniques such as polymerase chain reaction (PCR)].
- Order invasive diagnostic procedures when clinically indicated.
- Serum samples should be stored for further workup when indicated.

e) Decide whether empirical therapy is needed.

1.7 How should the evaluation be modified according to the severity of the risk?

Mucocutaneous barriers damage

Patients who have damage to mucosal barriers should be evaluated primarily for bacterial, fungal or viral infections. Posttransplant reintubation and higher steroid dosages are significant risk factors for pneumonia after transplantation.

Immunosuppression state

Patients in critical condition or with previous rejection treated with aggressive immunosuppression should be evaluated expediently and appropriate diagnostic techniques should be performed as rapidly as possible. Opportunistic pathogens, particularly viruses and fungi, should be investigated and empirical therapy promptly initiated if necessary.

Epidemiologic exposure

Nosocomial outbreaks
If a nosocomial outbreak is detected in a center with a transplant program (especially aspergillosis, legionellosis, VRE, etc.), particular care should be taken in these highly immunosuppressed patients. The microorganisms causing the outbreak should be covered when choosing the empirical treatment in the presence of a severe infectious episode.

Exposure to environmental pathogens or infected patients
If a patient is known to have been in contact with pathogens like tuberculosis or endemic fungi, specific cultures and serologic tests should be performed even when clinical symptoms are absent. A high index of suspicion is required to establish the diagnosis of unusual infections like *S. stercoralis*, which should be considered in any immunosuppressed patients with eosinophilia, recurrent skin lesions, multiple pulmonary infiltrates, ileus with or without perforation, abdominal pain, malabsorption, meningitis or bacteremia. Chronic carriage is normal among individuals environmentally exposed, and has been found to persist for up to 30 years.

Malaria, *Borrelia*, *Leptospira*, etc., should be investigated if appropriate risk factors are found.

1.8 What are the specific evaluation measures? (See Chapter 2 in Part 1)

Evaluation methods according to clinical presentation

Nonfocal infection
Patients with fever without signs and symptoms of focal infection should have blood and urine cultures for bacteria, fungi, viruses and mycobacteria, as well as CMV antigenemia. Endemic mycotic infections should be excluded in regimens where these fungi are common. Patients with systemic candidiasis may have negative blood cultures. Other possibilities, such as cryptic abscesses or anicteric viral hepatitis, should also be excluded. A serum sample should be sent to the laboratory for further workup if the fever persists despite empirical treatment and no pathogen is identified. Less common etiologies are to be investigated, such as EBV, Q fever, syphilis, *Legionella*, *Brucella*, *Cryptococcus*, *Toxoplasma*, *Leishmania*, parvovirus B19 infection.

If all tests are negative but the patient remains febrile, the possibility of noninfectious causes should be considered, such as cardiac failure, lymphoma, drug fever, rejection, hematoma, pulmonary emboli and splenic infarction. Moreover, acute adrenal insufficiency in transplant patients in stress situations, such as admission to an intensive care unit, sepsis or surgery, should be kept in mind.

Pneumonia
Imaging techniques. Although radiographic [chest radiography, computed tomography (CT)] manifestations are not pathognomonic of any etiology, some may suggest particular pathogens. Alveolar infiltrates predominate in nosocomial pneumonia (95% versus 37% in the remaining pneumonias); interstitial infiltrates (82%) and bilateral extension (82%) are typical of PCP (13% and 33%, respectively, compared with other pneumonias);

and nodules (62% versus 8%) and cavitation (38% versus 4%) predominate in *Aspergillus* pneumonia.

CT is more sensitive than simple chest radiography for the diagnosis of pulmonary complications in immunodepressed patients. It improves the information obtained from a plain chest radiography in 33% of the cases (increasing the number of visible nodules, showing cavitation or serving for guiding transparietal puncture).

Etiological diagnosis. Only 50% of the empirical treatments prescribed in a multicenter study for pneumonia in heart transplant patients were appropriate. Therefore, rapid diagnostic procedures that guide antimicrobial treatment are indicated. Overall, bronchoscopy is the diagnostic procedure used most commonly for obtaining respiratory samples. The diagnostic sensitivity of the different procedures varies with the etiology but, considering all microorganisms isolated, the sensitivities in the authors' experience are: for sputum examination, 47%; for bronchoalveolar lavage (BAL), 89%; for telescoping plugged catheterization, 70%; for bronchial washings, 46%; for transbronchial biopsy, 50%; for open lung biopsy, 50%; for transthoracic pulmonary needle aspiration, 100%; and for blood culture, 24%. Serum samples should also be taken both in the acute phase and 4–6 weeks later.

If a bacterial etiology is suspected and the patient is not receiving antimicrobial agents, a transtracheal aspirate may be performed (assuming the clinical condition of the patient permits it). The sputum (if available) should be examined and *Legionella* antigen sought in urine, as well as serology and blood cultures. If the stains of the transtracheal aspirate fail to show the etiologic agent or this technique cannot be performed, or an opportunistic infection is suspected, BAL or a transthoracic pulmonary needle aspiration should be performed depending on the radiologic appearance (the latter is better for peripheral lung nodules).

Urinary tract infections

UTIs are usually diagnosed with semiquantitative urinary culture in conventional culture media. If nonbacterial pathogens are suspected, more prolonged incubation and the use of specific media should be asked for (fungi, mycobacteria, etc.). Abdominal echography, intravenous urography and prostatic investigations may be needed. Blood cultures are also recommended if sepsis is suspected.

Skin lesions

The presence of skin lesions in a heart transplant patient should lead to a careful search for a primary infection site. The standard approach is to perform a punch biopsy, which should be sent for rapid histologic examination and cultures for bacteria, viruses and fungi. Direct stains (Gram, Ziehl, potassium hydroxide, Giemsa, Tzanck smears) and antigen detection (for example of S. *pyogenes*) may be done from the biopsy or the aspirate. Blood cultures should also be ordered.

Intravascular infections

When there is an infection related to a difficult to replace catheter, there are some simple techniques that may predict the involvement of the device without removing it, including quantitative culture of the exit site and of the hub, as well as using the lysis-centrifugation blood culture technique for samples obtained from venipuncture as well as through the catheter. If the patient is unstable, the catheter should be removed and the tip sent to the laboratory. Intravascular infections other than those that are catheter related may be difficult to diagnose, since they may present with few specific signs or symptoms.

Recurrent bacteremia may be the clue. Transesophagic echocardiography examination and indium-111-labeled white blood cell scan are helpful tools for investigating the presence of endocarditis.

Central nervous system
An acute brain infarction or bleeding occurring in the first 3 months posttransplant should be assumed to be caused by *Aspergillus* until proven otherwise. Since the mortality rate may exceed 90% in most series, these patients should be diagnosed and treated aggressively. A brain CT scan should be rapidly ordered, possibly with biopsy and histologic examination and culture, since this is the most reliable method of diagnosis. Extraneural sites should be looked for, as they may be more easily accessible for sampling. Serology may be helpful in *Toxoplasma* infections.

A lumbar puncture should be promptly performed when meningitis is suspected. Stains and antigen detection techniques may provide prompt results. Cultures for bacteria, mycobacteria and viruses will be done. If tuberculosis is suspected, measurement of adenosine deaminase in the CSF may be a useful adjunctive marker in centers with experience with this test (specificity 60–87%, sensitivity 90–100%).

Gastrointestinal infections
In addition to conventional stool cultures, an endoscopic procedure is frequently needed. Ulcerative hemorrhagic mucositis has been the most common finding of CMV disease at colonoscopy, with sharply demarcated areas of ulceration and necrosis. CMV inclusion bodies may be demonstrated in the biopsy specimen, although their absence does not rule out CMV disease. Antigenemia is usually positive.

Evaluation method according to each particular microorganism (see Chapter 2 in Part I)
The diagnostic yield of any procedure may be reduced after 1–2 days of treatment. However, this should not preclude an attempt at diagnosis.

Viruses
For HSV and VZV, a Tzanck smear or fluorescent stain should be performed; culture in viral media for 48–72 h. For CMV, microscopic examination of samples may show the characteristic intranuclear inclusions. Immunoperoxidase staining methods or DNA hybridization techniques are also helpful for rapid diagnosis. Shell vial cultures can usually confirm the diagnosis in 48–72 h. Respiratory viruses can also be rapidly detected in respiratory tract samples.

Bacteria
Blood cultures as well as cultures from any other available site are mandatory in the initial evaluation. Appropriate culture and staining media should be ordered when unconventional pathogens are suspected (*Mycoplasma*, *Legionella*).

For *Mycobacteria*, Ziehl or auramine stain and culture in liquid or solid media provide the diagnosis. If nontuberculous mycobacteria are suspected, this should be notified to the laboratory.

With *Nocardia*, Gram and modified Ziehl stains of respiratory samples, skin biopsies or CNS abscesses may disclose the characteristic appearance of *Nocardia* (delicate Gram-positive branching filamentous rods). *Nocardia* can be grown in conventional culture media if long incubation is provided.

Fungus

In the authors' series, 78% of the patients with aspergillosis were diagnosed a median of 6 days after symptoms appeared. The most useful technique was BAL, followed by needle aspiration of nodular lesions.

Candida spp. will grow in conventional culture media. Non-albicans species may take longer than the usual 18 h incubation period; here again, the suspicion should be notified to the laboratory. Differential media, such as CHROMagar®, may provide a rapid identification of species. Long incubation blood cultures are no longer necessary when a fungemia is suspected, since new systems (continuous agitation) allow the detection of fungemia in a median of 3 days.

For *P. carinii*, the diagnostic yield of induced sputum is lower in solid organ transplant patients than in patients with acquired immune deficiency syndrome (AIDS), probably due to the smaller organism burden in these patients. Bronchoscopy is the cornerstone of the diagnostic workup, but the efficacy of BAL is slightly increased with the addition of transbronchial biopsy. New microbiologic techniques, such as indirect immunofluorescence or DNA amplification, improve the detection of *P. carinii* and are relatively easy to perform, although they are more expensive than conventional stains (methenamine silver, Giemsa and toluidine blue O stain).

Parasites

Serologic tests and direct stains should be used to diagnose most common parasitic infections in this population. *Toxoplasma* has been cultured from BAL and endomyocardial biopsies, although this is not a common procedure.

Serologic testing may be useful [positive immunoglobulin (Ig) M titer, seroconversion or increased antibody levels in CSF or vitreous fluid relative to those in peripheral blood].

Regarding strongyloidiasis, eosinophilia may be a clue (although it may be absent). Examining stool specimens with concentration procedures (Harada–Mori test) for rhabditiform larvae makes the diagnosis. Several stool specimens should be examined.

Leishmaniasis is a fairly uncommon complication of solid organ transplant patients. Diagnosis is based on the identification and isolation of the organism from bone marrow or other tissues. Serologic tests may also be useful.

1.9 What new developments are going to impact on emerging organisms, recognition, evaluation and diagnosis of infection in heart transplant recipients?

Developments in clinical microbiology provide new diagnostic techniques that permit faster and more sensitive and specific diagnosis. Molecular techniques such as quantitative PCR for CMV and other microorganisms will impact on the approach to both therapy and prophylaxis of infectious complications in heart transplant patients. However, the clinical impact of most of these expensive and still cumbersome tests remains to be proven. These methods have already an important role in the analysis of epidemiologic data. Investigation of the susceptibility pattern of both fungi and viruses will soon become routine and will help to select appropriate therapy. The role of CMV and *Chlamydia pneumoniae* in the development of cardiac allograft arteriosclerosis (the primary cause of late death in heart transplant patients) needs further elucidation.

The most important goal to achieve is the close collaboration among all those involved in the care of a transplant patient, such as infectious diseases specialists, clinical microbiologists, cardiologists, surgeons and immunologists.

Emerging pathogens

The term 'emerging pathogens' refers to infections that have appeared recently in the population or that have been previously recognized but are rapidly increasing in incidence or geographic distribution, or to infections that have been known but adopt an unusual severity.

Recent technical advances now permit very debilitated patients to remain alive. Consequently, low-virulence pathogens can become problems in this setting. For example, it is interesting to note that 65% of dematiaceous fungal infections following organ transplantation reported in one review occurred in the 1990s, suggesting that such fungi are emerging pathogens. They are usually late infections (2 years after transplantation) and usually affect the skin and/or soft tissue. The predominant pathogen was *Exophiala* spp.

Other examples include VRE, MRS and azole-resistant *Candida* spp., pathogens that have emerged as a substantive problem in some transplant units. Hepatitis viruses and HIV could be considered emerging pathogens in this patient population.

Pathogens such as HHV-8, HHV-6, parvovirus B19, *Bartonella* and many others might well be related to more and more clinical manifestations in heart transplant patients. For example, recently a case of a cardiac transplant recipient with hepatic and splenic bacillary epithelioid angiomatosis manifesting as a fever of unknown origin has been reported. The clinical manifestations of HHV-6 are not clearly defined in this population. HHV-6 may cause a CMV-like syndrome, and in fact dual infection has been described. Other manifestations include febrile seizures, encephalitis, pneumonia, exanthema subitum and bone marrow suppression.

Finally, when xenotransplantation becomes a reality, there will need to be an awareness of new infections transmitted from animals.

2 REGARDING THE RISK FACTORS IN HEART TRANSPLANT RECIPIENTS

2.1 What are the main alterations in host defense mechanisms and what are the appropriate investigations to document them?

Heart transplant recipients need lifelong immunosuppression to avoid rejection of the allograft. Most regimens include cyclosporin, azathioprine and low-dose prednisone.

The use of steroids is associated with phagocytic neutrophil defects through various mechanisms. When high doses are administered, inhibition of specific antibody production and reduction of immunoglobulin levels may occur. This effect is maximal after 2–4 weeks. This is why, in the last decades, steroid-sparing regimens have been developed.

Azathioprine inhibits DNA and RNA synthesis, thus inhibiting both humoral and cellular immunity. It is a potent immunosuppressive agent with few cytotoxic effects, although it may be myelotoxic.

Cyclosporin A reduces the production and release of cytokines by T-lymphocytes. It diminishes the proliferation of activated and cytotoxic T-cells, while maintaining suppressor T-cell levels. It is not myelotoxic and its effects disappear rapidly when the drug administration is discontinued.

Tacrolimus is a newer immunosuppressive drug that is now used both as a primary immunosuppressive agent and as rescue therapy. It inhibits the production and release of interleukin-2 (IL-2), the expression of IL-2 receptors, and the activation of T-cells secondary to antigen stimulation, at a dose 100–1000 times lower than that of cyclosporin. Its use has been associated with lower rejection and infection rates than those seen after cyclosporin treatment. Tacrolimus appears to be more steroid sparing than cyclosporin. Unfortunately, it is nephrotoxic and neurotoxic, and may induce a generalized vasculitis.

Both tacrolimus and cyclosporin levels may be influenced by interactions with other drugs (see Chapter 7.1, section 2.2). The use of drugs that reduce their serum levels (rifampicin, sulfadiazine) may lead to rejection, and drugs that increase their serum levels (azoles, erythromycin, methylprednisolone and calcium antagonists) may produce severe nephrotoxicity (3–6% of heart transplant recipients surviving 3 years require hemodialysis). In addition, toxic levels of cyclosporin are reported to increase the susceptibility to certain infections such as invasive aspergillosis. In view of these interactions, treatment of pneumonia, tuberculosis, VRE or fungal infections, amongst others, is more difficult in the transplant recipient.

The new agent mycophenolate mofetil has been used in heart transplant recipients with frequent rejection episodes. It is a potent inhibitor of de-novo guanine nucleotide synthesis that selectively blocks lymphocyte proliferative responses. Mycophenolate is safe and well tolerated in cardiac transplant recipients, is less myelosuppressive than azathioprine, and appears to have at least as potent immunosuppressive properties as cyclosporin. Mycophenolate use has been associated in some series with the development of more common CMV infections.

As mentioned above, the main toxicities of the immunosuppressive agents are nephrotoxicity in the case of cyclosporin, and leukopenia in the case of azathioprine. Accordingly, serum levels of cyclosporin should be carefully monitored (serum trough levels at 100–300 ng/ml for the first month and 100–150 ng/ml thereafter) and the dose of azathioprine adjusted to a peripheral white blood cell count of 4000–6000/mm^3

Several studies have demonstrated a clear relationship between the rate of infectious complications and the immunosuppressive regimen. Most heart transplant patients require triple drug immunosuppression, although trough levels of cyclosporin are targeted lower after the first year.

2.2 What are the alterations due to iatrogenic factors?
In general, iatrogenic factors are similar in all types of solid organ transplant recipients and mostly refer to the immunosuppression treatment, the surgical procedure and the necessary period of admission to the intensive care unit. The length of this period is mainly determined by the appearance of postsurgical complications (bleeding, acute rejection, allograft dysfunction, etc.).

Moreover, skin and mucosal surfaces of patients receiving immunosuppressive drugs become atrophic and more susceptible to infection and colonization with multiresistant pathogens.

2.3. What is the influence of environmental factors?
Heart transplant patients may acquire several infections from the environment. The most common are given below.

Community
Common community-acquired infections include tuberculosis, influenza and other respiratory viruses (thus it is important to consider influenza vaccine for patients and contacts and the pneumococcal vaccine). Patients are recommended not to frequent public places in the first 6 months following transplantation, and to avoid contact with ill people.

Hospital
Various viral infections may be acquired in the hospital (e.g. influenza, RSV, other respiratory viruses). Nosocomial transmission of HBV during endomyocardial biopsy

procedures has recently been described (8% incidence in one center and 27% in one outbreak). These reports highlight the importance of strict hygienic precautions during intravascular diagnostic procedures. The most likely explanation was found to be indirect blood–blood contact between patients. Some authors also recommend performing biopsies on hepatitis B surface antigen (HBsAg)-positive and -negative patients in separate rooms. HBV was found also to be transmitted to heart transplant partners. Vaccination against HBV and routine monitoring for certain bloodborne infections should be considered in cardiac allograft recipients.

Prolonged hospital stay before operation and previous antimicrobials increase the colonization rate with multiresistant strains. Contact with other patients or with healthcare workers may permit infection with *P. carinii*, *M. tuberculosis*, MRSA, VRE and other multiresistant species.

Outbreaks of *Legionella* related to contamination of water supply have also been described. Construction works in hospital centers have been related to increased incidence of invasive aspergillosis.

Food
Listeria, *Salmonella*, *Brucella*, *Campylobacter*, *Pseudomonas* and *Aspergillus* spp. have been associated with food.

Region, country and travel
Endemic mycoses, hepatitis A, strongyloidiasis, malaria, recommended vaccinations (typhoid fever inactivated vaccine) are the most common factors.

2.4 What are the most significant factors that contribute to the risk of infection in heart transplant recipients?

Pretransplant conditions
Patients receiving a heart transplant are usually suffering from a chronic cardiopulmonary disease, which may have led to cachexia and repeated hospital admissions, with the resulting nosocomial aggressions. Prolonged intubation before and after transplantation and ventilator support confer a greater tendency for recurrent lung infections, which have been shown to be a significant cause of mortality in some series. Whether the patient is critically ill before transplantation and prior to sternotomy also increase the risk of early nosocomial infection. Pulmonary hypertension unresponsive to vasodilator challenge and preoperative requirement of hemodynamic support increase the risk for premature death following heart transplantation (30% mortality from infection in the 3 months after transplantation compared with less than 2% when these factors are not present).

Older age, use of a ventilator at the time of transplantation, induction therapy with OKT3, donor CMV-positive serology and donors of black race all have been found to increase early infections after heart transplantation.

Posttransplant conditions
In the early postsurgical period after transplantation anatomic barriers are severely altered by mechanical ventilation, surgical wound, chest tubes, intravascular devices, indwelling bladder catheter, and occasionally mechanical circulatory support. These risk factors are sustained for at least 1 week after operation and are extremely important for infection.

Heart transplant patients are at high risk for developing postsurgical major sternal wound infections and mediastinitis. Risk factors include the hospital environment, interval between admission and surgery, early chest reexploration, low cardiac output syndrome in adults, and the immature state of immune response in infants, amongst others.

Ventricular assistance has emerged as a risk factor for initial and cumulative infection episodes. In some series, up to one third of the patients on biventricular assist devices have died from sepsis, 59% have developed bacteremia, 28% have developed line infection, and 11% pump infection.

Age

A recipient age of 60 years or older has been identified in some studies as a significant risk factor for early death (i.e. within the first 3 months) after heart transplantation. This is due to an increased rate of infectious complications during the early postoperative period, and to nonheart-related organ system failure. On the other hand, a high early mortality rate is characteristic for all pediatric patients and particularly so for the youngest age group. In this setting, infection, as a cause of death, accounts for a significant minority early after transplantation, but by 3 years infection-related deaths are uncommon.

Type of immunosuppressive regimen
See section 2.1.

Primary allograft dysfunction or rejection requiring increased immunosuppression
Graft rejection is not easy to diagnose in patients receiving immunosuppressive therapy, and changes in serial electrocardiographic voltages are diagnostically unreliable. In adult patients, repeated transvenous endomyocardial biopsy is used routinely to obtain grafted tissue that can be examined histologically for signs of rejection at times when rejection is most likely. Endomyocardial biopsies pose a specific risk factor to heart transplant recipients. They are uncommonly related to bacterial infection, although a high rate of HBV transmission has been reported in some centers during such procedures.

Alteration of host defenses by microorganisms
CMV disease increases the risk of severe infectious complication in this population and has been recognized as a risk factor for opportunistic infections like *Aspergillus* or *P. carinii*. CMV has also been linked to rejection, atherosclerosis and death. Occasionally CMV disease may condition a profound neutropenia, with its well-described associated risks. However, this neutropenia is usually short and resolves soon after treatment is initiated. HIV or HCV infection are also risk factors for opportunistic infections.

2.5 What are the specific or nonspecific measures aimed at minimizing each of these factors?
See sections 3 and 4 for details.
- Preoperative donor and recipient screening for infectious diseases and exposures.
- Review of the patient's vaccination history.
- Donor–recipient antigen matching (not easily feasible).
- Careful surgical procedure and hospital management. Careful use of antimicrobials both for prophylaxis and perioperatively.
- Avoid drug interactions that may lower the dose of cyclosporin A and induce rejection (rifampicin forbidden) (see Chapter 7.1, section 2.2)
- Prevention of CMV disease (donor–recipient CMV serology matching, infusion of leukocyte-free blood products, surveillance cultures, preemptive ganciclovir therapy).

- Administration of antifungal prophylaxis against *Candida* with oral fluconazole to patients at high risk for systemic candidosis. Some centers consider prophylaxis against *Aspergillus* mandatory in cases of heart–lung transplantation.
- Administration of cotrimoxazole to prevent PCP. Patients not receiving cotrimoxazole prophylaxis are at higher risk of suffering infections caused by *Listeria, P. carinii* or *Nocardia*. Therefore, because of its benefits and relative absence of secondary effects, cotrimoxazole prophylaxis is mandatory.
- Avoid contact with highly contagious patients in common areas of the hospital (e.g. radiology department)
- Control of environmental risk factors (isolation from construction works, conventional barrier nursing care in an open ward, and rigorously enforced handwashing policies)
- Stimulate each transplant center to examine which risk factors may potentially be minimized.

2.6 Are there different levels of risk of infection recognized for heart transplant recipients?

Data show that the mortality rate from infection is around 15% in the first 30 postoperative days and 35% thereafter. At 6 months after surgery, over 70% of patients are free from infection. It would be desirable to be able to anticipate which patient is at higher risk of suffering a severe infection. Preoperative variables seem to be of limited value with respect to immunosuppressive treatment in predicting outcome, and no single or combination of variables is able to indicate patients with an event-free course. In some series, risk factors for mortality were postoperative acute kidney failure, prolonged cardiopulmonary bypass time and previous cardiac surgery. Infection was associated with steroid immunosuppression, cytolytic treatment (antilymphocytic antibodies for corticosteroid-resistant rejection), venous line placement for more than 7 days, and mechanical ventilation time. Older age was a poor prognostic factor in some series.

Patients mismatched for CMV or *Toxoplasma* are at high risk of severe disease.

Risk factors for fungal infection have not been clearly established in this population but higher needs for immunosuppression, CMV disease and other infections seem to promote aspergillosis in this population. Patients with frequent, long-lasting or severe rejection episodes are at higher risk of infection.

2.7 How does the level of risk impact on management?

Surveillance measures

Surveillance samples may be obtained from patients at risk for primary infections (CMV, *Toxoplasma*), mainly if prophylaxis is not implemented. Some authors recommend surveillance cultures of the respiratory tract while the patient is intubated, in search of *Aspergillus*, although the efficacy of such measures has not been proven. Whenever cases of *Aspergillus* infection are detected, air contamination should be checked.

When outbreaks of multiresistant Gram-negative (*Acinetobacter, Pseudomonas*) or Gram-positive (VRE, MRSA) microorganisms appear in a center with transplant programs, isolation measures should be implemented and nosocomial infection control measures closely followed. When cases of *L. pneumophila* infection are detected, surveillance cultures of the water supply are recommended.

Preventive measures (see section 4.1)

Most centers recommend prophylaxis in high-risk patients (e.g. primary CMV or *Toxoplasma* infection in serologically negative recipients of a serologically positive organ donor). Patients with corticosteroid-resistant rejection should receive prophylaxis against CMV. Patients with history of residence or travel to endemic *S. stercoralis* areas should undergo specific diagnostic testing and treatment before transplantation.

Therapeutic measures

When any infection (bacterial, viral, fungal or parasitic infection) of any site is suspected, management should be rapid and aggressive. Previously mentioned risk factors should be considered when choosing empirical therapy.

2.8 What new developments are going to impact on minimizing or suppressing the specific risk factors?

Patients requiring biventricular assistance devices may develop immunologic abnormalities that are associated with a poor outcome. Some authors suggest that the human leucocyte antigen (HLA)-DR expression on monocytes should be monitored (especially in case of infection). If persistent loss of HLA-DR+ monocytes is identified, restitution of monocytic function should be attempted by removal of inhibitory factors using plasmapheresis and/or administration of interferon-γ to improve the antimicrobial defense. However, this approach is still investigational. More studies with parametric survival analysis are needed. These studies can produce patient-specific predictions of a given event and of a patient's risk factor profile, or could identify surrogate markers (or predictors) of severe infections and/or other transplant-related complications (such as rejection episodes).

As long-term survival after cardiac transplantation improves, neoplastic complications are increasingly being discovered. Although lymphatic neoplasms predominate, the incidence of solid tumors has been estimated at 3.3% (50% of the frequency of lymphoproliferative disorders). Most patients with de novo solid malignancies have a significant smoking history. These tumors may have a rapid growth and early manifestation, which suggests a preexistent occult carcinoma. An aggressive and repetitive preoperative screening for occult malignancy during pretransplantation evaluation in heart transplant candidates who are heavy smokers should be considered.

3 REGARDING THE SURVEILLANCE OF HEART TRANSPLANT RECIPIENTS

3.1 What is the important pretransplant information to be gathered?

Pretransplant evaluation of the donor

- Donors with an active uncontrolled infection are usually rejected for transplantation.
- It is advisable to obtain tissue or to examine the donor to investigate possible infections and neoplasia.
- Culture of the transport fluids.
- Serology: detection of antibodies against HIV-1 and HIV-2 [enzyme-linked immunosorbent assay (ELISA)]; positive results will be confirmed by Western blotting and/or RNA-PCR; antibodies against human T-lymphotropic virus (HTLV) I, hepatitis A, HBV, HDV, HCV, CMV, EBV, *Toxoplasma*, HSV, VZV, syphilis (HHV-8 if available). Whenever possible, a serum sample should be stored in case further studies

are necessary. Some 26% of centers refuse to use HCV-positive organs, whereas the remainder restrict the use of HCV-positive organs to United Network of Organ Sharing (UNOS) status 1 recipients (critically ill patients in the intensive care unit waiting for transplantation) or HCV-positive candidates.

Pretransplant evaluation of the recipient

- Record of previous antimicrobial allergies, previous infections (upper and lower respiratory tract, diverticulosis, hepatitis, parasitic infections, diarrhea, genitourinary tract, herpes, osteomyelitis, etc.).
- Identification of active uncontrolled infection is a basis for exclusion. This includes any infection that cannot be controlled before the transplantation procedure.
- Assessment of previous exposures: travel or history of previous residential locations, transfusions, pet or animal contact, hobbies (gardening, farming), origin of the drinking water, contact with children, dietary habits (raw food, nonpasteurized milk derivatives, seafood) and exposure to tuberculosis [purified protein derivative (PPD), booster and chest radiography]. The second-step tuberculin test or booster allowed the authors to identify an extra 11% of patients susceptible to receive isoniazid. Anergy study (cutaneous tests for delayed-type hypersensitivity) may be helpful in negative patients, and antituberculous prophylaxis may be indicated in anergic patients with a negative PPD finding but a clear exposure history. Positive patients should submit samples for mycobacterial culture and receive prophylaxis. Previous immunizations should be investigated.
- Physical examination and complementary data: abdominal echography, thoracic CT scan, paranasal sinuses radiography, urine and feces analysis, study of nares colonization, mouth, urinary and gynecologic tract examination.
- Pretransplant serology: CMV, VZV, HSV, EBV, HBV, HCV, HIV, *T. gondii*, syphilis, *Leishmania* and endemic mycosis if previous exposure (HHV-8 if available).
- Whether HCV-positive donor organs should be used remains controversial.
- Screening for exposure to endemic mycoses before transplantation for recipients who have lived in endemic areas is also required. If either past medical history or serology is positive, azole administration is started immediately after transplantation and maintained indefinitely.
- Regarding parasitic infections, the authors advise the search of *S. stercoralis* infestation in patients with a recent or remote history of travel or residence in endemic areas. The Harada-Mori concentration technique of fecal specimens of asymptomatic recipients is recommended. All positive potentially infected patients should be treated with a course of ivermectin or albendazole before transplantation
- Vaccination: influenza, pneumococcal, HBV, *H. influenzae*; routine vaccination against VZV is not yet performed routinely in most transplant programs.

3.2 What are the surveillance measures to be taken in heart transplant recipients?

Posttransplant surveillance

The monitoring of cardiac transplant patients who present with suspicion of an infection should be started immediately (see section 1.6) and includes a careful history and physical examination, together with a thorough investigation of epidemiologic antecedents. The chronology of the infection after transplantation is essential since infectious episodes vary substantially from one posttransplant period to another.

The authors always consider the possibilities for viral, bacterial, mycobacterial, fungal and parasitic infections. A review of pretransplant serology of the recipient and donor should be undertaken regularly. The authors perform surveillance CMV antigenemia and a PPD and booster study, preferentially before transplantation. Positive patients should be followed with repeated samples for mycobacterial culture and should receive prophylaxis.

3.3 What are the other specific measures to be taken in heart transplant recipients?
Recipients of heart transplants infrequently become granulocytopenic, so that a protected environment is not required. Different studies have proved that isolation does not influence the incidence, type or location of infections after heart transplantation. Accordingly, an open ward is recommended using only routine handwashing practices.

3.4 What development(s) are to be expected for surveillance in heart transplant recipients?
Recent molecular biology methodologies may detect the presence of pathogens with higher sensitivity than culture and serologic methods. These methods may also be helpful in the analysis of outbreaks and nosocomial transmission. However, the efficacy of some surveillance methods for fungal organisms remains to be defined.

4 REGARDING THE PREVENTION OF INFECTION IN HEART TRANSPLANT RECIPIENTS

4.1 What approaches, if any, to the prevention of infection should be considered in heart transplant recipients?
Prevention of infection is a much better strategy than therapy in solid organ transplant patients. The strategies for posttransplant prophylaxis that are most commonly followed are listed below.

- Surgical prophylaxis should be routinely given (two or three doses of cefazolin). Surgery and postsurgical management should be carefully performed and ventilation, tubes and catheters withdrawn as soon as possible.
- Perioperative selective bowel decontamination and early administration of oral nystatin has been recommended before bone marrow, liver and intestinal transplantation by some investigators and clinicians. However, the efficacy of this measure has not been proven in heart transplantion. Patients who require prolonged care in the intensive care unit may especially benefit from it.
- Annual immunization with influenza vaccine or prophylaxis with amantadine after exposure to persons with influenza or during an epidemic is recommended in heart transplant recipients. The vaccine can be administered safely to this patient population, although it may be associated with low-level histologic rejection.
- VZV infection should be prevented in seronegative patients who have been in contact with patients with varicella or zoster. Hyperimmune globulins may be used in these cases.
- Due to the relatively benign nature of herpes simplex infections in most cases, the majority of authors prefer an 'early therapeutic' approach rather than widespread and long-term prophylaxis in heart transplant patients.
- The most important aspect of prophylaxis against viral infections is anti-CMV prophylaxis. Mismatched recipients should receive early prophylaxis, but the best strategy to follow in such patients remains controversial. Currently the use of ganciclovir

and γ-globulins for 4–6 weeks seems the most effective. In seropositive recipients, especially those receiving OKT3 or antithymocyte globulins, prophylaxis against CMV may be performed with either intravenous or oral ganciclovir. The latter approach should be used only if viral replication has been excluded. An alternative approach is to follow the clinical evolution closely and monitor for antigenemia, and to introduce preemptive therapy in the presence of clinical or laboratory signs of CMV infection (see Chapter 7.0).

- Antibiotic prophylaxis against bacterial infections is not indicated in most cases. As mentioned, antipneumococcal and anti-*H. influenzae* (group B) vaccines should be offered to this population even when no definitive evidence of efficacy is available. Pneumococcal vaccination may be repeated 5 years after the first shot.

- Tuberculosis is difficult to diagnose and to treat after solid organ transplantation. As mentioned above, the authors recommend isoniazid prophylaxis for all PPD-positive patients. In countries with a high rate of tuberculosis, the finding of scarred lesions on the chest radiograph should probably be considered equivalent to a positive tuberculin skin test. This approach is not universally shared, but in the authors' experience isoniazid is efficacious and well tolerated in heart transplant recipients.

- Regarding fungal infections, patients with previous exposure to endemic regional mycosis should receive prophylaxis with azole derivatives during the period of maximum immunosuppression. There is no clearcut information regarding the approach to take in patients with previous exposure to agents such as *Penicillium marneffeii*. With regard to the prevention of infection caused by invasive filamentous fungi of universal distribution, environmental procedures and air-cleaning systems are the most efficacious measures. However, in institutions where such measures are not available or clearly insufficient, the use of itraconazole prophylaxis during the first 6 months after transplantation may be useful. In the authors' institution there was a profound decrease in invasive aspergillosis after the implementation of itraconazole prophylaxis (400 mg daily) during the first 6 months after transplantation, although they are aware that the efficacy of such a measure has not been documented in well-designed prospective and randomized clinical trials.

- Most authors recommend prophylaxis against *P. carinii*, while others select only high-risk patients (i.e. those receiving high-dose immunosuppression or suffering from CMV infection). Cotrimoxazole remains the drug of choice, most commonly on a 3 days a week regimen, either alternative or consecutive, while some centers recommend 7 days per month. The authors give primary prophylaxis with one double-strength tablet every 12 h twice a week (e.g. Saturdays and Sundays). No case of PCP has occurred since this regimen was started, nor have infections with *Listeria* or *Nocardia* been observed. For patients unable to tolerate cotrimoxazole, other prophylactic regimens include pyrimethamine–sulfadoxine, atovaquone or aerosolized pentamidine or dapsone. However, breakthrough cases have been described and the latter has no efficacy against *T. gondii*. Prophylaxis should be started soon after operation and cover the period of highest incidence of PCP (the first 2–6 months posttransplantation). The occasional occurrence of PCP following discontinuation of prophylaxis at 6 months raises the question of extending chemoprophylaxis for 12–18 months in heart transplant patients, and certainly underscores the need to restart it in transplant recipients requiring high-dose immunosuppression (doses of prednisone greater than 10 mg/day). Since prophylaxis does not eradicate *P. carinii*, it is effective only as long as it is administered.

- *Toxoplasma*-seronegative recipients of grafts from positive donors should receive 6 weeks of pyrimethamine with folinic acid. As PCP may develop despite such a regimen, some recommend adding one double-strength tablet of cotrimoxazole 3 days a week to extend protection.

4.2 What are the future challenges and opportunities for reducing the risk of infection?

Studies are needed to establish the measures that are really effective in heart transplant patients since the indiscriminate use of prophylaxis may represent an ecologic threat. Since preventive measures vary among transplant centers, collaborative studies are mandatory to establish firm recommendations.

5 REGARDING THE TREATMENT OF HEART TRANSPLANT RECIPIENTS

5.1 What is the role of empirical therapy?

Decision to start empirical therapy

The steps required before initiation of empirical antimicrobial therapy may be summarized as follows:

1 A thorough clinical history regarding pertinent personal and epidemiologic antecedents is required.
2 A careful physical examination should be performed.
3 A tentative diagnosis of infection should be formulated (which site or organ is involved), as well as an appreciation of the clinical situation and the prospects for possible clinical deterioration.
4 A list of the microorganisms likely to be responsible for the episode should be made, taking into account the posttransplant period of the patient.
5 A well-planned approach to obtaining, transporting and processing the clinical samples is necessary to confirm the diagnosis. The sampling should ideally be performed before antimicrobial therapy is initiated.
6 Empirical therapy should then be started when the clinical situation dictates, particularly in patients with possible rapid clinical deterioration. Most presumptive viral infections can wait for the preliminary laboratory results. In contrast, potentially severe bacterial, mycobacterial and fungal infections do require prompt antimicrobial treatment.
7 Modifications of the empirical therapy have to be made after positive or negative microbiologic results have been received.

Choice of antimicrobials

Treatment of infection should include measures aimed at targeting the microorganisms with antimicrobial agents as well as measures such as removal or drainage of a focal source of infection, withdrawal of intravenous or bladder catheters, or even removal of prosthetic devices.

Supportive measures such as adequate organ perfusion (systolic pressure greater than 90 mmHg) and oxygen delivery (ventilator therapy) are essential and urine output should be kept over 30 ml/h by continuing fluid administration. If this cannot be achieved by volume infusion alone, inotropic and vasopressor therapy is indicated. Corticosteroid therapy should de considered only if adrenal insufficiency is suspected.

Antimicrobials are selected on the basis of the timing of infection after transplant, the site of infection and the resistance pattern of the expected pathogen(s). The choice of drugs should be based on the probable source of infection, the results of Gram staining of smears of appropriate clinical specimens, and the immune status of the patient.

For initial treatment of a suspected bacterial life-threatening sepsis a third- or fourth-generation cephalosporin or a ureidopenicillin with β-lactamase inhibitor is indicated. A carbapenem or fluoroquinolone is a reasonable alternative in hospitals with an increased rate of resistant Gram-negative bacilli. The use of an aminoglycoside should be avoided in patients on cyclosporin A and should be reserved for severe infections caused by *P. aeruginosa* or other resistant microorganims.

When methicillin-resistant staphylococci are suspected, treatment with vancomycin or teicoplanin (with or without an aminoglycoside) is often recommended. Potential nephrotoxicity of such regimens should be carefully monitored by repeated creatinine measurements in patients receiving cyclosporin.

For intraabdominal or other infections likely to involve anaerobes, empirical treatment should include a β-lactam active against anaerobes, such as ampicillin–sulbactam or amoxicillin–clavulanate, piperacillin–tazobactam or a carbapenem, each with or without an aminoglycoside. Alternatively, metronidazole or clindamycin can be administered in combination with an aminoglycoside.

When the source of bacteremia is thought to be in the biliary tract, the possibility of *Enterococcus* as an etiologic agent leads some clinicians to prefer penicillin derivatives such as piperacillin, piperacillin–tazobactam or ampicillin–sulbactam plus metronidazole, each with or without an aminoglycoside.

Empirical therapy of urinary tract infections or urinary-related sepsis must be selected with the knowledge that in some areas resistance of *E. coli* to amoxicillin and to cotrimoxazole is close to 50%, and resistance to fluoroquinolones may reach 20% of the isolates.

If meningeal involvement is suspected and the patient is not receiving cotrimoxazole prophylaxis, therapy should include ampicillin to cover *Listeria*.

Duration of treatment

First, empirical therapy should ideally be adapted to the etiologic agent as soon as possible. In circumstances in which no confirmation of etiology is available, the length of treatment depends on the evolution of the patient, the clinical syndrome and the potential etiology. The maximum length of empirical anti-CMV therapy is 14 days.

Regarding bacterial infections, most entities require 10–14 days of treatment, but severe pneumonia should be treated for no less than 3 weeks and postsurgical mediastinitis for a minimum of 4 weeks.

If antituberculous treatment is started but the diagnosis is not confirmed, therapy should be continued for 2 months or, if the suspicion is high enough, for a full cycle of 6–9 months. A cumulative minimal dose of amphotericin B 500 mg should be administered empirically on suspicion of *Candida* infection. Higher doses are warranted for suspicion of invasive *Candida* or aspergillosis or other invasive mycoses due to filamentous fungi. PCP should be treated for at least 3 weeks.

Events that direct change of empirical therapy

When results of cultures and antimicrobial susceptibilities are known, modifications of empirical treatment should be performed accordingly. When the clinical situation is stabilized, the empirical regimen can often be simplified, and therapy with a single antimicrobial agent is often adequate. Sequential intravenous and oral therapy may be appropriate in some circumstances.

In contrast, clinical deterioration, isolation of a resistant microorganism, or isolation of a microorganism that can be treated with a narrow-spectrum antimicrobial, allergic or toxic reactions, or drug interactions, may require a change of empirical-therapy.

Summary

In summary the following considerations should be taken into account before choosing an antimicrobial agent:

- Time after transplantation (< 1 month, 2–6 months, > 6 months with or without chronic allograft dysfunction).
- Site of infection (no clinically evident site, lower respiratory tract, CNS, etc.).
- Pace of progression (acute, chronic) and clinical situation of the patient.
- Expected pathogens.
- Selection of empirical therapy.
- Changes of empirical therapy and definitive treatment.

5.2 What is the appropriate approach to the heart transplant recipient with evidence of:

Upper respiratory tract infection?

Upper respiratory tract infections in the heart transplant patient are usually managed as in noncompromised hosts. Appropriate antimicrobial treatment for bacterial infections is amoxicillin–clavulanate, oral cephalosporins and, occasionally, fluoro-quinolones. The use of macrolides is usually precluded due to the interference with cyclosporin A.

Fungal sinusitis is uncommon but should be borne in mind in case symptoms are refractory to conventional therapy.

Lower respiratory tract infection?

Bacterial pneumonia in the heart transplant recipient varies widely in potential etiologies depending on the chronology of the infection and the severity of the clinical presentation. Pneumonia in the early postoperative period is frequently of bacterial origin. Microorganisms such as *S. pneumoniae*, *H. influenzae*, *P. aeruginosa*, Enterobacteriaceae or *S. aureus* are amongst the most common agents. The initial empirical choice should cover these pathogens and therefore be broad spectrum. *Pseudomonas* pneumonia is best treated with a combination of β-lactam agents with anti-*Pseudomonas* activity (such as ceftazidime) plus an aminoglycoside. When there is suspicion of methicillin-resistant *S. aureus* (MRSA) a glycopeptide should be included in the initial empirical choice. *Aspergillus* pneumonia may also appear in this period in patients with postoperative complications.

Pneumonia during the period of maximum immunosuppression (i.e. the intermediate period) is most frequently due to nonbacterial causes. Late pneumonia in the heart transplant patient is frequently a less severe disease, with clinical behavior similar to that in noncompromised patients.

There are no precise data regarding the length of therapy. The most severe cases should be treated for at least 2–3 weeks, depending on their clinical course. For nosocomially acquired pneumonia caused by *L. pneumophila*, *P. aeruginosa* or *Acinetobacter*, the authors recommend 3 weeks of therapy.

Gastrointestinal infection?

Stomatitis is caused predominantly by HSV in this patient population and should be treated with acyclovir if prophylaxis was not already given, since HSV stomatitis may impede the patient's well-being and nutrition. The gastrointestinal tract is also a frequent site of CMV infection after heart transplantation and, when diagnosed, therapy should include high-dose intravenous ganciclovir with or without hyperimmune globulin.

Candida infections should be treated with standard antifungals (fluconazole and, less commonly, amphotericin B).

Genitourinary tract infection?

The appropriate therapy, route and duration of administration for a UTI has been well defined in immunocompetent hosts. In heart transplant recipients, early postsurgical urinary tract infections are mostly related to bladder indwelling catheterization, and late UTI occur mainly in elderly men and women. Accordingly, unlike normal hosts, a single dose or a short course (1–3 days) of treatment is almost never indicated in heart transplant patients.

Complicated UTIs of patients requiring hospital admission should initially be treated parenterally until the etiology of the infection, clinical course and the availability of - adequate oral agents have been carefully evaluated. A 7–14–day course of trimethoprim–sulfamethoxazole, a fluoroquinolone or a third-generation cephalosporin is usually adequate. Complicated UTI also requires aggressive search for obstructive predisposing factors.

Cardiovascular system infection?

Two issues are of particular therapeutic importance: the treatment of bacteremic episodes and endocarditis. Bloodstream infections during the postoperative period are usually related to the invasive procedures and they originate in the intravenous catheters, the lung or the surgical wound. Bloodstream infections may be due to either Gram-positive or Gram-negative bacteria and their management is indistinguishable from that in other postsurgical situations.

Endocarditis is distinctly uncommon in the heart graft. Therapy will depend on the isolated microorganism. However, while cultures are pending, it is important to remember the overrepresentation of fungal endocarditis in heart transplant recipients when compared with bacterial causes. When established, fungal endocarditis may require the combination of surgical treatment and antifungal therapy.

Musculoskeletal infection?

With the exception of sternal osteomyelitis, bone infections are not common after heart transplantation. Osteomyelitis may occur as a consequence of metastatic bone involvement after bloodstream infections. Gram positive bacteria are more frequent than Gram-negative bacteria, and vertebral involvement is the most common site. Treatment requires etiologic evidence obtained by aspiration or biopsy, and should be administered for at least 6 weeks. Treatment should avoid the use of rifampicin in combination therapy, in order to minimize interference with cyclosporin metabolism.

Patients with postsurgical mediastinitis should promptly undergo surgery, and infected or necrotic edges of the sternum and mediastinal collections should be debrided. Reconstruction may be achieved by means of bilateral pectoralis myocutaneous flaps, which provide adequate coverage and vascular supply. Prolonged antimicrobial therapy is recommended.

Vertebral osteoporosis and even fractures are a common long-term complication of heart transplantation, and in the setting of fever vertebral pain may raise the suspicion of vertebral osteomyelitis.

Skin infection?

Skin and soft tissue infections are an expression of either local invasion of microorganisms due to the rupture of cutaneous barriers or of deep-seated or metastatic infections with secondary skin involvement. Lesions should always be aspirated and biopsied since they may be the first manifestation of disseminated *Nocardia* or fungal disease. Viral infections (particularly those caused by HVS or VZV) are to be treated with acyclovir.

Bacterial infections usually represent surgical wound infections or soft tissue infections related to the use of corticosteroids and secondary bacterial infection (transplant elbow).

Central nervous system infection?

The treatment of meningitis should be based on clinical grounds (i.e. patient characteristics, clinical presentation, skin lesions, etc.) and on microscopic examination of CSF sediment, which helps to predict the most frequent pathogen. The duration of treatment is 7 days in *H. influenzae* and *N. meningitidis*, 10–14 days in *S. pneumoniae*, and 21 days in *Listeria* and Gram-negative bacilli.

The coadministration of corticosteroids in acute purulent bacterial meningitis remains a controversial issue. Dexamethasone ($1.2 \ mg/m^2$ every 6 h for 4 days) appears to be safe in children, but sufficient data are lacking in adults. It might be reasonable to consider the use of dexamethasone if a high number of organisms are present in the CSF on microscopy or in adults who present with poor prognostic factors such as coma or stupor. Preventive treatment of contacts and carriers is indicated in clustering of meningococcal and *H. influenzae* meningitis. Phenitoin and manitol are recommended in severe bacterial meningitis.

Fungal cerebral abscesses are often resistant to therapy. Systemic administration of intravenous amphotericin B (conventional or lipid formulations) is the standard treatment. CT-guided stereotactic aspiration or an open craniotomy and drainage are recognized as adjunctive to medical therapy for diagnosis and therapeutic purposes. The role of local administration of amphotericin B and of new agents such as itraconazole or voriconazole is still unclear.

Sulfonamides are effective if rapidly administered for patients with a nonfungal brain abscess and should be initiated empirically until a specific etiology is established in cases not suspected of being caused by fungi.

Foreign body in place?

The most frequent foreign body-related infections in heart transplant recipients are bloodstream infections related to intravenous catheter infections. Only the infections caused by *Staphylococcus* spp. in hemodynamically stable patients can be given the chance of sterilization without catheter removal. The authors recommend that all other catheters be removed immediately, although it is recognized that more conservative approaches might be tried.

Recurrent bacteremias may indicate the infection of prosthetic pulmonary artery graft or pacemaker. Most often, these devices are to be surgically replaced in order to cure the patient.

5.3 What is the appropriate approach to a heart transplant recipient with evidence of a documented bacteremia, with or without site of infection?

Gram-positive bacteremia

In the early postoperative period, wound infections, catheter-related infections and mediastinitis must be excluded in patients with Gram-positive bacteremia. Superficial cultures of the catheter (skin and hubs) and lysis-centrifugation blood cultures should be obtained (one through the catheter and another through direct venous puncture) if difficult to substitute catheters are in place.

When *S. pneumoniae* bacteremia is diagnosed, pneumonia, meningitis and endocarditis should be excluded. If *L. monocytogenes* is isolated from blood, a lumbar puncture should be performed and therapy with high-dose ampicillin and gentamicin promptly initiated.

Specific therapy should be based on the isolated organism. There is no reason to continue with glycopeptides if methicillin-susceptible *Staphylococcus* spp. are recovered. In these cases oxacillin or cloxacillin are preferred.

Many enterococcal strains are now resistant to penicillins, streptomycin, gentamicin and even vancomycin. They may require teicoplanin (not always cross-resistance with vancomycin), chloramphenicol, doxycycline, fluoroquinolones or Synercid (a combination of quinupristine–dalfopristine).

Gram-negative bacteremia

Therapy will be based on the susceptibility pattern of the isolated microorganism. Intraabdominal, urinary tract, wound or catheter origins should be investigated.

Most bacteremic infections caused by *Pseudomonas aeruginosa* should be treated with a combination of a β-lactam drug and aminoglycoside.

Anaerobic infection

If the infection is exclusively caused by anaerobic microorganisms, penicillin, metronidazole or clindamycin may be used. In addition, a pyogenic collection that could be drained must be excluded.

Mixed or polymicrobial bacteremia

Most anaerobic infections are polymicrobial. In these cases, treatment should include ampicillin–sulbactam or amoxicillin–clavulanate, piperacillin–tazobactam, a carbapenem, cefoxitin each with or without an aminoglycoside or, alternatively, metronidazole or clindamycin together with an aminoglycoside. If aminoglycosides are used cyclosporin levels and creatinine clearance should be monitored.

Bacteremia with a defined primary site of infection

In this case the primary site will be treated, and in some cases it will define the choice of antimicrobial (for example, in meningitis an antibiotic that achieves adequate levels in CSF is required) and the length of the treatment.

Approach to heart transplant recipients with mycobacterial infection

In patients with tuberculosis, rifampicin should not be used in patients who are receiving cyclosporin A. In these cases, the authors prefer the use of isoniazid (INH) and ethambutol (EMB) with one or two more drugs (streptomycin, pyrazinamide or a fluoroquinolone). After an initial period of at least 2 months with three or four drugs, the authors recommend continued therapy with INH and EMB for no less than 18 months.

In patients with resistance to first-line drugs the treatment should include at least three to five drugs that are active in vitro, including second-line drugs. Therapy should be continued for at least 2 years. Combined treatment administered under direct supervision over a long period of time is essential for the cure of tuberculosis.

Treatment of infections caused by nontuberculous mycobacteria usually involves surgery and removal of prosthetic devices when possible. Irresectable lesions require antimicrobial agents which may vary from one species to another, and which may benefit from expert consultation. Because in vitro tests are usually time consuming and do not always correlate with clinical efficacy, treatment should be based on clinical studies and should include a prolonged course of a combination of two or more drugs with known activity.

5.4 What is the appropriate approach to the heart transplant recipient with evidence of a viral infection?

HSV infections involving the skin or mucous surface may be treated orally with either acyclovir or famciclovir in patients who are not severely ill. However, parenteral therapy is necessary for more severe infections. VZV can be treated with either systemic acyclovir or oral famciclovir in patients who are not severely ill.

Strategies for the treatment of CMV infection have been outlined above. Intravenous ganciclovir is the drug of choice and has been shown to be effective in different groups of immunocompromised patients. In the authors' experience, at least 60% of all heart transplant patients require intravenous ganciclovir sometime during their course. Some authors recommend the association of intravenous CMV-hyperimmune β-globulin. In certain patients granulocyte colony-stimulating factor (G-CSF) may be associated in order to avoid myelosupression during ganciclovir therapy. To date, ganciclovir resistant isolates of CMV have not posed major problems in heart transplant recipients.

Very little experience on the treatment of adenovirus pneumonia in cardiac transplant patients is available. Ribavirin and interferon-α or high doses of ganciclovir with intravenous immunoglobulins have been used.

Influenza virus infection may have severe consequences in the transplant population, with an increased incidence of pneumonia and neurologic complications, and may occasionally deserve therapy.

5.5 What is the appropriate approach to the heart transplant recipient with evidence of a fungal infection?

Candida fungemia can be treated with fluconazole, especially C. *albicans* fungemia in patients not previously treated with azole derivatives. With regard to invasive aspergillosis, conventional amphotericin B, liposomal preparations of amphotericin B and itraconazole are the therapeutic options. Patients who do not respond to conventional amphotericin B may benefit from itraconazole or a lipid-associated amphotericin B preparation. There are some suggestions that therapy with liposomal amphotericin B or itraconazole could be associated with a lower crude mortality rate than that associated with conventional amphotericin B. In addition, liposomal preparations of amphotericin B permit the use of higher doses with low nephrotoxicity.

Itraconazole has also been used as maintenance therapy in patients with invasive aspergillosis previously treated with amphotericin. The recommended administration schedule includes loading doses (600 mg daily for 4 days) and subsequent doses of at least 400 mg daily. The new formulation of itraconazole in cyclodextrin is better absorbed and should be used initially in the same dose. Cyclosporin levels should be monitored and itraconazole serum concentrations measured within 7 days of starting therapy.

Surgery should be considered in patients with invasive aspergillosis and presenting with hemoptysis, poor clinical response, isolated lesions, endocarditis, endophthalmitis, sinusitis, peritonitis and osteomyelitis.

In particularly severe cases, immunosuppression may be reduced, although this approach should be followed very carefully as it may lead to fatal rejection episodes. Endocavitary administration of amphotericin B has also been described. The administration of growth factors has been proven useful in selected severe cases, but it is not yet considered a conventional therapeutic strategy.

5.6 What is the appropriate approach to the heart transplant recipient with evidence of a parasitic infection?

The standard therapy for PCP is intravenous cotrimoxazole at a dose of 20 mg/kg daily. This agent provides the most rapid clinical response. Adverse reactions occur in 25% of cases and include skin rashes, creatinine and transaminase elevation, hyponatremia and bone marrow depression. Pentamidine iv is the alternative drug, although it may cause hypoglycemia, hyperglycemia, nephrotoxicity, pancreatitis and pancytopenia. Atovaquone is a new therapeutic option.

Treatment should be maintained for 14–21 days and clinical response is expected to occur after 3–4 days of cotrimoxazole or 5–7 days of pentamidine. Lack of response does not seem to be related to antimicrobial resistance. In cases of persistent temperature and worsening of respiratory status after 4–5 days of treatment, some authors switch to pentamidine, whereas others recommend adjunctive therapies, such as corticosteroids. There are no controlled trials assessing corticosteroid use in patients without HIV infection, although similar beneficial effects to those observed in HIV-infected patients with PCP might be expected. Respiratory isolation until completion of 10–14 days of therapy should be considered, at least in hospitals with a high proportion of immunocompromised patients.

The necessity to treat CMV infection when it appears as a copathogen with *P. carinii* in the respiratory secretions is controversial.

Toxoplasmosis is treated with pyrimethamine and folinic acid, with sulfadiazine or clindamycin.

Treatment of strongyloidiasis consists of thiabendazole or ivermectin. It is important to consider the possibility of relapses after therapy.

REFERENCES

Cisneros JM, Muñoz P, Torre-Cisneros J et al. Pneumonia after heart transplant: a multiinstitutional study. *Clin Infect Dis* 1998; **27**: 324–331.

Gentry LO, Zeluff B, Kielhofner MA. Dermatologic manifestation of infectious diseases in cardiac transplant patients. *Infect Dis Clin North Am* 1994; **8**: 637–645.

Gorensek MJ, Stewart RW, Keys TF, Mehta AC, McHenry MC, Goormastic M. A multivariate analysis of risk factors for pneumonia following cardiac transplantation. *Transplantation* 1988; **46**: 860–865.

Grossi P, De Maria R, Caroli A, Zaina MS, Minoli L. Infections in heart transplant recipients: the experience of the Italian heart transplant program. Italian Study Group on Infections in Heart Transplant. *J Heart Lung Transplant* 1992; **11**: 847–866.

Keating MR, Whilhelm MP, Walker RC. Strategies for prevention of infection after cardiac transplantation. *Mayo Clin Proc* 1992; **67**: 676–684.

Kirklin JK, Naftel DC, Levine TB et al. Cytomegalovirus after heart transplant. Risk factors for infection and death: a multiinstitutional study. *J Heart Lung Transplant* 1994; **13**: 394–404.

Merigan TC, Renlund DG, Keay S et al. A controlled trial of ganciclovir to prevent cytomegalovirus disease after heart transplant. *N Engl J Med* 1992; **326**: 1182–1186.

Muñoz P, Palomo J, Muñoz R, Rodrìguez H Creixéms M, Pelaez T, Bouza E. Tuberculosis in heart transplant recipients. *Clin Infect Dis* 1995; **21**: 398–402.

Muñoz P, Muñoz RM, Palomo J, Rodrìguez Creixéms M, Muñoz R, Bouza E. *Pneumocystis carinii* infections in heart transplant patients. Twice a week prophylaxis. *Medicine (Baltimore)* 1997; **76**: 53–61.

Smart FW, Naftel DC, Costanzo MR et al. Risk factors for early, cumulative and fatal infections after heart transplant: a multiinstitutional study. *J Heart Lung Transplant* 1996; **15**: 329–341.

Infections in Lung and Heart–Lung Transplant Recipients

Marian Michaels and Michael Green

Introduction

Infections remain a major cause of both morbidity and mortality after transplantation. While 40–50% of deaths after lung transplantation are attributed to infection, many more patients have infectious complications impacting on their quality of life after transplantation. This chapter reviews important aspects of infectious complications following lung or heart–lung transplantation.

I REGARDING THE CLINICAL PRESENTATION AND EVALUATION OF THE PATIENT

I.1 What are the clinically predominant modes of presentation of infection in lung and heart-lung transplant recipients?

To understand the manifestations of infection it is important first to consider the timing of presentation with respect to the transplant. Similar to the presentation of infections after other solid organ transplantation, the posttransplant period for patients undergoing lung or heart–lung transplantation can be divided into an early period (≤ 1 month), an intermediate period (1–6 months) and a late period (> 6 months). The differential diagnosis of infection varies within each of these time periods. Likewise, the underlying disease impacts on the presentation of infection and the types of infection that occur after thoracic organ transplantation. This is particularly true for individuals with cystic fibrosis (CF) who harbor a host of microbial agents in the lungs and upper airways that can impact on the posttransplant course.

Fever and a change in respiratory effort are the two most frequent and important presenting symptoms of infection after lung transplantation. The differential diagnosis of infection will vary depending on the time period in which it presents after transplantation; if the presenting symptom is a change in respiratory effort, then rejection of the pulmonary allograft must be in the differential diagnosis. A localizing source of infection is often found emanating from the pulmonary tree and is frequently accompanied by a change in sputum production and pulmonary function studies. While an etiologic agent can often be confirmed microbiologically, this is not always the case. Accordingly, it is always important to differentiate cases of infection from rejection, particularly for patients in whom a microbiologic pathogen cannot be identified.

Early period (first month after transplantation)

In the early period after transplantation, surgical complications or nosocomial exposures are the primary causes of infection, and patients often present with fever. Infections involving the surgical site most often are related to skin flora, although *Mycoplasma hominis* has been noted as a cause of mediastinitis following lung transplantation at some centers. Presentation in these settings often includes erythema and breakdown at the surgical site. Another potential surgical complication early after transplantation is infection at the site of anastomosis. Bacteria, yeast or fungi can cause this, especially if these organisms are found to colonize the airway of the donor or recipient before transplantation. Accordingly, specimens should be obtained at the time of transplantation from both the donor and recipient so that therapy can be specifically directed if pathogens are identified. Preoperative sputum cultures from the recipient will help direct empirical surgical prophylaxis, particularly if the patient has underlying CF.

Bacteremia is an important cause of fever that may develop early after lung transplantation in one of two major settings. First, patients develop bacteremia or candidemia in association with central venous catheters, which are typically present in the early posttransplant period. The second setting occurs in patients with underlying CF whose bloodstream is occasionally seeded with organisms that normally inhabit their airway (unpublished experience at the Children's Hospital of Pittsburgh). Other catheters can also be a nidus for infection. Patients who have a fever and who had, or still have, a bladder catheter in place should have their urine examined to rule out the presence of urinary tract infection (UTI). Fever can also be seen in association with infection of the airway. Mechanical ventilation, while often not prolonged, is a source of airway contamination and associated pneumonia. Examination of tracheal secretions by Gram staining for the presence of polymorphonuclear cells and predominant morphotypes is helpful. In addition, it can be difficult to differentiate diffuse pneumonia early after lung transplantation from diffuse alveolar damage associated with donor organ harvest trauma. The presence of fever favors infection in this setting.

In general, viruses infrequently cause infections early after transplantation. However, several exceptions to this rule are notable. Herpes simplex virus (HSV) reactivation can occur shortly after transplantation as a result of the stress of the operation and the heavy amount of immunosuppression required in the early posttransplant period. The presence of common community-acquired viruses, which the recipient may be incubating at the time of transplantation or exposed to nosocomially, may also cause infections in the early posttransplant period. Adenovirus infection is particularly aggressive in the new recipient of lungs and can lead to necrotizing pneumonitis. Influenza or respiratory syncytial virus (RSV) can also cause severe disease early after lung transplantation.

Intermediate period (1–6 months after transplantation)

The differential diagnosis of fever for patients presenting in the intermediate period can overlap with the early period if the patient is still in the hospital. Patients who continue to have central venous catheters in place remain at risk for catheter-associated infections. Likewise, individuals who require assisted ventilation are at risk for tracheitis or lower airway infection. In contrast to the early posttransplant period, pathogens that were latent in the donor or recipient can become active in the immunosuppressed transplant recipient and typically present during this intermediate period. In the former scenario, patients experience either a primary infection from the donor, which may be very severe, or reinfection of a donor strain of virus. In the latter scenario, patients experience reactivation of their own latent virus, which generally results in less severe disease.

Cytomegalovirus (CMV) and Epstein–Barr virus (EBV) are among the most important donor-transmitted viruses causing infection during this time period. Typically, the highest risk for disease occurs in the mismatched donor–recipient combination where the donor is seropositive and the recipient is naive to the virus. Both CMV and EBV can be transferred within the donor lungs or accompanying cells. Disease will often be heralded by fever and somatic complaints of fatigue followed by respiratory symptoms. In addition, changes in hematologic parameters such as leukopenia, atypical lymphocytosis and thrombocytopenia are common. Nodules in the lung radiographs are common in EBV-associated posttransplant lymphoproliferative disease (PTLD) after lung transplantation. Patients with PTLD may also present with skin nodules or gastrointestinal disturbance such as bleeding or pain. Previously, CMV pneumonitis was a common presenting symptom of primary CMV after lung transplantation. However, its incidence has decreased substantially with the use of antiviral prophylaxis and/or preemptive treatment strategies. To a lesser degree these organisms can lead to disease as secondary infections, either from reactivation of the host's latent viruses or from reinfection with a donor strain of virus.

Reactivation of other latent organisms can also occur (particularly from latently infected donor organs), including histoplasmosis, tuberculosis and toxoplasmosis. The latter is more common if a heart–lung transplant was performed. *Pneumocystis carinii* pneumonia (PCP) is more frequently found in recipients of lung transplants than of other solid organs if prophylaxis is not instituted. It also arises during this intermediate period. While the risk of PCP is highest during the first 1–2 years after transplantation, it never goes away completely.

Late period (>6 months after transplantation)

Fever appears to be a less common presenting symptom of infection in patients late after lung transplantation. However, late infections tend to be less well studied as patients are often at sites distant from the transplant center. Compared with other types of organ transplantation, lung transplant recipients have some unique types of late infection, particularly patients with chronic rejection or bronchiolitis obliterans. Rather than fever as a presenting sign, these patients often present with a decrease in pulmonary function along with an increase in sputum production or change of sputum quality and color. Of interest, microbial agents usually associated with individuals with CF are found in lung transplant recipients regardless of their underlying disease if they have bronchiolitis obliterans. These include *Pseudomonas aeruginosa*, *Alcaligenes xylosoxidans*, *Stenotrophomonas maltophilia* and *Aspergillus fumigatus*. The recovery of *Aspergillus* may represent asymptomatic colonization or disease. Manifestations of infection include localized or diffuse pneumonia, necrotizing pneumonitis with cavitation, and extrapulmonary dissemination. The other types of infection that may occur late in recipients of lung transplantation include opportunistic pulmonary infections with organisms such as *Nocardia* or *Cryptococcus*. PTLD can also occur late after transplantation, albeit less often than in the intermediate period. Also of note, PTLD late after transplantation is not always associated with EBV infection.

1.2 What are the predominant sites of infection?

The respiratory tract is the predominant site of infection in lung transplant recipients regardless of the timing after transplantation. Clinically important infections are usually found in the lower respiratory tract; however, sinusitis may be a cause of disease long after transplantation. Oropharyngeal reactivation of HSV can also occur, particularly when the patient is receiving high levels of immunosuppression (early after transplantation or after augmentation of immunosuppression to treat rejection).

Early after transplantation, local surgical wound infections can occur. Bacteremia is also found early after transplantation in association with the presence of central venous catheters or in patients with CF. *Burkholderia cepacia* is a serious cause of bacteremia and abscess formation after lung transplantation in patients with underlying CF. This has led many centers to consider colonization with this organism as a contraindication to lung transplantation. Less frequently patients with CF become bacteremic with *P. aeruginosa* or *A. xylosoxidans* after lung transplantation.

Lung transplant recipients are not at high risk for infections of the gastrointestinal tract. Patients who have been on prolonged antibiotics can subsequently develop *Clostridium difficile* colitis; also, EBV-associated PTLD can cause disease in the gastrointestinal system. Nosocomial or community-acquired gastrointestinal pathogens may be important, particularly in the pediatric age group, including rotavirus, adenovirus, *Salmonella* and *Shigella*.

The central nervous system (CNS) is infrequently a site of infection after thoracic organ transplantation. However, CNS infection due to *Aspergillus* may occur, particularly in patients who have chronic rejection or preceding CMV disease. Cryptococcal meningitis has also been reported in heavily immunosuppressed lung transplant recipients. Individuals who have a heart–lung block are at risk for transmission of *Toxoplasma gondii* within the donor heart, which frequently presents with CNS findings.

1.3 What are the predominant organisms that contribute (by site)?

Upper respiratory tract

The predominant pathogens isolated from the oropharynx after lung transplantation are *Candida* spp. and HSV. The risk for these organisms is particularly high in patients who are severely immunosuppressed. Accordingly, early after transplantation the authors recommend prophylaxis with mycostatin or clotrimazole troches to prevent oropharyngeal thrush and acyclovir to prevent reactivation of herpes stomatitis in a previously seropositive individual. Lung transplant recipients who demonstrate recurrent problems with these organisms receive more prolonged courses of these antimicrobial agents.

Sinusitis after lung transplantation is frequently caused by the same pathogens that cause sinusitis in immunocompetent patients, such as *Streptococcus pneumoniae*, *Haemophilus influenzae* and *Moraxella catarrhalis*. In addition, patients with underlying CF may develop sinusitis caused by organisms that typically inhabit their upper airways, such as *P. aeruginosa*. Consideration should be given to obtaining sinus culture and biopsy in patients who do not respond to antibiotics for radiographically proven sinusitis in order to look for antibiotic-resistant pathogens or *Aspergillus*.

Respiratory viruses that are circulating in the community or hospital, such as parainfluenza, RSV, influenza or adenovirus, can also cause upper respiratory tract infections in lung transplant recipients. Many of these community-acquired viruses, as well as *Streptococcus pyogenes*, may produce pharyngitis in these patients. However, the differential diagnosis of exudative pharyngitis after transplantation must also include EBV disease.

Lower respiratory tract

Many pathogens can cause lower respiratory tract infection or tracheitis in patients who have undergone lung transplantation. Patients with underlying CF frequently develop disease caused by the same pathogens that colonized their native lungs. While the new lungs do not have the physiologic defects associated with abnormal CF genes, they still remain at high risk for infection because of denervation, abnormal diaphragmatic movement or stenosis at the anastomotic sites, making pulmonary toilet difficult. Persistent colonization of the trachea and upper airway with organisms that colonized the native lung in CF patients can serve as a source of infection of the new lungs. Interestingly, lung transplant recipients who develop obliterative bronchiolitis after transplantation are also at high risk for these same types of pathogens, even if they do not have underlying CF.

In addition to the above pathogens, recurrent pneumococcal pneumonia has been found to occur in some lung transplant recipients. *Staphylococcus aureus* should also be considered in patients with high fever and effusions. Similarly, fungi (especially *A. fumigatus*), *Cryptococcus*, *Nocardia* and *P. carinii* should also be included as possible pathogens in lung transplant recipients who present with signs and symptoms of lower respiratory tract infection. Some of these pathogens, in particular *P. carinii*, can be readily prevented by means of prophylaxis (e.g. TMP–SMX). CMV and EBV can also present with lower respiratory tract symptoms, as can *Mycobacterium tuberculosis*, although the role of nontuberculous mycobacteria as a true pathogen is less clear. Early after transplantation, viruses such as adenovirus, influenza, parainfluenza or RSV may also cause serious and sometimes fatal lower respiratory tract infection.

Urinary tract

Gram-negative enteric organisms, *Candida* spp., enterococci or coagulase-negative staphylococci most often cause UTI. Viral pathogens that may affect the urinary tract include adenovirus, JC and BK viruses. Each of these viruses has been described as the cause of hemorrhagic cystitis. Although they have tended to be identified after bone marrow transplantation, and the latter two have not been described after lung transplantation, their presence is worth considering in a patient with sterile pyuria and hematuria. It is also worth noting that some viruses, including CMV and adenovirus, may be shed asymptomatically in the urine without disease implications.

Heart

The risk of infection of the heart and the types of pathogens that are found in a lung transplant recipient are dependent on whether or not the patient received a heart graft along with the lungs. Patients who are naive to *T. gondii* who receive a heart–lung bloc from a donor who had previous toxoplasmosis are at higher risk for this pathogen than is a recipient of lungs alone. Patients who undergo isolated lung transplantation are not at a higher risk for heart infections than other transplant recipients.

Gastrointestinal tract

A wide variety of pathogens are associated with infections of the gastrointestinal tract of lung transplant recipients. *C. difficile* (particularly if patients are on antibiotics for other infections) and rotavirus (common in children during the winter months) are among the most frequent gastrointestinal pathogens. *Giardia lamblia* and *Cryptosporidium* may cause more severe disease in transplant recipients than in immunocompetent family members with similar exposures, but are infrequent causes of disease after lung transplantation. EBV-associated PTLD should be strongly considered in lung transplant recipients with symptoms referable to the gastrointestinal tract, particularly if they were seronegative before transplantation. Finally, CMV may also cause disease of the gastrointestinal tract after lung transplantation.

Viral hepatitis is a potentially important problem following lung transplantation. Hepatitis C virus has been a particular problem for individuals who received transfusions or transplant grafts before the time of screening for this virus. Diffuse infection of the liver may be from CMV, EBV, HSV, varicella zoster virus (VZV), hepatitis B virus or adenovirus. In addition, discrete liver lesions can be found with EBV-associated PTLD or fungal disease.

Skin and soft tissue

Most wound infections after lung transplantation are caused by Gram-positive organisms such *S. aureus*, coagulase-negative staphylococci or *S. pyogenes*. Younger patients also appear to be at higher risk for wound infections due to Gram-negative organisms. In addition, *M. hominis* has been described as infecting wounds after lung transplantation.

Many types of pathogens may cause skin infections following lung transplantation. VZV, manifesting as either primary (chickenpox) or reactivation (zoster) infection, may be a nidus for secondary bacterial skin infections with *S. aureus* or *S. pyogenes*. Reactivation of HSV after transplantation is also common. Papillomavirus may be the cause of persistent and often severe warts in these patients that are often resistant to many therapeutic maneuvers. Finally, nodular skin lesions due to PTLD, *Aspergillus* and, less frequently, other fungi have also been diagnosed in lung transplant recipients.

Bloodstream

Central venous catheters are the most frequent source of bloodstream infections in lung transplant recipients. These infections are most often caused by coagulase-negative staphylococci, followed less frequently by other Gram-positive and Gram-negative bacteria. *Candida* spp. may also cause catheter-associated infections after transplantation, particularly in the setting of the intensive care unit, or previous use of broad-spectrum antibiotics. Recurrent pneumococcal bacteremia has been found in some lung transplant recipients without other underlying risks such as asplenia. The authors' institution has noted bacteremia early after lung transplantation in patients with underlying CF with organisms that colonized their lungs before transplantation, including *P. aeruginosa*, *A. xylosoxidans* and *B. cepacia*.

Central nervous system

Infections of the CNS occur infrequently after lung transplantation. When present, they carry a broad differential diagnosis of opportunistic pathogens. Cryptococcal meningitis is unusual in the young child but must be considered in the teenager or adult who has undergone lung transplantation. Patients who received a heart–lung bloc may have primary toxoplasmosis present with CNS disease. *Aspergillus* is of particular concern in individuals with underlying CF, or in those who develop bronchiolitis obliterans or CMV infection. Viruses are a less common cause of CNS disease; however, EBV-associated PTLD and, less often, CMV may present in this fashion.

1.4 How do the organisms vary according to various risk factors?

Multiple risk factors play a role in the severity of disease from organisms infecting patients who have undergone lung transplantation. The severity of the candidate's pre-transplant clinical status (including whether or not the patient is on a mechanical respirator or is malnourished) correlates with increased severity of infections after transplantation. The absence of preexisting immunity to specific pathogens also increases the severity of disease after transplantation. This is particularly true for donor-associated infections such as CMV, EBV or toxoplasmosis. Numerous studies have proven that seronegativity of the recipient of lungs or heart–lungs from a seropositive donor is a major risk factor for disease with each of these organisms. In addition, previous colonization with antibiotic-resistant bacteria or *Aspergillus* is a risk factor for these same microbial agents causing disease after lung transplantation, especially if underlying CF is present.

The intensity of immunosuppression affects the risk of infection after transplantation. Patients who require high amounts of baseline immunosuppression or multiple courses of augmented treatment of rejection are at greater risk for infections than those with relatively benign rejection histories. Typically, lung and heart–lung transplant recipients require triple drug baseline immunosuppression consisting of cyclosporin or tacrolimus used in combination with steroids and either azathioprine or mycophenolate mofetil. In addition to the baseline immunosuppression, steroid-resistant rejection is treated with antilymphocytic antibodies, which increase the risk for viral and fungal infections. Recipients who go on to develop obliterative bronchiolitis due to chronic rejection are at high risk for colonization and infection with *Aspergillus, P. aeruginosa, A. xylosoxidans* and *S. maltophilia*.

Technical complications of surgery such as stenosis at the site of the tracheal anastomosis may be associated with the development of bacterial infections distal to the area of stenosis due to impaired clearance of the airway. Similarly, phrenic nerve dysfunction after surgery leading to poor or absent movement of the diaphragm impairs airway clearance and is also a risk factor for bacterial pneumonia.

Nosocomial and environmental exposures are also risk factors for infection after lung transplantation. Construction in the hospital or breakdown in the water heating system can lead to environmental exposures to *Aspergillus* and *Legionella*. Nosocomial acquisition of circulating viruses or antibiotic-resistant bacteria is a risk for any hospitalized patient, but particularly for one whose immune system is compromised by transplantation. The presence of an indwelling catheter is a risk for bacterial and yeast infections. Finally, patients are at increased risk for specific infections if they are not receiving prophylaxis. For example, PCP should be high on the differential diagnosis of a lung transplant recipient who is not taking TMP–SMX as prophylaxis, and who presents with hypoxia and pneumonitis, particularly during the first 2 years after transplantation.

1.5 How does this differ from other conditions, from center to center, and from country to country?

Infections after lung transplantation differ from infections in recipients of other types of transplants by their more frequent involvement of the pulmonary tree. In addition, recipients of lung transplantation appear to have a higher risk of infection than other transplant recipients; this is probably related to their chronic requirement for higher amounts of immunosuppression to prevent rejection and possibly to an increase in lymphoid tissue brought over with the allograft. Both of these factors increase the risk of opportunistic infection and EBV disease. Only intestinal transplant recipients have a higher risk for EBV-associated PTLD.

Risks for and manifestations of infection after lung transplantation may also vary between centers and countries. These differences may be due to variations in immunosuppressive regimens and antiinfective prophylactic strategies. In addition, unique environmental exposures will lead to differences in the types of infection encountered at various centers. Individual transplant centers may have distinct antibiotic resistance patterns of bacteria that may be spread nosocomially. Patients who live in areas that are endemic for certain pathogens (e.g. *M. tuberculosis, Coccidioides immitis*) are at greater risk for acquiring these infections or reactivating their own latent pathogens after transplantation. Fewer lung transplant centers exist than centers performing kidney, liver or heart transplantation. Accordingly, patients may come from diverse geographic backgrounds; for this reason it is important to consider the environmental exposures from the individual's home as well as the transplant center when evaluating infections after transplantation.

1.6 What is the appropriate approach to the initial evaluation and diagnosis of infection in lung and heart-lung transplant recipients?

The initial evaluation of a lung transplant recipient must include a careful history and physical examination to help ascertain the cause and source of infection. Consideration of the time after transplantation at which the patient presents, medication history, illness exposures, donor–recipient serologic status for CMV and EBV, and whether or not the patient has current or recent rejection will help in developing a differential diagnosis. As with all patients, signs and symptoms will help to suggest the site of infection. The presence of a vascular catheter, urinary catheter or endotracheal tube should make one consider the potential for bloodstream infection, UTI or ventilator-associated pneumonia, respectively.

After completing a thorough history and physical examination, the clinician should obtain appropriate diagnostic tests including sputum, blood and urine cultures. Pulmonary function testing and pulse oximetry are of great importance if the patient has any symptoms suggestive of lower respiratory tract involvement. Strong consideration should be given to obtaining a chest radiograph on every lung or heart–lung recipient with fever and/or symptoms referable to the respiratory tract. Performance of bronchoalveolar lavage (BAL) should be undertaken in patients with changes on the chest radiograph who are unable to provide an adequate sputum specimen, or those with evidence of interstitial disease, as well as those with significant fever and changes in pulmonary function tests. Samples from the lavage should be sent for histological examination, Gram staining, and bacterial, viral and fungal culture. In addition the authors perform *Legionella*, *Mycoplasma* and *Mycobacterium* cultures on all bronchoalveolar specimens. Transbronchial biopsies are often necessary to determine whether or not rejection is concurrently present. This is particularly helpful if consideration is being given to decreasing immunosuppression to help the body overcome the infectious insult. Patients who are at high risk for EBV or CMV disease (donor–recipient mismatch and in the first year after transplantation) should have special studies to look for active disease from these viruses. It should be stressed that an adequate database is mandatory before instituting antimicrobial therapy, except under extreme conditions.

1.7 How should the evaluation be modified according to the severity of the risk?

Patients in extremis require a rapid workup and empirical treatment even if optimal sampling has not been carried out. Empirical therapy may be started after obtaining a sputum or tracheal aspirate for culture, rather than performing BAL on a lung transplant recipient who presents in the middle of the night with sudden deterioration in oxygen saturation and increasing pulmonary infiltration. Empirical therapy should be based on previous culture results as well as on pathogens known frequently to infect this population. Awareness of the local prevalence of antibiotic resistance is important when making this initial antibiotic decision. On the other hand, BAL and biopsy should be performed on a patient who is slowly deteriorating before instituting antimicrobial agents.

Evaluation of a patient is also influenced by risk for specific diseases. CMV studies such as CMV pp65 antigenemia and/or CMV polymerase chain reaction (PCR) testing should be undertaken when a recipient presents 1–12 months after transplantation with fever, malaise, and leukopenia, and is known to be mismatched for CMV. However, an alternate source of infection should be sought for a patient who is donor seronegative/recipient seronegative (D–/R–) for CMV, or who presents with symptoms within the first month following transplantation. Similar consideration should be given for EBV studies based on recipient pretransplant serologic status. Since EBV infection can occur from sources other than the lung donor (including blood products or saliva), all seronegative recipients of lung transplants are at risk for new acquisition of EBV infection and PTLD. Patients with bronchiolitis obliterans should be evaluated for the presence of fungal disease and/or infection with bacteria such as *P. aeruginosa*, *S. maltophilia* and *A. xylosoxidans*.

1.8 What are the specific evaluation measures? (see also Chapter 2 in Part I)
An overview of the evaluation of infection following lung transplantation by site of involvement and particular organism is shown in Table 7.4.1.

1.9 What new developments are going to impact on emerging organisms, recognition, evaluation and diagnosis of infection in lung and heart-lung transplant recipients?
New and/or emerging organisms are recognized either because they are truly new, or because of the availability of new diagnostic tests to recognize microbial agents that have long been present. Several human herpesviruses (HHV-6, HHV-7 and HHV-8) were recognized only in the relatively recent past, even though they are not truly new organisms. However, the availability of new tests to identify their presence provides the opportunity to understand their pathogenic potential after lung transplantation. Similarly, parvovirus B19 has only in recent years been recognized as causing red cell aplasia in solid organ transplant recipients.

The use of new and stronger immunosuppressants to prevent or treat rejection has led to the emergence of opportunistic diseases from organisms that are typically non-pathogens in less immunosuppressed patients. Examples include invasive disease caused by organisms such *Alternaria* or *Fusaria* after bone marrow transplantation. Atypical mycobacteria or *Scedosporium apiospermum* (asexual form of *Pseudallescheria boydii*) are microbial agents being found in BAL specimens after lung transplantation. Further clinical correlation, controlling for rejection and coinfections, is required to help determine whether these are emerging pathogens or simply colonizing agents. *S. maltophilia* and *A. xylosoxidans*, along with *P. aeruginosa*, are increasingly found in the sputum of lung transplant recipients with chronic rejection in association with increasing cough, respiratory effort and change in sputum; as such they may also be considered as emerging pathogens.

One of the most exciting new developments impacting on the recognition and evaluation of infection in lung transplant recipients has been the more rapid and sensitive tests for CMV. Classic culture techniques for CMV in the virology laboratory take 2–3 weeks to exhibit a cytopathic effect. The development of the rapid spin culture technique has decreased the culture time to within 72 h. The CMV pp65 antigenemia assay, as well as PCR techniques, provide earlier and more sensitive recognition of the presence of this virus. The decision of which diagnostic test for CMV should be used is dictated by the expertise of the local laboratory. In addition, the availability of quantitative PCR testing for multiple pathogens (e.g. EBV), more rapid growth techniques for organisms (e.g.

Table 7.4.1 Evaluation of infections in lung transplant recipients according to the site of infection and possible etiologic agent

Site of infection	Infectious syndrome (clinical features)	Predominant pathogens	Diagnostic investigation
Bloodstream	Bacteremia (fever with or without local signs of infection)	Streptococcus pneumoniae (recurrent) Coagulase-negative staphylococci Staphylococcus aureus Enterococcus spp. (nosocomial outbreaks in some institutions) Gram-negative bacilli (Escherichia coli, Klebsiella pneumoniae, Enterobacter spp., Pseudomonas aeruginosa) Candida spp.	Blood cultures (two sets drawn from separate sites and at least one set drawn from intravenous catheter)
Intravascular catheter-related infections	Pain, erythema, tenderness, discharge from catheter entry site	Coagulase-negative staphylococci Staphylococcus aureus Corynebacterium jeikeium Enterococcus spp. (nosocomial outbreaks in some institutions) Gram-negative bacilli Candida spp.	Swab of entry site Culture of catheter tip Blood cultures (consider drawing blood through each lumen of catheter and doing quantitative blood cultures)
Oral cavity	Stomatitis/mucositis (aphthous ulcers) Oral thrush (white plaques)	Herpes simplex virus Candida spp.	Direct examination and culture of specimen
Throat	Pharyngitis Tonsilitis (sore throat, odynophagia)	Streptococcus pyogenes Epstein–Barr virus Herpes simplex virus Adenovirus, rhinovirus, coronavirus Influenza virus, parainfluenza virus	Swab of pharynx Serology
Upper respiratory tract (ear, nose, sinus, nasopharynx, larynx, trachea)	Otitis media Otitis externa (earache, drainage, irritability)	Streptococcus pneumoniae Haemophilus influenzae Moraxella catarrhalis Pseudomonas aeruginosa	Consider empirical therapy for otitis media Tympanocentesis (in case of treatment failure)

Site	Clinical features	Organisms	Investigation
		Mycoplasma pneumoniae	Swab of external auditory canal (otitis externa)
	Sinusitis (tightness of sinus areas, headache, toothache, nasal obstruction, nasal voice)	Streptococcus pneumoniae Haemophilus influenzae Moraxella catarrhalis Aspergillus spp.. Mucor spp. Candida spp. Viruses (influenza, parainfluenza, rhinovirus, adenovirus)	Aspiration of sinus Biopsy (if no improvement after 72–96 h of empirical antibiotic therapy)
	Laryngitis (sore throat, hoarseness, otalgia)	Viruses (influenza, parainfluenza, adenovirus, respiratory syncytial virus) Streptococcus pyogenes Haemophilus influenzae	
	Tracheitis (stridor, dyspnea, cough)	Staphylococcus aureus Moraxella catarrhalis Pseudomonas aeruginosa Stenotrophomonas maltophilia Achromobacter xylosoxidans	Culture of tracheal secretions
Lower respiratory tract (bronchi, terminal airways, alveoli)	Bronchopneumonia Pneumonia (cough, dyspnea, chest pain, sputum, hemoptysis, pleural effusion)	Conventional infections: Gram-negative bacilli (Pseudomonas spp., Stenotrophomonas maltophilia, Burkholderia cepacia, Escherichia coli, Klebsiella pneumoniae, Acinetobacter spp.) Streptococcus pneumoniae Haemophilus influenzae Staphylococcus aureus Mycoplasma pneumoniae Virus (influenza, parainfluenza, respiratory syncytial virus) Opportunistic infections: Aspergillus spp. (very frequent in cystic fibrosis and bronchiolitis obliterans)	Chest radiography, CT, MRI Fiberoptic bronchoscopy with bronchoalveolar lavage Transbronchial biopsy Thoracocentesis Open lung biopsy

Site of infection	Infectious syndrome (clinical features)	Predominant pathogens	Diagnostic investigation
		Mucor spp. Scedosporium spp./Pseudallescheria boydii Nocardia asteroides Pneumocystis carinii Mycobacterium tuberculosis Atypical mycobacteria (? pathogenic role) Cytomegalovirus Epstein–Barr virus Adenovirus Varicella zoster virus Histoplasma, Coccidioides	Chest radiography, CT Sputum culture Fiberoptic bronchoscopy with bronchoalveolar lavage Percutaneous transthoracic aspiration Thoracocentesis
	Lung abscess	Bacteroides spp. Fusobacterium spp. Peptostreptococcus spp. Gram-negative bacilli Staphylococcus aureus Streptococci (Streptococcus milleri, group A streptococci, anaerobic streptococci)	
	Empyema	Streptococci (Streptococcus pneumoniae, group A streptococci, Streptococcus milleri, anaerobic streptococci) Staphylococcus aureus Haemophilus influenzae Gram-negative bacilli Bacteroides spp.	
Heart (in case of heart–lung transplantation)	Endocarditis Pericarditis	Staphylococcus aureus Enterococcus spp. Gram-negative bacilli Coagulase-negative staphylococci	Blood cultures Echocardiography Biopsy Culture of pericardial fluid

System	Infection	Organisms	Diagnostics
	Myocarditis	Viridans streptococci *Aspergillus* spp. *Candida* spp. *Toxoplasma gondii* Cytomegalovirus	
Urinary tract	Pyelonephritis Cystitis	Gram-negative bacilli (*Escherichia coli, Klebsiella* spp., *Proteus* spp., *Enterobacter* spp., *Pseudomonas aeruginosa*) *Enterococcus* spp. *Candida* spp. Adenovirus, BK and JC virus Cytomegalovirus (?viruria versus disease)	Urinanalysis Culture of urine Ultrasonography, CT (if suspicion of abscess)
Central nervous system*	Acute meningitis Subacute, chronic meningitis	*Listeria monocytogenes* *Cryptococcus neoformans* *Candida* spp. *Mycobacterium tuberculosis* *Coccidioides immitis* *Histoplasma capsulatum*	CT, MRI Lumbar puncture Aspiration or biopsy under stereotaxic CT guidance
	Focal brain diseases	*Aspergillus* spp. *Scedosporium* spp./*Pseudallescheria boydii* *Nocardia asteroides* *Listeria monocytogenes* *Toxoplasma gondii* (heart–lung transplant) Viruses (EBV, HSV, varicella zoster virus, cytomegalovirus, HHV-6, adenovirus, papillomavirus, JC virus)	
	Progressive dementia	JC virus (progressive multifocal leukoencephalopathy)	
Skin infection and soft tissue	Surgical wound infections	*Staphylococcus aureus* Coagulase-negative staphylococci *Enterococcus* spp. Gram-negative bacilli (Enterobacteriaceae, *Pseudomonas aeruginosa*)	Aspiration (needle) or swab of skin exudate

Site of infection	Infectious syndrome (clinical features)	Predominant pathogens	Diagnostic investigation
		Candida spp. *Mycoplasma hominis*	Aspiration (needle) or swab of skin exudate Skin biopsy (histology and culture) Serology
	Rash Cellulitis (pain, erythema, tenderness, necrosis in case of ecthyma gangrenosum)	Primary infections: *Staphylococcus aureus* Coagulase-negative staphylococci Gram-negative bacilli (*Pseudomonas aeruginosa, Escherichia coli, Klebsiella pneumoniae*) *Candida* spp. *Mucor* spp., *Rhizopus* spp. Mycobacteria Epstein–Barr virus	
	Papules, nodules (with or without myalgia and muscle tenderness)	Disseminated infections: *Candida* spp., *Fusarium* spp., *Alternaria* spp., *Aspergillus* spp. Gram-negative bacilli (*Escherichia coli, Pseudomonas aeruginosa, Aeromonas hydrophilia, Serratia marcescens*) Epstein–Barr virus, adenovirus	
	Ulcers, vesicles, hemorrhagic or crusted lesions (isolated or with dermatomal distribution)	Herpes simplex virus Varicella zoster virus Cytomegalovirus	
	Disseminated vesicles, hemorrhagic or crusted lesions	Varicella zoster virus, herpes simplex virus *Staphylococcus aureus*, streptococci	
	Skin necrosis	*Aspergillus* spp., *Mucor* spp.	
	Warts	Papillomavirus	
	Molluscum contagiosum	Poxvirus-related virus	

Gastrointestinal tract

Esophagus	Esophagitis (dysphagia, retrosternal pain)	Herpes simplex virus Candida spp., Aspergillus spp. Cytomegalovirus	Esogastroscopy Culture of endoscopic specimens
Small intestine, colon	Enteritis Colitis (nausea, vomiting, bloating, abdominal discomfort, cramp, pain, constipation, diarrhea)	Clostridium difficile (antibiotic-associated diarrhea) Cytomegalovirus Epstein–Barr virus Adenovirus Rotavirus (children) Cryptosporidium Giardia lamblia	Plain abdominal films Ultrasonography, CT or MRI Colonoscopy Biopsy Culture of endoscopic specimens Stool cultures Toxin detection
Liver	Hepatitis	Viral hepatitis (A, B, C) – reactivation in graft Epstein–Barr virus Cytomegalovirus Herpes simplex virus Adenovirus	Liver biopsy Serology

* Transplant patients have the same susceptibility to conventional pathogens of the central nervous system (meningitis: Streptococcus pneumoniae, Neisseria meningitidis, Haemophilus influenzae, Gram-negative bacilli; brain abscess: streptococci, Bacteroides spp., Staphylococcus aureus, Enterobacteriaceae) as the general population. Listed above are unique pathogens.

mycobacteria) and in-situ hybridization studies for pathologic specimens have all advanced the ability to recognize infections in lung transplant recipients.

Although these many new techniques bring a great promise of improved patient care, it is critical to evaluate each new technique and to understand its limitations. Increased sensitivity is not always superior, as it may be so sensitive that it is no longer clinically valuable – leading to treatment when none was required. The use of all diagnostic techniques should be based on sound clinical studies and used in the presence of good clinical judgement.

2 REGARDING THE RISK FACTORS IN LUNG AND HEART–LUNG TRANSPLANT RECIPIENTS

2.1. What are the main alterations in host defense mechanisms and what are the appropriate investigations to document them?

Similar to recipients of other types of organ transplant, recipients of lung or heart–lung transplants have their immunologic defenses against infections altered by the need to use potent immunosuppressive agents to prevent rejection of the new graft. These agents act most strongly on the cytotoxic T-cell arm of the immunologic system. Accordingly, the recipient is at increased risk for pathogens such as viruses, *Candida* spp. and fungi, which are normally controlled by these cells. Unlike some other transplant recipients, most lung or heart–lung transplant recipients continue to require triple drug immunosuppression, even long after transplantation. Accordingly, other arms of the immune system are altered by the use of corticosteroids and azathioprine or mycophenolic acid. These latter two agents may also produce neutropenia. Use of antithymocyte globulins or monoclonal antibodies for the treatment of steroid-resistant rejection produces a substantial alteration in the immune system and further increases the patient's risk for viral and fungal illnesses.

Unique to lung and heart–lung transplantation, anatomic barriers of the pulmonary tree can be disrupted at the anastomotic site, leading to poor clearance of secretions distal to the anastomosis and recurrent pneumonia. Likewise, damage to the phrenic nerve interferes with the normal diaphragm movement, and again decreases clearance of pathogens in the respiratory tree. The presence of a foreign body, such as an endotracheal tube, urinary catheter or vascular catheters, also interrupts the normal host barriers against microbial agents. Prolonged use of antibiotics can change the normal milieu of colonizing agents and allow for overgrowth of antibiotic-resistant bacteria or yeast. Finally, some infections, such as CMV or EBV, may decrease the host's immunologic reserves, putting the recipient at risk for subsequent fungal infection.

2.2 What are the alterations due to iatrogenic factors?

The major alterations in the lung transplant recipients' host defenses are due to iatrogenic factors. The use of immunosuppressive agents, the presence of foreign bodies and even the interruption of the anatomic barriers at operation are iatrogenic manipulations that increase the patient's risk of infection. Previously administered antimicrobial agents influence the antibiotic susceptibility of bacteria. This is particularly true for patients with underlying CF who have had a great deal of previous antibiotic exposures, often resulting in multi-resistant strains of *Pseudomonas*.

2.3 What is the influence of environmental factors?

Environmental factors within the hospital are important primarily as risks for nosocomial transmission of infections and are similar for most transplant recipients. In particular, transplant centers endemically colonized with vancomycin-resistant enterococci (VRE) and methicillin-resistant *S. aureus* (MRSA) are much more likely to have patients infected with these organisms after lung transplantation. Local construction has been associated with nosocomial transmission of *Aspergillus* if the construction is ongoing in areas where the transplant patients are located. Likewise, contamination of the water system with *Legionella* may lead to serious infection after transplantation. Finally, nosocomial infections can occur with seasonal community-acquired viruses such as RSV, influenza or rotavirus.

Community environmental factors are important after a person goes home, but need to be considered even before transplantation as they may predict which latent pathogens might be present and capable of reactivating under the influence of immunosuppression. Exposure to tuberculosis is particularly serious. Lung transplant recipients should be evaluated thoroughly for the presence of pathogens that have a potential for reactivation under immunosuppressive therapy during their initial pretransplant evaluation. Treatment and prophylaxis should be considered before or at the time that patients are to start immunosuppressive therapy. Different communities or countries will have different risks for contact with specific organisms such as *Babesia microtii*, *Plasmodium* spp., *C. immitis*, *Histoplasma capsulatum* or *M. tuberculosis*. In addition, food and water sources are important environmental risk factors to consider. Immunosuppressed individuals may be more susceptible to *Cryptosporidium* or *Giardia* contamination of water systems. In addition, recipients who consume raw or rare meats may be putting themselves at increase risk for disease from parasites that could be harbored within the food. Environmental exposures to animals should also be considered, such as the risk of *T. gondii* with cats or *Salmonella* with pet reptiles. Patient education can assist in decreasing many of these community environmental exposures.

2.4 What are the most significant factors that contribute to the risk of infection in lung and heart-lung transplant recipients?

The use of immunosuppressants is the most important factor contributing to the risk of infection after lung transplantation. Patients who have required augmentation of their immunosuppression because of frequent rejection, especially those who received anti-lymphocytic antibodies, are at the highest risk for infection. Other significant factors include technical complications during or after operation, use of indwelling catheters, donor and recipient mismatched serologic status for CMV and EBV, nosocomial exposures to pathogens, and acute and chronic rejection. In addition, the patient's underlying disease, particularly CF, has a major impact on the types of infectious agents that will be found after transplantation. Finally, the age of the patient impacts on the risk of infection and the likelihood of having preexisting immunity from natural infection or vaccination. For example, children are more likely to be immunologically naive to viruses such as EBV and CMV, and are thus at greater risk for disease after transplantation. Alternatively, some organisms (e.g. *Cryptococcus*) do not appear to cause disease in young children. Each of the above factors may affect the likelihood of acquiring infection, as well as its potential severity, after transplantation.

2.5 What are the specific or nonspecific measures aimed at minimizing each of these factors?

Measures can be taken to minimize many risk factors for infection after lung transplantation. First, it is important to evaluate candidates fully and to establish relative and absolute contraindications to transplantation. Many centers will not transplant patients with CF who have colonization with *B. cepacia* or panresistant pseudomonads. Delayed-type hypersensitivity testing will help to identify individuals with previous *M. tuberculosis* infection and allow for adequate treatment before transplantation. Updating vaccinations whenever possible is also a readily available method for minimizing infectious disease risks after transplantation.

Immunosuppressive doses should be maintained at levels aimed at avoiding rejection but minimized to the extent possible to prevent infectious complications. Prophylaxis or preemptive treatment strategies for patients who are CMV-mismatched appear to be helpful in lessening the severity of disease from this virus. In addition, prophylaxis against PCP and *Aspergillus* for patients with chronic rejection has been valuable in decreasing disease from these pathogens.

2.6 Are there different levels of risk of infection recognized for lung and heart-lung transplant recipients?

Several different factors can be identified that increase the risk for specific types of infections after lung transplantation. Patients with underlying CF who undergo lung transplantation are at higher risk for bacteremia shortly after transplantation with the microbes that previously colonized their lungs than recipients without underlying CF. For this reason, many centers opt to give a 10–14-day course of antibiotics after lung transplantation in this group of patients. *B. cepacia* is a particularly aggressive bacterium after transplantation, leading to invasive, often fatal, disease. Accordingly, a number of centers view this agent as a contraindication to lung transplantation. In addition, patients with CF almost uniformly have at least one episode of pneumonia or bronchitis diagnosed after transplantation, with the same agents that colonized their lungs before the operation.

Lung transplant recipients who are mismatched for CMV (D+/R–) are at very high risk for symptomatic CMV disease after transplantation, even when prophylaxis has been instituted. Likewise, lung transplant recipients mismatched for EBV are at higher risk than other organ transplant recipients (except for small bowel recipients) for EBV-driven PTLD. Recipients who are seronegative for EBV before transplantation also acquire primary infection from sources other than the lung donor. Accordingly, even patients whose donors are seronegative for EBV are at high risk for PTLD if they develop primary infection early after transplantation.

Individuals who develop chronic rejection after lung transplantation become colonized with many of the same microbial agents that colonize people with CF, including *A. fumigatus*, *P. aeruginosa*, *S. maltophilia* and *A. xylosoxidans*. Bronchitis or pneumonia may result from any of these organisms. In addition, disseminated invasive disease due to *Aspergillus* may also develop in these patients.

2.7 How does the level of risk impact on management?

Patients known to be at high risk for particular diseases can be followed closely for the development of problems and are ideal candidates for preventive strategies. Some centers provide prophylaxis against CMV disease in mismatched donor/recipient pairs, while other centers monitor these patients closely with either pp65 antigenemia assays or CMV PCR testing. In either case, knowing about the high-risk situation allows caretakers to follow closely if signs or symptoms of disease develop, and to initiate antiviral treatment promptly while awaiting confirmatory results from the laboratory. Patients at increased risk for EBV disease can also be followed closely to evaluate concerns for developing PTLD. While studies are ongoing to determine whether or not prophylaxis or preemptive treatment protocols will be beneficial against PTLD, knowing that a patient is at high risk allows caretakers to make efforts to minimize immunosuppression to the lowest levels possible and should allow them to diagnose these syndromes at earlier and more responsive stages of the disease.

Patients with underlying CF have perioperative prophylaxis tailored by the specific susceptibility patterns of microbial agents known to colonize their respiratory tract. Because these bacteria are known to colonize the sinuses and upper respiratory tracts of patients, studies are ongoing to determine whether or not aggressive sinus surgery will prevent recurrent bacterial pneumonia and bronchitis. In addition, itraconazole or aerosolized amphotericin B can be used as prophylaxis for individuals known to harbor *Aspergillus* prior to transplantation. Itraconazole prophylaxis against *Aspergillus* may also be given to individuals with bronchiolitis obliterans to avoid invasive fungal disease.

2.8 What new developments are going to impact on minimizing or suppressing the specific risk factors?

The ongoing development and use of newer and more specific immunosuppressive agents will impact positively on the risk for infection after lung transplantation. As these agents become more specific, they should decrease the risk of developing infections with opportunistic pathogens. However, if the newer agents are more potent but are still nonspecific in their effect on the immune system, they will have an adverse impact on risk of infection. Better prophylactic strategies against CMV and EBV disease, or the development of vaccines against these herpesviruses, would also have a significant impact on disease after transplantation. Improved diagnostic testing will impact on many infectious diseases by being able to identify pathogens more accurately and promptly.

3 REGARDING THE SURVEILLANCE OF LUNG AND HEART–LUNG TRANSPLANT RECIPIENTS

3.1 What is the important pretransplant information to be gathered?

Before transplantation all lung transplant candidates should have a thorough infectious disease evaluation. This evaluation is critical: to (1) identify potential contraindications to transplantation, (2) to identify risk factors for infection after transplantation, (3) to allow for appropriate preventive strategies, and (4) to educate the patients and their family about potential infectious disease risks. In particular, the pretransplant evaluation should identify infection or colonization with antibiotic-resistant bacteria. Many centers consider colonization with panresistant pseudomonads to be a contraindication to transplantation. Similarly, any colonization with *B. cepacia* is considered by many centers to be a contraindication to lung transplantation. Additional contraindications might include recent cancer, untreated tuberculosis and infection with human immunodeficiency virus (HIV). These latter two may represent relative contraindications, dependent on the candidate status and the philosophy of the individual center.

Candidates for lung transplantation often have prolonged waits for organs. Accordingly the authors recommend obtaining surveillance sputum cultures every 6 months, and even more frequently if the patient's name comes close to the top of the waiting list.

Infection with *M. tuberculosis* should be sought in all transplant candidates by performing PPD skin testing. Follow-up chest radiography, acid fast cultures and smears of sputum or gastric washes should be performed for patients with positive reactions. A history of previous infections is important to obtain. Patients with a history of symptomatic HSV may benefit from prophylaxis following transplantation. Previous varicella infection decreases the risk of infection after exposure to chickenpox. Immunization history should be reviewed, and lapsed immunizations updated (see below and section 4.1). This is of particular importance for pediatric lung transplant candidates.

Serologic evaluation to document previous infections is important, as individuals will often not have a history of specific viral infections. The authors' recommendations for pretransplant laboratory evaluation of infections are noted below (see section 3.2).

3.2 What are the surveillance measures to be taken when a patient presents for lung or heart-lung transplantation?

Surveillance cultures of sputum of candidates with underlying CF or purulent pulmonary disease are essential before lung transplantation. Cultures should be evaluated in a laboratory with experience in isolating microbes harbored by patients with CF and in performing antibiotic susceptibility tests. Patients with multiply antibiotic-resistant microbial agents may benefit from having the bacteria tested at a reference laboratory for synergistic combinations of antibiotics. In addition, evidence of mycobacterial and fungal infection should be sought on surveillance cultures.

Serologic status for a number of agents should be obtained routinely for all potential donors, including CMV, EBV, hepatitis B and C, and HIV. In addition, donors of heart–lung blocs should be tested for antibodies directed against *T. gondii*. Similarly, serology should be performed on the lung transplant candidate for these same agents. Candidate serology should also be obtained against HSV and VZV. Tests for evidence of protective antibody titers against measles, mumps and rubella will help to identify individuals who did not develop a protective response and who may benefit from repeat vaccination before transplantation.

Some centers perform environmental surveillance cultures for the presence of nosocomial pathogens such as *A. fumigatus* or *Legionella* spp. The authors' institution has not found fungal cultures to be of assistance, but evidence of *Legionella* contamination continues to be sought twice a year.

3.3 What are the other specific measures to be taken when a patient presents for lung or heart-lung transplantation?

The majority of surveillance testing should have been performed before the patient's arrival for lung transplantation. Occasionally, studies were not previously performed or more than 3 months have passed since the previous evaluation. In these circumstances, repeat testing of serology that had been negative will allow detection of newly acquired infections that may impact on prophylaxis. Cultures obtained from the donor trachea as well as the trachea of the patient at the time of transplantation help to guide perioperative antibiotic administration and may give valuable information about colonizing agents that may pose a problem after operation. Isolation policies should be consistent with the hospital infectious control practices. With the exception of using private rooms, the authors have not found a need to have specific isolation strategies (e.g. masks, gowns, laminar flow).

A candidate who presents with acute fever and illness on the day of transplantation requires a thorough infectious disease evaluation before continuing with the operation. Patients with acute viral illnesses at the time of maximum immunosuppression from transplantation may develop disseminated disease, with dire consequences.

3.4 What development(s) are to be expected for surveillance in patients undergoing lung or heart-lung transplantation?

Results of surveillance help to determine prophylaxis and follow-up strategies for patients undergoing lung transplantation. For example, results of surveillance sputum cultures help to direct initial postoperative antibiotic coverage. Likewise, results of donor–recipient CMV serologies allow for assessment of the level of risk for CMV disease after transplantation and permit individualization of preventive strategies.

4 REGARDING THE PREVENTION OF INFECTION IN LUNG AND HEART-LUNG TRANSPLANT RECIPIENTS

4.1 What approaches, if any, to the prevention of infection should be considered in patients undergoing lung or heart-lung transplantation?

Preventive efforts may be divided into pretransplant and posttransplant strategies, and further separated into short-term perioperative and more long-term prophylactic strategies. Many of these will be the same regardless of the type of transplant being performed. Before transplantation, immunizations should be updated. This is important both for live virus vaccines that may be contraindicated after transplantation because of immunosuppression and because only limited data are available about the effectiveness of vaccines when administered to immunosuppressed transplant recipients.

Immunizations for children should include diphtheria, tetanus, pertussis, hepatitis B, *Haemophilus influenzae* type b and polio. Children aged over 1 year should also receive measles, mumps, rubella and varicella vaccines. Transplantation within 1 month after the receipt of a live vaccine could lead to vaccine-associated disease and should be considered on a patient-by-patient basis. Finally, polysaccharide pneumococcal vaccine should be considered for individuals above 2 years of age.

Immunizations for adults should include updating tetanus and diphtheria vaccines, as well as hepatitis B vaccination. Measles, mumps, rubella and varicella vaccine should be given to individuals without previous immunity. Yearly influenza vaccine is recommended for all lung transplant candidates, recipients and their close contacts (see section 5.4). Pneumoccocal vaccine should also be considered.

Perioperative antibiotics should be used for 48–72 h in patients without previous bacterial colonization, and for 10–14 days in those with underlying CF. The authors generally recommend using two intravenous antibiotics active against the colonizing agents of patients with CF. Patients colonized with *Aspergillus* should also receive prophylaxis with intravenous or aerosolized amphotericin or itraconazole. Oral nystatin, mycostatin or clotrimazole troches are administered for the first 1–3 months after transplantation to decrease yeast colonization. In addition, oral acyclovir is administered to all patients who are seropositive for HSV to avoid reactivation early after transplantation.

Preventive strategies are recommended against the development of CMV disease after lung transplantation. These strategies have evolved over time and vary from center to center. The authors currently recommend 3–4 weeks of intravenous ganciclovir as prophylaxis for all patients except those who are CMV D–/R–. High-risk patients (D+/R–) are additionally followed with serial CMV pp65 antigenemia studies, and preemptive ganciclovir is administered if more than 10 positive cells are found per 200 000 cells counted. Other groups rely strictly on preemptive treatment. Ganciclovir is also administered as prophylaxis against CMV if immunosuppression is augmented for treatment of rejection. The high frequency of EBV-associated PTLD in high-risk lung transplant recipients (D+/R−) has led the authors to serially evaluate these patients with a quantitative competitive EBV PCR assay on peripheral blood lymphocytes. To date, the vast majority of experience correlating EBV viral load with disease has measured cell-associated virus. It is too early at this time to determine whether or not preemptive treatment (intra-venous ganciclovir and CytoGam) will decrease the incidence of EBV disease in this population. However, this strategy appears to be helpful in the intestinal transplant pop-ulation.

Lung transplant recipients are given TMP–SMX as prophylaxis against PCP. Patients who cannot tolerate this drug are offered aerosolized pentamidine or oral daily dapsone. While the risk for PCP is highest during the first 2 years after transplantation, the authors recommend continuing therapy lifelong since the risk is always increased com-pared with that in nontransplant individuals. Patients and their family members should receive influenza vaccines on a yearly basis. Also, patients who are not immune to chick-enpox should receive varicella zoster immune globulin (VZIG) within 96 h of exposure to active varicella.

Finally, because of the high incidence of *Aspergillus* colonization and disease for patients with chronic lung rejection, the authors recommend itraconazole prophylaxis for all individuals with bronchiolitis obliterans. Cyclosporin or tacrolimus levels must be monitored for patients receiving azole therapy. In addition, the erratic absorption of itra-conazole has led the authors to recommend periodic evaluation of the patient's blood level when on this drug.

4.2 What are the future challenges and opportunities for reducing the risk of infection?

The development of superior, more specific, antirejection medications will directly decrease the risk of infections by minimizing the number of opportunistic infections, and will indirectly decrease infections by preventing chronic rejection and its accompanying host of infectious agents.

Improved strategies and medications against fungi and viruses will be of great benefit in reducing the disease load from infections after lung transplantation. The continued disease toll from CMV and EBV presents great challenges to the future progress of lung transplantation. Opportunities to assess preventive treatment strategies in multicenter trials and vaccine development will be helpful in the future.

5 REGARDING THE TREATMENT OF LUNG AND HEART-LUNG TRANSPLANT RECIPIENTS

5.1 What is the role of empirical therapy?

The decision to initiate empirical therapy in a patient after lung transplantation is based upon the degree of illness and the likelihood of a particular infection. Empirical therapy should be withheld from patients with clinical evidence suggesting the presence of infec-tion due to a common community-acquired respiratory or gastrointestinal viral pathogen, such as rhinovirus or rotavirus. Alternatively, empirical therapy may be administered to an ill patient after taking an appropriate history, physical examination and cultures so that modification of therapy can be made based on culture results. For example, it would be appropriate to begin intravenous ganciclovir in a CMV-mismatched patient (D+/R−) who presents with fever, leukopenia, thrombocytopenia and pneumonitis 4 months after transplantation. However, therapy should be started only after obtaining the appropriate database, including viral cultures and CMV-specific studies.

The choice of antimicrobial agents is based on the patient's previous history of infections and knowledge of 'resistance' patterns for the patient and within a hospital, as well as the site of the suspected infection. It is important to limit the duration of antimicrobial therapy for empirically treated patients who have no positive cultures in an effort to minimize the development of antimicrobial resistance and secondary fungemia. However, a full course of treatment should be given for patients with positive cultures or for whom a site of infection is identified. A change of empirical therapy should be based upon clinical and/or microbiologic failure of initial treatment, recognition of antimicrobial resistance, or adverse interaction to the initial treatment. Every effort should be made to obtain a more detailed database before changing empirical therapy

5.2 What is the appropriate approach to the lung or heart-lung transplant recipient with evidence of:

Upper respiratory tract infection?

Sinusitis
Patients with mild illness and radiographic evidence of sinusitis, who do not have underlying CF, can be treated empirically with therapy against the typical sinus pathogens (e.g. *S. pneumoniae*, *H. influenzae* and *M. catarrhalis*). Initial treatment with amoxycillin or with amoxicillin–clavulanate (to cover for both penicillin-resistant pneumococcus and β-lactamase-producing organisms) is appropriate for patients who have not received antibiotics recently. Patients with CF should have therapy that covers *Pseudomonas* as well as the other above-mentioned organisms (e.g. levofloxacin). Patients who are moderately or severely ill or who do not improve with empirical therapy should be considered for culture of sinus aspirate and biopsy to identify antibiotic-resistant organisms or fungal sinusitis. Consideration of culture and biopsy should be undertaken more rapidly for patients with underlying CF. The role of sinus surgery before transplantation for patients with CF is being evaluated at several centers. However, it is not clear which type of surgery, if any, will be of benefit to reduce colonization and prevent infection.

Otitis media
Similar to the above recommendations for patients with sinusitis, empirical therapy may be initiated covering typical pathogens associated with middle ear disease (e.g. *S. pneumoniae*, *H. influenzae* and *M. catarrhalis*). A diagnostic tympanocentesis should be performed if the patient fails to improve after 3 days of empirical therapy.

Conjunctivitis
Bacterial and viral cultures should be obtained from transplant recipients with conjunctivitis. Topical or systemic antibacterial agents can be considered for patients with positive bacterial cultures.

Tonsillitis
The presence of exudative tonsillitis after lung transplantation should prompt consideration for primary EBV infection, adenovirus or yeast as well as for group A streptococci. A positive culture for group A streptococci should be treated with penicillin. *Candida* can usually be treated effectively with topical agents such as nystatin gargle or clotrimazole troches. Negative bacterial and yeast cultures or accompanying symptoms should

prompt a further evaluation for viruses, including EBV, adenovirus or other respiratory viruses (e.g. influenza).

Clinically, EBV infection is often manifest as an exudative tonsillitis which is not distinguishable from the classic appearance of tonsillar disease in immunocompetent patients with EBV-associated mononucleosis. Histologic evaluation of tonsillar tissue obtained from transplant recipients presenting in this manner may demonstrate a continuum of pathology, including acute EBV infection, mononucleosis and PTLD. The variability in the histologic grade observed is likely to be due to the rapidity of proliferation of EBV-infected B cells and the ability of the host to contain this process. The authors believe that patients presenting with EBV-associated tonsillitis are all on the same continuum of disease. Accordingly, the recommendation is to treat them all the same once it has been confirmed that the tonsillitis is EBV related. EBV serologies, as well as a monospot test, should be performed in these patients. Where available, the EBV viral load in the peripheral blood should also be determined.

Teeth and gingiva
Dental care is important in transplant recipients and the authors generally recommend dental evaluation of oral health before transplantation. Dental abscesses or gingivitis are relatively uncommon after transplantation. Dental consultation and radiographs of the periapical region or entire jaw should be obtained as clinically dictated. HSV should be considered in patients presenting with gingiva stomatitis. This is particularly important early after transplantation in a previously naive host.

Lower respiratory tract infection?
Lower respiratory tract infections are very common after lung transplantation. Patients who present with new symptoms of lower respiratory tract disease need to be evaluated for both infection and rejection. While patients should have chest radiography, it is important to recognize that acute cellular rejection of the lungs can also manifest as pulmonary infiltrates, especially early after transplantation. Accordingly, a low threshold must be maintained to perform BAL for cultures and transbronchial biopsy of the lung to rule out rejection. Gram staining should be performed on the BAL specimen, which should be cultured for bacteria, viruses, fungi, mycobacteria, *Mycoplasma* and *Legionella*. Histologic stains should also be performed to look for evidence of PCP and fungi. Biopsies of the lung tissue should be examined by an experienced pathologist to look for evidence of rejection, bronchiolitis obliterans and infection.

Empirical antibiotics should be withheld if possible until after an adequate specimen has been obtained for culture. In addition, augmented immunosuppression should be avoided until an infectious etiology can reasonably be ruled out as the cause of pulmonary decompensation. Once adequate specimens have been obtained, empirical therapy can be initiated based upon the timing of the patient's presentation and the risk of specific organisms (e.g. *Pseudomonas* in a patient with CF, or CMV in a mismatched patient). Specific antibiotic recommendations for empirical therapy should be based upon knowledge of the organisms that have been found in the individual patient's previous respiratory tract and on local resistance patterns for bacteria.

Gastrointestinal infection?
Gastrointestinal infections can occur after lung transplantation. The types of infections to consider may be modified by epidemiologic considerations. For example, *C. difficile* colitis should be high on the differential diagnosis of a patient who presents with bloody

diarrhea after prolonged and multiple antibiotic exposures. Rotavirus and other causes of viral gastroenteritis are common, particularly in young children. A low threshold should be present for obtaining an endoscopic evaluation of the gastrointestinal tract to rule out the presence of CMV, EBV-driven PTLD and other pathogens.

Genitourinary infection?

Patients who present with classic symptoms of UTI, such as frequency, urgency and dysuria, should have a urine culture and urinanalysis performed. Empirical antibiotics can be started if the urinanalysis is suggestive of bacterial infection, with modification of antibiotics made after culture results become available. Fungal infections (e.g. *Candida* spp.) may occur, especially in patients who have been on prolonged antibiotics and have recent urethral instrumentation. Consideration should be given to viral etiologies (e.g. adenovirus) if sterile pyuria is found. *M. tuberculosis*, JC and BK viruses should also be in the differential diagnosis. Children with pyelonephritis should undergo evaluation for the presence of vesicoureteral reflux at or near the end of therapy.

Cardiovascular infection?

Cardiovascular infections are more common after heart–lung transplantation than isolated lung transplantation. In particular, donor-associated infections, such as toxoplasmosis or CMV myocarditis, are more commonly found in recipients of heart or heart–lung grafts than other types of organs. There has not been an increase in documented episodes of myocarditis or endocarditis after lung transplantation. However, single case reports of *Fusarium* and *S. aureus* endocarditis after lung transplantation have been published. Patients who have a prolonged need for indwelling vascular catheters are at increased risk for developing catheter-associated line infections and infectious thrombophlebitis.

Musculoskeletal infection?

Mediastinitis can occur early after lung transplantation involving the sternum. After this period, musculoskeletal infections are uncommon and evaluation for these infections would be similar to that in any other patient with signs or symptoms suggestive of a myositis, osteomyelitis or suppurative arthritis.

Skin infections?

Skin infections are most often associated with a break in the normal barriers because of surgery or the presence of a foreign body (e.g. intravascular catheter or surgical drain). Culture and Gram staining of purulent material should be performed. Empirical antimicrobial therapy can be aimed at typical pathogens associated with infections of the skin (*S. aureus* or *S. pyogenes*). However, it should be noted that *M. hominis* was found to cause mediastinal wound infection after lung transplantation in one series. Gram staining of purulent material was negative but pinpoint colonies were noted on the anaerobic cultures, which were identified after transfer to *Mycoplasma* agar. Fungal infections may present with skin lesions. In addition, patients with EBV-associated PTLD may present with relatively benign-appearing skin lesions. Biopsy and culture should be entertained for suspicious lesions. Viruses such as VZV (either primary or reactivation) may produce skin lesions, as can HSV. Viral cultures can be obtained to confirm these viruses if not clinically apparent. In general, the authors strongly recommend hospitalization and intravenous acyclovir therapy for patients with primary varicella infection. Finally, papillomavirus infections manifest as warts may be prominent, and are often resistant to treatment after transplantation.

Central nervous system infection?

While CNS infections are not common after lung transplantation, they can be quite serious. When present, CNS infections are typically due to opportunistic pathogens including *T. gondii, Cryptococcus neoformans* or *A. fumigatus*. Viral infections of the CNS, in particular EBV-associated PTLD, and to a lesser extent CMV, may also occur. Patients do not appear to be at a substantially increased risk for community-acquired bacterial or viral meningitis. It should also be kept in mind that transplant recipients could develop noninfectious CNS disease on the basis of high-dose steroids, antilymphocyte antibody preparations, and cyclosporin or tacrolimus.

Foreign body in place?

Similar to other immunocompromised patients, lung transplant recipients are at increased risk for infections arising because of the presence of a foreign body. This is particularly true of intraluminal catheters. Unique to lung transplant recipients is the occasional need for a stent at the site of a collapsed bronchial anastomosis. Increased risk of infection may occur distal to the stent if it collapses, becomes dislodged or develops significant granulation.

Intraabdominal infections?

Intraabdominal infections are uncommon after lung transplantation. The finding of a mass in the abdominal cavity should lead to an aggressive evaluation to rule out PTLD.

5.3 What is the appropriate approach to the lung or heart-lung transplant recipient with evidence of bacteremia, with or without site of infection?

Gram-positive bacteremia

Antibiotic therapy should be initiated for lung transplant recipients with documented bacteremia after ensuring that an adequate number of cultures has been obtained to rule out the possibility of a skin contamination of the initial blood culture. It is important to consider risk factors for bacterial infection such as a recent transplant, the presence of a wound infection, or the presence of venous or arterial catheters. Vancomycin can be considered for initial coverage for Gram-positive bacteria. However, its use should be modified as soon as results of antimicrobial susceptibility testing are available. A primary site for infection should be sought. *S. pneumoniae* bacteremia has been found to recur in several thoracic organ transplant recipients who were over the age of 5 years at the authors' institution despite having normal serum immunoglobulin levels and splenic function. While the risk for recurrent bacteremia with this bacterium was not obvious, these patients appeared to have benefited from pneumococcal vaccination and penicillin prophylaxis.

Gram-negative bacteremia

Lung transplant recipients with underlying CF may develop bacteremia with Gram-negative organisms. In particular, the microbes that previously colonized the patient's lungs are likely to be the culprit. *B. cepacia* is particularly aggressive and may cause bacteremia and empyema after transplantation. Empirical therapy should be started with at least two classes of antimicrobial agents known to be effective against the patient's colonizing bacteria, such as an aminoglycoside and a ureido-penicillin. It is for this reason that it is important to obtain pretransplant surveillance sputum and perioperative bronchial samples. As above, therapy can be modified once susceptibility results are available. Unlike Gram-positive bacteremia, double antibiotic coverage against *Burkholderia* or *Pseudomonas* should be maintained. In general, *B. cepacia* is resistant to aminoglycosides but susceptible to TMP–SMX. In addition, empirical therapy with piperacillin–tazobactam or ciprofloxacin can be used while awaiting susceptibility data.

Anaerobic bacteremia
Anaerobic bacteremia is rare after lung transplantation but may occur, particularly in the presence of a pulmonary abscess. As noted above, a primary source of infection should be sought.

Mixed or polymicrobial bacteremia
Polymicrobial bacteremia may be found, although less often than a single infecting agent. Risk factors such as an intravascular groin catheter or a gastrointestinal source should be considered. Poor aseptic technique is too commonly found as the reason for either recurring line infections or polymicrobial bacteremia in young children who have undergone lung transplantation.

Bacteremia with defined primary site
Regardless of the recovered organism, identification of a defined primary site of infection is extremely important. All patients must have documentation of clearance of the bloodstream after the initiation of therapy. Patients with catheter-associated bacteremia, which does not clear with appropriate therapy, should have the catheter removed. The use of urokinase has been shown to increase the chance of saving a catheter in some patients with 'refractory' bacteremia and may be tried if the patient is clinically stable. Medical management alone may not be sufficient for patients who are bacteremic secondary to an abscess or empyema. These individuals may require drainage procedures.

5.4 What is the appropriate approach to the lung or heart-lung transplant recipient with evidence of a viral infection?
Viruses can cause substantial disease after lung transplantation, particularly during the early and intermediate periods. The approach and treatment vary depending on the infectious agent and timing of the infection.

Herpesviruses
HSV may cause substantial disease, including fatal pneumonitis if reactivation or primary infection occurs shortly after transplantation, during a period of maximum immunosuppression. For this reason, the authors recommend obtaining serology before transplantation and using acyclovir prophylaxis for the first 3 months after operation in all patients who have evidence of previous infection. Prophylaxis is reinstituted if individual patients have recurrent disease or if immunosuppression is being substantially augmented to treat rejection. Parents of the authors' pediatric candidates are also questioned about their history of oral herpes stomatitis and cautioned to use oral acyclovir if reactivation occurs. Patients who are receiving ganciclovir for CMV prophylaxis or treatment do not require additional acyclovir.

Varicella can cause primary or reactivation disease after lung transplantation. Pretransplant serology should be obtained for all candidates. Varicella vaccine is recommended for candidates who are seronegative and deemed to have at least 1 month of waiting time on the lung transplant list. One patient underwent lung transplantation the day after receiving varicella vaccine. Acyclovir was administered for 3 months without untoward effects, but the patient did not mount a detectable antibody response to varicella. If possible, patients who are seronegative for varicella and are exposed are given varicella immune globulin within 96 h of exposure. If varicella lesions develop, all patients are hospitalized and given intravenous acyclovir until no further crops of lesions appear and current lesions begin to crust (5–10 days).

CMV is still one of the most common and important viral infections after lung transplantation. Protocols for prophylaxis or preemptive treatment vary from center to center. Comparison of individual protocols at various centers would be difficult to perform because of multiple other confounders; accordingly, it is difficult to recommend one strategy over another. However, it is clear that mismatched patients (D+/R−) are at high risk for CMV disease and must be monitored and treated when infection occurs. Appropriate prophylaxis includes the use of ganciclovir with or without CMV hyperimmune globulin. CMV pp65 antigenemia studies or CMV quantitative PCR studies are used to monitor patients after transplantation. Serologic monitoring does not give timely enough information to prevent disease in most cases. In Pittsburgh, the authors use a combination of prophylaxis and monitoring. All patients who are seropositive or have a seropositive donor receive intravenous ganciclovir at full dose for 2 weeks and then half dose until week 4. CMV pp65 antigenemia studies are followed serially and a rise above 10 positive cells per 200 000 cells, indicating infection, leads to preemptive treatment with intravenous ganciclovir. Disease is also treated with intravenous ganciclovir for 14–21 days. CMV hyperimmune globulin is reserved for treatment of disseminated disease.

EBV causes significantly more disease after lung transplantation than after most other organ transplant procedures, ranging from a mononucleosis syndrome, lymphocytic bronchitis to disseminated lymphoproliferations. Patients who seroconvert against EBV within the first 6 months following transplantation have close to a 50% risk of developing EBV-associated PTLD. In contrast, patients who are seropositive for EBV before transplantation have little risk of subsequent development of EBV-associated PTLD. Protocols for prophylaxis and preemptive treatment using combinations of ganciclovir and hyperimmune globulin are being conducted. Treatment strategies vary from center to center but should include decreasing immunosuppression as much as possible. When decreased immunosuppression fails to cause regression of the EBV disease, additional treatment strategies have been used including ganciclovir, interferon, monoclonal antibodies, chemotherapy and lymphokine-activated killer (LAK) cells. Our center monitors at-risk patients serially with a quantitative competitive PCR assay. Patients with newly positive assays are fully evaluated for evidence of EBV disease by physical examination, computed tomography of the chest and abdomen (with or without the head) and biopsy of suspicious lesions. Decreased immunosuppression and ganciclovir are used initially if PTLD is diagnosed. Specific recommendations after failure to respond to decreased immunosuppression are limited owing to the absence of published comparative studies. Chemotherapy is generally reserved for the individual with histologically proven malignancy, or those with either rapidly progressive disease or failure to respond to all other manipulations.

Other herpesviruses such as HHV-6, HHV-7 and HHV-8 have been less well studied after lung transplantation. Treatment is supportive.

Respiratory viruses
Respiratory viruses are relatively common after lung transplantation but generally represent a significant cause of disease only in the early period. Adenovirus during the first

month after transplantation may lead to disseminated fatal disease. Intravenous ribavirin has been used anecdotally for severe adenovirus infections, primarily in recipients of bone marrow transplant recipients. Unfortunately, this anecdotal use does not provide much guidance regarding the efficacy of this therapy. Parainfluenza, influenza and RSV are likewise of main concern in the early perioperative period. Specific treatment is often not helpful in these cases. However, ribavirin should be considered for disease occurring within the first 3 months after transplantation. Yearly influenza vaccine is recommended for all lung transplant candidates, recipients and their close contacts.

Enteroviruses

Lung transplant recipients do not appear to be at increased risk for severe disease from enteroviruses. Diagnosis is by viral culture or PCR assay. Supportive care is usually all that is required, but if patients appear to be having severe disease immunosuppression should be decreased if possible.

Hepatitis viruses

Candidates being evaluated for transplantation should be tested serologically for evidence of previous infection and/or immunity to hepatitis A, B and C viruses. Those without immunity to hepatitis B virus should be given the vaccine series. In the authors' experience this vaccine has not worked well after transplantation. Patients with hepatitis C should be cautioned about the potential for disease advancement under immunosuppression. Studies looking at treatment with ribavirin and interferon show promise and should be considered both before and after transplantation under protocol conditions. Serial evaluation of liver function and hepatitis C viral load is necessary.

5.5 What is the appropriate approach to the lung or heart-lung transplant recipient with evidence of a fungal infection?

Candida

Candida spp. can cause noninvasive mucositis, dermatitis and cystitis in patients after lung transplantation, as well as invasive disease. Diagnosis is made by clinical examination, culture and Gram staining. Prophylaxis and treatment of oropharyngeal *Candida* is recommended with topical use of nystatin, mycostatin or clotrimazole troches early after transplantation. The authors continue with this therapy for at least the first month, and generally for several months in young children. More serious invasive disease should be treated aggressively. Fluconazole or intravenous amphotericin B should be administered promptly. If an azole is used, it is important to decrease the dose of cyclosporin or tacrolimus and to follow drug levels closely. Removal of intravascular catheters is necessary if associated with candidemia. Even after the removal, a full course of systemic treatment should be given to avoid relapse of *Candida*. Prolonged candidemia should prompt evaluation for other sites of infection, including echocardiography, ultrasonography of the kidneys and ophthalmologic examination. Additional use of 5-fluorocytosine may be required if prompt clearance is not achieved with first-line antifungal agents.

Aspergillus

Aspergillus is a major cause of morbidity and mortality after lung transplantation. A number of patients with underlying CF will be colonized with *Aspergillus* before transplantation. Determining whether it is pathogenic is often controversial; however, most centers recommend using prophylaxis with either itraconazole, intravenous amphotericin B or aerosolized amphotericin B. Invasive aspergillosis, in which the manifestations may range from a solitary pulmonary nodule to multiple nodules with visceral or CNS dissemination, should be treated with intravenous amphotericin B with or without adjunctive treatment of itraconazole, 5-fluorocytosine or rifampicin. Prolonged intravenous treatment is usually required for a minimum of 4 weeks, but often 8–12 weeks. These longer durations should be used for patients with disseminated disease. Liposomal formulations of amphotericin should be considered for patients with renal dysfunction. Invasive disease in one part of the body should prompt radiographic staging to look for other sites of involvement including the lung, liver, spleen and head. After successful treatment, lifelong suppressive oral therapy with itraconazole should be considered. Risks for invasive disease include antecedent CMV disease and bronchiolitis obliterans. Patients undergoing repeat lung transplantation due to bronchiolitis obliterans may also be at increased risk for invasive aspergillosis.

Cryptococcus

The risk of cryptococcal disease after lung transplantation is similar to that for other types of organ transplant procedures. It is particularly rare in children but may be seen in adolescents and adults who are immunosuppressed. Culture, cryptococcal antigen assays, histology and India ink stains are all useful in making the diagnosis of cryptococcal disease. Cerebrospinal examination is also important in evaluating infection of the CNS. Treatment can be with either fluconazole or amphotericin B with or without the addition of 5-fluorocytosine. Treatment is for a minimum of 8 weeks, but many would continue oral fluconazole indefinitely. Close clinical examination and serial cryptococcal antigen testing, if initially positive, can be useful in evaluating these patients.

Pneumocystis carinii

Lung transplant recipients are at higher risk for PCP than are other solid organ transplant recipients, with disease usually occurring between 1 and 12 months after transplantation. While the first 1–2 years is the highest risk period for PCP, disease can occur later, especially if immunosuppression is augmented. Prophylaxis with TMP–SMX is preventive. Accordingly, the authors recommend this prophylaxis indefinitely. Other centers use prophylaxis for the first 1–2 years and with augmentation of immunosuppression. Alternative drugs are inferior but can be used for patients unable to tolerate TMP–SMX, including dapsone and pentamidine. Patients with PCP should be treated aggressively with full-dose TMP–SMX and steriods. Patients who do not respond to TMP–SMX treatment should be given intravenous pentamidine.

Other fungi

Similar to other immunocompromised hosts, recipients of lung transplants are at risk for disease from other fungi. Reports of serious disease from fungi include C. *immitis*, H. *capsulatum*, *Fusarium* spp. and *Scedosporium* spp. Diagnosis is by culture, histology and serologic techniques. The specifics of the patient, the extent of initial disease and the rate of clearance will help to individualize treatment plans.

5.6 What is the appropriate approach to the lung or heart-lung transplant recipient with evidence of a parasitic infection?

Similar to other immunosuppressed individuals, lung transplant recipients are at risk for more severe disease from parasites. Diarrhea from *Cryptosporidium, Isospora* or *Cyclospora* can be refractory to treatment. The authors have had success with paramomycin for *Cryptosporidium* in a small bowel transplant recipient and other immunocompromised hosts. Patients who received both a heart and lung graft do have increased risk of toxoplasmosis if they were naive to this parasite and the donor had previous infection (D+/R–). Prophylaxis with pyrimethamine with adjunctive use of folinic acid should be considered in these high-risk patients. Treatment consists of pyrimethamine and sulfadiazine. In addition, folinic acid (leukovorin) should be administered to counteract the bone suppressive effects of pyrimethamine.

5.7 What is the role of nonantiinfective interventions (including reducing or altering immunosuppression) in the management of established infection?

Immunosuppression should be reduced if at all possible in lung transplant recipients who have moderate to severe infections. The decision to reduce immunosuppression will depend on the severity of the infection and the rejection history of the patient. Immunosuppression may not be able to be altered if concurrent rejection is present. In general, the authors attempt to keep levels of tacrolimus lower in patients who have had EBV-driven PTLD, CMV or invasive fungal disease. Patients with leukopenia may require modification of drugs such as azathioprine or mycophenolic acid. Granulocyte-stimulating factor should be given to patients with neutropenia and established infections.

REFERENCES

Boyle G, Michaels MG, Webber S et al. Post transplant lymphoproliferative disorders in pediatric thoracic organ recipients. *J Pediatr* 1997; **131**: 309–313.

Dummer JS, White LT, Ho M, Griffith BP, Hardesty RL, Bahnson HT. Morbidity of cytomegalovirus infection in recipients of heart or heart–lung transplants who received cyclosporine. *J Infect Dis* 1985; **152**: 1182–1191.

Egan JJ, Lomax J, Barber L et al. Preemptive treatment for the prevention of cytomegalovirus disease in lung and heart transplant recipients. *Transplantation* 1998; **65**: 747–752.

Fishman JA, Rubin RH. Infection in organ-transplant recipients. *N Engl J Med* 1998; **338**: 1741–1751.

Green M, Michaels M. Infections in solid organ transplant receptions. In: Long SS, Prober CG, Pickering LK, eds. *Principles and Practice of Pediatric Infectious Diseases* 1st edn. New York: Churchill Livingstone, 1997; 626–633.

Green M, Reyes J, Rowe D. New strategies in the prevention and management of Epstein Barr virus infection and posttransplant lymphoproliferative disease following solid organ transplantation. *Curr Opin Organ Transplant* 1998; **3**: 143 147.

Kramer MR, Marshall SE, Starnes VA, Gamberg P, Amitai Z, Thodore J. Infectious complications in heart–lung transplantation. Analysis of 200 episodes. *Arch Intern Med* 1993; **153**: 2010–2016.

Michaels MG, Green MD. Infectious complications of heart and lung transplantation in children. In: Franco KL, ed. *Pediatric Cardiopulmonary Transplantation*. Armonk, NY: Futura, 1997; 27–45.

Chapter 7.5 Infections in Intestinal Transplant Recipients

Michael Green and Marian Michaels

I REGARDING THE CLINICAL PRESENTATION AND EVALUATION OF THE PATIENT

1.1 What are the clinically predominant modes of presentation of infection in intestinal transplant recipients?

Fever is the most frequent and one of the most important symptoms of infection following intestinal transplantation. The post transplant period can generally be broken into early (≤ 1 month), intermediate (1–6 months) and late (> 6 months) periods. The differential diagnosis of fever and infection varies within each of these time periods and can be further refined by whether or not it is associated with localizing signs or symptoms (Table 7.5.1 and Chapter 7.0, Table 7.0.4). While many febrile illnesses are confirmed microbiologically, some infections may not be microbiologically defined (e.g. viral gastroenteritis, upper respiratory tract infection). In these cases it is imperative to differentiate between infectious enteritis and rejection of the intestinal allograft (see below).

Early transplant period

Infection in the early transplant period (during the first month) often involves surgical sites or is related to nosocomial exposures. For intestinal transplant recipients, intraabdominal infection as well as superficial or deep wound infections are among the most likely infectious explanations for early fever. In addition, these patients are likely to require central venous catheters (CVCs) for much of the early posttransplant period. The development of a catheter-associated bloodstream infection should be suspected for patients with fever whenever they have a CVC in place. The presence of an endotracheal tube in a febrile patient raises the question of ventilator-associated pneumonia. Although bladder catheters are usually in place for only a limited time following intestinal transplantation, the urine should be evaluated for the presence of urinary tract infection (UTI) in febrile intestinal transplant recipients (particularly early after transplant) because of their recent history of bladder catheterization. Finally, moderate to severe rejection of the intestinal graft is associated with the development of bacteremia. Accordingly, the finding of bacteremia due to Gram-negative enteric organisms raises the question of intestinal rejection and warrants endoscopic evaluation. Similarly, the identification of intestinal rejection in a febrile intestinal transplant recipient warrants evaluation for the presence of concomitant bacteremia.

Intestinal rejection may present as fever, alone or in combination with an increase in stool and/or stoma output. Frequently there is frank diarrhea, which may be guiaic positive or grossly bloody. The stool will often be positive for reducing substances, identifying the malabsorption of sugar during intestinal rejection. Alternatively, intestinal rejection

Table 7.5.1 Modes of presentation of infection by timing of presentation after intestinal transplantation

Timing of presentation	Type of infection	Frequency of infection
Early (0–30 days)	Surgical site	
	Intraabdominal	10%
	Superficial and deep wound	20–30%
	Catheter associated	
	Bloodstream	25%
	Urinary tract	10%
	Ventilator-associated pneumonia	10%
	Rejection-associated bacteremia	5–10%
Intermediate (1–6 months)	Catheter associated	
	Bloodstream	10–20%
	Rejection associated	10–15%
	EBV/PTLD associated	5%
	CMV	20–50% *
	EBV/PTLD	10–33% †
Late (> 6 months)	Catheter associated	
	Bloodstream	5–10%
	Rejection associated	10–15%
	EBV/PTLD associated	< 5%
	CMV	< 10%
	EBV/PTLD	< 5%
	Community-acquired infection	NA‡

* Incidence higher in adult intestinal transplant recipients.
† incidence higher in pediatric intestinal transplant recipients.
‡ Not applicable; varies by age and community exposures.

may present with a decrease in gastrointestinal output or even an ileus. This will usually be accompanied by an increase in abdominal girth. Intestinal rejection may be accompanied by nonspecific changes on radiography, including dilated loops of bowel and air fluid levels. A coincidental increase in gamma glutamyl transpeptidase (GGT) concentration without a change in bilirubin or alanine transaminase (ALT) levels may be noted. Leukocytosis with neutrophilia is often present. Concern for the presence of intestinal rejection warrants an endoscopic evaluation.

Intermediate time period

Although some overlap exists, the differential diagnosis of patients presenting with fever during the intermediate period (1–6 months) after intestinal transplantation differs from that in patients presenting in the early posttransplant period. The presence of a CVC places the intestinal transplant recipient at risk for catheter-associated bloodstream infections as long as the catheter remains in place. Likewise, patients remain at risk for rejection-associated bacteremia (and less commonly fungemia) during the intermediate period.

The major differences in the differential diagnosis in the intermediate versus the early period is the consideration of opportunistic pathogens, especially cytomegalovirus (CMV) and Epstein–Barr virus (EBV). Both of these viruses may cause a primary infection typically acquired from the donor in a recipient who is seronegative. Alternatively, secondary infection (either reactivation of the recipient's own latent viral strain or reinfection with a new strain from the donor or other source) occurs in a patient who is seropositive for CMV or EBV before transplantation.

While clinical syndromes associated with CMV are similar among many types of immunosuppressed patients, EBV disease and posttransplant lymphoproliferative disease (PTLD) are uncommon in patients who have not undergone transplantation. In general, the increased importance of EBV infection in this population is due to the effect of immunosuppressant agents aimed at preventing rejection in these patients. As a consequence, EBV-infected and immortalized B-lymphocytes may proliferate, leading to a wide range of clinical manifestations. EBV may present with a stereotypical viral syndrome consisting of fever, leukopenia, thrombocytopenia and atypical lymphocytosis, which is indistinguishable from the so-called CMV syndrome. The range of EBV disease also includes mononucleosis, PTLD and malignant lymphoma.

Both CMV and EBV most commonly present with gastrointestinal symptoms (diarrhea, occult or gross blood in stool) in intestinal transplant recipients. The clinical presentation of CMV and EBV is very similar in these patients. In particular, clinical manifestations of gastrointestinal involvement of these pathogens may not differ and also need to be differentiated from intestinal rejection as well as other enteric pathogens. Less commonly, the use of immunosuppression may also lead to reactivation and development of disease due to other latent pathogens (e.g. *Mycobacterium tuberculosis*, *Histoplasma capsulatum*) in the intermediate period.

Late period

Although less frequent, febrile episodes of infection continue to occur late (> 6 months) after intestinal transplantation. The continuing development of bloodstream infections, related either to the presence of CVC or to intestinal graft rejection late after transplant is a fairly unique finding that differentiates intestinal transplant recipients from those undergoing other solid organ transplant procedures. Bacteremia also may develop in association with PTLD involving the intestine. Infection due to community-acquired

Table 7.5.2 Evaluation of infections in intestinal transplant recipients according to the site of infection and the possible etiologic agent

Site of infection	Infectious syndrome (clinical features)	Predominant pathogens	Diagnostic investigations
Bloodstream	Bacteremia (fever with or without local signs of infection)	Coagulase-negative staphylococci Staphylococcus aureus Enterococcus spp. (nosocomial outbreaks in some institutions) Gram-negative bacilli (Escherichia coli, Klebsiella pneumoniae, Enterobacter spp., Pseudomonas aeruginosa) Candida spp.	Quantitative blood cultures (two sets drawn from separate sites and at least one set drawn from indwelling intravenous catheter) Endoscopic evaluation for presence of rejection or post-transplant lymphoproliferative disease
Intravascular catheter-related infections	Pain, erythema, tenderness, discharge from catheter entry site	Coagulase-negative staphylococci Staphylococcus aureus Enterococcus spp. Gram-negative bacilli Candida spp.	Swab entry site Culture of catheter Blood cultures (consider drawing blood from each lumen of the catheter)
Peritoneum	Peritonitis Intraabdominal abscess	Gram-negative bacilli (Enterobacteriaceae, Pseudomonas aeruginosa) Enterococcus spp. Anaerobic bacilli (Clostridium spp., Bacteroides spp.) Candida spp.	Culture of peritoneal fluid Ultrasonography CT/MRI
Gastrointestinal tract: Esophagus	Esophagitis (dysphagia, retrosternal pain)	Herpes simplex virus Candida spp. Aspergillus spp.	Esogastroscopy Culture of endoscopic specimens
Small intestine, colon	Enteritis Colitis (nausea, vomiting, bloating, abdominal discomfort, cramp, pain, constipation, diarrhea)	Cytomegalovirus Epstein–Barr virus Adenovirus Rotavirus (children) Clostridium difficile (antibiotic-associated diarrhea) Cryptosporidium Giardia lamblia Increased susceptibility to infections by Salmonella spp., Shigella spp., Yersinia spp. and Campylobacter spp.	Endoscopic evaluation with histologies Stool for viral and bacterial cultures, rotaviral antigen detection, and C. difficile toxin assay CMV antigenemia assay or PCR in peripheral blood EBV viral load in peripheral blood

Hepatobiliary tract:

Liver	Hepatitis	Viral hepatitis (B, C): reactivation in graft Cytomegalovirus Epstein–Barr virus Adenovirus Herpes simplex virus	Liver biopsy Serology
	Liver abscess	Gram-negative bacilli (Enterobacteriaceae, Pseudomonas aeruginosa, Acinetobacter spp.) Enterococcus spp. Candida spp. Staphylococcus aureus spp. Anaerobic bacilli (Bacteroides spp., Peptostreptococcus, streptococci, Fusobacterium)	Ultrasonography CT or MRI Aspiration under CT guidance for culture
Biliary tract	Cholecystitis Cholangitis	Aerobic Gram-negative bacilli (Enterobacteriaceae, Pseudomonas aeruginosa) Anaerobic bacilli (Bacteroides spp., Clostridium spp.) Enterococcus spp. Candida spp.	Cholangiography Ultrasonography CT, MRI Culture of biliary drainage fluid
Skin infection and soft tissue	Surgical wound infection	Staphylococcus aureus Coagulase-negative staphylococci Enterococcus spp., Gram-negative bacilli (Enterobacteriaceae, Pseudomonas aeruginosa) Candida spp.,	Aspiration (needle) or swab of skin exudate
	Rash Cellulitis (pain, erythema, tenderness, necrosis in case of ecthyma gangrenosum)	Primary infections: Coagulase-negative staphylococci Staphylococcus aureus Gram-negative bacilli (Pseudomonas aeruginosa, E. coli, Klebsiella pneumoniae) Candida spp. Mucor spp., Rhizopus spp., Absidia spp., Mycobacteria Human herpesvirus-6 and 7 (HHV-6, HHV-7)	Aspiration (needle) or swab of skin Skin biospy (histology and culture) Serology

Site of infection	Infectious syndrome (clinical features)	Predominant pathogens	Diagnostic investigations
	Papules, nodules (with or without myalgias and muscle tenderness)	Disseminated infections: Candida species, Fusarium species, Alternaria species Gram-negative bacilli (Escherichia coli, Pseudomonas aeruginosa, Aeromonas hydrophilia, Serratia marcescens) Epstein-Barr virus, adenovirus	
	Ulcers, vesicles, hemorrhagic or crusted lesions (isolated or with dermatomal distribution)	Herpes simplex Varicella zoster virus Cytomegalovirus	
	Disseminated vesicles, hemorrhagic or crusted lesions	Varicella-zoster virus, herpes simplex Staphylococcus aureus, streptococci	
	Skin necrosis	Aspergillus spp., Mucor spp.	
	Warts	Papillomavirus	
	Molluscum contagiosum	Poxvirus-related virus	
Upper respiratory tract: (ear, nose, sinus, nasopharynx, larynx, trachea)	Sinusitis (tightness of sinus areas, headache, toothache, nasal obstruction, nasal voice)	Streptococcus pneumoniae Haemophilus influenzae Moraxella catarrhalis Aspergillus spp., Mucor spp. Candida spp. Viruses (influenza, parainfluenza, rhinovirus, adenovirus)	Aspiration of sinus Biopsy (if no improvement after 72–96 h of empirical antibiotic therapy)
	Otitis media Otitis externa (earache, drainage irritability)	Streptococcus pneumoniae Haemophilus influenzae Moraxella catarrhalis Streptococcus pyogenes Staphylococcus aureus Pseudomonas aeruginosa Mycoplasma pneumoniae	Consider empiric therapy for otitis media Tympanocentesis (in case of treatment failure) Swab of external auditory canal (otitis externa)
Lower respiratory tract (bronchi, terminal airways, alveoli)	Bronchopneumonia Pneumonia (cough, dyspnea, chest pain sputum, hemoptysia, pleural effusion)	Conventional infections: Streptococcus pneumoniae Gram-negative bacilli (Escherichia coli, Klebsiella	Chest X-ray, CT, MRI Nasopharyngeal aspirate for viral culture and/or antigen

	Pathogens	Diagnosis
	pneumoniae, Pseudomonas aeruginosa, Acinetobacter spp.) Virus (influenza, parainfluenza, respiratory syncytial virus) Opportunistic infections: *Cytomegalovirus* *Pneumocystis carinii* *Mycobacterium tuberculosis* *Aspergillus* spp. (uncommon) *Candida* spp. (uncommon)	detection Sputum or endotracheal aspirate (if available) Fiberoptic bronchoscopy with bronchoalveolar lavage (if severe or atypical infection or if viral pneumonia is suspected) Transbronchial biopsy Thoracocentesis Open lung biopsy
Urinary tract Pyelonephritis Cystitis	Gram-negative bacilli (*Escherichia coli, Klebsiella* spp.., *Proteus* spp.., *Enterobacter* spp.., *Pseudomonas aeruginosa*) *Enterococcus* spp. *Candida* spp.	Urinanalysis Culture of urine Ultrasonography, CT (if suspicion of abscess) Consider voiding cytourethrography if clinical evidence of pyelonephritis
Central nervous system* Acute meningitis	*Listeria monocytogenes*	CT, MRI
Subacute, chronic meningitis	*Cryptococcus neoformans* *Candida* spp. *Mycobacterium tuberculosis* *Coccidioides immitis* *Histoplasma capsulatum*	Lumbar puncture
Focal brain diseases	*Aspergillus* spp. *Nocardia asteroides* *Listeria monocytogenes* *Toxoplasma gondii* Viruses (herpes simplex virus, varicella, cytomegalovirus, Epstein–Barr virus, human herpesvirus-6, adenovirus, papillomavirus, JC virus)	Aspiration or biopsy under stereotaxic CT guidance
Progressive dementia	JC virus (progressive multifocal leukoencephalopathy)	

* Intestinal transplant patients have the same susceptibility to conventional pathogens of the central nervous system (meningitis: *Streptococcus pneumoniae, Neisseria meningitidis, Haemophilus influenzae.* Gram-negative bacilli; brain abscess: streptococci, *Bacteroides* spp., *Staphylococcus aureus*, Enterobacteriaceae) as the general population. Listed above are unique pathogens.

pathogens involving the respiratory or gastrointestinal tract also presents during this time period. The causative pathogens are typically those associated with community-acquired diseases.

1.2 What are the predominant sites of infection?
The intraabdominal space and surgical wound are among the most frequent sites of infection early after intestinal transplantation. Similarly, UTI and pneumonia also occur early after transplantation. The bloodstream is the most important and among the most frequent sites of infection following intestinal transplantation. Bloodstream infection may be associated with the presence of CVC, rejection or PTLD of the intestine. These infections occur both early and late after intestinal transplantation. The gastrointestinal tract is another important and frequent site of infection in these patients. Infections of the gastrointestinal tract are most often caused by viral pathogens, the most important of which are CMV and EBV. Both CMV and EBV may be associated with focal or diffuse erythema and friability of the gastrointestinal mucosa as well as discrete ulcerative lesions within the gastrointestinal tract. Of interest, the ulcers of EBV may be larger and more pronounced and are more likely to be associated with gastrointestinal perforations. Both these viruses may present with 'typical' symptoms of gastroenteritis. The presence of bloody stools, particularly bloody diarrhea, should lead to a higher level of concern that one of these viral pathogens is present. However, infection due to adenovirus and rotavirus also occurs following intestinal transplantation, but is diagnosed more frequently in children undergoing this procedure. In general, infections of the gastrointestinal tract are more likely to occur after the first month posttransplant. An overview of these pathogens and their diagnostic evaluations is shown in Table 7.5.2 and is further discussed in section 1.6.

1.3 What are the predominant organisms that contribute (by site)?
The predominant organisms recovered from the bloodstream vary depending on whether the source of infection is the intestinal allograft or a CVC. In the former scenario, enteric bacteria, including members of the Enterobacteriaciae, enterococci and less commonly *Candida* spp. are typically recovered. Coagulase-negative staphylococci are the most common pathogens recovered from catheter-associated bloodstream infections. However, other Gram-positive cocci (including *Staphylococcus aureus* and enterococci) and less frequently Gram-negative enterics as well as *Candida* may cause catheter-associated bloodstream infections.

Enteric pathogens and *Candida* are also commonly recovered from patients with infections involving the intraabdominal space, urinary tract or surgical wound. *S. aureus* is also a common cause of wound infections in intestinal transplant recipients. Pneumonia is most often caused by *Streptococcus pneumoniae* or Gram-negative enterics (usually in association with mechanical ventilation). Uncommonly, *Aspergillus fumigatus* may also cause infection of lung. Of importance, regardless of the site of bacterial infection, the authors have observed a high prevalence of antibiotic resistant bacteria species recovered from intestinal transplant recipients.

Enteritis involving both the intestinal allograft and the native gastrointestinal tract is a frequent problem after intestinal transplantation. In the authors' experience, viruses, particularly CMV and EBV, are the most common pathogens seen in association with this syndrome. Enteritis due to rotavirus has been a fairly frequent cause of enteritis in children, but not in adults undergoing intestinal transplantation. Enteritis due to toxin-producing strains of *Clostridium difficile* also occurs fairly frequently in intestinal transplant recipients of all ages. The authors have not noted an increased susceptibility to infection due to *Salmonella*, *Shigella*, *Yersinia* or *Campylobacter*. However, enteritis due to *Cryptosporidium* has been diagnosed in several intestinal transplant recipients.

1.4 How do the organisms vary according to various risk factors?

Risk factors, such as the absence of preexisting immunity, exposure to specific pathogens and intensity of immunosuppression, affect the frequency and severity of disease due to specific pathogens in intestinal transplant recipients. This is well illustrated by CMV where donor and recipient serologic status before transplantation are major predictors of both the likelihood and severity of infection. CMV-negative recipients of organs from CMV-positive donors are not only at greatest risk of developing CMV disease but are also more likely to have severe and chronic symptoms. The importance of this risk has led us to make specific recommendations regarding the performance of intestinal transplantation on CMV D+IR− recipients (see section 2.5). In contrast, the risk of CMV disease is very low when both the donor and recipient are seronegative for CMV, especially if transplant centers use CMV-negative blood products or white blood cell filters with the transfusions to minimize exposure to this pathogen. The risk of CMV disease is also affected by the amount of immunosuppression the patient has received.

The likelihood and severity of EBV infection following intestinal transplantation also varies with the presence or absence of specific risk factors. Unlike CMV (and unique to recipients of intestinal transplantation), the frequency of EBV disease does not appear to vary by recipient status, except in EBV-seronegative recipients of EBV-seronegative donors where, in the authors' experience, the risk of developing EBV disease and PTLD is lower. Similar to CMV, patients who have been heavily immunosuppressed, especially those who required the use of antilymphocyte antibody preparations, are at a greater risk of developing EBV disease. Preliminary analysis of several studies has identified that younger age of the transplant recipient may also be a risk factor for the development of EBV disease. This observation has yet to be confirmed and explained. If there are any symptoms, the authors would strongly recommend obtaining intestinal biopsies. The finding of pathology leads the authors to 'treat' rather than 'preempt' the infection. However, in the absence of symptoms, 'preemptive therapy' would be used in the hope of preventing progression to symptomatic disease.

Several risk factors contribute to the likelihood of developing bacterial infections following intestinal transplantation. The presence of liver disease associated with the development of ascites is a risk for spontaneous bacterial peritonitis before transplantation. Patients who have experienced one or more episodes of spontaneous bacterial peritonitis before intestinal transplantation may be at increased risk of postoperative intraabdominal infection on the basis of increased technical difficulty of the transplant surgery. In addition, bacteria recovered from these patients are frequently antibiotic resistant. Rejection carries with it a risk of development of bloodstream infection with enteric pathogens in intestinal transplant recipients. Finally, intraluminal catheters increase the risk of infection at the site of catheterization.

1.5 How does this differ from other conditions, from center to center, and from country to country?

Infections in intestinal transplant recipients differ from those in other organ transplant recipients in a number of ways. Bloodstream infections are more common after intestinal transplantation than after other types of organ transplantation. The association of bacteremia and candidemia with the rejection of the intestinal allograft, as well as the more frequent and prolonged use of CVCs, probably explains this observation. The prolonged use of CVCs may be required for the provision of parenteral nutrition, for fluid replacement for patients with high gastrointestinal output, or for the provision of long-term antimicrobial therapy. Patients undergoing intestinal transplantation also differ from other organ transplant recipients in the frequency, severity and chronicity of CMV and EBV infections. This may be explained by their chronic requirements for a high level of immunosuppression, but may also be due in part to the lymphatic nature of the intestinal allograft.

Risks for and manifestations of infection in intestinal transplant recipients may also vary from center to center and from country to country. These variations are due in part to differences in immunosuppressive protocols and antiinfective prophylactic strategies. Environmental exposures also vary between centers. Patients undergoing transplantation in areas that are endemic for certain pathogens (e.g. *M. tuberculosis, Coccidioides immitis*) will be at greater risk of either acquiring these infections from their donors or developing reactivation of their own latent pathogens under the pressure of immunosuppression.

1.6 What is the appropriate approach to the initial evaluation and diagnosis of infection in intestinal transplant recipients?

The initial step in the evaluation of infection in intestinal transplant recipients is to obtain a careful history and perform a thorough physical examination, focusing on signs and symptoms that may suggest an underlying source of infection. Consideration of acute cellular rejection is always important in the differential diagnosis of fever and infection in these patients. The timing of presentation can help guide the diagnosis of infection (e.g. early presentation suggests wound or intraabdominal infection). Attention should be paid to the presence of intraluminal catheters as risk factors for bloodstream infection, UTI or ventilator-associated pneumonia. Donor and recipient serologic data for CMV and EBV should be reviewed, particularly if the patient is presenting in the intermediate or late period following transplantation.

After completing the examination and considering these factors, the clinician should obtain appropriate diagnostic tests including blood and urine cultures. A sputum specimen (if available) and chest radiograph should be obtained for patients with symptoms suggestive of lower respiratory tract infection. Appropriate virologic studies should be ordered [e.g. CMV pp65 antigenemia assay or polymerase chain reaction (PCR), CMV buffy coat, EBV PCR]. Stool for viral culture and rotaviral antigen detection should be obtained if the patient has gastrointestinal symptoms, especially in the pediatric intestinal transplant recipient. Computed tomography (CT) of the abdomen may be obtained for patients with clinical evidence of intraabdominal infection or for those with fever and leukocytosis without another apparent source. Nasopharyngeal aspiration for viral culture against respiratory viruses, as well as for the performance of antigen detection against RSV and influenza A, should be considered during annual seasonal epidemics of respiratory viruses [e.g. respiratory syncytial virus (RSV), unfluenza virus or parainfluenza virus]. Performance or bronchoalveolar lavage (BAL) should be considered for patients with abnormalities of the chest radiograph. In general, the use of nonspecific tests, such as the C-reactive protein or erythrocyte sedimentation rate, has not been helpful and is not recommended for these patients. A summary of the diagnostic evaluation by site of infection and type of pathogen is provided in Tables 7.5.2–7.5.5.

1.7 How should the evaluation be modified according to the severity of the risk?

The presence or absence of risk factors helps to guide the differential diagnosis. Of interest, the risk of infection does not appear to vary according to whether or not a patient

Table 7.5.3 Overview of the diagnosis and management of viral infections following intestinal transplantation

Organism	Frequency[*]	Diagnostic test	Treatment			Duration of therapy	Follow-up
			Primary	Secondary	Adjunctive		
HSV	Uncommon	Culture Tzanck smear	Acyclovir	Foscarnet	Decrease IS	Site dependent	Chronic acyclovir prophylaxis
CMV	Common	Culture pp65 antigen Histology	Ganciclovir	Foscarnet	Decrease IS CMV IVIG	Site dependent	Monitor pp65 Ag
EBV	Common	EBV PCR Histology Serology	Decrease IS		Ganciclovir IVIG	Individualized	Monitor EBV PCR Repeat imaging studies positive at outset
RSV	Adults: rare Children: uncommon	NP aspirate for antigen detection and culture	Supportive care Aerosolized	RSV IVIG Decrease IS	Decreased IS	Individualized	None
Influenza	Uncommon	NP aspirate for antigen detection and culture	Supportive care	Amantadine/rimantadine		Individualized	None
Parainfluenza	Adults: rare	NP aspirate for antigen	Supportive care			Individualized	None
Adenovirus	Uncommon	Viral culture Histology	Decrease IS	IV ribavirin[‡]	Decreased IS IVIG[†]	Individualized	None
Enterovirus	Adults: rare Children: uncommon	Viral culture	Decrease IS	Supportive care		Individualized	None
HBV	Rare	HBV serologies HBV PCR Histology	Lamivudine	Interferon		Indefinite	HBV PCR Serial liver function tests
HCV	Rare	HCV serologies	Interferon	IV ribavirin[§]		Indefinite	HCV viral load Serial liver function tests

* Rare, < 1%; Uncommon, 1–5%; Common, > 5%.
† Foscarnet is used for CMV infection when ganciclovir resistance is suspected or proven; experience in patients with HIV suggests that a synergistic benefit will be obtained from the combined use of both these agents when ganciclovir resistance is present.
‡ Use of this agent is based on anecdotal experience.
§ Recent data suggest that combined use of intravenous ribavirin with interferon may be of benefit in hepatitis C.
IS, immuno suppression; IV, intravenous; IVIG, intravenous immunoglobulin; Ag, antigen; NP, nasopharyngeal.

Table 7.5.4 Overview of the diagnosis and management of fungal infections following intestinal transplantation

Organism	Frequency[a]	Diagnostic tests	Treatment[d]			Duration of therapy	Follow-up
			Primary	Secondary	Adjunctive		
Candida Noninvasive (mucositis, dermatitis and) cystitis	Common	Clinical examination culture Gram stain	Nystatin Clotrimazole	Topical Ampotericin [b] Fluconazole[c,h]		Dependent on rate of clearance	Clinical examination Repeat urine analysis / cultures
Invasive	Common	Culture Gram stain Histology	Amphotericin B[e] Fluconazole[c,f]	5-Fluorocytosine[g]	Removal of central lines	Dependent on the rate of clearance: minimum of 14 days	Dependent on clinical scenario
Aspergillus	Uncommon	Culture Gram stain Histology Radiographic staging[h]	Amphotericin B[b]	Itraconazole[c,i,j] 5-Fluorocytosine[g]	Surgical resection	Dependent on the rate of clearance: minimum of 4 weeks, usually 8–12 weeks	Dependent of clinical scenario
Cryptococcus	Adults: uncommon Children: rare	Culture Antigen test India ink stain Histology CSF examination	Amphotericin B[e] Fluconazole[c,f]	5-Fluorocytosine**		Minimum of 6–8 weeks Many would continue with fluconazole indefinitely	Clinical examination Antigen testing Repeat culture of appropriate source (sputum, CSF, urine) Radiography if relevant
Others (*Histoplasma, Mucor, Fusarium,*	Rare	Culture Histology Antigen testing (when appropriate)	Amphotericin B[e]	Azole therapy (for susceptible organisms)[c]	Surgical debridement	Dependent on rate of clearance	Clinical examination Antigen testing Repeat culture of

appropriate
source (sputum,
CSF, urine)
Radiography if
relevant

*Blastomycetes,
Altenaria, etc.)*

a Common, > 5%; uncommon, 1–5%; rare, < 1%.

b Topical amphotericin B for bladder wash for noninvasive candiduria; ultrasonography of kidneys recommended to determine that no invasive disease is present.

c Azole use must be accompanied by close follow-up of levels of cyclosporin or tacrolimus.

d In general, tacrolimus dosing should be cut in half when using a standard dose of fluconazole.

e Amphotericin B lipid formulations are used if renal failure is present.

f Fluoroconazole is an alternative first-line drug for invasive disease if the species is known to be sensitive to fluconazole and the patient is clinically stable.

g 5-Fluorocytosine should not be used alone but is synergistic when used in conjunction with amphotericin B.

h Radiographic staging includes CT of head, chest and abdomen.

i Itraconazole can be used long term for patients who have been treated for invasive aspergillosis, but in general is not recommended as a first-line therapy.

j Itraconazole absorption can be erratic; accordingly, monitoring of itraconazole levels is recommended. Adjustment of cyclosporin or tacrolimus dosage should be individualized.

Table 7.5.5 Overview of the diagnosis and management of parasitic infections following intestinal transplantation

Organism	Frequency	Diagnostic tests	Treatment		Adjunctive	Duration of therapy	Follow-up
			Primary	Secondary			
Pneumocystis carinii	Rare	Cytology of broncho-alveolar lavage fluid Lung biopsy	Trimethoprim	Pentamidine	Corticosteroids	2–3 weeks	None
Toxoplasma gondii	Rare	Serologic testing Histology	Pyrimethamine	Pyrimethamine Clindamycin	Folinic acid	4–6 weeks beyond resolution of signs and symptoms	Clinical surveillance for recurrence
Strongyloides stercoralis	Rare	Stool for ova and parasites Serology	Thiabendazole	Ivermectin		≥ 7 days	Monitor serologic response
Cryptosporidium	Uncommon	Stool for ova and parasites Histology	Paromomycin	Azithromycin Bovine colostrum	Reduced IS	2–4 weeks	Endoscopic surveillance
Isospora and Cyclospora	Rare	Stool for ova and parasites Histology	Trimethoprim–sulfamethoxazole	Pyrimethamine		10–21 weeks	Serial stool for ova and parasite
Entamoeba	Rare	Stool for ova and Parasite	Mild/moderate intestinal disease: metronidazole plus iodoquinol or paromomycin	Severe intestinal or hepatic abscess: Metronidazole followed by iodoquinol or paromomycin		Individualize parasite	Stool for ova
Babesia	Rare	Thick and thin blood	Clindamycin Clindamycin		Exchange transfusion	≥ 7 days	None

| *Malaria* | Rare | smear
Serology
Thick and thin blood smear | + quinine
All *Plasmodium* spp. except chloroquine resistant *P. falciparum*: chloroquine phosphate or quinidine gluconate
Chloroquine-resistant *P. falciparum*: quinine sulfate plus tetracycline, plus pyrimethamine with sulfdoxine, or plus clindamycin | Mefloquine | Supportive care | Varies by regimen | None |

receives an isolated intestinal transplant, a combined liver–intestinal transplant, or a multivisceral transplant. This is probably explained by the fact that the immunosuppressive regimens are very similar for each of these three procedures. The only exception to this might be an increased risk of intraabdominal infections in multivisceral transplant recipients. The latter finding is explained by the increased technical complexity of this procedure.

D–/R– patients for CMV are at reduced risk for symptomatic CMV disease. While CMV may still develop in such patients, an extra effort should be made to identify an alternate source of infection. In contrast, D+/R– patients are at high risk for CMV disease, especially if the timing is appropriate and the patient has a history of augmented immunosuppression. These patients may benefit from empirical antiviral treatment while waiting for results of diagnostic tests. As noted above in section 1.4, with the exception of the D–/R– patient, the risk of EBV/PTLD does not appear to differ according to the donor–recipient serostatus against EBV.

1.8 What are the specific evaluation measures?
An overview of the evaluation of infection following intestinal transplantation by site of involvement and pathogen is shown in Tables 7.5.2 and Chapter 2 in Part I.

1.9 What new developments are going to impact on emerging organisms, recognition, evaluation and diagnosis of infection in intestinal transplant recipients?
New and/or emerging organisms are recognized following organ transplantation primarily for one of two reasons. The first explanation is the availability of new diagnostic tests. The recent discovery and subsequent development of diagnostic tests for 'new' viral pathogens, including human herpesviruses (HHV-6, HHV-7, HHV-8) and parvovirus B19, has offered the opportunity to determine the potential role of these viruses in organ transplant recipients. Investigators have begun to explore whether one or more of these 'new' viruses are the cause of previously unexplained febrile episodes or laboratory abnormalities following organ transplantation. For example, parvovirus B19 is now recognized as causing red cell aplasia in solid organ transplant recipients. Likewise, HHV-6 may cause neutropenia or delayed engraftment in bone marrow transplant recipients. However, the full extent and impact of infections due to these newer viruses has not been determined in solid organ transplant recipients.

The second explanation for the recognition of new or emerging pathogens affecting transplant recipients is the use of increasingly potent immunosuppressants, rendering patients susceptible to what otherwise might be saprophytic organisms. This has been most frequently observed in patients undergoing bone marrow transplantation who have developed invasive infection with unusual fungi such as *Alternaria* or *Fusaria*. This may also be relevant to intestinal transplant recipients, who require higher levels of immunosuppression than most other solid organ transplant recipients. Accordingly, recognition of the importance of these 'emerging' pathogens in patients undergoing intestinal transplantation may develop with increasing experience with this procedure.

The concept of measuring and/or monitoring of viral loads promises to have an important impact on the diagnosis of infection in intestinal transplant recipients. The measurement of EBV viral load in the peripheral blood using PCR has recently been introduced as a method of diagnosing patients with EBV-associated PTLD. In addition, it is hoped that serial measurements of the EBV viral load will be able to identify patients who are infected and at risk of developing disease before they manifest symptoms, and allow a preemptive intervention to prevent progression to disease. In a similar fashion, assays designed to measure CMV pp65 antigen levels in the peripheral blood also provide a determination of viral load. As with EBV, the CMV viral load (as measured by the pp65 antigenemia assay or quantitative CMV PCR) is positive in patients with symptomatic disease. The CMV pp65 antigenemia assay also becomes positive before the onset of symptomatic infection and is the basis of a proposed preemptive strategy (see section 4.1).

The development of new immunosuppressive agents and combinations will likely have a dramatic effect on the diagnosis and management of infections in intestinal transplant recipients. Historically, the introduction of newer agents has altered the pattern and severity of infections following transplantation. This is illustrated by the increased risk of viral and fungal infections for patients receiving antilymphocyte antibody products. More recently, the use of mycophenolic acid has been associated with an increased risk of developing symptomatic CMV infection and perhaps with an increased likelihood of developing recurrent CMV disease. These changes in the timing and manifestations of infection are often not apparent at the time of licensure of the new immunosuppressant agent. Accordingly, clinicians involved in the care of organ transplant recipients need to be aware that the spectrum of infectious complications may be altered for patients receiving new immunosuppressant agents and regimens.

2 REGARDING THE RISK FACTORS IN INTESTINAL TRANSPLANT RECIPIENTS

2.1 What are the main alterations in host defense mechanisms and what are the appropriate investigations to document them?

Patients undergoing intestinal transplantation experience two main alterations in host defense mechanisms. The first is the breakdown of normally protective anatomic barriers because of surgery or the presence of foreign bodies (including intraluminal catheters and surgical drains). This may also occur at the epithelial surface of the gastrointestinal tract in association with the presence of acute cellular rejection or PTLD.

The second alteration in host defenses is a consequence of the use of immunosuppressive agents to prevent rejection. Although these agents are intended to limit the ability of recipient T cells to recognize and react to the intestinal allograft, the lack of specificity of these agents leads to an increased risk of infections caused by pathogens that are normally controlled by cytotoxic T cells (e.g. CMV, EBV, *Candida* spp.). Additionally, the use of immunosuppressants (e.g. corticosteroids) can affect other arms of the immune system and may be associated with the development of neutropenia (e.g. azathioprine or mycophenolic acid). Most intestinal transplant recipients receive a triple drug immunosuppressant regimen consisting of tacrolimus, corticosteroids and mycophenolic acid. As noted above, this regimen is similar for recipients of isolated intestine, combined liver–intestine or multivisceral transplantation.

In general, investigations are not performed to document alterations in host defenses in intestinal transplant recipients. However, a complete blood count should be obtained to evaluate the patient for the presence of neutropenia.

2.2 What are the alterations due to iatrogenic factors?

Essentially all alterations to host defense mechanisms in intestinal transplant recipients are due to iatrogenic factors. The use of immunosuppressive agents and the presence of foreign bodies are two of the most frequent iatrogenic factors affecting host defense mechanisms in these patients. Although there is variation between centers, intestinal transplant recipients currently typically receive triple drug immunosuppression consisting of tacrolimus, mycophenolic acid and steroids. In addition, previous and continuing exposure to antimicrobial agents increases the risk of developing infections with multiply resistant organisms and/or superinfection with yeast or other fungi. In general, these risks are very similar for all solid organ transplant recipients.

2.3 What is the influence of environmental factors?

Environmental factors influence the risk of infection following intestinal transplantation, particularly within the hospital setting. The presence of local construction may lead to environmental exposure to *A. fumigatus*, or contamination of the hospital water supply with *Legionella* may lead to outbreaks of this pathogen in transplant recipients. Exposure to other hospitalized patients with contagious diseases, such as *M. tuberculosis* and vancomycin-resistant enterococci (VRE), also affects the likelihood of acquiring infection. The risk of infection in intestinal transplant recipients may also be influenced by community-based environmental factors. A prime example of this would be the presence of seasonal epidemic pathogens (e.g. respiratory syncytial virus (RSV), influenza virus, rotavirus) within the community. Examples of environmental factors within a geographic region or country are exposures to endemic fungi (e.g. *C. immitis*, *H. capsulatum*) or vector-associated pathogens (malaria, *Borrelia*), which vary between regions or countries. In general, the impact of these environmental factors is similar for all solid organ transplant recipients, including intestinal transplant recipients.

2.4 What are the most significant factors that contribute to the risk of infection in intestinal transplant recipients?

The most important factors contributing to the risk of infection after intestinal transplantation are the level of immunosuppression, the presence of rejection, technical events occurring during operation, development of technical complications after operation, donor and recipient serologic status against CMV, use of indwelling catheters and nosocomial exposures to pathogens. In addition, the age of the transplant recipient is an important factor contributing to infection in intestinal transplant recipients. This latter risk may be explained by the underlying immaturity of the immune system in pediatric patients, and also by the increased likelihood that pediatric transplant recipients will not have had exposure and subsequent development of immunity to a variety of pathogens, most notably CMV and EBV. Finally, the small size of the pediatric patient may predispose them to technical complications of surgery, which may lead to postoperative infections. Each of these factors may affect the likelihood of acquiring, as well as the potential severity of, infection due to specific pathogens.

2.5 What are the specific or nonspecific measures aimed at minimizing each of these factors?

Measures can be taken to minimize the risk for some of the factors contributing to infection following intestinal transplantation. Every effort should be made to keep the level of immunosuppression adequate to prevent rejection without overimmunosuppressing the patient.

The availability of an effective vaccine against CMV would be an excellent protective measure against the absence of preexisting immunity to this virus. Unfortunately, it is unlikely that an effective vaccine will be available in the near future. In the absence of active immunization, passive immunization against CMV using high-titered intravenous immunoglobulin (e.g. CytoGam®) is available. While the prophylactic use of this product has been shown to offer some protection in adult renal and liver transplant recipients, it has been least effective in high-risk CMV-seronegative recipients (R–) of CMV-seropositive donors (D+). The authors currently use CMV intravenous immunoglobulin (IVIG) in combination with a 3-month course of ganciclovir (initially given intravenously followed by oral dosing) for the prevention of CMV in D+/R– patients (see section 4.1).

While there is no way to control the serologic status of the intestinal transplant recipient, centers can limit donor acceptability on the basis of CMV status. Because of the frequency, severity and chronicity of primary CMV disease in D+/R– intestinal transplant recipients, the University of Pittsburgh no longer performs CMV-mismatched isolated intestinal transplants. However, this rule is not extended to patients requiring a liver–intestine transplant as they may not survive long enough to wait for a 'low-risk' donor.

Data from a severe combined immune deficiency (SCID) mouse model suggest that the use of IVIG-containing antibodies against EBV may also provide protection against EBV disease in organ transplant recipients. On the basis of this and the authors' clinical experience, they also use IVIG in combination with intravenous ganciclovir as part of the preemptive strategy against EBV/PTLD (see section 4.1).

Technical complications are undesirable but are at times unavoidable in association with organ transplantation. This is particularly true of intestinal transplantation because it is the newest of the organ transplant procedures. Accordingly, transplant teams have less total surgical experience and the optimal techniques for this procedure may not be completely established. The identification of a finite number of 'centers of excellence' on a regional, national or global level for the performance of this procedure may help to limit technical complications.

To minimize the risk of infection after intestinal transplantation, the clinical team in charge of the patient must be aware of any technical events that occur during the operation. A prolonged course of antimicrobial prophylaxis should be considered in the event of a high-risk complication (e.g. bowel perforation). Additional measures to minimize the risk of infection in intestinal transplant recipients should include the removal of all indwelling cannulas and drains as soon as possible following the transplant procedure. For patients who will require the long-term presence of CVCs, attention should be paid to catheter care. Every effort should be made to minimize the number of times that the catheter is 'entered'. Patients and their caretakers should be enstructed in the proper technique for caring for CVCs when patients are to be discharged home with them. Finally, excellent infection control technique should be taught and enforced on the transplant unit to minimize the likelihood of nosocomial spread of infection. Strict adherence to handwashing should be emphasized for all members of the clinical care team. Of interest, the routine use of laminar flow rooms or strict 'gown and gloves' isolation is not necessary for intestinal transplant recipients. Single-room isolation is recommended for the early posttransplant period.

2.6 Are there different levels of risk of infection recognized for intestinal transplant recipients?

There appear to be several differences in the risk of acquiring infections for recipients of intestinal transplantation compared with patients undergoing other types of solid organ transplantation. Transplantation of a CMV D+/R– patient creates an extremely high-risk scenario for the development of symptomatic, chronic and invasive CMV disease. This risk exceeds that observed in CMV-mismatched patients undergoing other types of organ transplantation, as well as that seen in CMV D+/R+, D–/R+ or D–/R– intestinal transplant recipients.

An extremely high risk of developing symptomatic EBV disease and PTLD has also been recognized after intestinal transplantation, particularly among pediatric patients.

Unlike CMV, the risk of acquiring EBV disease appears to be independent of the presence of preexisting immunity against EBV in children undergoing intestinal transplantation. While the risk may be diminished in the D–/R– recipient, these low-risk patients may still acquire EBV from either blood products or exposure to EBV-infected secretions from close contacts. The risk of developing EBV/PTLD in these pediatric recipients exceeds the risk observed both in adult intestinal transplant recipients and in children undergoing other types of organ transplantation. To date, the reason for the excess risk of EBV-associated PTLD in pediatric intestinal transplant recipients (including EBV-seropositive patients) has not been identified. Finally, the risk of EBV/PTLD does not appear to differ according to whether a patient receives an isolated intestine, combined liver–intestine or a multivisceral transplant.

2.7 How does the level of risk impact on management?

Patients who are known to be at high risk of developing infection are the most likely candidates for preventive strategies (see sections 1.4, 2.5 and 2.6). Depending on the philosophy of the intestinal transplant center, programs may choose to use virologic monitoring for CMV (pp65 antigenemia or CMV PCR) or EBV (quantitative PCR of blood) to identify patients at risk of developing disease and to intervene with preemptive therapy. Alternatively, transplant centers may choose to provide prophylaxis to all high-risk patients. The duration of prophylaxis may be modified based on the level of risk of acquiring symptomatic disease due to a pathogen. Regardless of which preventive strategy a transplant center chooses, use of empirical therapy for symptomatic patients at high risk of developing a specific infection should be considered pending the results of diagnostic studies (see section 4.1).

2.8 What new developments are going to impact on minimizing or suppressing the specific risk factors?

The development of new and more specific immunosuppressive agents will likely have a major impact on the risk of infections following intestinal transplantation. The availability of such agents should diminish both the rate of rejection-associated bloodstream infections as well as the likelihood of developing opportunistic infections. The development of effective vaccines against CMV and EBV might also impact positively on the infectious sequelae of intestinal transplantation. Identification of alternative, effective, chemoprophylactic or immunoprophylactic regimens to be used as primary prophylaxis or as the basis of preemptive therapy against CMV and EBV would clearly reduce the risk of infection following intestinal transplantation. The adaptation of cellular therapy against CMV and EBV for intestinal transplant recipients should allow these patients to enjoy some of the benefits experienced by bone marrow transplant recipients where these strategies are already in place. Finally, increased experience with intestinal transplantation should lead to improvements in technical aspects of this surgery and a subsequent decrease in infectious complications.

3 REGARDING THE SURVELLANCE OF INTESTINAL TRANSPLANT RECIPIENTS

3.1 What is the most important pretransplant information to be gathered?

A thorough infectious disease history should be taken from all candidates for intestinal transplantation as part of the pretransplant evaluation. Particular attention should be paid to a previous history of infection with antibiotic-resistant organisms (e.g. vancomycin-resistant *Enterococcus faecium*, multiply resistant *Klebsiella pneumoniae*), tuberculosis and endemic fungi (e.g. *H. capsulatum*, *C. immitis*). Candidates for intestinal transplantation should undergo purified protein derivative (PPD) skin testing. A chest radiograph should be obtained and evaluated for the presence of lesions that may be consistent with quiescent tuberculosis. A previous history of varicella and herpes simplex infection should also be sought. The immunization status should also be reviewed thoroughly, particularly for pediatric intestinal transplant recipients. If possible, missing immunizations should be given before transplantation.

3.2 What are the surveillance measures to be taken when a patient presents for intestinal transplantation?

The serologic status of the donor against donor-associated pathogens should be obtained routinely. For intestinal transplantation, this should at a minimum include testing for CMV, EBV, hepatitis B and C viruses (HBV, HCV) and human immunodeficiency virus (HIV). These serologies should also be determined for the intestinal transplant recipient. Additionally, serologic testing of the recipient should include varicella and herpes simplex virus (HSV). A surveillance stool culture might be obtained from the recipient at the time of transplant to screen for the presence of multiply antibiotic-resistant organisms and to provide guidance for empirical therapy following intestinal transplantation. Unfortunately, effective strategies to eradicate colonization with these organisms are not currently available. Some centers perform environmental surveillance cultures for the presence of nosocomial pathogens including *A. fumigatus* and *Legionella* spp.

3.3 What are the other specific measures to be taken when a patient presents for intestinal transplantation?

In general, no other specific measures are necessary for the patient presenting for intestinal transplantation. However, a full infectious disease evaluation should be performed for the intestinal transplant candidate who has fever or other symptoms suggestive of infection at the time that an organ becomes available.

4 REGARDING THE PREVENTION OF INFECTION IN INTESTINAL TRANSPLANT RECIPIENTS

4.1 What approaches, if any, to the prevention of infection should be considered in intestinal transplant recipients?

Preventive strategies can be separated into short-term, perioperative prophylaxis as well as more long-term prophylactic strategies. The authors currently recommend the use of intravenous antibiotics to cover enteric organisms for the first 3–5 days after intestinal transplantation. Acceptable regimens might include the combination of ampicillin and cefotaxime or piperacillin–tazobactam. Use of oral nonabsorbable antibiotics is also recommended to decontaminate the gut in the early postoperative period. The authors currently use a combination of an oral aminoglycoside, colistin and amphotericin B for the first 2 weeks after intestinal transplantation and until there is endoscopic as well as histologic evidence of a good epithelial barrier against invasion of intestinal microorganisms. Prolonged use of oral decontamination beyond this relatively brief time period is discouraged because in the authors' experience it is associated with the development of antimicrobial resistance. Oral vancomycin is also discouraged because its use has been associated with acquisition of VRE.

Preventive strategies are recommended against the development of CMV disease in intestinal transplant recipients. The authors currently favor the use of ganciclovir prophylaxis in intestinal transplant recipients. Their prophylactic strategy for high-risk, CMV D+/R− patients has evolved over time. Currently they use intravenous ganciclovir for the first 14–21 days following transplant (or until the patient has adequate absorptive function of the intestinal graft), followed by oral ganciclovir to complete the first 3 months after transplantation. In addition, these high-risk mismatched patients also receive high-titered CMV-specific intravenous immunoglobulin (CytoGam®) according to published dosing schedules for liver transplant recipients. For intestinal transplant recipients at lower risk of developing CMV disease (CMV D−/R−, D+/R+ and D−/R+), the authors currently use 14 days of intravenous ganciclovir. An alternate approach would be to monitor at-risk patients with serial measurements of pp65 antigenemia or quantitative CMV PCRs, with the introduction of ganciclovir for patients crossing a predetermined threshold for treatment.

The high frequency and severity of EBV infections in intestinal transplant recipients has prompted the authors to introduce 'experimental' strategies aimed at preventing or modifying disease due to this virus in intestinal transplant recipients. They currently monitor the EBV viral load in the peripheral blood using a quantitative competitive EBV PCR assay. Patients with viral loads exceeding predetermined cutoffs (which will vary by the type of assay and the pretransplant serologic status of the patient) are treated preemptively. Currently, a combination of intravenous CytoGam® and ganciclovir is used as preemptive therapy. CytoGam® is preferred to 'generic' IVIG because of the lot-to-lot consistency of anti-EBV antibodies with this product. Patients are started on intravenous ganciclovir and receive three 100 mg/kg doses of CytoGam® when the EBV viral load exceeds predetermined cutoffs. At the authors' institution, this is $\geq$ 40 genome copies per 10^5 peripheral blood lymphocytes for EBV-seronegative and $\geq$ 200 for EBV-seropositive recipients. Where possible, the amount of immunosuppression is decreased, although this is not possible for patients presenting with concurrent increases in EBV viral load and rejection. Patients are continued on the intravenous ganciclovir and undergo measurement of the EBV viral load every 2–3 weeks. Three additional doses of CytoGam® are given each time that the follow-up viral load exceeds the initial cutoffs for therapy.

Monitoring is continued for the first 2–3 years following intestinal transplantation. However, a recent analysis of data revealed that the vast majority of patients who will require preemptive therapy have an initial increase in EBV viral load during the first 6 months after intestinal transplantation. The introduction of this strategy has resulted in an approximately 40% decline in the incidence of EBV-associated disease in the authors' intestinal transplant program. Despite this improvement, the rate of EBV continues to be high, and better preemptive strategies need to be identified for patients with increased viral loads.

Intestinal transplant recipients should also receive trimethroprim–sulfamethoxazole as prophylaxis against the development of *Pneumocystis carinii* pneumonia. Because of the chronically high levels of immunosuppression required in these patients, the authors recommend lifelong use of the preventive strategy. Finally, intestinal transplant recipients who are seronegative against varicella zoster virus (VZV) should receive zoster immune globulin (ZIG) within 96 h of any exposure to active varicella.

4.2 What are the future challenges and opportunities for reducing the risk of infection?

Finding solutions to two major challenges would provide important opportunities for reducing the risk of infection after intestinal transplantation. The first is to develop improved antirejection therapy, leading to a decreased rate of rejection and improved graft function. This should lead to a decrease in bloodstream infections, both in association with the presence of rejection and because improvement in graft function should decrease the need for CVCs. Ideally, new antirejection therapies would be more specific than current regimens and thus minimize the likelihood of some opportunistic infections.

The second major challenge is to identify and develop better strategies for the prevention of EBV disease in intestinal transplant recipients. One potentially important possibility would be the adaptation of cellular therapy using EBV-specific cytotoxic T cells for preemptive therapy, as has been demonstrated in bone marrow transplant recipients. However, to date, a number of theoretical and technical problems have prevented the implementation of this approach for solid organ transplant recipients in general, and for intestinal transplant recipients in particular.

5 REGARDING THE TREATMENT OF INTESTINAL TRANSPLANT RECIPIENTS

5.1 What is the role of empirical therapy?

Decisions regarding the use of empirical therapy are made based upon the timing of presentation of infection and the presence or absence of risk factors. Empirical therapy is appropriately started in the intestinal transplant recipient with fever after performance of a careful clinical evaluation including obtaining appropriate specimens for culture. However, empirical therapy should be withheld from patients with clinical evidence suggesting the presence of infection due to common respiratory or gastrointestinal viral pathogens (e.g. rhinovirus, rotavirus). This is particularly true in pediatric transplant recipients in whom these infections are more common. Empirical therapy should still be considered for febrile patients with known severe intestinal rejection (an alternative cause for fever) because of its association with bloodstream infections. The choice of antimicrobial agents should be made to cover enteric and typical 'catheter' pathogens. Knowledge of prior 'resistance' patterns for a given patient and within a hospital also helps to guide the choice of antibiotics. It is important to limit the duration of antimicrobial therapy for empirically treated patients who have no positive cultures in an effort to minimize the development of antimicrobial resistance and secondary fungemia. However, a full course of treatment should be given for patients with positive cultures or for whom a site of infection is identified. A change in empirical therapy may be indicated if a patient fails to respond to initial empirical therapy or experiences a clinical deterioration.

5.2 What is the appropriate approach to the intestinal transplan recipient with evidence of:

Upper respiratory tract infection?

Sinusitis
Patients with mild illness and radiographic evidence of sinusitis may be treated empirically with therapy against the typical sinus pathogens (e.g. S. pneumoniae, H. influenzae, M. catarrhalis). A microbiologic sample with biopsy to rule out fungal sinusitis should be considered for patients who are moderately or severely ill, or for those who show no improvement on empirical therapy.

Otitis media
Patients with otitis media should be started on empirical therapy against typical pathogens associated with middle ear disease (e.g. S. pneumoniae, H. influenzae, M.

catarrhalis). Failure to improve on empirical antibiotics should prompt diagnostic tympanocentesis.

Conjunctivitis

Bacterial and viral viral cultures should be obtained from intestinal transplant recipients with evidence of conjunctivitis. The use of topical or systemic antibacterial agents should be considered for patients with bacterial cultures positive for typical pathogens including *S. pneumoniae*, *H. influenzae* and *M. catarrhalis*.

Tonsillitis

The presence of exudative tonsillitis should prompt consideration of infection due to *Streptococcus pyogenes* (group A streptococcus) as well as viral pathogens including EBV and adenovirus. Exudative tonsillitis may also be caused by *Candida* spp. Patients presenting with this condition should initially undergo a throat culture to look for the presence of group A streptococcus and yeast.

A positive culture for group A streptococcus should prompt treatment with penicillin. Patients with positive throat cultures for yeast without evidence of fungal esophagitis can usually be treated with oral nystatin. However, failure to respond to this therapy warrants consideration of the use of fluconazole.

The presence of tonsillitis in patients without evidence of group A streptococci or *Candida* raises the possibility of EBV infection. Clinically, this is often manifest as an exudative tonsillitis which is not distinguishable from the classic appearance of tonsillar disease in immunocompetent patients with EBV-associated mononucleosis. Histologic evaluation of tonsillar tissue obtained from transplant recipients presenting in this manner may demonstrate a continuum of pathology including acute EBV infection, mononucleosis and PTLD. The variability in the histologic grade observed is likely to be due to the rapidity of proliferation of EBV-infected B cells and the ability of the host to contain this process. The authors believe that patients presenting with EBV-associated tonsillitis are all on the same continuum of disease. Accordingly, it is recommended that they are treated the same once it has been confirmed that the tonsillitis is EBV related. EBV serologies as well as a monospot test should also be performed in these patients. Where available, the EBV viral load in the peripheral blood should also be determined. Finally, a throat culture for viruses should be sent to look for the presence of adenovirus or other respiratory viruses (e.g. influenza).

Teeth and gingiva

Dental abscesses and gingivitis occur uncommonly in intestinal transplant recipients. Patients with clinical evidence of a dental infection should be evaluated by a dentist. The diagnosis of HSV should be considered for patients with gingivitis. A viral culture should be obtained from these patients.

Lower respiratory tract infection?

A chest radiograph should be obtained from all patients who present with evidence of a lower respiratory tract infection. A sputum specimen should be sought from older children and adult intestinal transplant recipients. However, young children are usually incapable of providing usable sputum specimens. Patients with community-acquired lower respiratory tract infection with radiographic evidence of typical bacterial pneumonia may be started empirically on therapy aimed at covering usual bacterial pathogens (e.g. *S. pneumoniae*, *M. pneumoniae*). Empirical therapy should be expanded to include coverage against nosocomial pathogens and enteric bacteria for patients who are currently or have recently been in an intensive care setting. Performance of a BAL should be considered in patients with atypical radiographic findings or those with more severe disease to rule out opportunistic pathogens (e.g. *P. carinii*, *Legionella* spp., CMV). Finally, CT of the chest and performance of a lung biopsy should be considered for patients with radiographic evidence of nodular disease.

Gastrointestinal infection?

Gastrointestinal symptoms are extremely common following intestinal transplantation. Noninfectious explanations, including rejection of the intestinal allograft or poor absorptive function of the graft because of dysmotility or allograft scarring, are the most likely reasons for these symptoms. However, gastroenteritis due to bacterial (e.g. C. *difficile*) or viral (e.g. CMV, EBV, rotavirus) infection is also common in intestinal transplant recipients. Routine evaluation of patients with new onset of gastrointestinal symptoms should include bacterial cultures for pathogens as well as performance of a C. *difficile* toxin assay. Stool evaluation for ova and parasites could be considered for patients presenting from the community, but is probably not necessary for those whose symptoms develop in hospital. Stool should be sent for antigen detection against rotavirus (especially in pediatric patients) as well as for viral cultures. Clinicians caring for intestinal transplant recipients should have a low threshold for obtaining an endoscopic evaluation of the gastrointestinal tract to rule out the presence of rejection, CMV, PTLD or other pathogens. Radiographic imaging studies are not typically helpful in the diagnosis of intraluminal gastrointestinal infections.

Genitourinary infection?

A urine culture and enhanced urinanalysis should be obtained from all patients who present with signs and symptoms suggestive of a UTI (e.g. dysuria, frequency, hematuria). The use of empirical antibiotics against typical urinary tract pathogens may be considered for patients with classic symptoms after obtaining these studies. Consideration should be given to viral (e.g. adenovirus) or fungal (e.g. *Candida* spp.) pathogens as alternative explanations for urinary tract symptoms. Evaluation for the presence of vesicoureteral reflux should be considered for children with evidence of pyelonephritis at or near the end of therapy. Patients found to have significant reflux may benefit from chronic antimicrobial prophylaxis. Those with high-grade reflux should undergo urologic consultation.

Cardiovascular infection?

äCardiovascular infections are uncommon in intestinal transplant recipients. Evaluation for these infections is similar to that for any other patient with signs or symptoms suggestive of an infection involving the cardiovascular system (e.g. blood culture, echocardiography).

Musculoskeletal infection?

Musculoskeletal infections are uncommon in intestinal transplant recipients. Evaluation for these infections would be similar to that for any other patient with signs or symptoms suggestive of an infection involving this system.

Skin infection?

Skin infections are most likely associated with the presence of a foreign body (e.g. intravascular catheter, surgical drain) or with extension of infection from the surgical wound. Culture of any purulent material should be performed. Antimicrobial therapy should be aimed at typical pathogens associated with infections of the skin (e.g. *S. aureus*, group A streptococci). Viral pathogens are an additional cause of skin infections in intestinal transplant recipients. The most common viral pathogens would be VZV (causing either primary varicella or shingles) or HSV. Viral cultures and a Tzanck preparation should be obtained from patients presenting with vesicular lesions in order to differentiate between these two pathogens. Empirical treatment with acyclovir should be initiated pending results of viral cultures. In general, the authors strongly recommend hospitalization and the use of intravenous acyclovir for patients who present with primary varicella infection.

Central nervous system infection?
Infection of the central nervous system (CNS) is an uncommon but important complication following intestinal transplantation. Intestinal transplant recipients do not appear to be at an increased risk of developing bacterial meningitis. However, they are at risk for cryptococcal meningitis (although this is rare in pediatric patients). Additional CNS pathogens include *A. fumigatus* and viruses (e.g. CMV, EBV, enterovirus). It is important to consider drug-associated toxicity for patients presenting with CNS symptoms since both cyclosporin and tacrolimus, as well as high-dose steroids and antilymphocyte antibody preparations, have CNS side effects.

Foreign body in place?
Foreign bodies are a likely source of infection in intestinal transplant recipients presenting with symptoms and signs of infection. This is particularly true of intraluminal cannulas. Accordingly, culture specimens should be obtained from involved sites.

Intraabdominal infection?
Intraabdominal infections occur somewhat frequently following intestinal transplantation. Infections of this space are typically due to a postoperative event or technical complication. An additional source of infection within the intraabdominal space would be a gastrointestinal perforation, which may occur as a sequela of severe rejection or of PTLD. Typical pathogens include enteric bacteria and *Candida* spp.

5.3 What is the appropriate approach to the intestinal transplant recipient with evidence of bacteremia, with or without site of infection?
Antimicrobial therapy should be initiated in intestinal transplant recipients with documented bacteremia. The initial use of vancomycin should be considered for patients with Gram-positive bacteremia. However, therapy should be modified if results of antimicrobial susceptibility testing allows the use of an alternate agent. A third-generation cephalosporin (e.g. cefotaxime) or an advanced-generation penicillin (e.g. piperacillin) alone or in combination with an aminoglycoside should be initiated in intestinal transplant recipients with Gram-negative bacteremia. The initial use of more broad-spectrum agents (including carbapenems and quinolones) should be reserved for patients with more severe illness or those with a history of colonization or disease with multiply antibiotic-resistant bacteria. Cephalosporin use should be avoided in patients with proven bacteremia due to *Enterobacter* spp. because of their inherent ability to derepress a chromosomal β-lactamase enzyme. Anaerobic pathogens have infrequently been recovered from the blood of intestinal transplant recipients. Recovery of an anaerobic pathogen should prompt the use of an appropriate agent (e.g. metronidazole, clindamycin).

Recovery of multiple pathogens requires the clinician to choose antimicrobial agents to cover all isolated organisms.

Regardless of the recovered organism, determination of a defined primary site of infection may also help to guide the management of bacteremic patients. For all patients, documentation of clearance of the bloodstream is an important marker of response to therapy. For patients with catheter-associated bacteremia, the catheter should be removed if the patient is very ill or remains bacteremic despite appropriate therapy. Some studies have shown that the use of urokinase may increase the likelihood of saving a catheter in some patients with 'refractory' bacteremia. However, this approach has not been uniformly accepted. Medical management alone may not be sufficient for patients who are bacteremic in association with the presence of an abscess. These patients may need to undergo an incision and drainage procedure. Uncommonly, patients who are bacteremic in association with severe allograft rejection have required decontamination of the graft with oral nonabsorbable antibiotics in order to clear the bloodstream infection.

5.4 What is the appropriate approach to the intestinal transplant recipient with evidence of a viral infection?

The treatment of viral infections following transplantation of the intestine varies according to which viral pathogen is responsible. In general, pathogens are similar for recipients of any type of solid organ transplant procedure. An overview of strategies for diagnosis, management and follow-up for many of the potential viral pathogens seen following intestinal transplantation is shown in Table 7.5.3.

5.5 What is the appropriate approach to the intestinal transplant recipient with evidence of a fungal infection?

The treatment of fungal infections following transplantation of the intestine varies according to which fungal pathogen is present, where it is found in the body, and whether or not it is invasive. In general, the approach to fungal infections is similar to that for recipients of many types of solid organ transplant procedure. An overview of strategies for diagnosis, management and follow-up for many of the potential fungal pathogens seen following intestinal transplantation is shown in Table 7.5.4.

5.6 What is the appropriate approach to the intestinal transplant recipient with evidence of a parasitic infection?

Parasitic infections occur rarely in intestinal transplant recipients. Although these patients are at high risk of developing *P. carinii* pneumonia, in the authors' experience this is completely preventable through the use of chronic prophylaxis with trimethoprim–sulfamethoxazole. It is worth noting that a few cases of cryptosporidiosis have been documented in intestinal transplant patients. The approach to diagnosis and management of parasitic infections in intestinal transplant recipients is reviewed in Table 7.5.5.

5.7 What is the role of nonantiinfective interventions (including reducing or altering immunosuppression) in the management of established infection?

In general, attempts to decrease the level of immunosuppression should be made in any intestinal transplant recipient who is experiencing a moderate to severe infection. This step should be considered carefully if the patient is simultaneously diagnosed with rejection. For patients who have received an isolated intestinal allograft, strong consideration should be given to decreasing or stopping immunosuppression despite the simultaneous presence of rejection, as these patients can be managed on intravenous hyperalimentation even if they experience graft failure. In fact, one should consider removal of isolated intestinal graft for severe nonresponsive viral and/or fungal infections rather than subject the patient to ongoing immunosuppression in this circumstance. This decision is not as clear for recipients of combined liver–intestin transplantation, for whom the decision to allow the hepatitic allograft with subsequent elective retransplantation is not a viable option.

In addition to modification of immune suppression and to adjunctive therapies noted in previous sections, clinicians caring for intestinal transplant recipients should consider the use of granulocyte colony-stimulating factor (G-CSF) in patients with neutropenia (secondary to either pathogen or treatment) during treatment of infections.

REFERENCES

Bueno J, Green M, Kocochis S et al. Cytomegalovirus infection after intestinal transplantation in children. *Clin Infect Dis* 1997; **25**: 1078–1083.

Finn L, Reyes J, Bueno J, Yunis E. Epstein–Barr virus infections in children after transplantation of the small intestine. *Am J Surg Pathol* 1998; **22**: 299–309.

Fishman JA, Rubin RH. Infection in organ-transplant recipients. *N Engl J Med* 1998; **338**: 1741–1751.

Green M, Michaels M. Infections in solid organ transplant recipients. In: Long SS, Prober CG, Pickering LK, eds. *Principles and Practice of Pediatric Infectious Diseases*, 1st edn., New York: Churchill Livingstone, 1997: 626–633.

Green M, Reyes J, Nour B, Tzakis A, Todo S. Early infectious complications of liver–intestinal transplantation in children: preliminary analysis. *Transplant Proc* 1994; **26**: 1420–1421.

Green M, Reyes J, Rowe D. New strategies in the prevention and management of Epstein–Barr virus infection and posttransplant lymphoproliferative disease following solid organ transplantation. *Curr Opin Organ Transplant* 1998; **3**: 143–147.

Green M, Cacciarelli TV, Mazariegos GV et al. Serial measurement of Epstein–Barr viral load in peripheral blood in pediatric liver transplant recipients during treatment for posttransplant lymphoproliferative disease. *Transplantation* 1998; **66**: 1641–1644.

Manez R, Kusne S, Green M et al. Incidence and risk factors associated with the development of cytomegalovirus disease after intestinal transplantation. *Transplantation* 1995; **59**: 1010–1014.

Reyes J, Bueno J, Kocochis S et al. Current status of intestinal transplantation in children. *Pediatr Surg* 1998; **33**: 243–254.

Sigurdsson L, Reyes J, Putnam PE et al. Endoscopies in pediatric small intestinal transplantation recipients: five year experience. *Am J Gastroenterol* 1998; **93**: 207–211.

Chapter 7.6 Infections in Pancreas Transplant Recipients

Michael Green, Marian Michaels and Velma Scantlebury

I REGARDING THE CLINICAL PRESENTATION AND EVALUATION OF THE PATIENT

1.1 What are the clinically predominant modes of presentation of infection in pancreas transplant recipients?

Infections are a frequent and important problem following pancreatic transplantation. Nearly all recipients of pancreatic transplant have undergone or will undergo a kidney transplant. Accordingly, there is a fair degree of overlap in infectious complications seen between patients undergoing these two procedures, although it is generally believed that patients undergoing simultaneous kidney–pancreas transplant are at a higher risk of infection than those undergoing an isolated kidney transplant. Taking this overlap into consideration, infectious complications in pancreatic transplant recipients can be divided into four categories:

1 Infections associated with immunosuppressive therapy.
2 Infections characteristic of renal transplantation in patients with nondiabetic renal disease.
3 Infectious complications that are unique to pancreatic transplantation.
4 Infectious complications related to diabetes.

Infectious complications falling into each of these four categories tend to follow a similar time pattern as that seen after most solid organ transplant procedures (see Chapter 7.0). This time pattern can generally be broken into early (first month), intermediate (1–6 months) and late (> 6 months) periods. The differential diagnosis of fever and infection varies within each of these time periods and can be further refined by whether or not it is associated with localizing signs or symptoms. Most febrile illnesses can be confirmed microbiologically following pancreatic transplantation.

Early period

Infection in the early posttransplant period (first month) often involves surgical sites or is related to nosocomial exposures. For pancreas transplant recipients, intraabdominal infection as well as superficial or deep wound infections are among the most likely infectious explanations for early fever. The incidence of all three of these sites range from 10% to 50%. Of these, a superficial infection at the wound site (e.g. stitch infection) is the most common infection in the early postoperative period. Since this procedure is typically undertaken in patients as part of a combined kidney–pancreas transplant or in patients who have already received a kidney transplant, infection of the urinary tract is another frequent site of infection. Accordingly, the urine should be evaluated for the presence of urinary tract infection (UTI) in these patients and the presence of urosepsis should be considered in any febrile pancreatic transplant recipient with a positive urine culture. The risk of UTI may be increased at or near the time of bladder catheterization. Bloodstream infection can also be seen early after transplant. This may be explained by the presence of a central venous catheter (CVC) for part of the early posttransplant period or by urosepsis. The presence of an endotracheal tube in a febrile patient raises the question of ventilator-associated pneumonia.

While the majority of infections diagnosed during the early time period are attributable to bacterial pathogens, fungi (in particular *Candida* spp.) are also frequently associated with the infectious syndromes noted to occur. In addition to these infections, recipients of pancreatic transplantation may experience herpes simplex virus (HSV) infections during the first month after transplant. Most of these episodes are due to reactivation of the recipients latent HSV virus and typically are relatively mild.

Intermediate period

The differential diagnosis of patients presenting with fever during the intermediate time period (1–6 months) after pancreatic transplantation differs from that in patients presenting in the early posttransplant period. The urinary tract continues to be an important site of infection, particularly in recipients of combined kidney–pancreas transplants. This risk is increased if the pancreas transplant was carried out with bladder drainage of pancreatic exocrine secretions. However, the most frequent causes of infection in the intermediate period are opportunistic pathogens, especially cytomegalovirus (CMV) and rarely Epstein–Barr virus (EBV). Both CMV and EBV may cause a primary (acquisition in a recipient who is seronegative) or secondary (reactivation of the recipient's own latent viral strain or reinfection with a new strain in a patient who is seropositive for CMV or EBV before transplantation) infection. Accordingly, disease due to CMV occurs much more frequently than that due to EBV. Disease from CMV may present as a nonspecific viral syndrome or, on occasion, with evidence of tissue-invasive disease. Disease related to EBV presents with a wide variety of symptoms from a nonspecific viral syndrome to high-grade malignant lymphoma. Less commonly, the use of immunosuppression may also lead to reactivation and development of disease due to other latent pathogens (e.g. *Mycobacterium tuberculosis*, *Histoplasma capsulatum*) in the intermediate time period.

Late period

Although less frequent, infectious complications continue to occur late (> 6 months) after pancreatic transplantation. The presence of vesicoureteral reflux at the site of the ureteral implantation is associated with an ongoing risk of graft pyelonephritis in recipients of combined or sequential kidney–pancreas transplantation. Similarly, the use of bladder drainage of pancreatic exocrine secretions has also been associated with persistent risks for late UTI in pancreatic transplant recipients. Of interest, at least one series reported a 5% incidence of late-onset nonurinary tract infections (e.g. osteoarticular infections) in pancreatic transplant recipients. These infections are relatively unique compared with those in recipients of most other types of solid organ transplant and are likely due to the presence of severe diabetic neuropathy and microangiopathy. *Staphylococcus aureus* and streptococcal species are the most common pathogens in patients with osteoarticular disease. Similarly, late-onset bacteremia in association with diabetic foot ulcers occurred in 14% of pancreas–kidney transplant recipients reported in one series. The role of immunosuppression in the pathogenesis of this type of bacteremia is unknown, and it is not clear whether an alternate explanation may be found in the fact that diabetics who undergo pancreatic transplantation have severe enough disease also to require a kidney transplant. Accordingly, this group of patients is more likely to have severe accompanying vascular and neurologic complications of diabetes which predispose to foot infections. Late infections have also been reported due to varicella zoster virus (VZV) and have typically been manifest as reactivated zoster (i.e. shingles). Finally, late presentation of EBV-associated posttransplant lymphoproliferative disease (PTLD) may also occur in these patients.

1.2 What are the predominant sites of infection?

Superficial and deep surgical site infections, often involving the intraabdominal space as well as the urinary tract, are the most frequent sites of infection early after pancreatic transplantation. The latter of these is more likely to be involved in patients undergoing simultaneous kidney–pancreas transplant. Bloodstream infection (typically associated with either urosepsis or the presence of an intravascular catheter) and pneumonia also occur early after transplantation. An increased frequency of infections involving bones and joints, as well as the urinary tract have been reported late after transplant. Finally, infection of the skin due to HSV early and VZV late occur fairly frequently in pancreas transplant recipients.

1.3 What are the predominant organisms that contribute (by site)

Gram-positive bacteria (including enterococci, coagulase-negative staphylococci and *S. aureus*) are frequently recovered from both superficial and deep surgical site infections. The high prevalence of Gram-positive organisms may be explained in part by the use of topical and systemic prophylactic antibiotics against Gram-negative pathogens. Gram-negative enterics (including *Escherichia coli* and other species of Enterobacteriaceae) are frequently associated with surgical site infections, but less often than Gram-positive bacteria. *Candida* spp. are also recovered, alone or in combination with bacteria, from surgical site infections. The finding of *Candida* spp. in deep wound or intraabdominal infections has been associated with a significant decline in graft and patient survival.

Pathogens associated with UTI following pancreatic transplantation are similar to those seen in normal individuals. Gram-negative enteric bacteria, enterococci and *Candida* spp. are most commonly recovered from these patients, although UTIs due to coagulase-negative staphylococci have also been reported.

The predominant organisms recovered from the bloodstream vary somewhat by whether the source of infection is urosepsis, a CVC or a complication of diabetes. Bloodstream pathogens associated with urosepsis are identical to those seen in patients with UTI. Gram-positive bacteria (including coagulase-negative staphylococci, *S. aureus* and enterococci) as well as *Candida* spp. are most frequently seen in catheter-associated bloodstream infections. *S. aureus* is the most frequent cause of bacteremia seen in association with diabetic complications. Finally, *S. aureus* and streptococcal species are the most likely pathogens to be recovered from osteoarticular infections.

The predominant organisms found in osteoarticular infections have been *S. aureus* and streptococcal species. Similar pathogens have been implicated in bacteremia with diabetic foot ulcers in pancreatic transplant recipients.

1.4 How do the organisms vary according to various risk factors?

Risk factors, such as the absence of preexisting immunity, exposure to specific pathogens and intensity of immunosuppression affect the frequency and severity of disease due to specific pathogens in pancreatic transplant recipients. This is well illustrated by CMV, where donor and recipient serologic status before transplantation is a major predictor of both the likelihood and severity of infection. CMV-negative recipients of organs from CMV-positive donors are not only at the highest risk of developing CMV disease but are also more likely to have severe symptoms. In contrast, the risk of CMV disease is very low when both the donor and recipient are seronegative for CMV, especially if transplant centers use CMV-negative blood products or white blood cell filters with the transfusion to minimize exposure to this pathogen. The risk of CMV disease is also affected by the amount of immunosuppression the patient has received. Numerous studies have correlated an increased risk of severe and invasive CMV disease with augmented immunosuppression, particularly the use of antilymphocyte antibody preparations. More recently, the use of mycophenolate mofetil has also been associated with an increased incidence of CMV disease.

The likelihood and severity of EBV infection following pancreas transplantation also varies with the presence or absence of specific risk factors. Unlike CMV, EBV disease tends to occur only in patients experiencing primary EBV infection. Similar to CMV, patients who have been heavily immunosuppressed, especially those who required the use of antilymphocyte antibody preparations, are at a greater risk of developing EBV disease.

Several risk factors contribute to the likelihood of developing bacterial infections following pancreas transplantation. Some, but not all, studies have identified a higher incidence of surgical site infections for patients who have been on peritoneal dialysis before transplantation. Many studies have found an association between the duration of the operation and the risk of surgical site infections. This risk for infection has been found following other types of solid organ transplantation as well, and probably reflects the increased likelihood for the development of a technical complication in patients who have more prolonged and complex surgery. The method of drainage of pancreatic exocrine secretions is also a major risk factor for the development of infection following pancreatic transplantation. Bladder drainage appears to be associated with an increased likelihood of UTI. In contrast, primary enteric drainage of the pancreatic exocrine secretions has been associated with an increased risk of intraabdominal infection. However, recent technical advances appear to have improved on the latter problem and an increasing number of pancreatic transplants are being performed with enteric drainage.

Finally, the presence of intraluminal catheters increases the risk of infection at the site of catheterization. This is particularly true of prolonged requirements for indwelling catheterization of the bladder in recipients of combined kidney–pancreas transplants where the risk of urosepsis appears to be correlated to the duration that the catheter is left in place.

1.5 How does this differ from other conditions, from center to center, and from country to country?

Infections in pancreatic transplant recipients differ from those in other organ transplant recipients in a number of ways. Although a great deal of overlap exists between the infectious complications seen in patients undergoing pancreas and kidney transplant (primarily because most pancreas recipients also receive a kidney graft), there is an increased risk of intraabdominal infections in these patients. In particular, infection within or near the pancreas is more common in these patients. Kidney–pancreas transplant recipients with bladder drainage of pancreatic exocrine secretions have a greater risk of developing UTI than patients undergoing isolated kidney transplantation. Because all patients receiving a pancreas transplant have a previous history of diabetes, these patients differ from most other solid organ transplant recipients in their tendency to develop infections related to diabetic neuropathies and microangiopathies. Accordingly, pancreatic transplant recipients are relatively unique in developing late osteoarticular infections or bloodstream infections secondary to diabetic ulcers. These patients also tend to require more immunosuppression than some other types of solid organ transplant recipients increasing the risk of developing infections with CMV and other opportunistic pathogens.

Risks for and manifestations of infection in pancreatic transplant recipients may also vary from center to center and from country to country. These variations are due in part to differences in surgical technique, immunosuppressive protocols and antiinfective prophylactic strategies. Environmental exposures also vary between centers. Patients undergoing transplantation in areas that are endemic for certain pathogens (e.g. *M. tuberculosis*, *Coccidioides immitis*) will be at greater risk of either acquiring these infections from their donors or developing reactivation of their own latent pathogens with the presence of immunosuppression.

1.6 What is the appropriate approach to the initial evaluation and diagnosis of infection in pancreas transplant recipients?

The initial step in the evaluation of infection in pancreas transplant recipients is to obtain a careful history and perform a thorough physical examination focusing on signs and symptoms that may suggest an underlying source of infection. The timing of presentation can help to guide the differential diagnosis (e.g. early infection involves superficial or deep surgical site infection, or UTI). Attention should be paid to the presence of intraluminal catheters as risk factors for bloodstream infection, UTI or ventilator-associated pneumonia. Donor and recipient serologic data for CMV and EBV should be reviewed, particularly if the patient is presenting in the intermediate or late period following transplantation.

After completing the examination and considering these factors, the clinician should obtain appropriate diagnostic tests. Standard workup should include blood and urine cultures as well as a sputum specimen (if available) and chest radiography for patients with symptoms suggestive of lower respiratory tract infection. Appropriate virologic studies should be ordered [e.g. CMV pp65 antigenemia assay or CMV polymerase chain reaction (PCR), viral cultures of the buffy coat, EBV PCR]. For CMV, the decision to use one assay versus another is based on the expertise of the individual laboratory. Stool to identify viruses such as adenovirus, enteroviruses or rotavirus should be sent for culture or antigenic detection. In addition, stool specimen for *Clostridium difficile* toxin should be obtained if the patient has gastrointestinal symptoms. While less common in a hospital-acquired infection, stool can be examined for gastrointestinal pathogens such as *Salmonella*, *Shigella*, *Yersinia* and *Campylobacter*. A nasopharyngeal aspirate for viral culture against respiratory viruses, as well as for the performance of antigen detection against RSV and influenza A, should be considered during the respiratory infection season. Performance of bronchoalveolar lavage (BAL) should be considered for patients with abnormalities of the chest radiograph.

1.7 How should the evaluation be modified according to the severity of the risk?

The presence or absence of risk factors help to guide differential diagnosis. D–/R– patients for CMV are at reduced risk for symptomatic CMV disease. While CMV may still develop in such patients, an extra effort should be made to identify an alternate source of infection. In contrast, D+/R– patients are at high risk for CMV disease, especially if the timing is appropriate and the patient has a history of augmented immunosuppression. These patients may benefit from empirical antiviral treatment while awaiting the results of diagnostic tests.

1.8 What are the specific evaluation measures?
An overview of the evaluation of infection following pancreatic transplantation by site of involvement and pathogen is shown in Table 7.6.1 (see also Chapter 2 in Part I).

1.9 What new developments are going to impact on emerging organisms, recognition, evaluation and diagnosis of infection in pancreas transplant recipients?
New and/or emerging organisms are recognized following organ transplantation primarily for one of two reasons. The first explanation is the availability of new diagnostic tests. The recent discovery and subsequent development of diagnostic tests for 'new' viral pathogens, including human herpesviruses (HHV-6, HHV-7, HHV-8) and parvovirus B19, has offered the opportunity to determine the potential role of these viruses in organ transplant recipients. Investigators have begun to explore whether one or more of these 'new' viruses are the cause of previously unexplained febrile episodes or laboratory abnormalities following organ transplantation. For example, parvovirus B19 is now recognized as causing red cell aplasia in solid organ transplant recipients. Likewise, HHV-6 may cause neutropenia or delayed engrafment in bone marrow transplant recipients. Also of concern is the emergence of papillomavirus (BK) infection in combined kidney–pancreas transplant recipients. However, the full extent and impact of infections due to these newer viruses have not been determined in solid organ transplant recipients.

The second explanation for the recognition of new or emerging pathogens affecting transplant recipients is the use of increasingly potent immunosuppressants, rendering patients susceptible to what otherwise might be saprophytic organisms. This has been observed most frequently for patients undergoing bone marrow transplantation who have developed invasive infection with unusual fungi such as *Alternaria* or *Fusaria*. This may also be relevant to pancreatic transplant recipients, who require higher levels of immunosuppression than most other solid organ transplant recipients. Accordingly, recognition of the importance of these emerging pathogens in patients undergoing pancreatic transplantation may develop with increasing experience with this procedure.

The concept of measuring and/or monitoring of viral load promises to have an important impact on the diagnosis of infection in pancreatic transplant recipients. Assays designed to measure CMV pp65 antigen levels in the peripheral blood provide a determination of CMV viral load. The CMV viral load (as measured by the pp65 antigenemia assay or quantitative CMV PCR) is positive in patients with symptomatic disease. The CMV pp65 antigenemia assay also becomes positive before the onset of symptomatic infection, and is the basis of a proposed preemptive strategy. The measurement of EBV viral load in the peripheral blood using PCR has also recently been introduced as a method of diagnosing patients with EBV-associated PTLD. In addition, it is hoped that serial measurements of the EBV viral load will be able to identify patients who are infected and at risk of developing disease before they manifest symptoms, and allow a preemptive intervention to prevent progression to disease.

The development of new immunosuppressive agents and combinations will likely have a dramatic effect on the diagnosis and management of infections in pancreatic transplant recipients. Historically, the introduction of newer agents has altered the pattern and severity of infections following transplantation. This is illustrated by the increased risk of viral and fungal infections for patients receiving antilymphocyte antibody products.

Table 7.6.1 Evaluation of infections in pancreas transplant recipients according to the site of infection and the possible etiologic agent

Site of infection	Infectious syndrome (clinical features)	Predominant pathogens	Diagnostic investigations
Bloodstream	Bacteremia (fever with or without local signs of infection)	Coagulase-negative staphylococci Staphylococcus aureus Enterococcus spp. (nosocomial outbreaks in some institutions) Gram-negative bacilli (Escherichia coli, Klebsiella pneumoniae, Enterobacter spp., Pseudomonas aeruginosa) Candida spp.	Blood cultures (two sets drawn from separate sites and at least one set drawn from intravenous catheter)
Intravascular catheter-related infections	Pain, erythema, tenderness, discharge from catheter entry site	Coagulase-negative staphylococci Staphylococcus aureus Corynebacterium jeikeium Enterococcus spp. (nosocomial outbreaks in some institutions) Gram-negative bacilli Candida spp.	Swab of entry site Culture of catheter tip Blood cultures (consider drawing blood through each lumen of catheter and doing quantitative blood cultures)
Hepatobiliary tract: Pancreas	Pancreatic abscess	Staphylococcus aureus Enterococcus spp. Streptococci Gram-negative bacilli (Enterobacteriaceae, Pseudomonas aeruginosa, Acinetobacter spp.) Candida spp. Anaerobic bacilli (Bacteroides spp., Peptostreptococcus, streptococci, Fusobacterium)	Ultrasonography CT or MRI Aspiration under CT guidance for culture

Site of infection	Infectious syndrome (clinical features)	Predominant pathogens	Diagnostic investigations
Liver	Liver abscess	Gram-negative bacilli (Enterobacteriaceae, Pseudomonas aeruginosa, Acinetobacter spp.) Enterococcus spp. Candida spp. Staphylococcus aureus Anaerobic bacilli (Bacteroides spp., Peptostreptococcus, streptococci, Fusobacterium)	Ultrasonography CT, MRI Aspiration under CT guidance for culture
	Hepatitis	Viral hepatitis (B, C); reactivation in graft Epstein–Barr virus Cytomegalovirus Herpes simplex virus, varicella zoster virus Adenovirus Coxsackievirus	Liver biopsy Serology
Biliary tract	Cholecystitis Cholangitis	Aerobic Gram-negative bacilli (Enterobacteriaceae, Pseudomonas aeruginosa) Anaerobic bacilli (Bacteroides spp., Clostridium spp.) Enterococcus spp. Candida spp.	Cholangiography Ultrasonography CT or MRI Culture of biliary drainage fluid
Gastrointestinal tract:			
Esophagus	Esophagitis (dysphagia, retrosternal pain)	Herpes simplex virus Candida spp., Aspergillus spp. Cytomegalovirus	Esogastroscopy Culture of endoscopic specimens
Small intestine, colon	Enteritis Colitis (nausea, vomiting, bloating, abdominal discomfort, cramp, pain, constipation, diarrhea)	Clostridium difficile (antibiotic-associated diarrhea) Cytomegalovirus Epstein–Barr virus Adenovirus Strongyloides stercoralis	Plain abdominal films Ultrasonography CT or MRI Colonoscopy Biopsy

System/Site	Clinical presentation	Pathogens	Diagnosis
		Cryptosporidium Giardia lamblia	Culture of endoscopic specimens Stool cultures Toxin detection
Peritoneum	Peritonitis Intraabdominal abscess	Gram-negative bacilli (Enterobacteriaceae, Pseudomonas aeruginosa) Streptococcus pneumoniae Enterococcus spp. Anaerobic bacilli (Clostridium, Bacteroides) Candida spp.	Ultrasonography CT or MRI Culture of peritoneal fluid
Upper respiratory tract (ear, nose, sinus, nasopharynx, larynx, trachea)	Otitis media Otitis externa (earache, drainage, irritability)	Streptococcus pneumoniae Haemophilus influenzae Moraxella catarrhalis Pseudomonas aeruginosa Mycoplasma pneumoniae	Consider empirical therapy for otitis media Tympanocentesis (in case of treatment failure) Swab of external auditory canal (otitis externa)
	Sinusitis (tightness of sinus areas, headache, toothache, nasal obstruction, nasal voice)	Streptococcus pneumoniae Haemophilus influenzae Moraxella catarrhalis Aspergillus spp., Mucor spp. Candida spp. Viruses (influenza, parainfluenza, rhinovirus, adenovirus)	Aspiration of sinus Biopsy (if no improvement after 72–96 h of empirical antibiotic therapy)
Lower respiratory tract (bronchi, terminal airways, alveoli)	Bronchopneumonia Pneumonia (cough, dyspnea, chest pain, sputum, hemoptysia, pleural effusion)	Conventional infections: Gram-negative bacilli (Pseudomonas spp., Stenotrophomonas maltophilia, Burkholderia cepacia, Escherichia coli, Klebsiella pneumoniae, Acinetobacter spp.) Streptococcus pneumoniae Haemophilus influenzae Staphylococcus aureus	Chest radiography, CT, MRI Fiberoptic bronchoscopy with bronchoalveolar lavage Transbronchial biopsy Thoracocentesis Open lung biopsy

Site of infection	Infectious syndrome (clinical features)	Predominant pathogens	Diagnostic investigations
		Mycoplasma pneumoniae	
		Virus (influenza, parainfluenza, respiratory syncytial virus)	
		Opportunistic infections:	
		Aspergillus spp.	
		Mucor spp.	
		Nocardia asteroides	
		Pneumocystis carinii	
		Mycobacterium tuberculosis	
		Atypical mycobacteria (?pathogenic role)	
		Cytomegalovirus	
		Epstein–Barr virus	
		Adenovirus	
		Varicella zoster virus	
		Histoplasma, Coccidioides	
Skin infection and soft tissue	Surgical wound infections	*Staphylococcus aureus*	Aspiration (needle) or swab of skin
		Coagulase-negative staphylococci	exudate
		Enterococcus spp.	
		Gram-negative bacilli (Enterobacteriaceae,	
		Pseudomonas aeruginosa)	
		Candida spp.	
	Rash	**Primary infections:**	Aspiration (needle) or swab of skin
	Cellulitis	Coagulase-negative staphylococci	exudate
	(pain, erythema, tenderness, necrosis	*Staphylococcus aureus*	Skin biopsy
	in case of ecthyma gangrenosum)	Gram-negative bacilli (*Pseudomonas aeruginosa,*	(histology and culture)
		Escherichia coli, Klebsiella pneumoniae)	Serology
		Candida spp.	
		Mucor spp., *Rhizopus* spp.	

Site / clinical manifestation	Microorganisms	Diagnostic tests
Papules, nodules (with or without myalgia and muscle tenderness)	Mycobacteria Epstein–Barr virus Disseminated infections: Candida spp., Fusarium spp., Alternaria spp. Gram-negative bacilli (Escherichia coli, Pseudomonas aeruginosa, Aeromonas hydrophilia, Serratia marcescens) Epstein–Barr virus, adenovirus	
Ulcers, vesicles, hemorrhagic or crusted lesions (isolated or with dermatomal distribution)	Herpes simplex Herpes zoster Cytomegalovirus	
Disseminated vesicles, hemorrhagic or crusted lesions	Varicella zoster virus, herpes simplex Staphylococcus aureus, streptococci	
Skin necrosis	Aspergillus spp., Mucor spp.	
Warts	Papillomavirus	
Molluscum contagiosum	Poxvirus-related virus	
Urinary tract		
Pyelonephritis	Gram-negative bacilli (Escherichia coli, Klebsiella spp., Proteus spp., Enterobacter spp., Pseudomonas aeruginosa) Enterococcus spp.	Urinanalyses Culture of urine Ultrasonography, CT (if suspicion of abscess)
Cystitis	Coagulase-negative staphylococci Staphylococcus aureus Candida spp. Adenovirus, JC and BK viruses	
Central nervous system*		
Acute meningitis	Listeria monocytogenes	CT, MRI Lumbar puncture Aspiration or biopsy under stereotaxic CT guidance
Subacute, chronic meningitis	Cryptococcus neoformans Candida spp. Mycobacterium tuberculosis	

Site of infection	Infectious syndrome (clinical features)	Predominant pathogens	Diagnostic investigations
	Focal brain disease	*Coccidioides immitis* *Histoplasma capsulatum* Aspergillus spp. Nocardia asteroides Listeria monocytogenes Viruses (EBV, HSV, varicella zoster, cytomegalovirus, HHV-6, adenovirus, papillomavirus, JC virus)	
	Progressive dementia	JC virus (progressive multifocal leukoencephalopathy)	

* Transplant patients have the same susceptibility to conventional pathogens of the central nervous system (meningitis: *Streptococcus pneumoniae*, *Neisseria meningitidis*, *Haemophilus influenzae*, Gram-negative bacilli; brain abscess: streptococci, *Bacteroides* spp., *Staphylococcus aureus*, Enterobacteriaceae) as the general population. Listed above are unique pathogens.

More recently, the use of mycophenolic acid has been associated with an increased risk of developing symptomatic CMV infection, and perhaps with an increased likelihood of developing recurrent CMV disease. These changes in timing and manifestations of infection are often not apparent at the time of licensure of the new immunosuppressant. Accordingly, clinicians involved in the care of organ transplant recipients should be aware that the spectrum of infectious complications may be altered for patients receiving new immunosuppressive agents and regimens.

2 REGARDING THE RISK FACTORS IN PANCREAS TRANSPLANT RECIPIENTS

2.1 What are the main alterations in host defense mechanisms and what are the appropriate investigations to document them?

Patients undergoing pancreatic transplantation experience two main alterations in their host defense mechanisms. The first alteration is the breakdown of normally protective anatomic barriers because of surgery or the presence of foreign bodies (including intraluminal catheters and surgical drains). This may also occur at the epithelial surface of the bladder in patients who have undergone bladder drainage of pancreatic exocrine secretions. Chronic exposure to these secretions may lead to injury to the urogenital mucosa. In addition, the alkanization of the urine as a result of this drainage may enhance the risk of bacteriuria and predispose to UTI.

The second alteration in host defenses is a consequence of the use of immunosuppressive agents to prevent rejection. Although these agents are intended to limit the ability of recipient T cells to recognize and react to the pancreatic allograft, the lack of specificity of these agents leads to an increased risk of infections caused by pathogens that are normally controlled by cytotoxic T cells (e.g. CMV, EBV, *Candida* spp.). Additionally, the use of immunosuppressants can affect other arms of the immune system (e.g. corticosteroids) and may be associated with the development of neutropenia (e.g. azathioprine or mycophenolic acid). In general, investigations are not performed to document alterations in host defenses in pancreatic transplant recipients. However, a complete blood count should be obtained to evaluate the patient for the presence of neutropenia.

2.2 What are the alterations due to iatrogenic factors?

As noted above, essentially all alterations to host defense mechanisms in pancreatic transplant recipients are due to iatrogenic factors. The use of immunosuppressive agents and the presence of foreign bodies are two of the most frequent iatrogenic factors affecting host defense mechanisms in these patients. In addition, previous and continuing exposure to antimicrobial agents increases the risk of developing infections with multiply resistant organisms and/or super infection with yeast or other fungi. In general, these risks are similar for all solid organ transplant recipients.

2.3 What is the influence of environmental factors?

Environmental factors influence the risk of infection following pancreatic transplantation, particularly within the hospital setting. The presence of local construction can lead to environmental exposure to *Aspergillus fumigatus*, or contamination of the hospital water supply with *Legionella* can lead to outbreaks of this pathogen in transplant recipients. Exposure to other hospitalized patients with contagious diseases [e.g. *M. tuberculosis*, vancomycin-resistant enterococci (VRE)] also affects the likelihood of acquiring infection. The risk of infection in pancreatic transplant recipients can also be influenced by community-based environmental factors. A prime example of this would be the presence of seasonal epidemic pathogens [e.g. respiratory syncytial virus (RSV), influenza virus] within the community. Examples of environmental factors within a geographic region or country are exposures to endemic fungi (e.g. *C. immitis*, *H. capsulatum*) or vector-associated pathogens (malaria, borreliosis) which vary between regions or countries. In general, the impact of these environmental factors is very similar for all solid organ transplant recipients, including pancreas transplant recipients.

2.4 What are the most significant factors that contribute to the risk of infection in pancreas transplant recipients?

äMultiple factors contribute to the risk of infection after pancreatic transplantation. These include the level of immunosuppression, type of drainage of pancreatic exocrine secretions, technical events occurring during surgery, development of technical complications after surgery, donor and recipient serologic status against CMV, use of indwelling catheters (especially bladder catheters), the severity of diabetic neuropathy and microangiopathy as well as nosocomial exposures to pathogens. Each of the above factors may affect both the likelihood of acquiring infection and the potential severity of disease due to specific pathogens. Pancreatic transplantation has not been performed widely in pediatric populations; accordingly, the impact of age in the development of infectious complications has not been well studied. However, it is likely that older recipients may be at greater risk for late infections.

2.5 What are the specific or nonspecific measures aimed at minimizing each of these factors?

Measures can be taken to minimize the risk for some of the factors contributing to infection following pancreatic transplantation. Increasing efforts are being made to evaluate the most effective approach to drainage of pancreatic exocrine secretions. Indwelling catheters, particularly bladder catheters, should be removed as soon as possible after transplantation. Every effort should be made to keep the level of immunosuppression adequate to prevent rejection without overimmunosuppressing the patient.

The availability of an effective vaccine against CMV would be an excellent protective measure against the absence of preexisting immunity to this virus. Unfortunately, it is unlikely that an effective vaccine will be available in the near future. In the absence of active immunization, passive immunization against CMV using high-titered intravenous immunoglobulin (e.g. CytoGam®) is available. While the prophylactic use of this product has been shown to offer some protection in adult renal, intestinal and liver transplant recipients, it has been least effective in high-risk CMV-seronegative recipients (R–) of CMV-seropositive donors (D+). Data from a severe combined immune deficiency (SCID) mouse model suggest that the use of intravenous immunoglobulin (IVIG)-containing antibodies against EBV may also provide protection against EBV disease in organ transplant recipients.

Technical complications are undesirable but are at times unavoidable in association with organ transplantation. This is particularly true of pancreatic transplantation where chronic exposure to pancreatic exocrine secretions may predispose to anastomotic leaks. In addition, pancreatic transplantation is a relatively new procedure, for which the demand is growing. As a consequence, the procedure is being performed by many centers with only a limited experience. Technical complications often occur during the 'learning curve' for each of these new centers. The identification of a finite number of centers of excellence on a regional, national or global level for the performance of this procedure may help to limit technical complications.

Because of the extremely high rate of superficial and deep surgical site infections that develop in pancreas transplant recipients, several centers have begun to evaluate the optimal regimen to provide perioperative prophylaxis for these patients. Unfortunately, these efforts have not led to a uniformly accepted strategy at this time. Some centers, including the authors' own, use irrigation containing both antibacterial and antifungal agents at the time of surgery to limit contamination from the duodenum which is attached to the pancreas graft. The continuous use of low-dose, daily trimethoprim–sulfamethoxazole has been shown to reduce the incidence of both UTI and *Pneumocystis carinii* pneumonia (PCP) in renal transplant recipients. Accordingly, the use of this approach in pancreas transplant recipients is also likely to be of value.

Finally, excellent infection control technique should be taught and enforced on the transplant unit to minimize the likelihood of nosocomial spread of infection. Strict adherence to handwashing should be emphasized for all members of the clinical care team.

2.6 Are there different levels of risk of infection recognized in pancreas transplant recipients?

The major differences in risk of developing infections after pancreatic transplantation appear to be related primarily to the type of drainage procedure undertaken for pancreatic exocrine secretions. Patients who receive bladder drainage are at increased risk of developing UTI. Patients who receive enteric drainage have been reported to be at increased risk of developing intraabdominal infections. However, recent studies suggest that the latter complication rate may be diminishing in more current experience.

The second major difference in risk of developing infection in these patients relates to the CMV antibody status of the donor and recipient. CMV-negative recipients of organs from a CMV-positive donor are at a high risk of developing CMV disease. This is particularly true if the patient requires augmented immunosuppression to treat rejection following transplantation. On the other hand, CMV-negative recipients of CMV-negative donors are at a much lower risk of developing CMV disease. Patients who are seronegative for EBV before transplantation are at a relatively high risk of developing EBV disease and PTLD. However, this is a very uncommon occurrence in adults. Patients who are EBV seropositive before pancreatic transplantation are at a low risk of developing EBV disease.

2.7 How does the level of risk impact on management?

Patients who are known to be at high risk of developing infection are the most likely candidates for preventive strategies. Depending on the philosophy of the pancreatic transplant center, programs may choose to use virologic monitoring for CMV (pp65 antigenemia or CMV PCR) to identify patients at risk of developing disease and to intervene with preemptive therapy. Alternatively, transplant centers may choose to provide prophylaxis to all high-risk patients. The duration of prophylaxis might be modified based upon the level of risk of acquiring symptomatic disease due to a pathogen. Potential advantages of monitoring with preemptive therapy include the cost-effective benefit of treating only those patients identified as being at risk of developing CMV disease. This strategy also avoids the need for intravenous access and the unnecessary exposure of all patients to ganciclovir. Limitations include the difficulty in obtaining specimens from patients once they have left the transplant center, as well as a current lack of specific guidelines for the use of this approach. The use of prophylaxis avoids these pitfalls. However, it requires the use of ganciclovir for all patients who are themselves or whose donors are CMV seropositive. Regardless of which preventive strategy a transplant center chooses, use of empirical therapy for symptomatic patients at high risk of developing a specific infection should be considered pending the results of diagnostic studies.

2.8 What new developments are going to impact on minimizing or suppressing the specific risk factors?

The development of new and more specific immunosuppressive agents will likely have a major impact on the risk of infections following pancreatic transplantation. The availability of such agents should diminish the likelihood of developing opportunistic infections. Further improvements in the technical aspects of bladder and enteric drainage should diminish the risk of both UTI and intraabdominal infections in these patients. The development of an effective vaccine against CMV might also impact positively on the infectious sequelae of pancreatic transplantation. Identification of alternative, effective chemoprophylactic or immunoprophylactic regimens to be used as primary prophylaxis or as the basis of preemptive therapy against CMV would clearly reduce the risk of infection following pancreatic transplantation.

3 REGARDING THE SURVEILLANCE OF PANCREAS TRANSPLANT RECIPIENTS

3.1 What is the important pretransplant information to be gathered?

A thorough infectious disease history should be taken from all candidates for pancreatic transplantation as part of their pretransplant evaluation. Particular attention should be paid to a previous history of infection with antibiotic-resistant organisms (e.g. vancomycin-resistant *Enterococcus faecium*), multiply resistant *Klebsiella pneumoniae*), tuberculosis and endemic fungi (e.g. *H. capsulatum*, *C. immitis*). Candidates for pancreatic transplantation should undergo purified protein derivative (PPD) skin testing. A chest radiograph should be obtained and evaluated for the presence of lesions that may be consistent with quiescent tuberculosis. A previous history of varicella and herpes simplex infection should also be sought. Because of the relationship between diabetic complications (neuropathy and vasculopathy) and increased risk of infections, the candidate's diabetic status should thoroughly reviewed. For example, a history of diabetic foot ulcers may increase the risk of bacteremia after pancreatic transplantation. Successful pancreatic transplantation leading to an euglycemic state should arrest but not correct the risk for further vasculopathy and neuropathy. Consideration should be given to providing appropriate immunizations to these candidates. These should include updating previous tetanus and diphtheria immunizations, completing a hepatitis B virus vaccine series, and providing influenza and pneumococcal vaccines.

3.2 What are the surveillance measures to be taken when a patient presents for pancreas transplantation?

The serologic status of the donor against potentially transmissable pathogens should be routinely obtained. For pancreatic transplantation, this should at a minimum include testing against CMV, EBV, hepatitis B and C virus (HBV, HCV) and human immunodeficiency virus (HIV). These serologies should also be determined for the pancreas transplant recipient. In addition, serologic testing of the recipient should include VZV and HSV. It is important to rule out the presence of a UTI when the patient presents for transplantation. Also, patients on peritoneal dialysis should be evaluated for the presence of occult intraabdominal or catheter-tract infections. All organisms found should be treated promptly as these occult infections have progressed to clinically important infections after pancreatic transplantation. Some centers perform environmental surveillance cultures for the presence of nosocomial pathogens including *A. fumigatus* and *Legionella* spp.

3.3 What are the other specific measures to be taken when a patient presents for pancreatic transplantation?

In general, no other specific measures are necessary for the patient presenting for pancreatic transplantation. However, a full infectious disease evaluation should be performed for the pancreas transplant candidate who has fever or other symptoms suggestive of infection at the time that an organ becomes available. Single room isolation is optimal in the immediate postoperative period. The need for further isolation (e.g. laminar air flow, gown and glove isolation) has not been proven to provide additional benefit beyond traditional infection control techniques (excellent handwashing).

4 REGARDING THE PREVENTION OF INFECTION IN PANCREAS TRANSPLANT RECIPIENTS

4.1 What approaches, if any, to the prevention of infection should be considered for pancreas transplant recipients?

Preventive strategies can be separated into short-term, perioperative prophylaxis as well as more long-term prophylactic strategies. The authors currently recommend the use of intravenous cefazolin for the first 24–48 h following pancreatic transplantation. In addition, the surgical site is irrigated with saline containing amphotericin B, a second-or third-generation cephalosporin and an aminoglycoside. While there are no published data to support this latter approach, it has been used successfully at several centers. Low-dose, daily trimethoprim–sulfamethoxazole is provided as UTI prophylaxis for the first 2 months following transplantation. Subsequently, this medication is given three times per week to prevent the development of PCP for at least the first year following transplant.

The development of preventive strategies against CMV disease in pancreatic transplant recipients is worthy of consideration. Unfortunately, consensus on the relative benefits of chronic viral load monitoring and preemptive antiviral therapy with ganciclovir, compared with the use of oral or intravenous ganciclovir prophylaxis for some or all at-risk patients, is not currently available. Both strategies have been used for pancreatic transplant recipients at the University of Pittsburgh. The apparent limitation to monitoring is the potential for failing to obtain surveillance specimens from patients and thus missing the opportunity to treat CMV infection preemptively. While uniform provision of antiviral prophylaxis avoids this problem, application of this strategy may result in unnecessary cost and exposure of pancreatic transplant recipients to intravenous or oral ganciclovir. Further, the optimal route and duration of ganciclovir prophylaxis has not been established in these patients. Accordingly, the authors recommend that each center review its own experience with CMV as well as the availability of laboratory support for both monitoring and diagnosis of CMV and the logistical support available to maintain a monitoring program before deciding on a strategy for patients. It is hoped that randomized multicenter studies will provide more definitive guidance to the question of prevention of CMV in pancreatic transplant recipients in the near future.

Finally, many centers use low-dose oral acyclovir for HSV-positive patients for the first 3 months following pancreatic transplantation in an effort to prevent reactivation of the recipient's latent HSV infection. Similarly, varicella zoster immune globulin (VZIG) should be provided within 96 h of exposure to varicella for pancreas transplant recipients with negative VZV titers.

4.2 What are the future challenges and opportunities for reducing the risk of infection?

Finding solutions to two major challenges would provide important opportunities for reducing the risk of infection after pancreatic transplantation. The first challenge is to develop improved antirejection therapy leading to a decreased rate of rejection and improved graft function. Ideally, these new antirejection therapies would be more specific than current regimens and thus minimize the likelihood of some opportunistic infections.

The second major challenge is avoiding technical complications related to this surgery in order to minimize the high rate of surgical site infections. Many of these infections are related to the status and condition of the patient pretransplant (e.g. preexisting steroid use). In particular, improvements in the approach to enteric drainage of pancreatic exocrine secretions should lead to minimization of both UTI and intraabdominal infections.

Finally, there is no doubt that the development of successful strategies for islet cell transplantation would be a worthwhile and better alternative to pancreatic transplantation. It certainly would avoid most of the infectious issues associated with the drainage of the pancreas, and would essentially reduce these patients back to 'kidney transplant' recipients from an infectious disease viewpoint.

5 REGARDING THE TREATMENT OF PANCREAS TRANSPLANT RECIPIENTS

5.1 What is the role of empirical therapy?

Algorithms for the use of empirical therapy may be designed based on the timing of presentation of infection and the presence or absence of risk factors. Empirical therapy is appropriately started in pancreatic transplant recipients with fever after performance of a careful clinical evaluation including obtaining suitable specimens for culture. However, empirical therapy should be withheld from patients with clinical evidence suggesting the presence of infection due to common respiratory or gastrointestinal viral pathogens (e.g. rhinovirus, rotavirus). The choice of antimicrobial agents should be made to cover the bacteria typically associated with the most likely site of infections. In general, empirical antibacterial coverage should have activity against enteric and typical 'catheter' pathogens. Choices might include piperacillin–tazobactam, fluroquinolones or cefepime. The latter drug may be preferable to ceftazidime because of its alleged decreased tendency to cause derepression of chromosomally located β-lactamases. Knowledge of previous 'resistance' patterns for a given patient and within a hospital also helps to guide the choice of antibiotics. It is important to limit the duration of antimicrobial therapy for empirically treated patients who have no positive cultures in an effort to minimize the development of antimicrobial resistance and secondary fungemia. However, a full course of treatment should be given to patients with positive cultures or for whom a site of infection is identified. A change in empirical therapy may be indicated if a patient fails to respond to initial empirical therapy or experiences a clinical deterioration.

In general, empirical use of systemic antifungal agents is discouraged because of the nephrotoxicity of amphotericin and drug–drug interactions of the azole antifungal agents with immunosuppressants. Exceptions to this might include patients known to be colonized at one or more sites.

Empirical antiviral therapy against CMV may be initiated in patients presenting at an appropriate time (e.g. intermediate period) with a compatible clinical syndrome. An adequate evaluation for CMV should be obtained before the initiation of therapy.

5.2 What is the appropriate approach to pancreas transplant recipients with evidence of:

Upper respiratory tract infection?

Sinusitis

Patients with mild illness and radiographic evidence of sinusitis may be treated empirically with therapy against the typical sinus pathogens (e.g. *S. pneumoniae*, *H. influenzae*, *M. catarrhalis*). A microbiologic sample with biopsy to rule out fungal sinusitis should be considered for patients who are moderately or severely ill or who show no improvement on empirical therapy.

Otitis media

Patients with otitis media should be started on empirical therapy against typical pathogens associated with middle ear disease (e.g. *S. pneumoniae*, *H. influenzae*, *M. catarrhalis*). Failure to improve on empirical antibiotics should prompt diagnostic tympanocentesis.

Conjunctivitis

Bacterial and viral cultures should be obtained from pancreas transplant recipients with evidence of conjunctivitis. The use of topical or systemic antibacterial agents should be considered for patients with bacterial cultures positive for typical pathogens including *S. pneumoniae*, *H. influenzae* and *M. catarrhalis*.

Tonsillitis

The presence of exudative tonsillitis should prompt consideration of infection due to *Streptococcus pyogenes* (group A *Streptococcus*) as well as viral pathogens including EBV and adenovirus. Exudative tonsillitis may also be caused by *Candida* spp. Patients presenting with this condition should initially undergo a throat culture to look for the presence of group A streptococcus and yeast.

A positive culture for group A *Streptococcus* should prompt treatment with penicillin. Patients with positive throat cultures for yeast can usually be treated with nystatin. However, failure to respond to this therapy warrants consideration of the use of fluconazole.

The presence of tonsillitis in patients without evidence of group A streptococci or *Candida* raises the possibility of EBV infection. Clinically, this is often manifest as an exudative tonsillitis which is not distinguishable from the classic appearance of tonsillar disease in immunocompetent patients with EBV-associated mononucleosis. Histologic evaluation of tonsillar tissue obtained from transplant recipients presenting in this manner may demonstrate a continuum of pathology including acute EBV infection, mononucleosis and PTLD. The variability in the histologic grade observed is likely to be due to the rapidity of proliferation of EBV-infected B-cells and the ability of the host to contain this process. The authors believe that patients presenting with EBV-associated tonsillitis are all on the same continuum of disease. Accordingly, they recommend treating them all the same once it has been confirmed that the tonsillitis is EBV-related. EBV serologies as well as a monospot test should be performed in these patients. Where available, the EBV viral load in the peripheral blood should also be determined. Finally, a throat culture for viruses should be sent to look for the presence of adenovirus or other respiratory viruses (e.g. influenza).

Teeth and gingiva

Dental abscesses and gingivitis occur uncommonly in pancreatic transplant recipients. Patients with clinical evidence of a dental infection should be evaluated by a dentist. The diagnosis of HSV should be considered for patients with gingivitis. A viral culture should be obtained from these patients.

Lower respiratory tract infection?

A chest radiograph should be obtained from all patients who present with evidence of a lower respiratory tract infection. A sputum specimen should be sought from patients with a productive cough. Patients with community-acquired lower respiratory tract infection with radiographic evidence of typical bacterial pneumonia may be started empirically on therapy aimed at covering usual bacterial pathogens. Patients presenting acutely are more likely to have *S. pneumoniae*, *S. aureus* or *Staphylococcus pyogenes* infection. Alternatively, a more subacute presentation suggests *M. pneumoniae*. *Legionella* spp. are uncommon but important causes of community-acquired pneumonia. Empirical therapy should be expanded to include coverage against nosocomial pathogens and enteric bacteria for patients who are currently or have recently been in an intensive care setting. Performance of BAL should be considered in patients with atypical radiographic findings such as interstitial patterns or those with more severe disease to rule out opportunistic pathogens (e.g. *P. carinii*, *Legionella* spp., CMV). Finally, computed tomography (CT) of the chest and performance of a lung biopsy should be considered for patients with radiographic evidence of nodular disease.

Gastrointestinal infection?

Gastrointestinal symptoms are a relatively uncommon following pancreatic transplantation. Gastroenteritis due to bacterial (e.g. *C. difficile*) or viral (e.g. CMV, EBV, rotavirus) infection may occur in these patients. Routine evaluation of patients with new onset of gastrointestinal symptoms should include bacterial cultures for pathogens such as *Salmonella*, *Shigella*, *Yersinia*, *Campylobacter* and *E. coli*, as well as performance of a *C. difficile* toxin assay. Stool evaluation for ova and parasites could be considered for patients presenting from the community, but is probably not necessary for patients whose symptoms develop in the hospital. Stool should be sent for viral cultures. Clinicians caring for pancreas transplant recipients with persistent or more severe gastrointestinal symptoms should consider obtaining an endoscopic evaluation of the gastrointestinal tract to rule out the presence of CMV or EBV/PTLD.

Genitourinary infection?

UTI are among the most frequent infectious complications seen in pancreatic transplant recipients. A urine culture and urinanalysis should be obtained from all patients who present with signs and symptoms suggestive of infection. The use of empirical antibiotics against typical urinary tract pathogens may be considered for patients with classic symptoms after obtaining these studies. Consideration should be given to viral (e.g.

adenovirus, JC or BK virus) or fungal (e.g. *Candida* spp.) pathogens as alternative explanations for urinary tract symptoms. Evaluation for the presence of severe vesicoureteral reflux should be considered for patients with evidence of graft pyelonephritis. Modification in chronic antimicrobial prophylaxis may be necessary for patients who develop infections with bacteria that have become resistant to trimethoprim–sulfamethoxazole.

Cardiovascular infection?
Cardiovascular infections are uncommon in pancreatic transplant recipients. Evaluation for these infections would be similar to that in any other patient with signs or symptoms suggestive of an infection involving the cardiovascular system (e.g. blood culture, echocardiography).

Musculoskeletal infection?
Osteoarticular infections are more common in pancreatic transplant recipients than in those receiving other types of solid organ transplant. Most likely these are a complication of the underlying severe diabetes. The presence of this complication should be considered in all febrile pancreatic transplant recipients, as well as in patients presenting with limp or other musculoskeletal complaints. Evaluation for these infections would be similar to that in other patients with signs or symptoms suggestive of an infection involving this system.

Skin infections
Skin infections are most likely associated with the presence of a foreign body (e.g. intravascular catheter, surgical drain) or with extension of infection from the surgical wound. Culture of any purulent material should be performed. Antimicrobial therapy should be aimed at typical pathogens associated with infections of the skin (e.g. *S. aureus*, group A streptococci). Viral pathogens are a fairly frequent cause of exanthems and skin lesions in pancreas transplant recipients. The most common viral pathogens are VZV (causing either primary varicella or shingles) or HSV. Viral cultures should be obtained from patients presenting with vesicular lesions in order to differentiate between these two pathogens. Empirical treatment with intravenous acyclovir should be initiated for patients whose clinical picture is consistent primary varicella. Oral therapy with acyclovir or alternative antiviral agents is appropriate for the treatment of HSV or zoster.

Central nervous system infection?
Infection of the central nervous system (CNS) is an uncommon but important complication following pancreas transplantation. These patients do not appear to be at an increased risk of developing bacterial meningitis. However, they are at risk for cryptococcal meningitis. Additional CNS pathogens include *A. fumigatus* and viruses (e.g. CMV, EBV, enterovirus). It is important to consider drug-associated toxicity for patients presenting with CNS symptoms since both cyclosporin and tacrolimus, as well as high-dose steroids and antilymphocyte antibody preparations, have CNS side effects.

Foreign body in place?
Foreign bodies are a likely source of infection in pancreatic transplant recipients presenting with symptoms and signs of infection. This is particularly true early after transplantation when the patients may have required the use of intraluminal cannulas. Accordingly, culture specimens should be obtained from involved sites.

Intraabdominal infection?

Intraabdominal infections occur frequently following pancreatic transplantation. Infection in this site most likely represents technical complications (e.g. anastomotic leak) or a deep wound infection. Evaluation should consist of CT with contrast of the abdomen to define localized collections. Exploratory laporatomy may be necessary and should be encouraged both to identify specific pathogens and to drain large collections. Small collections may be able to be managed with percutaneous drainage.

5.3 What is the appropriate approach to the pancreas transplant recipient with evidence of bacteremia, with or without site of infection?

Antimicrobial therapy should be initiated for pancreas transplant recipients with documented bacteremia. The initial use of vancomycin should be considered for patients with Gram-positive bacteremia. However, therapy should be modified if results of antimicrobial susceptibility testing allows the use of an alternative agent. A third-generation cephalosporin (e.g. cefotaxime) or an advanced-generation penicillin (e.g. piperacillin or piperacillin–tazobactam) alone or in combination with an aminoglycoside should be initiated in pancreas transplant recipients with Gram-negative bacteremia. The initial use of newer agents (including carbapenems and newer quinolones), whose spectrum of antimicrobial activity tends to be more preserved, should be reserved for patients with more severe illness or those with a history of colonization or disease with multiply antibiotic-resistant bacteria. Cephalosporin use should be avoided in patients with proven bacteremia due to *Enterobacter* spp. because of their inherent ability to derepress a chromosomal β-lactamase enzyme. The new agent cefepime is reported to be less derepressing for chromosomal β-lactamase genes. Anaerobic pathogens have infrequently been recovered from the blood of pancreatic transplant recipients. Recovery of an anaerobic pathogen should prompt use of an appropriate agent (e.g. metronidazole, clindamycin). Recovery of multiple pathogens requires the clinician to choose antimicrobial agents to cover all isolated organisms.

Regardless of the recovered organism, determination of a defined primary site of infection may also help to guide the management of bacteremic patients. For all patients, documentation of clearance of the bloodstream is an important marker of response to therapy. For patients with catheter-associated bacteremia, the catheter should be removed if the patient is very ill or remains bacteremic despite appropriate therapy. The use of urokinase may increase the likelihood of saving a catheter in some but not all patients with 'refractory' bacteremia. Although several small studies support this approach, the efficacy of the use of urokinase has not been proven. Medical management alone may not be sufficient for patients who are bacteremic in association with the presence of an abscess. These patients may need to undergo an incision and drainage procedure.

5.4 What is the appropriate approach to the pancreas transplant patient with evidence of a viral infection?

The treatment of viral infections following transplantation of the pancreas varies according to which viral pathogen is causing the infection. In general, these are similar for recipients of any type of solid organ transplant. An overview of strategies for diagnosis, management and follow-up for many of the potential viral pathogens seen following pancreas transplantation are shown in Table 7.6.2.

Table 7.6.2 Overview of the diagnosis and management of viral infections following pancreatic transplantation

Organism	Frequency*	Diagnostic tests	Treatment			Duration of therapy	Follow-up
			Primary	Secondary	Adjunctive		
HSV	Uncommon	Culture Tzanck smear	Acyclovir	Foscarnet[†]	Decrease IS	Site dependent	Chronic acyclovir prophylaxis
CMV	Common	Culture pp65 antigen Histology	Ganciclovir	Foscarnet[†]	Decrease IS CMV-IVIG	Site dependent	Monitor pp65 Ag
EBV	Uncommon	EBV PCR Histology Serology	Decrease IS		Ganciclovir IVIG (?)	Individualized	Monitor EBV PCR Repeat imaging studies if positive at outset[‡]
RSV	Rare	NP aspirate for antigen detection and culture	Supportive care	Aerosolized ribavirin	RSV IVIG Decrease IS	Individualized	None
Influenza virus	Uncommon	NP aspirate for antigen detection and culture	Supportive care	Amantadine/rimantadine	Decrease IS	Individualized	None
Parainfluenza virus	Rare	NP aspirate for culture	Supportive care		Decrease IS	Individualized	None
Adenovirus	Rare	Viral culture Histology	Decrease IS	IV ribavirin[§]	IVIG[§]	Individualized	None
Enterovirus	Rare	Viral culture	Decrease IS	Supportive care		Individualized	None
HBV	Rare	HBV serologies HBV PCR Histology	Lamivudine	Interferon		Indefinite	HBV PCR Serial liver function tests
HCV	Rare	HCV serologies HCV viral load	Interferon	IV ribavirin[§]		Indefinite	HCV viral load Serial liver function tests

* Rare, < 1%; Uncommon, 1–5%; common, > 5%.

[†] Foscarnet used for CMV infection when ganciclovir resistance is suspected or proven; experience from patients with HIV suggests that a synergistic benefit will be obtained from the combined use of both of these agents when ganciclovir resistance is present.

[‡] Follow-up radiographic studies of affected sites such as lung or abdominal masses should be followed serially.

[§] Use of this agent is based on anecdotal experience.

IS, immunosuppression; IV, intravenous; IVIG, intravenous immunoglobulin; NP, nasopharyngeal; Ag, antigen.

Table 7.6.3 Overview of the diagnosis and management of fungal infections following pancreatic transplantation

Organism	Frequency[a]	Diagnostic tests	Treatment — Primary	Treatment — Secondary	Adjunctive	Duration of therapy	Follow-up
Candida Noninvasive (mucositis, dermatitis and) cystitis	Common	Clinical examination culture Gram stain	Nystatin Clotrimazole	Topical Amphotericin B[b] Fluconazole[c, h]		Dependent on rate of clearance	Clinical examination Repeat urine analysis / cultures
Invasive	Common	Culture Gram stain Histology	Amphotericin B[e] Fluconazole[c, f]	5-Fluorocytosine[g]	Removal of central lines	Dependent on the rate of clearance: minimum of 14 days	Dependent on clinical scenario
Aspergillus	Uncommon	Culture Gram stain Histology Radiographic staging[h]	Amphotericin B[e]	Itraconazole[c, i, j] 5-Fluorocytosine[g]	Surgical resection	Dependent on the rate of clearance: minimum of 4 weeks, usually 8–12 weeks	Dependent of clinical scenario
Cryptococcus	Adults: Uncommon Children: rare	Culture Antigen test India ink stain Histology CSF examination	Amphotericin B[e] Fluconazole[c, f]	5-Fluorocytosine[g]		Minimum of 6–8 weeks Many would Many would continue with fluconazole indefinitely	Clinical examination Antigen testing Repeat culture of appropriate source (sputum, CSF, urine) Radiography if relevant

| Others (Histoplasma, Mucor, Fusarium, Blastomycetes, Altenaria, etc.) | Rare | Culture Histology Antigen testing (when appropriate) | Amphotericin B[e] | Azole therapy (for susceptible organisms)[c] | Surgical debridement | Dependent on rate of clearance | Clinical examination Antigen testing Repeat culture of appropriate source (sputum, CSF, urine) Radiography if relevant |

a   Common, > 5%; uncommon, 1–5%; rare, < 1%.

b   Topical amphotericin B for bladder wash for noninvasive candiduria; ultrasonography of kidneys recommended to determine that no invasive disease is present.

c   Azole use must be accompanied by close follow-up of levels of cyclosporin or tacrolimus.

d   In general, tacrolimus dosing should be cut in half when using a standard dose of fluconazole.

e   Amphotericin B lipid formulations are used if renal failure is present.

f   Fluconazole is an alternative first-line drug for invasive disease if the species is known to be sensitive to fluconazole and the patient is clinically stable.

g   5-Fluorocytosine should not be used alone but is synergistic when used in conjunction with amphotericin B.

h   Radiographic staging includes CT of head, chest and abdomen.

i   Itraconazole can be used long term for patients who have been treated for invasive aspergillosis, but in general is not recommended as a first-line therapy.

j   Itraconazole absorption can be erratic; accordingly, monitoring of itraconazole levels is recommended. Adjustment of cyclosporin or tacrolimus dosage should be individualized.

Table 7.6.4 Overview of the diagnosis and management of parasitic infections following pancreatic transplantation

Organism	Frequency	Diagnostic tests	Treatment Primary	Treatment Secondary	Adjunctive	Duration of therapy	Follow-up
Pneumocystis carinii	Rare	Cytology of bronchoalveolar lavage fluid Lung biopsy	Trimethoprim	Pentamidine Atovaquone	Corticosteroids	2–3 weeks	None
Toxoplasma gondii	Rare	Serologic testing Histology	Pyrimethamine + sulfadiazine	Pyrimethamine + clindamycin	Folinic acid	4– weeks beyond resolution of signs and symptoms	Clinical surveillance for recurrence
Strongyloides stercoralis	Rare	Stool for ova and parasites Serology	Thiabendazole	Ivermectin		≥ 7 days	Monitor serologic response
Cryptosporidium	Rare	Stool for ova and parasites Histology	Paramomycin	Azithromycin	Reduced IS	2–4 weeks	Endoscopic surveillance
Isospora and *Cyclospora*	Rare	Stool for ova and parasites Histology	Trimethoprim– sulfamethoxazole	Pyrimethamine		10–12 days	Serial stool for ova and parasites
Entamoeba	Rare	Stool for ova and parasites	Mild/moderate intestinal disease: metronidazole plus iodoquinol or paramomycin Severe intestinal or hepatic abscess: metronidazole followed by iodoquinol or paramomycin			Individualize	Stool for ova and parasites
Babesia	Rare	Thick and thin blood smear Serology	Clindamycin Clindamycin + quinine	Exchange transfusion		≥ 7 days	None

Malaria	Rare	Thick and thin blood smear	All *Plasmodium* spp. except chloroquine-resistant *P. falciparum*: Chloroquine phosphate or quinidine gluconate Chloroquine-resistant *P. falciparum*: quinine sulfate plus tetracyline, plus pyramethamine with sulfadoxine, or plus clindamycin	Mefloquine	Supportive care	Varies by regimen	None

5.5 What is the appropriate approach to the pancreas transplant patient with evidence of a fungal infection?

The treatment of fungal infections following transplantation of the pancreas varies according to which fungal pathogen is present, where it is found in the body, and whether or not it is invasive. In general, the approach to fungal infections is similar to that for recipients of many types of solid organ transplant. An overview of strategies for diagnosis, management and follow-up for many of the potential fungal pathogens seen following pancreas transplantation are shown in Table 7.6.3.

5.6 What is the appropriate approach to the pancreas transplant patient with evidence of a parasitic infection?

Parasitic infections occur rarely in pancreas transplant recipients. Although these patients are at high risk of developing PCP, in the authors' experience this is completely preventable through the use of prophylaxis with trimethoprim–sulfamethoxazole. The approach to diagnosis and management of parasitic infections in pancreas transplant recipients is reviewed in Table 7.6.4.

5.7 What is the role of nonantiinfective interventions (including reducing or altering immunosuppression) in the management of established infection?

In general, attempts to decrease the level of immuno suppression should be made in any pancreas transplant recipient who is experiencing a moderate to severe infection. This step should be considered carefully if the patient is simultaneously diagnosed with rejection. However, since patients can survive despite removal of the pancreatic graft, its removal (as well the renal allograft) should be considered for severe nonresponsive viral and/or fungal infections, rather than subjecting the patient to ongoing immunosuppression.

In addition to modification of immuno suppression and to adjunctive therapies noted in previous sections, clinicians caring for pancreatic transplant recipients should consider the use of of granulocyte colony-stimulating factor (G-CSF) in patients with neutropenia (secondary to either pathogen or treatment) during treatment of infections.

REFERENCES

Benedetti E, Gruessner AC, Troppmann C et al. Intra-abdominal fungal infections after pancreatic transplantation: incidence, treatment and outcome. *J Am Coll Surg* 1996; **183**: 307–316.

Everett JE, Wahoff DC, Statz C et al. Characterization and impact of wound infection after pancreas transplantation. *Arch Surg* 1994; **129**: 1310–1317.

Fishman JA, Rubin RH. Infection in organ-transplant recipients. *N Engl J Med* 1998; **338**: 1741–1751.

Kuo PC, Johnson LB, Schweitzer EJ, Bartlett ST. Simultaneous pancreas/kidney transplantation – a comparison of enteric and bladder drainage of exocrine secretions. *Transplantation* 1997; **63**: 238–243.

Lumbreras C, Fernandez I, Velosa J, Munn S, Sterioff S, Paya CV. Infectious complications following pancreatic transplantation: incidence, microbiological and clinical characteristics, and outcome. *Clin Infect Dis* 1995; **20**: 514–520.

Smets YFC, van der Pijl JW, van Dissel JT, Ringers J, de Fijter JW, Lemkes HHPJ. Infectious disease complications of simultaneous pancreas kidney transplantation. *Nephrol Dial Transplant* 1997; **12**: 764–771.

Index

Page numbers in *italics* refer to tables